Welner's Guide to the Care of Women with Disabilities

Welner's Guide to the Care of Women with Disabilities

Editors

Sandra L. Welner, M.D.†

Department of Obstetrics and Gynecology
University of Maryland Medical Center
Baltimore, Maryland

Florence Haseltine, Ph.D., M.D.

National Institute of Child Health and Human Development
Bethesda, Maryland
Founder of the Society for Women's Health Research

Editorial Assistant

Bliss Temple
Disability Advocate

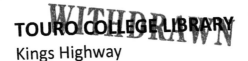
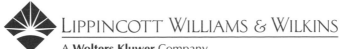

LIPPINCOTT WILLIAMS & WILKINS
A **Wolters Kluwer** Company

Philadelphia • Baltimore • New York • London
Buenos Aires • Hong Kong • Sydney • Tokyo

Acquisitions Editor: Timothy Y. Hiscock
Developmental Editor: Maureen Iannuzzi
Production Editor: Emily Lerman
Manufacturing Manager: Ben Rivera
Cover Designer: Christine Jenny
Compositor: Lippincott Williams & Wilkins Desktop Division
Printer: Maple Press

© 2004 by LIPPINCOTT WILLIAMS & WILKINS
530 Walnut Street
Philadelphia, PA 19106 USA
LWW.com

Printed in the USA

Library of Congress Cataloging-in-Publication Data

Welner's guide to the care of women with disabilities / edited by Sandra L. Welner, Florence Haseltine.
   p. ; cm.
  Includes bibliographical references and index.
  ISBN 0-7817-3532-7 (alk. paper)
   1. Women with disabilities—Health and hygiene. 2. Women with disabilities—Medical care. 3. Health services accessibility. I. Title: Guide to the care of women with disabilities. II. Welner, Sandra L. III. Haseltine, Florence.
  [DNLM: 1. Disabled Persons. 2. Women's Health. 3. Activities of Daily Living. 4. Health Services Accessibility. 5. Needs Assessment. WA 309 W457 2004]
  RA564.88.W45 2004
  613'.04244'087—dc22

                               2003060705

10 9 8 7 6 5 4 3 2 1

11/29/04

Patients inspired *Welner's Guide to the Care of Women with Disabilities*, and this first edition is dedicated to those who inspired me to ask questions. Now, caregivers are physicians, nurses, and paraprofessionals. But traditionally, families have nurtured and inspired the disabled to a healthier, more fulfilling future. My family filled the void that medical care could not, and helped me to find the stamina and spirit to make light out of darkness.

I dedicate *Welner's Guide to the Care of Women with Disabilities* with the hope that the pearls within will cement the unique and necessary partnership of patients, family supports, and their medical care providers, so that all of those disabled may hold onto dreams of a tomorrow in a world that is theirs to discover, and theirs to make a better place.

Sandra L. Welner, M.D.
Silver Spring, Maryland

I dedicate this book, in part, to my children, Anna Haseltine Chodos and Elizabeth Jean Haseltine Chodos, because the world is their future.

—Florence Haseltine

Contents

Contributing Authors

Rodney A. Appell, M.D.
Professor
Department of Urology
Baylor College of Medicine
Houston, Texas

Joyce B. Atchison, M.Ed.
Adjunct Faculty
Department of Communications Disorders
St. Cloud State University
St. Cloud, Minnesota

Matteo Balzarro, M.D.
Clinical Research Fellow
Department of Urology
Baylor College of Medicine
Houston, Texas

Ahmet A. Baschat, M.D.
Assistant Professor
Fellow, Division of Maternal Fetal Medicine
Department of Obstetrics and Gynecology
University of Maryland Medical Center
Baltimore, Maryland

Jean Cassidy, R.D.
Clinical Dietitian
Boulder Manor Progressive Care Center
Boulder, Colorado

Ling-Ling Cheng, M.D.
Assistant Professor
Department of Physical Medicine and
  Rehabilitation
The Johns Hopkins University School of
  Medicine
Baltimore, Maryland

M.E. Csuka, M.D., F.A.C.P.
Associate Professor
Department of Medicine
Medical College of Wisconsin
Milwaukee, Wisconsin

Juliana K. Cyril, Ph.D., M.P.H.
Centers for Disease Control and Prevention
Atlanta, Georgia

Philip D. Darney, M.D., M.Sc.
Professor
Department of Obstetrics, Gynecology, and
  Reproductive Sciences
University of California, San Francisco;
Chief
Department of Obstetrics and Gynecology
San Francisco General Hospital
San Francisco, California

Barbara J. de Lateur, M.D., M.S.
Professor
Department of Physical Medicine and Rehabilitation
The Johns Hopkins University School of Medicine;
Chief of Service
Department of Physical Medicine and Rehabilitation
Johns Hopkins Bayview Medical Center
Baltimore, Maryland

Eleanor A. Drey, M.D.
Clinical and Research Fellow in Family Planning
Clinical Instructor
Department of Obstetrics, Gynecology, and
  Reproductive Sciences
San Francisco General Hospital
San Francisco, California

Barbara Duncan
Rehabilitation International
Albany, California

Michelle M. Duprey, J.D.
New Haven, Connecticut

Dwight L. Evans, M.D.
Ruth Meltzer Professor and Chairman
Department of Psychiatry
University of Pennsylvania School of Medicine and
  Health System
Philadelphia, Pennsylvania

Roger B. Fillingim, Ph.D.
Associate Professor
Public Health Services and Research
University of Florida College of Dentistry;
Staff Psychologist
Department of Psychology
Gainesville VA Medical Center
Gainesville, Florida

Jo Ann Ford, M.R.C.
Substance Abuse Resources and Disability Issues
Wright State University School of Medicine
Dayton, Ohio

Margaret K. Glenn, Ed.D.
College of Human Resources and Education
West Virginia University
Morgantown, West Virginia

Bonnie L. Gracer, M.A., M.S.W.
Alexandria, Virginia

Patricia C. Gregory, M.D.
Assistant Professor
Department of Physical Medicine and Rehabilitation
The Johns Hopkins University School of Medicine;
Associate Medical Director, Comprehensive
*　Inpatient Rehabilitation Unit*
Department of Physical Medicine and Rehabilitation
The Good Samaritan Hospital
Baltimore, Maryland

Carol A. Howland, M.S.
Assistant Professor
Department of Physical Medicine and
*　Rehabilitation;*
Senior Investigator
Center for Research on Women with Disabilities
Baylor College of Medicine
Houston, Texas

Rosemary B. Hughes, Ph.D.
Assistant Professor
Department of Physical Medicine and
*　Rehabilitation*
Baylor College of Medicine
Houston, Texas

Rebecca D. Jackson, M.D.
Associate Professor
Department of Internal Medicine
Division of Endocrinology, Diabetes, and
*　Metabolism*
The Ohio State University
Columbus, Ohio

Iqbal H. Jafri, M.D.
Assistant Professor
Department of Rehabilitation
Robert Wood Johnson Medical School;
Department of Rehabilitation Medicine
JFK Medical Center
Edison, New Jersey

Wanda K. Jones, Dr.P.H.
Deputy Assistant Secretary for Health (Women's
*　Health)*
Office on Women's Health
US Department of Health and Human Services
Washington, DC

Amalia C. Kelly, M.D.
Associate Professor
Department of Obstetrics and Gynecology
Columbia University;
Associate Attending Physician
Department of Obstetrics and Gynecology
New York Presbyterian Hospital
New York, New York

Li Li, Ph.D.
Center for Community Health
UCLA—NPI
Los Angeles, California

Kirk A. Ludwig, M.D.
Assistant Professor
Department of Surgery
Duke University Medical Center
Durham, North Carolina

Kathy Martinez
Deputy Director
World Institute on Disability
Oakland, California

Maureen Moomjy, M.D.
Clinical Assistant Professor
Department of Obstetrics and Gynecology
Cornell-Weill Medical College—New York
*　Presbyterian;*
Attending Physician
Department of Obstetrics and Gynecology
Cornell-New York Hospital—New York Presbyterian
New York, New York

Dennnis C. Moore, Ed.D.
Substance Abuse Resources and Disability Issues
Wright State University School of Medicine
Dayton, Ohio

W. Jerry Mysiw M.D.
Bert C. Wiley Professor of Physical Medicine and
*　Rehabilitation*
Associate Professor
Department of Physical Medicine and Rehabilitation
The Ohio State University
Columbus, Ohio

Margaret A. Nosek, Ph.D.
Department of Physical Medicine and Rehabilitation
Baylor College of Medicine
Center for Research on Women with Disabilities
Houston, Texas

Rhoda Olkin, Ph.D.
Professor
Department of Clinical Psychology
California School of Professional Psychology at
*   Alliant International University*
Alameda, California

Elisabeth H. Quint, M.D.
Clinical Associate Professor
Department of Obstetrics and Gynecology
University of Michigan
Ann Arbor, Michigan

Natalie E. Roche, M.D.
Director of GYN Service
Department of Obstetrics and Gynecology
New Jersey Medical School
University of Medicine and Dentistry of New Jersey
Newark, New Jersey

Judith G. Rogers, O.T.R./L
Pregnancy, Birthing, and Parenting Specialist
Through the Looking Glass
Berkeley, California

Laura E. Ryan M.D.
Clinical Assistant Professor
Department of Internal Medicine
Division of Endocrinology, Diabetes, and Metabolism
The Ohio State University
Columbus, Ohio

Theresa B. San Agustin, M.D.
Gaithersburg, Maryland

Mayra C. Santiago, Ph.D., F.A.C.S.M.
Associate Professor
Department of Kinesiology
Temple University
Philadelphia, Pennsylvania

Ferne B. Sevarino, M.D.
Professor
Department of Anesthesiology
Yale University School of Medicine;
Chief
Section of Obstetrical Anesthesiology
Yale-New Haven Hospital
New Haven, Connecticut

Jeffrey P. Staab, M.D., M.S.
Assistant Professor of Psychiatry
Departments of Psychiatry and
*   Otorhinolaryngology—*
*   Head and Neck Surgery*
University of Pennsylvania;
Director of Clinical Services
Department of Psychiatry
Hospital of the University of Pennsylvania
Philadelphia, Pennsylvania

Heather B. Taylor, Ph.D.
Assistant Professor
Department of Physical Medicine and
*   Rehabilitation*
Baylor College of Medicine
Houston, Texas

Bliss Temple
Disability Advocate

JoAnn M. Thierry, M.S., M.S.W.
Behavioral Scientist
Centers for Disease Control and Prevention
Atlanta, Georgia

Christi V. Tuleja, M.S., O.T.R.
Parenting Equipment Specialist
National Resource Center for Parents with
*   Disabilities*
Through the Looking Glass
Berkeley, California

Margaret A. Turk, M.D.
Professor
Department of Physical Medicine and
*   Rehabilitation*
SUNY Upstate Medical University
Syracuse, New York

Kris Vensand
Encinitas, California

Carl P. Weiner, M.D., M.B.A.
Professor
Department of Physiology
Department of Obstetrics, Gynecology, and
*   Reproductive Sciences*
University of Maryland School of Medicine
Baltimore, Maryland

Gerson Weiss, M.D.
Professor and Chair
Department of Obstetrics and Gynecology and
   Women's Health
UMD—New Jersey Medical School
Newark, New Jersey;
Attending Physician
Department of Obstetrics and Gynecology
Hackensack University Medical Center
Hackensack, New Jersey

Sandra L. Welner, M.D.
Assistant Professor
Department of Obstetrics and Gynecology
University of Maryland Medical Center
Baltimore, Maryland

Beverly Whipple, Ph.D., R.N., F.A.A.N.
Professor Emerita
Rutgers, The State University of New Jersey
Medford, New Jersey

Kirsten Bass Wilkins, M.D.
Colon and Rectal Surgery Fellow
University of Medicine and Dentistry of
   New Jersey—Robert Wood Johnson
   Medical School
New Brunswick, New Jersey

Ilene R. Zeitzer, M.A.
President, Disability Policy Solutions
Washington, DC

Preface

Welner's Guide to the Care of Women with Disabilities, and the subspecialty it charts, is born and develops, in a way, much like the life and academic inspiration of its Chief Editor, the late Sandra Welner, M.D. Only a decade ago, the disabled patient remained completely disenfranchised from the health care landscape. Sensitivity to the needs of the disabled patient was limited to the construction of wide bathroom stalls and accommodating elevators. The absence of vehicles for communicating the special needs of the disabled perpetuated a reality that the best health care in the world was still unavailable to many. Furthermore, organized health care responded only to a consumer community in which voices of the disabled were not influential.

Now, the new millennium witnesses increasing recognition of the unique health care challenges confronting the disabled, and even hospital and clinic programs exist specifically to cater to their needs. Dedicated caregivers have discovered that sensitivity, creativity, and responsiveness to the abilities and strengths of the disabled, in an individualized and tailored fashion, provide far more optimistic outcomes and improved quality of life to a surprisingly large and increasingly integrated population sector.

Yet, even as physicians and their assistants, nurses, hospital administrators, and patient advocates become more sensitive to the health needs of the disabled, very little information is available to guide their competent care. It is clear that a reference text that enables clinicians to adapt to the special needs of their patients is long overdue. *Welner's Guide to the Care of Women with Disabilities* is dedicated to the patients who deserve the best that medicine has to offer, and to the devoted physicians and health care providers who attend to them.

A number of specialists have demonstrated their commitment to the disabled for years, and their study and experience are shared in this landmark first edition. The guide addresses issues as fundamental as physical examination, nutrition, exercise, sexuality, victimization, and access to care, as well as specific disabilities such as neurologic impairment, rheumatologic illness, blindness, and deafness. Primarily, however, *Welner's Guide* focuses on the management of medical problems that warrant special consideration in the disabled woman. Pain, osteoporosis, anesthesia, incontinence, infertility, depression and psychotropics, substance abuse, and hormonal management are among the areas drawing particular illumination.

Nurtured to its completion by the progressive publishing vision of Lippincott Williams & Wilkins, *Welner's Guide to the Care of Women with Disabilities* is the culmination of the trademark indomitable tenacity of its creator and Editor-in-Chief, Sandra L. Welner, M.D.

Dr. Welner was a compassionate, creative, energetic, humble, and old-school obstetrician/gynecologist who devoted her early career to the study of infertility by publishing influential research on Pergonal, for example, which influences treatment planning to this day. When she suffered an anoxic brain injury in 1987, the meteorically rising Dr. Welner immediately confronted life as a person with severe coordination deficits, visual impairment, and neurologic abnormalities that would dash her dreams of a life of helping patients and of devising solutions for future generations of obstetricians and gynecologists.

Or would they?

To the amazement of anyone who witnessed the gravity of her losses, Dr. Welner, through tooth-spitting determination and the devoted support of her family, regained independence after nearly five years of arduous neurologic rehabilitation that in certain instances amounted to relearning the simplest of functions that all of us can understandably take for granted.

Along the way, Dr. Welner employed every strength she could salvage—from her determination, to her perceptual memory, to her artistic sense, to her creative sensitivity, to her acute capacity to listen, with wisdom and long-range sensibility. It was this open-mindedness that, for her, registered her experience as a disabled patient and the terrible shortcomings in health care for the disabled.

In the spirit of her memorable initiative, Dr. Welner's subsequent voracious study of the disabled woman's needs eventually won her the opportunity to open and direct the first primary care program for women with disabilities at the National Rehabilitation Hospital in Washington, DC. A program that was before its time, the experience enabled Dr. Welner to inspire and personally guide the development of similar programs in major medical centers around the United States, and to respond to the needs of different states to develop guidelines for the care of the disabled among their populations. In so doing, Dr. Welner self-funded many of her initiatives, including original research—not waiting for the pace of the rest of the world to dictate her quest for solutions.

Noting how difficult it was for many disabled patients to be positioned comfortably for examination and respectful treatment, Dr. Welner again employed her irrepressible initiative to develop the first universally accessible examination table. The company she inspired, Welner Enabled, was founded specifically to address the unique challenges confronting the disabled who seek routine medical care, and manufactures the Welner Table for hospitals, clinics, and doctors' offices around the United States.

Ultimately, Dr. Welner's charismatic lecturing, at conferences and before groups of all sizes around the world, inspired substantial interest in responding to the needs of the newly appreciated disabled patient. With no appropriate reference text available, and fielding an endless stream of e-mail and letter requests from colleagues and patients far and wide, Dr. Welner then embarked on commissioning the first guide for the care of women with disabilities. As was the case for her other progressive ideas, Dr. Welner's vision was not immediately recognized for its significance, and its potential benefit to society and to health care.

That is, until Lippincott Williams & Wilkins sensed the pivotal importance of providing guidance to caregivers with increasing appreciation for the disabled patient. *Welner's Guide to the Care of Women with Disabilities* brings together an impressive collection of specialists, covering, in depth, important problems that uniquely confront the disabled. The Guide also provides pearls of experience from Dr. Welner's practice, morsels of an irreplaceable expertise that educated and shaped medical care until the very moment of her untimely death in a tragic accident in her home.

Assessment and treatment of the disabled requires the type of out-of-the-box problem-solving that fulfilled the dreams of space exploration, DNA mapping, and the computer revolution. It further mandates that we follow the enduring example of Dr. Welner to search for the answers with resolve and rigor, notwithstanding our intellectual and experiential shortcomings at this stage. Far greater handicaps could not stop Dr. Welner. Her legacy of commanding relevance will live on in the future editions of *Welner's Guide to the Care of Women with Disabilities*, in lessons of compassion, appreciation of how much each of us can contribute as physicians, and how any human life can be enhanced, with all of its potentials, may return precious and incalculable rewards to the society that nurtures her.

May her spirit guide each of you to use this book in health, and with speedy recovery to your patients.

Michael Welner, M.D.
President, Welner Enabled
New York, New York

Acknowledgments

The person whom I most acknowledge is Dr. Sandra Welner, who had a vision that persons with disabilities needed individualized care. She and I were both trained as gynecologists, and I knew her first as a determined resident. After she became disabled, I knew her as a determined advocate for women's health. This book incorporates her spirit, as well as her ideas.

I also acknowledge in general persons with disabilities. Their presence in my life has enriched it, and made me aware of the problems Dr. Welner saw. Four individuals whom I met at critical points in my life represent them. The first was a girl of about 6 or 7 years. I think her name was Helen. She had osteogenesis imperfecta, and she challenged me to climb trees. Granted, we were in the desert and the trees were not big. She was in casts and scooted on her bottom. She was irritated that her casts itched.

In my teens, I lived across the street from a boy who developed meningitis and had become mentally retarded. Billy rode the school bus. My assignment was to make sure he went to his special education class when I went to my special education class. Mine was for kids who had difficulty reading (now I would be labeled dyslexic and hyperactive).

Later, as a resident, I was privileged to have Dr. Charles Krauthammer, now a well-known syndicated columnist, as a medical student on rotation in obstetrics and gynecology. He was recovering from an accident and adapting to his disability, and my interactions with him are strongly seared into my brain. After I worked with Dr. Welner, another problem was brought to my attention. Solving it involved inventing a product and marketing the product. Through this I met a man who works with me today, Mr. Frank Warner.

While editing this volume, I also met a wonderful and dedicated young woman, Bliss Temple, who wants to help persons with disabilities by exploring her personal experiences and her knowledge. Since Bliss is starting a career and I am somewhat more senior, I am encouraged that she and people like her will continue Dr. Welner's work.

Florence Haseltine, Ph.D., M.D.
National Institute of Child Health and Human Development
Bethesda, Maryland
Founder of the Society for Women's Health Research

*Welner's Guide to the Care of
Women with Disabilities*

Introduction

Wanda K. Jones

"Disability" is defined many ways, and some people think they know one when they see one. However, not all disabilities are readily visible, and some people with visible physical disabilities lead fuller, more complete lives than people who have no disabilities. This book provides a comprehensive overview of health issues among disabled women, looking across the lifespan and examining contributing cultural and socioeconomic factors.

Perhaps the most comprehensive definition of disability is used by the Survey of Income and Program Participants of the Census Bureau. It defines "disability" as limitations in specific functional activities, activities of daily living, and instrumental activities of daily living, as well as the use of special aids, the presence of certain conditions related to mental functioning, and questions pertaining to the ability to work (1). The National Health Interview Survey of the National Center for Health Statistics, Centers for Disease Control and Prevention, uses a simpler definition: a limitation in a major activity, caused by a chronic health condition (1).

Almost 30 million women in the United States, or 21%, are disabled (1). Severe functional limitations are estimated to affect about 65%, and about 21% require personal assistance (2).

The proportion of white, non-Hispanic, and black women who are disabled mirrors that of the total population, whereas about 14% of Asian or Pacific Islander women and 15% of Hispanic women (who may be of any race) report some level of disability. The aging of the U.S. population also has implications for the number of women (and men) living with activity limitations–because the prevalence of disability increases with age, and more women than men survive into old age (2).

Ideally, health and social services systems strive to help the disabled individual maintain independence and maximize quality of life. Too often, however, barriers in either or both systems obviate achievement of these goals. Women who are disabled report that far too many facilities or services are not accessible to them, even facilities that appear to have met the requirements of the Americans with Disabilities Act. Examples include any type of services provided in space that is converted from a residence (the entry and "public" space may be accessible, but certain rooms may not be); equipment (e.g., mammography machines, dental chairs, examination tables) that requires assistance in transferring the patient or demands a position that is physically impossible for some disabilities; office equipment and furniture that cannot accommodate a wheelchair; and inadequate or inappropriate materials or assistance for the blind or hearing impaired. Furthermore, one third of disabled women in one study reported being denied care because of their disability (3).

At any given age, women with disabilities need the same preventive services as their nondisabled peers. Whether it is a gynecologic exam, pap test, contraceptive or sexually transmitted disease (STD) discussion, colon or breast cancer screening, or immunization, providers should make *NO* assumptions about the woman's health needs based solely on the nature and extent of her disability. However, certain other considerations may pertain. The woman who is physically disabled and whose movement is limited may be at significant risk for osteoporosis at any age. Pain management may need to be integrated with other treatments, even when the provider's experience may tell her that pain should not be an issue. Women who are disabled are no less at risk for physical or sexual violence than any other woman, and these issues should be carefully explored, with the caregiver out of the room, at every encounter with the health or social services system. Physical examinations should include an oral health assessment—brushing and flossing and other basics of oral hygiene may be inadequate in women with severe tremor, facial tics or spasms, paralysis, or limited range of motion. And every physical examination or social services assessment should include assessment for nutritional status and depression, substance abuse, or other mental health issues.

Women with disabilities who are young to midlife may have menstrual cycles and be fertile, despite their cognitive or physical limitations; their sexual urges and responsiveness may equal those of nondisabled women. They may want children, and their ability to conceive and carry a pregnancy to term may not be affected significantly by their disability. However, they may be vulnerable to sexual abuse or assault by caregivers and others who would exploit their limited ability to defend themselves. If sexually active, women with disabilities also are at risk for STDs, and little is known about the capacity of women who are disabled to negotiate condom use or otherwise reduce their risk. Any provider of care to women who are disabled must be willing to discuss the woman's sexual health needs and to work with her to ensure appropriate contraception (if desired by the woman), test for STDs, and support her informed decision making regarding her sexual health.

Treatment of chronic diseases, pregnancy, or cancer among disabled women may require more intensive oversight or even special adaptations to accommodate life-sustaining therapies that are part of the woman's usual routine. Physiatrists, physician specialists in the care of persons with disabilities, should be included as part of the medical management team whenever conditions arise unrelated to the disability. Although they may not be prepared to manage obstetric or gynecologic needs, physiatrists can serve as a resource for the woman to the appropriate providers. Few primary care providers have the expertise to diagnose or treat mental illness or substance abuse adequately in any population, let alone the disabled. Management of health issues for persons with disabilities, particularly women, requires an interdisciplinary team of providers; ideally, they are connected further with the social services system to ensure that nonmedical issues do not impede efforts at achieving optimal health status and quality of life.

At the federal level, during his presidency, George W. Bush directed agencies to examine their programs, policies, statutes, and regulations to determine whether any should be revised or modified to ensure full community integration of the disabled. Information about the Administration's "New Freedom Initiative" can be found at *www.hhs. gov/newfreedom* or at *www.disabilitydirect. gov*. Research on a variety of health, rehabilitation, and outcomes issues for the disabled is conducted by several federal agencies: the U.S. Department of Education (*http://ed. gov*), the Centers for Disease Control and Prevention (*www.cdc.gov*), and the National Institutes of Health (*www.nih.gov*) of the U.S. Department of Health and Human Services. The National Women's Health Information Center, sponsored by the U.S. Department of Health and Human Services' Office on Women's Health, is a commercial-free information gateway for women with disabilities. The Web site (*www.4woman. gov*) and toll-free numbers (1-800-994-9662, or TDD 1-888-220-5446) provide access to numerous federal and other resources. The Women with Disabilities section, launched in August 1999, receives more than 3,000 visitors per month, consistently placing it among the top-ten pages (out of almost 3,500) on the site.

This book provides a concise overview of the physical and mental health assessment issues for women with disabilities. Most importantly, it puts these issues in the context of a whole woman, albeit one with some level of disability. Many women with disabilities have claimed their place in society as mothers, employers, employees, and advocates. They have worked hard to overturn old notions of burden, pity, and even shame that once kept people who are disabled behind closed doors and drawn curtains. The more we understand the unique needs of women with disabilities, and the often simple ways we can address them, we will achieve an accessible society that truly will allow *every* woman to achieve her full potential.

ACKNOWLEDGMENT

I am grateful to Lyndy A. Potter, MA, for her expert reviews and helpful comments on numerous drafts of this introduction and to her husband, Hugh, who referred her to me when I described this project to him.

REFERENCES

1. Jans L, Stoddard S. *Chartbook on women and disability in the United States*. U.S. Department of Education, National Institute on Disability and Rehabilitation Research. Washington, DC: Publication number H133D50017-96.
2. U.S. Department of Commerce, Economics and Statistics Administration, U.S. Census Bureau. Americans with Disabilities 1997. Household economic studies. Current Population Reports 2001; P70-73. Accessed June 27, 2003. *www.census.gov/hhes/www/disability/html*.
3. Nosek MA, Rintala DH, Young ME, et al. *National study of women with physical disabilities*. Houston, TX: Baylor College of Medicine, Center for Research on Women with Disabilities, 1997.

1

Health Care Challenges for Clinicians and Clinical Researchers

Margaret A. Turk

Providing high-quality health care for persons with disabilities has challenged both providers and consumers for a long time. Once the challenge may have been met just by providing information for insurers, education for providers, and adjustments for accessibility. However, changes in the health care environment now impose layers of bureaucracy that require providing extensive supporting information and/or meeting specific standards for documentation, mastering insurance coverage (federal, state, and private), meeting facility policies, scheduling a facility or consumer with limited time availability, expending enormous amounts of time by office staff and insurance policy holders to obtain treatment authorization, continuing education for professionals, meeting complex privacy requirements, and making adjustments for accessibility. Adding to the complexity, more knowledgeable consumers now appropriately demand more information and involvement in choices for their health care. Information is accumulating regarding the health needs of persons with disabilities, including recognition of disability-specific health issues and identification of general secondary conditions. Gender-specific health concerns—in particular, the health of women with disabilities—is an area of keen interest for consumers, clinicians, researchers, and policy analysts. Consumers with disabilities are excellent advocates and are demanding parity with the general consumer in general, preventive, and specialty health care.

These changes create a very exciting as well as demanding time for clinicians. As a clinician and researcher for more than 25 years, I have observed a significant growth in our understanding of the health issues of women with disabilities and contributed to that clinical knowledge base. Technologic and biomedical advancements have offered better diagnostic and interventional options, and epidemiologic studies present information to assist clinicians in identifying aging and secondary conditions and considering possible lifelong disability management strategies. Yet despite all of these advancements, high-quality health care for women with disabilities remains inconsistent and difficult to achieve. This chapter will discuss four conceptual areas that are issues for clinicians and clinical researchers working for and with women with disabilities: knowledge base, health insurance, accessibility, and patient partnerships.

KNOWLEDGE BASE: THE INDEX OF SUSPICION

For years, the words *health* and *disability* rarely were used together; in fact, for the most part this concept continues to elude recognition in general medical education. Consequently there are many often-asked questions by students and practitioners regarding a woman with a disability. Can a woman with cerebral palsy be healthy? Does she consider herself healthy? Does she receive routine preventive health care, and does her primary care physician offer it to her? Are there general women's health issues that are important for her? What are the aging and secondary conditions that she might experience? Will she lose considerable function over time? Why has she had hip and back pain for the past year? Does she need physical therapy–or possibly an individualized exercise program? What are the modifications in procedures required for accessibility? Are there equipment changes that could be made considering new technology or her long-term functioning issues? Can she increase her personal care assistance time? Will her insurance cover her needs?

Each of these questions has been asked of or by me during the course of a routine clinical experience. Because of the expanding literature available, each of these questions can be answered in context and has been addressed in a variety of publications. However, it is the "index of suspicion" that directs the practitioner to ask these questions. There is now recognition that there are both specific and generalized disability health issues that should be addressed with women patients with disabilities. The physician or other health care provider who offers service to women with disabilities should begin to direct their ongoing education regarding these issues or should begin networking with practitioners knowledgeable in these areas. In fact, patients can be the conduits for information for their practitioners.

These questions are the base for clinical texts and research. Now there is more information published regarding clinical experience and anecdotal information, yet some of this information may not be accurate and even may be refuted by recent research. Much of the information available in this text and in other publications has been the result of recent research. Most of the initial clinical research has been descriptive in nature, with identification of health issues, recognition and discussion of etiologies or risk/protective factors, and report of multiple case outcomes. There is also much more research dedicated to women's health in general, and some of this information can be broadened to a disability population. More recent research is dedicated to interventions and outcomes. Although there is much more published information available, how it can be applied to women with disabilities and to certain types of disabilities is not always completely clear.

A typical question asked by women with disabilities is "What can I do to prevent and/or treat this health condition?" Often the answer is not as straightforward as it might seem. Having the index of suspicion, sorting through your own clinical experience, interpreting leading-edge information within the context of the situation, and being able to communicate this information to patients is often a complex and difficult task.

HEALTH INSURANCE: DIRECTING THE PLAN

Health insurance and managed care have had substantial impact on the health and health care of women with disabilities. As has been noted through analysis of the National Health Interview Survey on Disability data, women with three or more functional limitations often have no or limited coverage. Nationally, these women usually receive few or no preventive health opportunities. These are usually not the women with whom practitioners most often interact.

The more common clinical experience is trying to order needed diagnostic or interventional procedures, equipment, or support services for women with disabilities with managed or limited insurance plans. Even federal or state assistance programs limit or direct plans of treatment. Some examples of requests for prior approval or denials for coverage include the following: newer techniques (e.g., botulinum toxin injection for spasticity management), preventive activities (e.g., access for routine exercise), alternative medicine options (e.g., massage), advanced technology equipment to enhance function (e.g., ultralightweight wheelchairs), perceived unnecessary testing (e.g., spine magnetic resonance imaging to consider a syrinx as a cause of pain for a woman with a spinal cord injury), ongoing support services (e.g., personal assistant services), and inpatient rehabilitation (e.g., hospital-based rehabilitation for a medically complex condition with a complex rehabilitation plan). Each of these scenarios requires an approval or appeals process necessitating not only a letter documenting medical need but also including published research supporting the requested coverage.

Many in this list may be prescribed because of leading-edge knowledge, not yet known or embraced by the plan medical directors or their physician reviewers. Some other examples may invoke long-held beliefs refuted or at least not supported in the literature (e.g., supported standing to decrease osteoporosis). This then requires a clear understanding of the existing evidence for prescription and an organized approach. For the physician, this means developing an infrastructure of time and personnel to write the letters and collect the publication listings. For the policy owner, this means understanding their policy, self-advocating with the company, and assisting the physician's office with the documentation. For both, this requires a commitment to the process, with no guarantee of success.

There have been studies to review the cost of health care for persons with disabilities through federal and state programs. Most studies show a collective high cost; however, one also should recognize that a very small percentage (usually less than 5%) of the recipients account for this cost. Nonetheless, the response to this has been a variety of measures aimed at curbing costs of perceived high-cost items. Although it is reasonable to take action to limit extraneous and unnecessary costs, increasing documentation to include forms of 20 pages or more plus the routine expected physician encounter documentation may not be the most effective solution.

ACCESSIBILITY: REFERRAL, INSURANCE, AND ENVIRONMENT

Although the Americans with Disabilities Act (ADA) requires environmental accessibil-

ity in health care provision, there is some inconsistency in its implementation. The clinician working with women with disabilities knows that accessibility means ability to refer to other practitioners having a disability knowledge base, prescription or referral with insurance coverage, environmental access to offices or facilities, and procedural modifications. What may be a relatively easy scheduling task requires more planning and discussion for successful completion concerning a woman with a disability.

In our office and associated programs, it is customary to provide background information or to make additional phone calls to clinicians or facilities to prepare them for an initial encounter with a person with a disability. Because of this policy, we have had more successful encounters but also have been more aware of possible difficulties. Many of our patients also make preparations and provide education for these events. This is not to say that we have had no problems or unsuccessful referrals, but we have learned from these. We have been able to develop a listing of accessible and "friendly" clinicians, facilities, and programs. Also, we have offered and been requested to provide education regarding these accessibility issues, often with the assistance of our patients.

THE OFFICE VISIT: A PARTNERSHIP

My view of health care for those with disabilities has at its core the need for a partnership between the patient and the physician. This requires responsibility, time, and infrastructure, all of which are more easily said than done. As noted, the present health economy climate demands efficiency and specific documentation. Also, procedures are more highly valued (by society in general and the insurers) than cognitively directed tasks. For primary care physicians, this often translates into time-limited visits; nonreferral for specialty care; or continual triage to specialists, which limits coordination. For the specialist, it can mean only a focused view of a problem, superspecialization, multiple visits for the patient, and procedurally directed care. However, there continue to be practitioners who avail themselves of new knowledge, attempt to spend as much time as is necessary to understand the problem, understand the need for coordinated care, avoid stereotypes of the capabilities of persons with disabilities, appreciate the issues of accessibility, and have some infrastructure to assist with disability-related issues. However, there is not a large cadre of these practitioners nationwide and often not within individual communities.

The consumer plays a strong role in this dyad. Being an informed consumer is an important ingredient in a successful patient—doctor relationship. This also supports choice by the consumer regarding their care providers. Consequently, it is right and appropriate that a consumer with or without a disability will choose to change providers to have their needs met. However, multiple changes over a year will not support a coordinated care approach, which is needed for persons with multiple or extraordinary needs. Therefore, depending on your community, choices may be limited, and priorities regarding health care needs may direct choices (as will insurance plans in some cases). Possibly a better understanding of the barriers clinicians have in providing care can assist the consumer in choices. Thus, consumers need to juggle priorities for health care, personal desired attributes for their practitioner, and stipulations of their chosen (or relegated) health insurance, which is not an easy task.

For both the physician and patient, there is the acceptance of responsibility for successful interactions. The physician or practitioner maintains an appropriate level of knowledge, skills, and attitudes, which allows an open exploration of the health and medical issues of persons with disabilities. The patient is ready at each visit to provide key information to the practitioner, which may require written or electronic material prepared before the visit, and both are willing to be taught by the other.

CONCLUSION

Traversing the landscape of health care is a difficult task for all concerned. Physicians and health care practitioners have a larger and larger knowledge base to maintain, and often their education and training experiences have given them limited or inappropriate contact with the issues or concerns of people with disabilities. Health insurance and access to care for women with disabilities is a national concern and difficult to battle at a local level. Despite the ADA, health care facilities, especially for procedures, may not be designed for persons with disabilities and their staff may not be educated in sensitive and appropriate responses. Yet it is the partnership that the consumer and patient have that can enhance the quality of health care provision.

For me, this has been a time for rethinking, reprioritizing, and reorganizing. Providing high-quality health care in this environment is difficult and challenging. It often seems there are more failures than successes. The successes, however, can be at a variety of levels: service, education, policy, or research. Each one is enthusiastically acknowledged by our team and allows us to meet the next challenge.

2

Employment Issues for Women with Disabilities: Opportunities, Programs, and Outreach Efforts

Ilene R. Zeitzer and Barbara Duncan†

PROLOGUE

"What are you going to do now?"

"I'm a doctor."

"You *were* a doctor. You can't be one anymore. You're disabled!"

The above exchange actually took place between the editor of this book, Dr. Sandra Welner, and her treating physician after Dr. Welner developed a disabling condition. It would be easy enough to dismiss this incident as past history or the failings of one ignorant member of the medical community, but even as these words are being written, one can be certain that some medical professional is uttering a similar negative message to a woman with a disability.

Why does the medical community persist in seeing disability as some deviation from the norm that, as such, is an overwhelming tragedy? Such a negative attitude prevents the medical profession from viewing men or women with disabilities as interested in, or capable of, any normal desires or activities whether they involve sexuality, reproductive rights, or employment, among others. Perhaps it is because the medical community for too long has viewed disability as something to be fixed or cured rather than as a variation on the human theme.

In his book, *No Pity: People with Disabilities Forging a New Civil Rights Movement*, author Joseph P. Shapiro quotes Judy Heumann, a well-known disability leader who, in the Clinton Administration, served as the Assistant Secretary for the Office of Spe-

cial Education and Rehabilitative Services in the Department of Education. She said, "Disability only becomes a tragedy for me when society fails to provide the things we need to lead our lives—job opportunities or barrier-free buildings, for example. It is not a tragedy to me that I'm living in a wheelchair" (1).

Whatever the reason that the medical profession has projected these views, physicians and medical caregivers must recognize the essential role that they play in how a woman deals with her disability. By the very nature of their profession and expertise, physicians and caregivers are likely to be the first person(s) to interact with the woman or girl with a disability. Hence, they play a pivotal role in the adjustment process for women who develop disabling conditions, as well as for girls and young women who are born with a disability or develop one in childhood. The message that they give is likely to have a profound effect on the individual's self-image—her sexuality, her competency, and her self-worth. The purpose of this chapter is to help physicians and medical caregivers send a positive message, especially when the patient who now has a disabling or chronic condition asks, "Can I still work?" or when the adolescent girl asks, "Will I ever be able to have a career like my peers?"

THE IMPORTANCE OF WORK

The authors of this chapter had the pleasure of being involved with organizing the International Leadership Forum for Women with Disabilities, held June 15–20, 1997, in the Washington, DC area. Conceived as a follow-up to the United Nations Fourth World Conference on Women in Beijing, the forum attracted 614 women from 80 countries. The vast majority of the participants were women with disabilities, primarily from developing countries. At the forum, a major research and evaluation project was carried out that used a variety of methods including personal interviews, focus groups, and individual workshop evaluations to capture information from the participants about several issues including what they saw as priorities. Despite the great diversity of cultures, nationalities, and languages, the women participants overwhelmingly identified economic empowerment and education as their key priorities. Their models for employment varied greatly from self-employment to jobs in the open labor market to forming collectives or cooperatives, but the underlying goal was always the same—employment leading to economic security.

It was perhaps a bit surprising to the women from the industrialized countries that their sisters in the developing world put as high a value on employment as do most Western societies, but it merely served to prove the importance of work in all societies. In Western societies, a woman's employment or profession often defines her social status. In any case, whether out of financial necessity or merely social interaction, the truth is that work is an integral part of life in all communities. The corollary is that an individual's inability to participate in the workforce frequently results in her being marginalized and often consigned to the fringes of society. All too often, girls with disabilities in developing countries are denied access to basic education, a situation that further exacerbates their social isolation and economic deprivation in adulthood. In Western societies, girls with disabilities do have access to education, but teachers and society at large still may convey a message of low expectations for them.

Polls and research conducted in the United States overwhelmingly confirm that even for people with severe disabilities, work is a fre-quently mentioned goal. Over the last 10 years, the National Council on Disability has funded several polls conducted by Louis Harris and Associates, all of which confirm that of the people with severe disabilities who are interviewed, routinely 70%–80% of those interviewed who are not working say they want to work, at least part-time (2).

PROBLEMS OF WORKING WITH A DISABILITY

Despite a recent sustained period of unprecedented economic growth and stability that saw historically low levels of unemployment and the creation of many new jobs, about 70% of people with disabilities still are not working—a percentage that has persisted for at least a decade. For women with disabilities, the percentage is even worse—about 75% are unemployed.

The explanations for the low levels of employment of people with disabilities are varied, generally untested, and too complex to be discussed in great depth here. It is believed that one of the chief disincentives is the absence of a national, universal health care system that instead relies on a system linked to employment. The vast majority of Americans who have health insurance, and there are 43 million who do not, have it through their employer. Hence, when they lose their job, perhaps because of developing a disabling condition, they also lose their health care coverage unless they can afford to pay both their contributions and those of their employer—which is unlikely.

If the person with a disability finds a job with a new employer, he or she is likely to find that the employer's insurance carrier will not provide coverage or will do so at very high rates because of preexisting-condition clauses. If the individual with a disability is receiving Social Security Disability Insurance (SSDI) benefits, she must wait 24 months before becoming eligible for Medicare, the federal health insurance program. Understandably, individuals who have had to wait for 2 years to be eligible for such benefits may be reluctant to jeopardize them by returning to work.

PUBLIC LAWS AND PROGRAMS THAT CAN HELP WITH EMPLOYMENT

Americans with Disabilities Act

These low levels of employment persist despite the passage in July 1990 of the Americans with Disabilities Act (ADA), the sweeping civil rights law that mandates equal access for people with disabilities in virtually all domains of American society such as employment, telecommunications, transportation, and public accommodations. The employment aspects of the ADA require that employers with 15 or more employees provide reasonable accommodations to workers with disabilities unless doing so would produce an undue hardship. "Undue hardship" for the employer is an individual concept typically defined by the size of the company, often based on gross revenues.

The importance of the ADA to the employee or applicant with a disability cannot be overstated. It took some time, but now most employers and/or their Human Resources departments "get it" and are willing to provide reasonable accommodations to workers who develop a disability or impairment. Most accommodations cost business less than $500, whereas failing to provide an accommodation eventually may end up in court and cost the employer a great deal more. However, it would be grossly misleading to overstate the litigious side of the ADA. Rather, the vast majority of complaints filed with the Equal Employment Opportunity Commission, which has oversight and compliance authority for the employment section of the ADA, are settled through helping to negotiate a reasonable accommodation. The precept of the ADA is "educate and negotiate and litigate only as a last resort."

Although the ADA does seem to be helping people stay in jobs after they develop a disabling condition, there has been little evidence thus far that it is having much effect in increasing employment of people who are out of the labor force. The law mandates a level playing field in hiring and promotions; for example, applicants with disabilities often find that it is hard to prove that they were not hired because they are disabled rather than because a nondisabled person was more qualified. In any case, the ADA remains a powerful legal tool that women with disabilities can use to broker the accommodations they need to work.

Family and Medical Leave Act

The Family and Medical Leave Act (FMLA) also could be helpful to a woman who develops a disabling condition that, at least temporarily, precludes her working. Passed in 1993, the FMLA provides job protection by requiring employers to hold the job for up to 12 weeks of leave in a 12-month period when the employee is unable to work because of her own serious health condition or that of a close family member. It must be noted that this is *unpaid* leave, so the protection is simply against dismissal during this time period. Nevertheless, for the woman whose condition is still uncertain or who requires a long recuperative period, the FMLA can at least ensure that she has a job to come back to if she wishes to do so.

Vocational Rehabilitation System

The vocational rehabilitation (VR) program is one of the oldest public programs to help people with disabilities. Every state has a VR program, but overall administration is through the Rehabilitation Services Administration (RSA) of the Department of Education, which provides close to 80% of the funds for the programs with state budgets making up the difference. State VR programs can provide a variety of help to a woman with a disability who wants to enter the workforce or to return to it. For example, state VR counselors can help a client set career goals, obtain specialized training, learn new skills, pay for a university education, pay for adaptive equipment, adapt a car or van, pay for attendant care services, and so forth.

State VR programs are required to serve those with the most severe needs first. In addition, many programs have significant backlogs of clients waiting for services. Nevertheless, any woman who acquires a chronic or disabling condition or impairment that would be improved by training or adaptive equipment should schedule an appointment with her state VR office to see how they might help. State VR programs also can provide for training or retraining to help people with disabilities return to the community or to live more independently, such as by learning homemaking skills.

Centers for Independent Living

The first Center for Independent Living (CIL), established in Berkeley, California, was an outgrowth of the independent living movement that began there in the 1960s. Originally begun by people with disabilities, it quickly proliferated so that there are now several hundred CILs nationwide. They are funded through discretionary grant programs to the states and administered by RSA in the Department of Education. CILs are consumer-run and provide a variety of services to help individuals with disability live independently in the community. CILs typically help with such services as housing assistance, transportation, referrals for personal attendant services, mobility training, and other needs associated with daily living in the community. In addition, some CILs also take an active role in employment-related activities to help prepare individuals with disabilities for the job market by providing help in job-seeking skills, preparing resumés, using the Internet, interviewing techniques, and so forth. The National Council on Independent Living, based in Arlington, VA, is the national member organization for CILs and can provide contact information for centers in each state.

Social Security Administration's Work Incentive Programs

As mentioned earlier, the Social Security Administration (SSA) provides cash benefits to individuals with disabilities who meet the definition of disability and whose disability prevents them from working. There are actually two SSA disability programs. The Disability Insurance (DI) program is the contributory program paid for by workers and employers through the Federal Insurance

Contributions Act, more commonly known as FICA taxes. Most workers think of their FICA taxes as paying for their Social Security retirement pensions, which is true, but a portion of the tax also goes toward funding the DI program for workers who become disabled before reaching retirement age and to funding survivor benefits. The other disability program is called the Supplemental Security Income (SSI) program. SSI pays benefits to elderly, blind, or disabled individuals, including children under age 18 with disabilities, who have limited income and resources. SSI benefits are flat-rated, paid to the individual, and financed through general revenues, whereas DI benefits are financed through payroll contributions and paid to the worker and dependent family members, and the benefit level is related to the level of previous earnings.

Typically, SSI beneficiaries have never worked or worked so little that they do not qualify for the DI program. In addition, about 16% of individuals currently on the disability rolls are concurrent beneficiaries, meaning that their earnings under the DI program were so low that they also meet the income and assets test for the SSI program and therefore receive benefits from both programs, perhaps with some offset. In addition, some states supplement the federal SSI benefit. Despite the differences in the two programs, the definition of disability for both DI and SSI is the same and quite strict. Essentially, the definition is as follows: inability to engage in any substantial gainful activity (SGA) because of medically determinable physical or mental impairment(s) that has lasted, or that can be expected to last, for a continuous period of not less than 12 months or to result in death.

SGA typically is determined using an earnings guideline that, in 2003, is more than $800 a month for nonblind claimants and more than $1,330 a month for blind claimants. For blind SSI applicants, SGA is not a factor. For DI benefits, there is usually at least a 5-month waiting period before receipt of the first check (as early as the sixth month) after determination of eligibility. The first DI benefit check is retroactive to the date that onset of disability is determined, up to a limit. However, there is no waiting period for SSI benefits but neither is there any retroactivity. Finally, SSI recipients are eligible immediately for Medicaid benefits, the means-tested health insurance program, whereas DI beneficiaries become eligible for Medicare coverage after a 24-month waiting period.

It may seem strange that a program that pays benefits to individuals whose disability prevents them from working then would offer incentives to those same individuals to try working. However, the U.S. Congress always felt that the door should be left open to people with severe disabilities who want to work. In recent years, there has been a decided effort, often led by people with disabilities themselves or their advocates, to spur public programs to do more to encourage work through creation of more and better incentives. At the end of 1999, Congress passed landmark new legislation (Public Law 106-170) that created even greater incentives for disability beneficiaries to try working.

Ticket to Work Program

This legislation introduces greater consumer choice through providing a ticket to almost every DI and SSI disability beneficiary (16 to 18 year olds and beneficiaries whose conditions are considered likely to improve medically will not receive a ticket). Use of the ticket is strictly voluntary, but if a beneficiary wants to try working, she can "shop" employment networks (called ENs) or the state VR agencies to see if they can help her with her vocational goals. The ENs are one of the new aspects of this legislation. Previously, SSA disability beneficiaries who wanted to try working had to go to the state VR agency, and, as mentioned, they often have large backlogs. Under the ticket, ENs are SSA-approved service providers who may be either private organizations or companies or public programs.

If the EN believes it can help the individual and they agree on the course of services to be provided, the individual deposits her ticket with the EN. If the EN is successful in helping the client go to work and leave the rolls, the EN can receive outcome payments equal to 40% of the average disability benefit for every month that its client works, up to 60 months. Alternatively, the EN can choose a milestone/outcome payment for any client. State VR agencies also can take a beneficiary's ticket and choose whatever payment method they prefer.

The Ticket program is being phased in nationally over a 3-year period that began January 2001. Beneficiaries living in the first group of 13 rollout states already have received their tickets in the mail. Distribution in the second group of states is in process, and the last group, which includes Puerto Rico, Virgin Islands, Guam, and Samoa, will be completed in 2004. Tickets have no expiration date and no dollar amount assigned to them. Once a beneficiary actually deposits a ticket with an EN, she has 60 months before it expires. However, at any point the ticket user can suspend use of the ticket, in which case benefits resume. During the time a beneficiary is using a ticket, SSA may not perform any continuing disability reviews (CDRs). CDRs normally are conducted periodically on all disability beneficiaries to determine their continued medical eligibility. Of course, if a beneficiary suspends use of the ticket, she is again subject to having a CDR. As of May 2003, more than 4 million tickets have been mailed out to disabled beneficiaries in 34 states (including some states that are just starting), and about 16,500 of those beneficiaries have decided to deposit their tickets with ENs to get help with their employment goals. Interested readers should go to the Web site at *www.ssa.gov/work*.

Expanded Availability of Health Care Services

The new law also includes several improvements to Medicare and Medicaid coverage that became effective on October 1, 2000. Among the new provisions are the following:

Part A Medicare coverage has been extended another 4.5 years to Social Security disability beneficiaries who work. This is in addition to the previous 4 years of coverage that already was provided.

States have been given new options and funding for Medicaid coverage. These options permit states to liberalize the limits on income and resources that people with disabilities may have and still be eligible for Medicaid coverage without paying for it. Even if the person with a disability is working and is no longer eligible for disability benefits because her medical condition has improved, the state has the option to allow such individuals to buy into Medicaid.

The law requires the Department of Health and Human Services (HHS) to award grants to states to develop and operate programs to support individuals with disabilities who work and to do public awareness campaigns about them. In addition, HHS is funding grants for demonstration projects for states to provide Medicaid-type coverage to working individuals with severe disabilities.

There are many other incentives provided under the new Ticket program that are too detailed to discuss here, but among them is a new position, being piloted in SSA field offices around the country, called the Employment Support Representative (ESR). ESRs will be trained intensely in all SSA employment support provisions. They will help beneficiaries return to work by serving as a technical resource for other SSA employees and will reach out to the community that serves people with disabilities.

In addition to the Ticket program, there are many other work incentives for SSA disability beneficiaries who want to try working. What follows is a brief description of most of them.

Trial Work Period

As the name implies, a trial work period (TWP) allows SSDI beneficiaries who still have a disabling impairment to try working and to keep any amount of earnings, no matter how high, and their benefit check as well. The TWP is 9 months (not necessarily consecutive) plus an additional 3 months grace period within a rolling 60-consecutive-month period. Any month with earnings of $570 counts as a trial work month, and for self-em-

ployed people who earn less than $570 a month, the determination of TWP is any month with 80 hours worked in the business.

Extended Period of Eligibility

The Extended Period of Eligibility work incentive ensures that even after exhaustion of the cash benefits paid under the TWP, disability beneficiaries have an extended period of eligibility of 36 consecutive months where cash benefits resume again if they fail at their work attempt. As long as they continue to have a disabling impairment, if their earnings in that month fall below the SGA level, their cash benefits are resumed without a waiting period or need to reapply for benefits.

Continuation of Medical Coverage

Former DI beneficiaries who have not medically improved but who work and perform SGA continue to be covered under Medicare. After the 24-month waiting period for Medicare eligibility and following the last month of the TWP, former DI beneficiaries working at the SGA level receive, premium-free, an additional 93 consecutive months of hospital and medical insurance coverage.

Impairment-Related Work Expenses

Impairment-related work expenses (IRWEs) apply to both SSDI and SSI beneficiaries who work but who have costs of certain impairment-related items and/or services they need to enable them to work. Some examples would include the costs of attendant care services to help the individual get ready for work in the morning such as help with bathing, dressing, and eating or services performed in the work setting. Another type of IRWE is transportation costs, such as for driver assistance, special taxicabs or accessible vehicles, or the cost to modify a personal vehicle. IRWEs are deducted from gross earnings to determine countable earnings for purposes of work at the SGA level. The individual may not claim IRWEs if she is being reimbursed by another source such as Medicare, Medicaid, or the VR system. IRWEs must be needed to work and must be because of the disabling impairment, but they also may be used for personal use.

Blind Work Expenses

Blind work expenses (BWEs) are applied in a manner similar to IRWEs in that they are deducted from earned income, but they do not have to be related to the blindness. Some examples of BWEs are federal, state, and local taxes; Social Security (FICA) taxes; and child care expenses.

SSI Employment Supports

Space does not permit for a more in-depth discussion of the employment supports that are specific to the SSI disability program. For the purposes of this discussion, it is sufficient just to mention that there are many incentives, in addition to some of the ones already cited, that are aimed specifically at promoting and supporting SSI recipients who want to work. For example, under a Plan for Achieving Self-Support (PASS), SSI recipients can set aside income and/or resources for a specified time toward a work goal. Sections 1619(a) and 1619(b) help continue cash or medical coverage for SSI recipients who are working; the Student Earned Income Exclusion helps students who are on SSI and work part-time keep more of their benefit check; and the Earned Income Exclusion works in a similar way for nonstudents who work but are receiving SSI. Readers wanting to know more about all SSA work incentives should contact their local SSA field office or go to SSA's Web site at *www.ssa.gov/work*.

In addition to the public programs already mentioned, there are numerous other sources of public and private help with various aspects of working with a disability. For example, there are low-cost loans available for the purchase of a van, specialized computer equipment, and adaptive equipment. There are many organizations that provide guide dogs or assist dogs and the necessary training. State VR programs can pay for many of these items; readers also should check local advocacy organizations and Independent Living Centers for help. The Bush Administration's New Freedom Initiative provides grants to states for technology loans for people with disabilities.

In conclusion, women with disabilities have many options available to help them work and be part of the mainstream of life. Next to family members, medical and treating professionals are in the best and most influential position to help young girls and women with disabilities achieve their full potential. The best way practitioners can do this is by projecting positive expectations and by referring them to other specialists who can assist them with their goals.

POOR PROGNOSES AND DIRE PREDICTIONS

The following are a few examples of women with physical disabilities who were given particularly negative views by medical and mental health practitioners about their potential for education and employment. These talented women, like Judy Heumann, were able to draw on their inner resources and forge ahead in spite of their doctors' opposition; many others have not had the chance to develop the strong self-image and self-reliance necessary to do so.

Doctor to parent of adolescent with cerebral palsy, circa late 1960s in New York:
"These children only end up as vegetables; they won't get jobs. They'll just end up in institutions."

"I impotently tried to comfort my mother using the same words she used on me in previous clinic visits. 'Mommy, don't listen to him', I pleaded, tugging at her arm. 'It isn't true. He's old. He doesn't know what he's saying. You said so yourself. That's why he's not head of the clinic anymore . . .'"

"That day, I watched the fight go out of her and be replaced by despair. My mother had focused the past 15 years on caring for me, encouraging me, prodding me on against the experts' so-called objective reality."

Because her mother died shortly after this exchange, she did not have the satisfaction of watching her daughter, Denise Sherer Jacobson, prove the experts wrong. The above quotes are excerpted from Denise's best selling book, *The Question of David: A Disabled Mother's Journey through Adoption, Family and Life*. (3) It is worth noting that at the time of the doctor's comments, that precarious stage known as adolescence, Denise's comic wit and academic excellence were already apparent to her family and teachers. Denise, a writer; her husband Neil, a bank vice president; and their son David, now an adolescent, live in California.

Doctor to adolescent with mobility impairment, circa mid-1960s, in New Orleans:
"There is no college you could function in, you are not being realistic."

After hearing this prognosis and receiving a letter from the Dean of Women recommending against her attempting campus life, Susan Daniels accepted her merit scholarship from Marquette University, and, for good measure, went on to earn a Master's and a Ph.D. Her ascending career in academia and government most recently included a Presidential appointment as the Deputy Commissioner of the Social Security Administration.

Interviewed for this paper, Susan was clear about what doctors' roles in advising about employment prospects should be: *"They should focus on differential diagnosis and treatment of medical problems, that is what they know. If their specialization is bones, that is what they should offer opinions about, B-O-N-E-S."*

She clarified, by describing a hypothetical situation, where a woman was seeing a doctor due to kidney problems. If asked about work implications, the doctor should not offer the opinion, "You can't work because of your kidneys," but instead should advise, "You need to plan on approximately 10 hours a week for dialysis." In other words, the decision about ability to work should as often as possible remain with the worker, and the doctor's comments should be directed to affected physical capacities. In this way, the woman's belief in her ability to continue working could be supported rather than shaken by the weight of professional opinion.

Psychological Counselor to college student with mobility impairment, circa 1960s in Chicago:
"If you take an advanced degree, you will emasculate every man you meet."

Sue Suter ignored his expert opinion, went on to finish her advanced degree and reports that neither her husband nor anyone else she dated, nor men she has worked with seemed to be thusly affected. Interviewed for this paper, the former head of the Illinois State Rehabilitation agency said she felt lucky that, for the most part, her family had not let the low expectations of the medical and academic communities get in the way of their belief in her abilities. Now president of the Center for International Rehabilitation in Chicago and Washington, Sue has been able to

introduce more modern and realistic world-views about the employment prospects of people with disabilities in both her state and federal level positions.

Doctor to parents of blind girl, circa 1970 in California:
"Religion will play a strong part in her life, more so than that of other girls."

Believing that their doctor had expertise in all matters, Kathy Martinez, age 7, and her parents began planning for her life as a nun. At age 10, when Kathy won a competition for a part in the Hollywood production of "Lassie" and was able to contribute substantially to the family income, they began to consider other possibilities. During adolescence, Kathy and her family started to meet blind adults who were employed in various careers and these role models were instrumental in expanding their expectations.

Graduating with a B.A. in Communications, Kathy has traveled to at least a dozen countries to train disabled individuals in leadership development, and was recently named deputy director of the World Institute on Disability, a public policy center. As often as she can, she visits primary schools to talk to both disabled and nondisabled children about the wide variety of careers they can all aspire to.

It is interesting to note that from New York to Louisiana, from Illinois to California—all across the country, the medical community was uniform in its opinion that these girls and young women had quite limited futures and little or no employment potential. Their opinion remained constant regardless if applied to girls with polio, blindness, cerebral palsy, or other mobility impairment. We hope that this book will help to retire that undifferentiated world-view of disability and replace it with one respectful and supportive of diversity and difference along the human continuum.

REFERENCES

1. Shapiro JP. *No pity: people with disabilities forging a new civil rights movement.* New York: Times Books, Random House, Inc., 1993
2. National Organization on Disability. *Survey of Americans with Disabilities.* Washington, DC: Louis Harris & Associates, 1998 (and previous years 1986 and 1994).
3. Jacobson DS. *The question of David: a disabled mother's journey through adoption, family and life.* Berkeley: Creative Arts Book Company, 1999.

3

Americans with Disabilities Act and the Women's Health Provider: What the Women's Health Provider Needs to Know about the ADA, Case Law Ramifications of Noncompliance, and the Like

Michelle M. Duprey

In the United States approximately 54 million Americans live with a disability. Many often are surprised to hear that people with disabilities are the largest minority group in the country. During the twentieth century medical advancements helped individuals to survive traumatic accidents or catastrophic illness or live with disability from birth or as they aged. Although medical advances moved swiftly to improve the lives of those with disabilities, laws and society have been slow to follow. In 1973 the Rehabilitation Act (1), or Rehab Act, was signed into law providing that all recipients of federal funding must not discriminate based on disability. It was followed quickly by the Individuals with Disabilities Education Act (2). It was not until July 26, 1990, when the Americans with Disabilities Act (ADA) (3) was signed into law, that disability civil rights moved to the consciousness of most Americans—including health care providers. This chapter will provide a brief overview of the ADA, examples of how the ADA has been used to provide more accessible health care services, and resources available to provide technical assistance.

BASICS OF THE AMERICANS WITH DISABILITIES ACT

The ADA cannot be summed up in a sentence or two; in fact, there is still a great deal of the legislation that remains ambiguous and awaits resolution by the courts. Essentially, the ADA makes it illegal for covered entities to discriminate against persons with disabilities and in many cases requires either an accommodation for persons with disabilities or modification to policies, practices, or procedures to ensure equal access to the entity's programs and services. Arguably the most valuable part of the ADA is its requirements for new construction and renovations performed after July 26, 1992 (4). The construction guidelines provide accessibility requirements for things such as ramps, doors wide enough to maneuver a wheelchair through, handicapped parking, accessible bathrooms, and signage. The construction guidelines are part of the regulations for Title III, and Title II entities can choose to follow the ADA Accessibility Guidelines or similar guidelines called UFAS. The ADA is divided into five sections, or titles, covering a myriad of entities. Table 3-1 explains how the law is divided.

TABLE 3-1. *Five titles of the Americans with Disabilities Act*

Section of the Americans with Disabilities Act	Topic	What entities are covered
Title I	Employment	*All employers with 15 or more employees*
Title II Subtitle A	Public services	*All state and local governments*
Title II Subtitle B	Public transportation	*Transportation provided by a public entity*
Title III	Public accommodations	*Private entities such as restaurants, theaters, stores, and health care facilities*
Title IV	Telecommunications	*Telecommunication service providers*
Title V	Miscellaneous provisions	*Entities covered under Titles I through IV*

Health care providers should become familiar with their obligations under Title I, Title II (if they are a program or service of the state or local government), and Title III. For example, a doctor's office with two physicians, a physician assistant, two nurses, and a secretary need only be concerned with Title III because their office is considered a place of public accommodation. A county hospital run by the local government with 50 employees would be covered by Title I because they have more than 15 employees and by Title II because their services are a program of a local government. Both scenarios bring with them a different level of obligation. State and local governments have a much higher level of obligation to accommodate persons with disabilities than a place of public accommodation that is covered only by Title III.

Most public and private entities are extremely concerned with the costs associated with accommodating and serving persons with disabilities and do not provide an appropriate level of service for persons with disabilities because of those costs. With each level of obligation under the ADA, there may be a cost; in most cases, the cost of serving and accommodating persons with disabilities is minimal. In some cases, the excessive cost overrides the obligation to serve persons with disabilities; in other cases, the cost of accommodating persons with disabilities is not assumed by the person with the disability but is assumed by all, whether by taxpayers or customers of the public accommodation. In many cases, for private entities the costs of complying with the ADA are tax deductible. (Two tax incentives are available to businesses to help cover the cost of making access improvements. The first is a tax credit that can be used for architectural adaptations, equipment acquisitions, and services such as sign language interpreters. The second is a tax deduction that can be used for architectural or transportation adaptations. Request IRS Publications 535 and 334 for further information on tax incentives, or request Form 8826 to claim your tax credit.)

COMPLIANCE WITH THE AMERICANS WITH DISABILITIES ACT

When serving the needs of patients the most important aspects of compliance with the ADA for health care providers relate to physical access, program access, and nondiscriminatory delivery of services. These issues are often most difficult for Title III entities or places of public accommodations, which include doctors' offices, radiology facilities, laboratories where patients have tests, and hospitals.

Title II entities, owned or operated by a government entity, have more stringent requirements under the ADA and more difficult issues. All Title II entities with 50 or more employees must appoint an ADA coordinator to oversee ADA compliance. Any health care provider with ADA questions related to a Title II facility should contact the ADA coordinator for assistance. Because most health care providers are not Title II entities, we will focus on the obligations of Title III, for places of public accommodation, in this chapter.

Title III of the ADA requires places of public accommodations to do the following:

1. Provide goods and services in an integrated setting, unless separate or different measures are necessary to ensure equal opportunity.

The requirement is designed to ensure that people with disabilities are not segregated from the nondisabled patrons or, in the health care setting, from other patients. Most of the activity under this section has been when establishments or arenas require people with disabilities to sit or dine in a specific area. This requirement under Title II has led to the U.S. Supreme Court's landmark decision in *Olmstead v. L.C.* (5) where it was determined that a state cannot institutionalize someone with a disability, in a nonintegrated setting, when that individual would be better served in the community.

This section precludes a health care provider from segregating persons with disabilities unless they need to do so to provide equal opportunity to access the program or service offered. For example, a health care provider cannot ask all persons with disabilities to use a side entrance and wait in a private waiting room because persons with certain types of disabilities make other patients uncomfortable. Alternatively, if the only part of the building accessible for persons with disabilities was the private waiting room, such segregation would be permissible to provide equal opportunity to receive care from the health care provider (6).

2. Eliminate unnecessary eligibility standards or rules that deny individuals with disabilities an equal opportunity to enjoy the goods and services of a place of public accommodation.

This requirement is straightforward. The best example of an unnecessary eligibility standard that denies individuals with disabilities equal opportunity is when a place of public accommodation requires a driver's license to pay a bill by check. This clearly would discriminate against a person who is blind. Al-though many requirements may be a violation of the ADA, safety requirements are permissible under the ADA and may be imposed if they are based on actual risk and are not speculative (6).

3. Make reasonable modifications in policies, practices, and procedures that deny equal access to individuals with disabilities, unless a fundamental alteration would result in the nature of the goods and services provided.

A public accommodation must make reasonable modifications in its policies, practices, and procedures to accommodate individuals with disabilities. A modification is not required if it would "fundamentally alter" the goods, services, or operations of the public accommodation. For example, a department store may need to modify a policy of only permitting one person at a time in a dressing room if an individual with mental retardation needs the assistance of a companion in dressing. Modifications in existing practices generally must be made to permit the use of guide dogs and other service animals.

Specialists are not required to provide services outside of their legitimate areas of specialization. For example, a doctor who specializes exclusively in burn treatment may refer an individual with a disability, who is not seeking burn treatment, to another provider. A burn specialist, however, could not refuse to provide burn treatment to, for example, an individual with the human immunodeficiency virus (HIV) (6).

This issue was highlighted in 1998 by the U.S. Supreme Court in the case of *Abbott v. Bragdon* (7). The "Supreme Court held that a health care professional who was concerned about the risk of transmitting a disease [HIV] from patient to provider had a duty under the ADA to assess the risk based on 'objective, scientific information available to him and others in his profession.' The dentist in *Bragdon* failed to present any medical or scientific evidence to demonstrate that filling the cavity of an HIV-positive patient is safer in a hospital than in an office setting. The dentist did not even know whether the hospital where the procedure was to be performed actually had the infection control measures that he claimed were essential" (8).

4. Furnish auxiliary aids when necessary to ensure effective communication, unless an undue burden or fundamental alteration would result.

This requirement by far is the most vexing for health care professionals and has led to a significant amount of litigation. A public accommodation must provide auxiliary aids and services when they are necessary to ensure effective communication with individuals with hearing, vision, or speech impairments. "Auxiliary aids" include such services or devices as qualified interpreters, assistive listening headsets, television captioning and decoders, telecommunications devices for deaf persons (TDDs), videotext displays, readers, taped texts, brailled materials, and large-print materials.

The auxiliary aid requirement is flexible. For example, a brailled medical information and instruction form is not required if the physician or nurse reads the information to patients who are blind. Standard forms or materials can be dictated onto an audiocassette and provided with a tape player to patients who are blind; this keeps staff free to do other work, allows for independence for the individual who is blind; and gets the necessary information to the patient (6).

Health care professionals, particularly smaller offices, often are surprised that they are obligated to provide auxiliary aids to individuals seeking their services. All health care providers should find out where to get a sign language interpreter in their area, the process established to book an interpreter, and an idea of the associated costs. In most parts of the country there is a shortage of interpreters; you may need to book an interpreter up to 2 weeks in advance.

Generally, it is illegal for a health care provider to require a patient to bring their own interpreter, and in most cases it is unacceptable to expect a family member or friend to interpret medical information for a patient who is deaf. Health care providers do not always need to provide interpreter services to meet their ADA duty to provide effective communication with patients with hearing impairments. The nature of the communication is critical. If it is merely a brief interaction, written notes might suffice. A qualified sign language interpreter is vital, however, when discussing medical procedures or surgery or when informed consent is an issue. The patient's literacy level is also a consideration. Sign language is not English translated into signs—it is a separate language. Therefore some individuals who sign may have difficulty communicating in written English. The health care provider should consider all factors and decide the best way to communicate with the patient; often the patient is the best resource regarding what accommodation works best for them.

Auxiliary aids that would result in an undue burden (i.e., "significant difficulty or expense") or in a fundamental alteration in the nature of the goods or services are not required by the regulation. However, a public accommodation still must furnish another auxiliary aid, if available, that does not result in a fundamental alteration or an undue burden (6). For most health care providers, providing a sign language interpreter will not result in an undue burden.

5. Remove architectural and structural communication barriers in existing facilities where readily achievable.

Removal of architectural barriers is the most well-known requirement of the ADA. Most people think of a wheelchair-ramped entrance when someone talks about accessibility. Simply put, the ADA requires that physical barriers to entering and using existing facilities must be removed when "readily achievable." Readily achievable means "easily accomplishable and able to be carried out without much difficulty or expense." The difficult part of this particular obligation is what is readily achievable will be determined on a case-by-case basis in light of the resources available to the public accommodation (6). Whereas a national health care chain may have a substantial amount of resources available to make their facilities accessible, a physical therapist working on their own may not. This is exemplified best by the settlement in *DRA v. Kaiser Foundation Health Plan, Inc. & Kaiser Foundation Hospital*, where a group of persons with disabilities sued because of the lack of access to its facilities, health care services, and programs. Allegations included inaccessible examination tables, inaccessible doors, and rooms that could not accommodate a wheelchair. As a result Kaiser agreed to appoint an ADA coordinator, evaluate their facilities, and buy new equipment (9).

Examples of barrier-removal measures include the following:

- Installing ramps
- Making curb cuts at sidewalks and entrances
- Rearranging tables, chairs, vending machines, display racks, and other furniture
- Widening doorways
- Installing grab bars in toilet stalls
- Adding raised letters or braille to elevator control buttons

First priority should be given to measures that will enable individuals with disabilities to "get in the front door," followed by measures to provide access to areas providing goods and services. Barrier-removal measures must comply, when readily achievable, with the alterations requirements of the ADA Accessibility Guidelines. If compliance with the guidelines is not readily achievable, other safe, readily achievable measures must be taken, such as installation of a slightly narrower door than would be required by the guidelines (6).

One common mistake health care providers make is assuming that because they rent their office space it is not their obligation to ensure their facilities are accessible. This in most cases in incorrect. The lease should state who is responsible for making the facility accessible. If the lease is silent on this issue, as in most cases, then the burden to make the facil-

ity accessible will fall on both the landlord and the renter. If the health care provider is a program of a state or local government, they cannot rent space that is inaccessible and it is illegal for them to contract with any entity that discriminates based on disability.

6. Provide readily achievable alternative measures when removal of barriers is not readily achievable.

The ADA requires the removal of physical barriers, such as stairs, if it is "readily achievable." However, if removal is not readily achievable, alternative steps must be taken to make goods and services accessible.

Examples of alternative measures include the following:

- Providing goods and services at the door, sidewalk, or curb
- Providing home delivery
- Retrieving merchandise from inaccessible shelves or racks
- Relocating activities to accessible locations

Extra charges may not be imposed on individuals with disabilities to cover the costs of measures used as alternatives to barrier removal. For example, a health care provider may not charge a wheelchair user extra for home delivery when it is provided as the alternative to barrier removal (6).

7. Maintain accessible features of facilities and equipment.

Although maintaining accessibility features seems like a simple requirement, it often is where public accommodations run into problems. For instance, not shoveling snow from a wheelchair ramp, storing equipment or products in a seldom-used accessible bathroom, or not plugging in a text telephone are all examples of poor maintenance of the accessibility features.

8. Design and construct new facilities and, when undertaking alterations, alter existing facilities in accordance with the ADA Accessibility Guidelines issued by the Architectural and Transportation Barriers

Compliance Board and incorporated in the final Department of Justice Title III regulation.

All newly constructed places of public accommodation and commercial facilities must be accessible to individuals with disabilities to the extent that it is not structurally impracticable. The new construction requirements apply to any facility occupied after January 26, 1993, for which the last application for a building permit or permit extension is certified as complete after January 26, 1992. Full compliance will be considered "structurally impracticable" only in those rare circumstances when the unique characteristics of terrain prevent the incorporation of accessibility features (e.g., marshland that requires construction on stilts).

The architectural standards for accessibility in new construction are contained in the ADA Accessibility Guidelines issued by the Architectural and Transportation Barriers Compliance Board, an independent federal agency. These standards are incorporated in the final Department of Justice Title III regulation. Elevators are not required in facilities with less than three stories or with fewer than 3,000 square feet per floor, unless the building is a shopping center, shopping mall, professional office of a health care provider, or station used for public transportation.

Alterations after January 26, 1992 to existing places of public accommodation and commercial facilities must be accessible to the maximum extent feasible. The architectural standards for accessibility in alterations are contained in the ADA Accessibility Guidelines. An alteration is a change that affects usability of a facility. For example, if during remodeling, renovation, or restoration, a doorway is being relocated, the new doorway must be wide enough to meet the requirements of the ADA Accessibility Guidelines. When alterations are made to a "primary function area," such as the lobby or work areas of a bank, an accessible path of travel to the altered area, and the bathrooms, telephones, and drinking fountains serving that area, must be made accessible to the extent that the added accessibility costs are not disproportionate to the overall cost of the original alteration. The added accessibility costs are disproportionate if they exceed 20% of the original alteration. Alterations to windows, hardware, controls, electrical outlets, and signage in primary function areas do not trigger the path-of-travel requirement (6).

OVERVIEW OF AMERICANS WITH DISABILITIES ACT ACCESSIBILITY GUIDELINES FOR NEW CONSTRUCTION AND ALTERATIONS

New construction and alterations must be accessible in compliance with the ADA Accessibility Guidelines. The Guidelines contain general design ("technical") standards for building and site elements, such as parking, accessible routes, ramps, stairs, elevators, doors, entrances, drinking fountains, bathrooms, controls and operating mechanisms, storage areas, alarms, signage, telephones, fixed seating and tables, assembly areas, automated teller machines, and dressing rooms. They also have specific technical standards for restaurants, medical care facilities, mercantile facilities, libraries, and transient lodging (such as hotels and shelters).

The guidelines also contain "scoping" requirements for various elements (i.e., it specifies how many, and under what circumstances, accessibility features must be incorporated). Following are examples of scoping requirements in new construction:

- At least 50% of all public entrances must be accessible. In addition, there must be accessible entrances to enclosed parking, pedestrian tunnels, and elevated walkways.
- An accessible route must connect accessible public transportation stops, parking spaces, passenger loading zones, and public streets or sidewalks to all accessible features and spaces within a building.
- Every public and common-use bathroom must be accessible. Only one stall must be accessible, unless there are six or more

stalls, in which case two stalls must be accessible (one of which must be of an alternate, narrow-style design).

- Each floor in a building without a supervised sprinkler system must contain an "area of rescue assistance" (i.e., an area with direct access to an exit stairway where people unable to use stairs may await assistance during an emergency evacuation).
- One TDD must be provided inside any building that has four or more public pay telephones, counting both interior and exterior phones. In addition, one TDD must be provided whenever there is an interior public pay phone in a stadium or arena; convention center; hotel with a convention center; covered shopping mall; or hospital emergency, recovery, or waiting room.
- One accessible public phone must be provided for each floor, unless the floor has two or more banks of phones, in which case there must be one accessible phone for each bank.
- At least 5% of fitting and dressing rooms (but never less than one) must be accessible.

Following is an example of specific scoping requirements for new construction of special types of facilities, such as medical care facilities:

- In medical care facilities, all public and common use areas must be accessible. In general-purpose hospitals and in psychiatric and detoxification facilities, 10% of patient bedrooms and toilets must be accessible. The required percentage is 100% for special facilities treating conditions that affect mobility and 50% for long-term care facilities and nursing homes.

Technical and scoping requirements for alterations are sometimes less stringent than those for new construction. For example, when compliance with the new construction requirements would be technically infeasible, one accessible unisex bathroom per floor is acceptable (6).

WHO IS COVERED BY THE AMERICANS WITH DISABILITIES ACT?

The most difficult part of complying with the ADA, as evidenced by all the legal wrangling of this issue, is determining whether someone requesting an accommodation under the ADA meets the definition of disability as defined by the statute. Most people wrongly assume that having a health condition or diagnosis or receipt of workers' compensation or Social Security benefits automatically entitles them to coverage under the ADA. Instead, the ADA is based on an individual assessment of a person's impairment and whether it substantially has impaired a major life activity. The ADA has three different definitions of disability, and at least one must be met to be covered by the ADA. According to the ADA, an individual with a disability is a person who meets one of the following criteria:

- Has a physical or mental impairment that substantially limits one or more *major life activities*
- Has a record of such an impairment
- Is regarded as having such an impairment

Examples of physical or mental impairments include, but are not limited to, such contagious and noncontagious diseases and conditions as orthopedic, visual, speech, and hearing impairments; cerebral palsy; epilepsy; muscular dystrophy; multiple sclerosis; cancer; heart disease; diabetes; mental retardation; emotional illness; specific learning disabilities; HIV disease (whether symptomatic or asymptomatic); tuberculosis; drug addiction; and alcoholism. Homosexuality and bisexuality are not physical or mental impairments under the ADA. "Major life activities" include functions such as caring for oneself, performing manual tasks, walking, seeing, hearing, speaking, breathing, learning, and working. Individuals who *currently* engage in the illegal use of drugs are not protected by the ADA when an action is taken on the basis of their current illegal use of drugs.

AMERICANS WITH DISABILITIES ACT RESOURCES AVAILABLE FOR HEALTH CARE PROVIDERS

If much of what has been discussed in this chapter might be overwhelming, there are a few resources available to assist you and answer any question you may have regarding the ADA. Below is a list of Web sites one should consult, particularly because there are very few attorneys intricately familiar with the ADA.

- The Department of Justice's Web site contains all the regulations for Title II and Title III entities (*www.ada.gov*).
- The construction requirements can be found at the Access Board's Web site at *www.access-board.gov*.
- For assistance in employment matters, consult the Equal Employment Opportunity Commission at *www.eeoc.gov* or the Office of Disability Employment Policy at *www. dol.gov/odep/*.
- A general disability resource out of the White House is *www.disabilityinfo.gov*. Their site also includes tax information that may be useful to a Title III entity.

- Other useful disability sites that focus on disability culture and ADA are the National Organization on Disability (*www.nod.org*), American Association of Persons with Disabilities (*www.aapd.com/*), and the online disability publication (*www.icanonline. org*).

You also can call a national network of ADA Technical and Accessible Information Technology Centers at 1-800-949-4232 or the Department of Justice ADA Hotline at 1-800-514-0301 (voice) or 1-800-514-0383 (TTY).

REFERENCES

1. 29 U.S.C. 701 *et seq.*
2. 20 U.S.C. 1400 *et seq.* formerly called P.L. 94-142 or the Education for all Handicapped Children Act of 1975.
3. 42 U.S.C. 12101 *et seq.* or P.L. 101-336.
4. ADA Accessibility Guidelines, 28 C.F.R. 36 Appendix A. See also *www.access-board.gov*.
5. 527 U.S. 581, 119 S.Ct. 2176.
6. *ADA Title III Highlights*, U.S. Department of Justice.
7. 524 U.S. 624 (1998).
8. *National Disability Law Reporter*, Highlights, May 1, 2001;19(5):12.
9. *Disability Law Reporter*, Highlights, May 3, 2001;20 (4):7.

4

The Blind or Visually Impaired Patient Seeking Health Care

Kathy Martinez

The purpose of this chapter is to provide health care professionals, particularly gynecologists, with guidance and advice on how to interact appropriately with their female patients who are blind or visually impaired. As a health care professional, you realize your responsibility to your patient involves providing treatment and conveying information in a means she can incorporate into her own experience. These same principles a thoughtful health care provider would follow in serving any patient apply equally to women who are blind or visually impaired. What may differ are the techniques and practices for doing so.

As with many patients, women who are blind may avoid seeking medical treatment out of fear or anxiety. Beyond this, however, women who are blind or have visual impairments, like other women with disabilities, sometimes avoid getting health care because of two additional barriers: lack of access to information and concern that health care providers may lack basic awareness regarding blindness or visual impairment and how these do and do not relate to their medical needs.

Therefore, in addition to her normal "white coat" anxiety, she may worry about how she will be dealt with as a person who is blind. As a general matter, you, the health care professional, are the expert on what she needs to know and what treatment she needs. However, she is the expert on how she needs to obtain that information and treatment. Even if she has been without sight for only a short time, the condition is not the same for her as it might be for you if you temporarily closed your eyes. Things that you think might worry her (things you imagine would worry you if you were blind, such as a slight step) may pose no problem at all. Similarly, things you might take for granted, such as where a chair is located, may be information your blind patient requires.

In dealing with these two threads—information she needs and information you need—we will present numerous examples, each using a familiar baseline and then introducing what might be different for a patient who is blind. To illustrate, let us take the most basic interaction: talking to each other. When addressing most patients, you establish eye contact. If your seeing patient does not respond to such contact you might think she is not listening or is experiencing certain emotions or fears; you then may deal with the situation accordingly. As you continue talking, you might expect her to nod as feedback to show she understands you. When addressing your patient who is blind, however, eye contact may not take place. She may hold her head down or never nod. You would be wrong to assume the usual things when you do not have eye contact or do not receive the usual feedback cues. You will want to give and should expect to receive other kinds of cues—probably verbal ones. You may need to ask more questions, such as, "Are you with me?" "Do you understand the treatment?" You even may want to let your patient know that it is perfectly all right to interrupt with questions or comments.

BASIC PRINCIPLES

A number of specific health professional–patient situations will be covered in this chapter. Because certain basic principles will recur, however, let us deal with these first.

1. Her condition of blindness is secondary to her condition as your female patient—that is, she is a patient with a medical problem first and only incidentally a blind person. In fact, even if she manifests symptoms of depression or anxiety, it would be extremely unwise to assume that the underlying cause has anything to do with her blindness.

2. No one technique is appropriate when dealing with all women who are blind or visually impaired, just as no single approach would work for dealing with all female patients.

Thus, the fundamental principle is when in doubt, ask. For instance, when being escorted in your facility, some women who are blind, even those using canes, will wish to take your arm (probably just above the elbow); others (especially those with guide dogs) may wish to follow you.

STEREOTYPES TO AVOID

1. She may not see, but she is not deaf. You do not need to talk in an extra loud voice.

2. Because she is blind, she is not a child or a dog and should not be called "Dear" or "Honey" or told she is a "good girl." Even if you normally speak to patients in such terms (which you may consider caring and reassuring terms), remember that your blind patient all too often may have been spoken to in such terms by people who have no right to claim such intimacy. She may view such expressions as condescending.

3. If she is accompanied by another person, it is inappropriate to address that person instead of the patient as if she is not there or cannot speak for herself. Many blind people have gone into a restaurant with a friend and have heard the waitress ask her companion, "Does she take sugar in her coffee?" That is inappropriate.

4. Despite film portrayals over the past few decades, she is neither more nor less sexually active than other women.

5. As with most people, women who are blind do not like their private space violated. As a health care professional you are particularly aware of this because in giving treatment you often must touch your patient, thereby violating her personal space. Do not touch your blind patient without her permission: do not grab, pull, or push her. To orient her in the spatial environment, you must use words or place her hand on an object such as a chair or table; you might need to ask her if you may demonstrate how to put on an examining gown, for example.

USEFUL TERMS

Blind: Although usually applied to a person with no vision, this is not an inappropriate term and few people will be offended or embarrassed by its use.

Visually impaired: Although sometimes used as a term for any person with vision loss, this term is most appropriate for persons who have some vision.

HER LEGAL RIGHTS AS A BLIND PERSON

Your blind patient has the same legal rights as any other patient, but implementing them may involve some additional civil rights considerations.

1. She has the right to receive all information relating to her condition or treatment any patient would, but because this information often may be available only in print, attention must be paid to ensuring that its contents are communicated effectively. Examples may include informed consent forms, lab reports, or other documents. Similarly, she may not be in a position to fill out print questionnaires. Effective communications in any of these situations involves the accurate, timely, and private giving or receiving of information verbally, by telephone, by e-mail, or some other mutually agreed-on appropriate means. Privacy may be an especially delicate consideration here. It is

not appropriate to ask her to stand at a reception desk and disclose personal health information with an entire waiting room of people present.

2. She has the right to ready access to her mobility aids, just as a patient who wears glasses ordinarily has the right to their immediate availability when needed. Typical mobility aids for a blind person would be a guide dog, a white cane, or a personal telescopic device. Many concerns exist around the access rights of people with guide dogs. Ordinarily, guide dogs are allowed to accompany their handlers in any place of public accommodation, including a medical or other professional facility except where specific and objective circumstances indicate otherwise. Generalized fears about sanitation or transmission of disease are unfounded; in fact, dogs have been permitted in hospital birthing rooms. As a matter of both commonsense and law, you can rely on the dog's handler to know what will be too stressful for the dog and what may be too stressful for her. She is no more inclined than you are to expose her dog, herself, other patients, or you to any risk. If you have specific concerns, the rule, as always, is to discuss them openly to work things out.

The other major mobility aid your patient is likely to use is the white cane. Many sighted people feel they are doing a blind person a service by relieving them of their need to use the cane and taking charge of their movement. This is not generally a good idea. The cane is not a badge of shame or a mark of inferiority, and your patient is skilled in using it in getting around. Of course, there is no harm in politely offering an arm; however, this is not a substitute but an augmentation to use of the cane for most people.

TYPICAL SITUATIONS AND CONCERNS WHEN DEALING WITH A PATIENT WHO IS VISUALLY IMPAIRED

Having laid down these basic guidelines, the remainder of this chapter sets forth tips that will assist you in your relationship with a patient who is blind or visually impaired.

"What assistance may I offer?" Or "What help do you need from me?" By asking these or similar questions, you seldom can go wrong.

When a sighted patient enters the office, she goes to the reception desk, makes herself known, signs in, and fills out any necessary paperwork. When a blind patient enters the office, she may have little idea where anything (the receptionist's desk, the waiting room, its chairs) may be. The receptionist, or person greeting patients, should identify themselves as well as where the check-in counter is. He or she should ask if the patient needs help finding the appropriate place on the sign-in sheet for her signature. (Some women who are blind carry writing guides, which can be placed over the line where the signature goes; some may wish you to put some kind of guide-a-card or envelope above the line where they must sign; others want the card below. Other women will just need to know where the line is. As with so many things, it is a matter of individual preference.) Ask the patient if she will need help filling out any necessary forms. Remember, if she does not have privacy in providing information, she may feel too embarrassed to disclose crucial information.

When the sighted patient moves from lobby or desk area to the waiting room, she finds a chair and sits down. When the blind patient moves from lobby or desk area to the waiting room, she may need assistance in finding a seat. Often the person calling out names of patients when time to go to the examining room will be different from those at the desk who may seat her initially.

Whoever will bring the blind patient back to the entrance should ask what kind of guiding assistance she needs. Some women prefer to be guided by holding their guide directly above the elbow. Remember to warn her when passing through doorways or when there are steps or a change in terrain. Other people simply will follow the guide. This may be the case with guide dog users or women who have some sight.

When the sighted patient's name is called, she rises and follows someone to an examining room. When the blind patient's name is called, she may have no clue where she is supposed to go. The person calling names may need to approach and guide her as described earlier.

When the sighted patient enters the examining room, she glances around, is given instructions, and prepares for the health professional's visit. When the blind patient enters the examining room, she may need information about its layout: is there a patient's chair, a doctor's desk, an examining table? Describe its set-up and show her where she will be sitting to wait for the doctor. If she is to wait on the examination table, orient her as to where she will sit by showing her the step she must climb to reach the table. If the patient must put on a gown before her examination, give her the gown, describing how it is to be worn and how it fastens. Does it tie in front or back? Is it a wrap-around style? If a number of women dress and undress together in a common area, let her know if there is an option for a private space. She may be as reluctant as anyone to undress in public and should know about her options.

With a sighted patient, when the examiner arrives, he or she introduces himself or herself and proceeds with the examination. With a blind patient, when the examiner arrives he or she should have been alerted that he or she is seeing a blind person so the patient won't have to explain everything all over again from the undignified position of lying on an examining table.

What happens next? Once again, the blind patient is very similar to any other: the basic rule is to let the person know what is going to happen next in a nonpatronizing way.

You may need to provide more details; for instance, she may wish to feel the thermometer or speculum. Although any instruments used in the examination may need to be resterilized, it is important that your blind patient know what will be happening to her and with what. However, like some of your patients, she may feel that the less she knows the better. As always, when in doubt, ask. If more invasive procedures are necessary, describe

them and how and what the patient will feel while those procedures are in progress.

When the examination is finished, the sighted patient dresses, returns to the waiting room or reception desk, makes any additional arrangements, and leaves. When the examination is finished, the blind patient probably can dress herself but may not remember how to return to other areas of the facility. Someone should escort her after giving her enough time to dress and collect her things in private. Remember, too, that she may need to have information read to her. Be sure to ask how she wants to do this: she may have her own writing implement and only need someone to read something to her such as directions for taking medicine, future appointment times, and so on. Ask her how she wants to handle this; it is not a good idea to assume that your writing everything down and handing it to her will be adequate. If extensive information is provided, such as brochures and background information, your blind patient likely does not expect you to sit down with her to read them. It will be helpful, however, if you can assist her in determining how she can obtain the information in a manner most convenient to everyone.

As health care costs increase, more and more patients are asked to conduct their own home tests or obtain samples for analysis by an outside facility. This process, although perhaps exacting, poses relatively little difficulty for your sighted patient. She collects the material (urine, saliva, feces), puts it in the tube and envelope, addresses it, and sends the packet. When a blind patient takes a test at home and sends the data to a lab, it may not be as easy. Often home tests involve measuring things—putting them in tubes up to line X, adding water to line Y, and finally sealing a tube or packet—all without touching anything. This is almost impossible for your blind patient if she has no one at home to assist her. Often asking even a close friend to perform such functions can be embarrassing; she may have no one she wishes to tell about what treatment she is receiving or why she is conducting such a test, and the collection process is very personal. As a result, to assist her, such tests may need to be conducted by staff in the office.

Much of the commonsense that applies to the office visit applies to a hospital visit as well. When a blind patient is admitted to the hospital for inpatient procedures, she will need to be escorted places, examined, and given information. The advice provided earlier is applicable: when in doubt, ask; give verbal feedback; and don't be condescending.

If a blind or visually impaired patient is to have surgery, ensure all relevant staff are aware of the situation, especially the anesthetist. Often eye contact is a sign that the anesthesia is wearing off. For blind patients with amblyopia, this is not a good indicator.

The blind person may not be the patient; he or she may be a spouse, relative, significant other, or good friend visiting your patient: As with any concerned visitor, a blind visitor may seek to monitor the care being given to or otherwise render assistance for his or her relative or friend who is the hospital patient. Here, too, the visiting blind person has the same rights as other visitors. The visitor may need your assistance in seeing that his or her needs as a concerned party are met. She or he may be entitled to know what is in the patient's chart so that she or he may better ask questions and see that appropriate care or treatment is being given. She or he may need to seek the assistance of nearby staff at a nurse's station. The visiting blind person may seek and require the same kinds of orientation and verbal information that a blind patient herself might require.

CONCLUSION

You probably have noticed that when listing what happens for your sighted patient, the list is much shorter than what is written about things that may occur for your blind patient. This is not to imply that a huge burdensome sequence of different steps must be taken when dealing with women who are blind. Nothing is more powerful than the familiar. As a health professional, you know that your patients are likely to feel much more comfortable and relaxed on second and subsequent visits than she does on her first one. The same holds true for your patient who is blind. On her subsequent visits, she also is more likely to be more at ease; she will remember more about where things are, such as where waiting room chairs are in relation to the reception desk, where the examining table is in relation to the patient's chair, and the like. You also will be more at ease as you get to know her; as with your other patients, you'll ask about her children or her job as you casually mention the new coat hook on the back of the door.

Although the environment and procedures in your office may be routine to you, they are often uncommon for the patient. As a health care professional, you witness many of these "first times." Whereas the unfamiliar is uncomfortable for all of us, the level of discomfort probably will be greater for the patient. Problems may arise: your blind patient may speak irritably if you try to help her in what she considers an inappropriate manner—remember she often deals with well-meant but inappropriately offered assistance. Your encounter with another blind person may provide a completely different experience as in encounters with any two individuals. Nonetheless, if you have made your best effort to be sensitive and thoughtful, your relationship with your patient who is blind will be as rewarding for you and nurturing to her as your relationship with anyone for whom you provide treatment and care.

5

Health Care and Deafness: Deaf Professionals Speak Out

Theresa B. San Agustin, Joyce B. Atchison, and Bonnie L. Gracer

Communication is at the heart of good health care. Triage, intakes, medical histories and decisions, instructions for home care and medication regimens, prenatal care, psychotherapy, or drug counseling–all are dependent on the successful exchange of information between health care professionals and the individuals who come to them for treatment.

Communication also is at the heart of deafness. Impairments to the auditory nerve, cochlea, and other physiologic components of hearing may preclude or hinder the capacity of a person who is deaf or hard of hearing to hear and understand sounds. Those impairments, however, have no bearing on a person's natural urge to share thoughts, feelings, love, joys, fears, cost estimates, and everything else, including medical information. The decision about *how* one will cross that communication bridge becomes, ultimately, a question of logistics. It is a very personal decision and is one that each person who is deaf or hard of hearing must make, based on his or her unique skills, preferences, talents, desires, and needs.

Paths to communication are broad. Some people who are deaf or hard of hearing try to maximize the use of whatever hearing they have by using hearing aids, cochlear implants, and assistive listening devices. Others have embraced the richness of American Sign Language (ASL), a form of manual communication that has its own linguistic structure and grammatic base. Others use manual signs in strictly English word order. Some people who are deaf arrive on our shores from other countries, and use Russian, French, Israeli, British, Chinese, or other signed languages. Speech-reading (also known as lip-reading) is another means of enhancing communication. Cued speech combines speech-reading and hand cues to help distinguish sounds that look alike on the lips. Many people who are deaf or hard of hearing use a mixture of these and other communication methods.

Regardless of the patient's communication modality, the key to bridging effective communication is to exude respect, openness, courtesy, curiosity, and a willingness to learn. These qualities, above all else, will make it work. Communication is a two-way street. For example, for a deaf person to speech-read, he or she must be able to see the doctor. That means the lights must be turned on and the doctor's face must be visible.

This chapter provides glimpses into real-life situations where health care and deafness intersect. In some of the anecdotes, you will observe doctors modeling flawless communication in seemingly impossible situations. In others, you will observe doctors who were caught unprepared and fumbled the experience–and as a result, communicated ineffectively with the deaf people who came to them for care. You also will meet the women and girls whose stories provide important lessons for health care professionals.

These are all true stories. Unless otherwise stated, each one was experienced personally by one of the authors, witnessed by one of us in a professional capacity (our professions include medicine, education, and social work), or shared with us by deaf or hard of hearing colleagues who experienced it personally. Stories told in the first-person narrative were experienced by one of the authors personally. Each story is followed by our discussion and commentary. We share these stories in the hope that they will be helpful to you in your practice. All proper names are fictitious. Of course, each situation is different, and each individual has different needs. When in doubt, request direction from the person with whom you wish to communicate.

communication with deaf and hard-of-hearing individuals. Research has shown that the most skilled lip-reader in the most favorable conditions (quiet, good lighting, no visual barriers) understands, at most, 25% of what is said (1). Many words in the English language look exactly the same on the lips, such as baby/maybe, time/dime/type, peanuts/penis, forty/fourteen, and eight/AIDS. Now add to that pain, sedation, and fear, and you will see the importance of taking the time to ensure effective communication with people who are deaf or hard of hearing.

THE STORIES

Son-of-a... What? The Limitations of Lip-Reading

Seventeen-year-old Suzie rang the nurse's station again–the third time that morning. She could barely breathe and was in extreme distress. This time, instead of a nurse, the doctor came to her bedside. "How are you feeling?" the doctor asked. "Son of a bitch," he said. Startled, Suzie stared at the doctor. Maybe she had heard wrong. "I'm sorry to keep pushing the buzzer, but I can't breathe." The doctor leaned over to examine Suzie and then wrote "SOB" in his chart. That night Suzie's father came to visit. Suzie broke down crying, telling him about the doctor calling her a son of a bitch. "He even wrote it in his chart!" The father went to the nurse's station and demanded an explanation. The nurses pulled Suzie's chart and, sure enough, "SOB" was written in clear, bold letters. "Oh," the nurse laughed, realizing what had happened, "SOB stands for 'shortness of breath.'" "Well then, what did that doctor say to my daughter?" the father demanded. The nurses called the doctor, who replied, "Oh, I asked if she was suffering much." After some confusion and a trip to the bathroom mirror, they realized that "suffering much" lip-reads very much like "son of a bitch."

Lip-reading is an inexact science, and generally is, by itself, an insufficient means of

Pencil and Paper Operations

Maria was experiencing severe abdominal pain. She had requested a sign language interpreter when making her appointment and the secretary had agreed. On arrival, however, the secretary explained that "[the doctor] said interpreters are an unnecessary expenditure. This is a routine appointment, and he will use pen and paper."

Although hesitant to proceed in this manner, Maria decided to see the doctor anyway. On examining Maria, the doctor realized this was no routine appointment. Maria needed immediate surgery, so he wrote: "Drive to hospital right away. We must take out growth in stomach. You need operation tomorrow."

Maria, an immigrant from Guatemala who spoke English as a third language behind Spanish and American Sign Language, did not understand the note. She needed surgery because her stomach was growing? She knew she was not pregnant and had not gained any weight recently. Confused, she shared this information with the doctor, who in turn could not understand why Maria was discussing pregnancy or weight at a time like this. The doctor, exasperated, wrote, "The hospital will explain what is going on." Maria did not understand the idiom "going on," but went to the hospital anyway. So Maria, far from home, underwent cancer surgery without ever having had a clear understanding of what was "going on."

When it is clear that one communication method is not working (e.g., Maria's answers did not make sense), it is the doctor's responsibility to find a more effective method. This is particularly true when the medical situation is critical. A good way to ascertain whether a person who is deaf or hard of hearing understands what you have just said is to ask them to repeat it. The best way to ascertain the most effective mode of communication is to request guidance from the deaf or hard-of-hearing person with whom you wish to speak and then comply with that person's request. In this case, Maria had requested an interpreter.

Medical and Legal Consequences of Not Providing an Interpreter

The U.S. Department of Justice, Civil Rights Division, Disability Rights Section reports the following (2):

> The Department reached an agreement with the Davis Hospital and Medical Center in Layton, Utah resolving a complaint that the hospital failed to provide a sign language interpreter to two deaf individuals, a patient and his wife. It was alleged that because of the lack of an interpreter the couple received inadequate information about the patient's cancer care and treatment options. Because of this failure, the couple did not know how to administer the medication properly at home and complications developed, requiring the patient to return to the hospital. The lack of effective communication also meant that the patient did not know of the terminal nature of his condition and that he was denied the opportunity to talk to family members and friends before he died. In addition to paying $130,000 in damages to the patient's wife, the hospital agreed to establish a comprehensive program to provide appropriate auxiliary aids and services to patients, their families, and their companions who are deaf or hard of hearing and annual training to hospital personnel and affiliated physician.

The Americans with Disabilities Act (ADA) requires that doctors provide effective communication to patients who are deaf or hard of hearing. It is in the doctor's best interest to ensure effective communication.

Provide *qualified* interpreters (when necessary for effective communication). The U.S. Department of Justice regulations implementing the ADA define a "qualified interpreter" as "an interpreter who can interpret effectively, accurately and impartially both receptively and expressively, using any necessary specialized vocabulary" (28 CFR Part 36, Section 36.104). Staff who can sign a little are not qualified (even those who can sign a lot are not qualified, unless they are professional interpreters). They may not be able or willing to interpret effectively, accurately, or impartially and will not be bound by the Registry of Interpreters for the Deaf (RID) Code of Ethics (see Appendix II of this chapter). Family members (including hearing children who can sign) cannot be impartial and are not qualified.

Treating people with respect and showing good-faith efforts to communicate effectively are helpful in avoiding charges of civil rights violations. Providing annual training to your staff on treating people with disabilities, complying with the ADA, and providing effective communication are all steps in the right direction. (See Appendix I for organizations and Web sites that can help you get started.)

Role of the Sign Language Interpreter

When Maya arrived at the hospital, she was relieved to find that her interpreters were waiting for her. When the nurse checked her vital signs and asked her questions, the interpreter interpreted and communication flowed smoothly. The nurse left.

*Eventually the doctor came in. Pointing to Maya, she asked the interpreter, "What's wrong with her?" The interpreter started to interpret the doctor's question for Maya, but was cut off by the doctor, who told her to stop. Pointing at the interpreter, she said, "I'm asking **you!**"*

Maya said, "Please speak to me, not to the interpreter." The doctor replied, "I don't tell you how to do your job, so don't tell ME how to do MY job!" At that point the interpreter stopped interpreting and explained to the doctor that his role was merely to facilitate communication, not to become involved in the conversation. He further explained that he had just met Maya and did not know anything about her. Furious, the doctor ordered the interpreter out of the room, saying he was "obstructing the examination process."

Speak with deaf people directly. The interpreter is a professional who shows up for the job and meets the deaf person at the time of the appointment. Interpreters are bound by a professional code of ethics that prohibits them from becoming involved in the content of the conversation. Their job is to facilitate the flow of communication between the deaf person and the doctor. Let the interpreters interpret. That is why you are paying them.

The Breast Exam

Knowing Amalia was deaf, the doctor arranged for an interpreter and planned to demonstrate the exam visually prior to examination to ensure that Amalia would understand fully. Amalia was shocked, however, when the doctor used the female interpreter as a model in his visual demonstration of the breast exam. The interpreter, embarrassed and humiliated, walked out of the room.

The role of the interpreter is to interpret, not to be used as an anatomic model or participate in the interaction in any way. The interpreter understandably felt violated. Although visual displays can be useful when working with people who are deaf, what happened here was grossly inappropriate. More appropriate visual displays could include captioned videos on breast examinations, patient education pamphlets, or plastic models of a human breast.

A Deaf Surgical Patient

I was anxious. The ward nurse said I had to take out my hearing aids before entering the operating room. How would I hear last-minute instructions and questions from the doctors? Finally, I requested (and received)

permission to wear my hearing aids and my glasses. The surgical staff, alerted to my concerns, went out of its way to make sure I could hear. When they needed me to understand something, they pulled down their surgical masks so I could lip-read. Being able to hear the reassuring words of the doctors and nurses helped me to relax just before surgery. After I was sedated and under anesthesia, they removed my hearing aids and glasses— but as I awoke to the nurses' voices in the recovery room, they were already back on.

The doctors thought of everything—even making sure I could communicate immediately with recovery room staff.

These are all very simple accommodations that hospital staffs easily can make for their patients who are deaf or hard of hearing.

Make sure people who are who are deaf or hard of hearing have easy access to their glasses or contact lenses. Deaf people use eyes to "hear." If we cannot see (for whatever reason), it is harder, if not impossible, to hear and understand what is being said.

A Positive Experience in Childbirth

"Honey, I think I am having contractions!" Oh no! Glenn had just come down with a nasty case of the flu and was miserably sick in the upstairs bathroom. This was our first baby—what was I going to do? I needed him there with me to coach me through my labor and delivery!

Glenn was in no shape to take me to the hospital. We called my girlfriend, who agreed to be the stand-in coach. My doctor had noted my hearing impairment in my medical chart, and when I arrived in labor, the doctors and nurses on call knew what to do. Rather than speak to me through the intercom, they came to my bedside when I rang the buzzer. They spoke normally, made direct eye contact, and pulled down their face masks so I could lip-read. They allowed me to wear my eyeglasses and hearing aids so I could see and hear what was going on.

The hospital staff also made sure my TV was set up with captions when I arrived in my room, and that the telephone was fitted with a volume control handset. Glenn managed to arrive just before our daughter was born. Thrilled, he signed to me, "It's a girl!" I could hear my baby crying as they carried her from the nursery to my room. What a wonderful, sweet sound!

All hospitals should be prepared to meet the needs of patients who are deaf or hard of hearing. The medical staff at this hospital showed great flexibility and care.

In this situation, the key to success was preparedness. The doctor had prepared his staff ahead of time, so that when his deaf patient arrived, everything was in place.

The Hospital Intercom System

Whenever I was hospitalized for surgery or the birth of my children, I always informed the hospital staff on my arrival that I was hard of hearing and a lip-reader. They then noted it on their charts. I made sure that the nursing team knew that they needed to come to my room for a face-to-face conversation when I used my call light. The bedside intercom system was useless for me. I needed to communicate directly with them regarding my symptoms, discomfort, or needs and hear and lip-read their responses. This extra effort of the staff was greatly appreciated during my hospital stays, and effective communication always was achieved. I also requested a television set with closed-captioning, as well as volume control and TTY (teletypewriter) on my room telephone so I could call family and friends during my hospital stay.

Please do not try to communicate with people who are deaf or hard of hearing over the intercom system. Intercoms are based on audition. Use visual communication with people who are deaf or hard of hearing.

Please make this clear to nurses on duty. People who are deaf may press the intercom button when in need of assistance because that is their only means of communication with the nursing station. However, they cannot hear the response and therefore do not respond. Then the nurses get frustrated and an-gry with the patient. When alerted via intercom by a patient who is deaf or hard of hearing, nurses and doctors need to respond by physically visiting the person.

The Neurologist

A hit-and-run driver had collided with my car and left me injured and in extreme pain. I had gone to the university health center where a physical therapist, ignoring my protestations of pain, had continued to press against newly injured muscles. The pain was so severe that I experienced a minor episode of semi-consciousness. This had never happened to me before. When I called to tell my internist about this, he referred me to a neurologist.

Exhausted, scared, and in pain, I arrived at the neurologist's office confident that I was in good hands. After all, this neurologist had come highly recommended by my doctor. Inside the examining room, however, I learned otherwise.

The neurologist insisted on turning out the lights before talking to me. He also turned his back on me while giving directions, with the lights turned out. "I am deaf," I told him repeatedly. "I need to see your face when you talk. Can you please turn the lights on, give me the instructions, and then turn off the lights?" This went on for quite a while, the doctor forging ahead and me objecting. He was in a hurry. He seemed disinterested. He did not take a full medical history. Finally, he obliged my request. "By the way," he muttered as we walked into the hall, "you probably have epilepsy." Then he turned into the file room and disappeared. Epilepsy? His lips were barely in view, and the background noise from staff typewriters was distracting. I was upset and exhausted. Next thing I knew, the nurse was handing me consent forms for a computerized tomography or computerized axial tomography (CAT) scan, which would have required injecting iodine into my bloodstream. Then the nurse started leading me into the CAT scan room. It was all happening so fast. Not trusting this doctor, I decided to leave the office. Later, after consulting with another doctor and reading the medical literature, I realized that iodine could have been fatal given my medical history. I also found out that I do not have epilepsy.

There are many medical examinations that require darkness. Darkness is not the issue. What matters is attitude. My ophthalmologist, for example, knows the routine: first directions, then lights. He knows the routine because he listened with respect when I explained my situation and because he was willing to make reasonable adjustments to the way he normally does things.

The neurologist discussed earlier, however, was less willing. Perhaps he was in a hurry. Perhaps he was unaccustomed to being told what to do by a patient. Perhaps he was not used to communicating with someone who is deaf or hard of hearing. Whatever the reasons, by not taking a complete enough history, he could have killed me with that injection. Also, by prematurely introducing the possibility that I might have a new disability, he caused unnecessary stress and fear.

Group Health

The health maintenance organization (HMO) doctor had a number of deaf people on his caseload, and for some reason they were all calling in for appointments. He told his secretary to arrange for an interpreter to come to the clinic, and he scheduled all of the deaf people on the same day—at the same time of day.

When they arrived, the doctor invited all the deaf people into a very large room. He then proceeded to move around the room, addressing each person in succession. There was no privacy whatsoever: "You–Mr. James, right? You are HIV negative. Mrs. Baskin? Where are you? You have a peptic ulcer. Mrs. Li, you are pregnant."

Fifteen year-old Jasmine approached the doctor and whispered, "Excuse me...doctor? In sex education we learned about, uhh, sexually transmitted diseases. How can I protect myself from that?" Much to Jasmine's horror,

the doctor went into explicit detail in a loud voice, with the interpreter interpreting, right in front of everyone. "Shhh, doctor, please not so loud," she begged. The doctor replied, "Oh, they are all deaf anyway, what difference does it make?" A number of the people who were hard of hearing had heard parts of the conversation. The deaf people, their eyes glued to the doctor and interpreter, had seen the entire interaction.

Unconcerned, the doctor finished his rounds and left. Jasmine and the others looked at each other in horror and embarrassment. They left feeling violated, their confidentiality having been completely dismissed by the doctor. Word spread of the incident in the deaf community. Complaints were filed against the doctor, and the HMO lost a lot of business.

Always respect confidentiality.

Have High Expectations

I was 9 years old when my family immigrated to the United States from the Philippines. My parents brought me to see an audiologist as soon as we settled into our new home. Announcing that I had a profound hearing loss, the audiologist told my parents that I would "never be able to graduate high school." My parents were reduced to tears. They told the audiologist that since I was four, I had wanted to be a pediatrician (just like my aunt). The audiologist smirked and walked out of the room. My parents felt belittled and dismissed. Years later, I am a medical doctor and was an honors student throughout high school.

Never underestimate individual potential. Individuals without disabilities may not be familiar with *how* people with disabilities maneuver around their disabilities. This audiologist, for example, may have assumed that because *he* could not figure out how someone could graduate high school without being able to hear, it must not be possible.

Consult with deaf and hard-of-hearing adults, teenagers, and children. People are proud of their successes and ingenuity. They will be happy to share strategies and ideas.

Smiles at the Dentist

I don't like dentists poking my teeth with sharp metal objects, so when I moved to a new city 11 years ago, finding a dentist was not my highest priority. However, one day an advertisement arrived in my mailbox for a dental clinic near my home. While looking at the new patient coupon, my eyes wandered and then fixed on the following statement: "For the hearing impaired, call us on our TDD (telecommunication device for the deaf) line. Dr. Murphy can speak in sign language to make your visit more comfortable." I was shocked. Sign language, a TTY...wow! In spite of myself, I called to make an appointment. The TTY was answered immediately, by a real person (usually it is hidden away in a storage room or set to auto-answer).

When I arrived for my appointment the following week, the receptionist greeted me with a smile and looked directly at me as she spoke. When it was my turn, the dental assistant motioned to me while calling my name. He also looked directly at me and smiled. Dr. Murphy practiced his sign language with me (he is not fluent, but he tries). He treated me with respect, and because of that, I have been seeing him ever since.

The beauty of this story is its utter normalcy. The author arrived in a new town and received an advertisement for dental services. She followed up, was treated by the dentist, and went home. With the exception of a few minor modifications by staff, this visit was much the same as any other routine dental appointment.

The ease with which she was able to call the dentist's office is worth noting. Deaf people use a telecommunications device called a TTY (teletypewriter) to talk on the telephone. The TTY is like a typewriter with a visual screen, so that individuals can type instead of speak and see instead of hear. There are several ways to use a TTY. The fastest and easiest way is if both parties to the call have a TTY. This was the case with Dr. Murphy.

Generally doctors are not required by the ADA to have TTYs if they don't normally allow patients to make or receive phone calls from their office. Instead, the ADA requires telephone companies to set up telecommunications relay services. The relay center provides a third party that has a TTY and can receive both voice and TTY calls. In most states, dialing 711 will connect you to the relay service. For general information on relay service, see the Web site *http://ftp.fcc.gov/cgb/dro/trsphonebk.html*. For a state-by state list of relay numbers and more information on their use, see *http://ftp.fcc.gov/cgb/dro/trs/con_trs.html*.

If Dr. Murphy had not had a TTY, the author could have called the relay center on her TTY. The relay center then would have called Dr. Murphy's office, voiced to the receptionist what the patient was saying on her TTY, and then typed the receptionist's response back to the patient. This is acceptable and legal. Actually *having* a TTY, however, made Dr. Murphy's practice that much more welcoming.

The Emergency Room

Well, there I was, alone and scared, in the emergency room. After signing in, I asked the nurse timidly, "Would you mind waving to me when it's my turn? I don't hear too well." This is what came out.

Not, "I am deaf, can you please get me a sign language interpreter?" Never mind that I am extremely familiar with the ADA and am an advocate for deaf people in medical and other settings. Never mind that I spent 2 years taking graduate courses on deafness and sign language. Never mind that I had been using sign language interpreters on a regular basis for 4 years.

No, because in my moment of personal crisis all of that went out the window, and I was reduced to "not hearing too well," an inadequate descriptor that had been applied to me in my childhood. Fortunately, emergency room staff at the hospital were educated and knew exactly what to do. The woman taking attendance immediately asked, "Do you want an interpreter?"

It had not even occurred to me to ask, but I said "Yes, please." An interpreter arrived 20 minutes later. So when the doctor examined me in the open, noisy emergency room, I understood what he was saying. My fears diminished as he talked and explained what had happened. The nurse stopped by later, put her hand on my leg, and said warmly, "You'll be okay." She made sure I could see her lips. (Just in case, my interpreter was there to tell me what she was saying.) All I had to worry about was getting better—not straining to lip-read, not piecing together fragments of words and trying to guess what they meant.

This is the model to follow. The hospital was prepared. Staff had been trained in advance. The hospital had an emergency contract with a local sign language interpreting agency, so that they could provide interpreters whenever needed–day or night. The nurses and doctors treated me with respect.

Cochlear Implants

Although profoundly deaf from birth, Tasneem has found her cochlear implant to be very successful. Tasneem now can hear her daughter's voice (although understanding what she is saying remains difficult). The transition from no hearing to improved hearing took some time, however. In the beginning, she felt somewhat disoriented, and it was during this period that a fluke slip on the ice landed her in the emergency room. She had banged her head badly. The emergency room staff took an x-ray, was not satisfied, and proceeded to prepare Tasneem for a magnetic resonance imaging (MRI) scan. Luckily, Tasneem was conscious enough to remember that because of her cochlear implant (which uses magnets), she could not have an MRI. By explaining the situation and refusing the MRI, Tasneem was able to prevent further injury.

Be aware that cochlear implants use magnets, so people with cochlear implants cannot receive MRIs.

Sudden Deafness

"I woke up with a BANG." Thus begins the story of 45-year-old Alexa, who, with perfect hearing and no prior health problems, awoke one morning to find her whole world changed. When she tried to get up out of bed, she was knocked back down by a sudden wave of vertigo. Her left ear felt like it was filled to the rim with sand or water, and she had no hearing in her left ear.

Panicked that she might be having a stroke or have an auditory nerve tumor, she called a friend (who happened to be an audiologist). This friend calmed her down. Alexa then contacted her internist. Her internist referred her to an ear, nose, and throat (ENT) doctor, who insisted she come to his office immediately. It was a Saturday.

Alexa, who at this point was nauseated and unable to locate the floor, arrived at the doctor's office highly anxious and agitated. Although she could no longer hear in one ear, there was no silence–instead there was a new, relentless onslaught of loud noise. The shrill, roaring, hissing, and whining noises simply would not let up. An otherwise calm and stable person, Alexa described herself as "losing her mind."

Five years later, Alexa remains profoundly deaf in her left ear. She still experiences tinnitus—every minute of every day—but she credits her ENT with helping her to adjust to her new reality. Her doctor, she reports with gratitude and relief, understood that tinnitus has both physiologic and emotional components. New research indicates that tinnitus affects emotions. Alexa and her ENT discussed the need for medication to help her calm down while her brain accommodated to the constant noise. Alexa also sought assistance from a psychopharmacologist, with the blessing of her ENT and internist. She was treated with respect—and she was treated effectively.

Now an advocate for others with acquired hearing loss, Alexa hears stories of people whose doctors told them "there's nothing we can do," or "you have to learn to live with it." Some people with tinnitus have tried to commit suicide. Alexa urges doctors to recognize and treat the emotional component of sudden hearing loss, tinnitus, and vertigo. These three symptoms often accompany one another.

Vertigo can have an impact on the person's ability to work, play, and function in general and can place the person at risk for falls. Neurologic assessments (e.g., observing the person change from a seated to a standing position, getting up from a chair, walking 10 feet, turning, returning, and sitting again) can be useful in identifying persons at risk for falls (3).

Finally, it is important to recognize that individuals who lose their hearing as adults have not grown up deaf—in most instances they do not know sign language or read lips, do not know deaf people, and are surrounded by hearing people who expect them to be able to hear. The sudden (or gradual) change from hearing to hard of hearing and/or deaf can strain relationships at home, work, and the community. Family members, friends, and colleagues must change old habits; for example, they no longer can talk to a newly deafened person from another room. Late-deafened individuals will need to learn how to navigate the world in a new way. It is important that doctors and health care professionals refer them to associations and support groups (see Appendix I). There, they can meet others with similar experiences and learn about assistive and alerting devices (e.g., flashing fire-lights; volume-amplified phones; and, for mothers, flashing lights that alert them to their babies' cries) and other solutions to everyday problems.

HEALING AND HURT ON A DEAF INPATIENT PSYCHIATRIC WARD

The following two vignettes took place on the same psychiatric ward for deaf adults. In the first instance ("Can Deaf People Hear Voices?"), the author was able to understand sign language, and thereby work effectively with a deaf person who was experiencing hallucinations. In the second ("Lip-Faced"), a lack of communications accessibility resulted in extreme frustration and hurt.

Can Deaf People Hear Voices?

Mary's signing was fast, animated, and passionate. She put forth her arguments with clarity and vigor. Fascinated, I watched the conversation from afar. I felt slightly ashamed. Eavesdropping, I had always been taught, was not polite. Finally, I approached somewhat shyly, not wanting to interrupt. "Excuse me," I said. "It's time for our appointment." "Okay," she said carefully, looking at me and ending her conversation. We were alone in the room. She had been hallucinating.

Lip-Faced

The nurse spoke to her, using her lips only. Kim was furious and lost control. She ripped apart the room, tearing posters from the walls and toppling chairs. "What's wrong?" I asked in sign language. "Talk, speak, lips-her,"* she responded, red-faced. Suddenly the nurse grabbed Kim and locked her in the isolation room.

Because lip-reading is so limited in its effectiveness, it can lead to frustration. In this situation, the nurse had been working on an all-deaf ward for more than 25 years, but had not taken the time to learn anything more than the alphabet in sign language, and even that was halting. The hospital did not have interpreters on site, and because all of the clients were deaf, communication was effective only with staff members who could sign well. One way or another, it is the responsibility of the health care professionals to ensure communication works.

---

*[American Sign Language has its own syntax and is primarily a manually based language. The use of a hyphen (i.e., in the phrase "oral-her" indicates an American Sign Language grammatic construction)].

CONCLUSIONS

The ADA requires that health care providers communicate effectively with people who are deaf or hard of hearing. Even without the legal requirements, providing effective communication is good business. Everybody benefits when doctors and patients communicate clearly. Doctors avoid unnecessary medical mistakes. Patients are better informed and more able to comply with medical instruction.

The U.S. Department of Justice has a toll-free ADA Information Line that health care professionals (and others) may call to discuss communication requirements (see Appendix I).

Some final thoughts:

Be prepared. Train your staff ahead of time. Do not be caught unaware. Know the names and phone numbers of interpreting agencies near you. Emergency rooms should contract for emergency services with interpreting agencies so that if a deaf person shows up with an emergency, emergency personnel can contact the agency without delay and the agency can respond immediately. Collaborate with other health care providers near you. Work together to serve the deaf community. Consider hiring one or more interpreters for your staff. When not interpreting, interpreters can do administrative or other work. If you need assistance finding qualified interpreters, contact RID at 301-608-0050. RID maintains a list of interpreters throughout the country and even internationally.

Be practical. Face the person. Do not turn away in the middle of a sentence. Keep your hands, coffee cups, and other objects away from your face and lips. Ensure adequate lighting. Minimize or eliminate background noise. Meet in a quiet area. Talk in a strong, audible voice. Use normal inflection and normal mouth movements. Make and maintain eye contact. Unless otherwise directed, do not whisper or shout.

Be flexible, open-minded, and willing to learn. Request guidance from the deaf or hard-of-hearing individual as to what means of communication will be most effective.

Use qualified interpreters. Contract with a professional agency or with professional interpreters. Do not use family members, friends, and staff who "know a little sign language"–they are not qualified.

Communicate with your staff. Make sure that appropriate staff know that you have a patient who is deaf or hard of hearing and how to communicate with that individual. Write this information clearly in the medical chart–on the cover, attached to or above the person's bed, and wherever else it is necessary. Keep it brief and to the point. For example: "John is deaf and reads lips"; "sign language (or oral) interpreter required"; "Liana cannot hear over intercom–visit bedside"; or "communicate by writing."

Be mindful of cultural and linguistic diversity. Deaf people from other countries may not know American Sign Language. They may not know how to read the English alphabet.

Be flexible about policies, practices, and procedures. Make reasonable modifications to your policies, practices, and procedures to permit service animals into medical facilities. Just as visually impaired individuals use "seeing eye dogs," many deaf and hard-of-hearing people use "hearing ear dogs." These are working animals, not pets.

Follow up by telephone or e-mail. At the end of this chapter is a list of relay centers across the United States. In many areas, simply dialing 711 will connect you with your state relay. Relay operators translate calls from TDD users into voice, and vice versa, allowing communication with the deaf and hard-of-hearing patients without a special telephone for the hearing person. Talk directly to the deaf person while the relay operator facilitates your conversation. All states are required by law to provide relay services for the deaf and hard of hearing.

Respect privacy. When a woman who is deaf or hard of hearing is changing in the examination room, for example, she will not hear a knock at the door. However, the doctor and interpreter should not just walk in unannounced. Be creative in getting the person's attention. Some ideas include turning the lights on and off a few times, sticking a note under the door, or opening the door a crack and waving. Better yet, establish a routine beforehand with the woman, so there is no confusion or embarrassment.

Have high expectations. Instill confidence. Encourage aspirations. Speak respectfully. (Avoid the term "deaf and dumb," for example; it is offensive.) Provide substantive information so people who are deaf or hard of hearing can make informed decisions.

Remember. People who are hard of hearing or deaf who speak well often are overlooked. People forget they cannot hear. Please, please, please remember.

Confirm understanding. Double-check. Make sure the person understood what you said.

Educate and empower. Provide information about technologies (i.e., assistive and alerting devices) that can enhance hearing and alertness through visual and tactile signals. Refer people to associations and self-help groups.

Be thorough. At least 200 genetic syndromes are associated with deafness and hearing loss (4). Do not dismiss complaints by saying "you'll get used to it" or "you'll be fine." Examine each person as an individual.

Consider learning a few basic signs. Even if all you can do is fingerspell your name, people who are deaf or hard of hearing who sign will appreciate your efforts. Your recognition of and willingness to use sign language demonstrate openness and acceptance. Here are two books to get your started: *Learning American Sign Language* by Humphries and Padden (Englewood Cliffs: Prentice Hall, 1992) and *A Basic Course in American Sign Language* by Humphries, Padden, and O'Rourke (Silver Spring, MD: TJ Publishers, 1980) (5). Of course, the best way to learn sign language is to interact with deaf people.

ACKNOWLEDGMENTS

The authors respectfully acknowledge the health care providers and deaf and hard-of-hearing women and girls whose experiences, described here, provide lessons for us all. To protect privacy, we do not mention them by name. In addition, we gratefully acknowledge the following individuals for their feedback on drafts of this chapter: Sharon Barnartt, Jane G. Blumenfeld, Myron I. Blumenfeld, Carol Cohen, Ernie Hairston, Louise Tripoli, and Brian Millin. Our publisher, Lippincott Williams & Wilkins, provided invaluable assistance. Specifically, the authors thank Bliss Temple for reviewing drafts and providing feedback and Maureen R. Iannuzzi, Anne Snyder, and Lloyd Unverferth of Lippincott Williams & Wilkins for their assistance in making this chapter come to fruition. Finally, the teachings of the late professor Irving Kenneth Zola, z'l, of Brandeis University, provided the inspiration for the format of this chapter–he taught that the sociologic observation of one's personal experiences, as told through stories, can be a powerful pedagogic tool.

REFERENCES

1. Kaplan H, Bally SJ, Garretson C. *Speechreading: a way to improve understanding*, 2nd ed. Washington, DC: Gallaudet University Press, 1985.
2. *Enforcing the Americans with Disabilities Act (ADA): A Status Report from the Department of Justice.* January–March, 2001, Issue 1.
3. Tierney LM, McPhee SJ, Papadakis MA, et al, eds. *Current medical diagnosis and treatment 1993.* Norwalk, CT: Appleton & Lange, 1993.
4. Konigsmark BW, Gorlin RJ. *Genetics and metabolic deafness.* Philadelphia: WB Saunders, 1976.
5. Humphries T, Padden C, O'Rourke TJ. *A basic course in American Sign Language.* Silver Spring, MD: TJ Publishers, 1980.

SELECTED READINGS

Barnett S. Clinical and cultural issues in caring for deaf people. *Fam Med* 1999;31(1):17–22.
Chermak G, Msiek F, Craig CH. *Central auditory processing disorders: new perspectives.* San Diego: Singular Publishing Group, Inc., 1997.
Collins J. Medical stress—deaf women as patients. *Deaf Worlds* 1996;1(12):8–11.

Costello E. *Signing: how to speak with your hands* (Illustrations by Louis Lehman). New York: Random House–Bantam Books, 1983.

Ebert DA, Heckerling PS. Communicating with deaf patients. Knowledge, beliefs, and practices of physicians. *JAMA* 1995;273:227–229.

Frishberg N. *Interpreting: an introduction.* Silver Spring, MD: Registry of Interpreters for the Deaf, Inc., 1990.

Gold J. Deaf patients sue to get interpreters. *Silent News* 1998;30(4):1.

Greenberg J. *In this sign.* New York: Holt, Rinehart and Winston, 1970.

Haffner L. Translation is not enough—interpreting in a medical setting. *West J Med* 1992;157:255–259.

Harvey MA. *Psychotherapy with deaf and hard-of-hearing persons: a systemic model.* Hillsdale, NJ: Lawrence Erlbaum Associates, Inc., 1989.

Herring R, Hock I. Communicating with patients who have hearing loss. *N J Med* 2000;97(2):45–49.

Hines J. Communication problems of hearing-impaired patients. *Nurs Stand* 2000;14(19):33–37.

Hochman F. Health care of the deaf—toward a new understanding [editorial; comment]. *J Am Board Fam Pract* 2000;13(1):81–83.

Humphries T, Padden C. *Learning American Sign Language.* Englewood Cliffs, NJ: Prentice Hall, 1992.

Jackson CB. Primary health care for deaf children: part II. *J Pediatr Health Care* 1990;4:39–41.

Knutson JK, Lansing CR. The relationship between communication problems and psychological difficulties in persons with profound hearing loss. *J Speech Hear Disord* 1990;55:656–664.

Lotke M. She won't look at me. *Ann Intern Med* 1995;123 (1):54–57.

Luey HS, Glass L, Elliot H. Hard-of-hearing or deaf: issues of ears, language, culture, and identity. *Social Work* 1995; 40(2):177–182.

MacKinney TG, Walters D, Bird GL, et al. Improvements in preventive care and communications for deaf patients: results of a novel primary health care program. *J Gen Intern Med* 1995;10(3):133–137.

McEntee MK. Deaf and hard-of-hearing clients: some legal implications. *Social Work* 1995;40(2):183–187.

McEwen E, Aston-Culver H. The medical communication of deaf patients. *J Fam Pract* 1988;26:289–291.

McGinnis C. Tinnitus self-help groups: how, and why, they work. *Hear J* 2001;54(11):49–50.

Myers LL, Thyer BA. Social work practice with deaf clients: issues in culturally competent assessment. *Soc Work Health Care* 1997;26(1):61–76.

Niparko J, Kirk KI, Mellon NK, et al, eds. *Cochlear implants: principles and practices.* Philadelphia: Lippincott Williams & Wilkins, 2000.

Public Law 101-336. The Americans with Disabilities Act of 1990.

Porter A. Sign-language interpreter in psychotherapy with deaf patients. *Am J Psychother* 1999,53(2):163–176.

Raifman LJ, Vernon M. New rights for deaf patients; new responsibilities for mental hospitals. *Psychiatr Q* 1996; 67(3):209–220.

Rennie D. Communicating with deaf patients [letters]. *JAMA* 1995;274:794–795.

Roberts C, Hindley P. Practitioner review: the assessment and treatment of deaf children with psychiatric disorders. *J Child Psychol Psychiatr* 1999;40(2):151–167.

Ruth R, Hamill-Ruth R. A multidisciplinary approach to management of tinnitus and hyperacusis. *Hear J* 2001;54(11):26–32.

Santelli B, Poyadue FS, Young JL. *The parent to parent handbook: connecting families of children with special needs.* Baltimore: Paul H. Brookes Publishing Company, 2001.

Smith MC, Hasnip JH. The lessons of deafness: deafness awareness and communication skills training with medical students. *Med Educ* 1991;25:319–321.

Spradley TS, Spradley JP. *Deaf like me.* New York: Random House, 1978.

Tamaskar P, Malia T, Stern C, et al. Preventive attitudes and beliefs of deaf and hard-of-hearing individuals. *Arch Fam Med* 2000;9(6):518–526.

Weber RD. Hearing impaired patients. Legal obligation to treat and pay for interpreters. *Mich Med* 1999;98(6):10.

Witte TN, Kuzel AJ. Elderly deaf patient's health care experiences. *J Am Board Fam Pract* 2000;13(1):17–22.

Zazove P, Doukas DJ. The silent health care crisis: ethical reflections of health care for the deaf and hard-of-hearing persons. *Fam Med* 1994;26:387–390.

Zazove P, Neimann LC, Gorenflo DW, et al. The health status and health care utilization of deaf and hard-of-hearing persons. *Arch Fam Med* 1993;2:745–752.

APPENDIX I

Organizational Resources

Alexander Graham Bell Association for the Deaf

3417 Volta Place, NW
Washington, DC 20007-2778
202-337-5220 (Voice/TTY)
www.agbell.org

American Speech Language Hearing Association

10801 Rockville Pike
Rockville, MD 20852
800-498-2071
www.asha.org

American Tinnitus Association

P.O. Box 5
Portland, OR 97207-0005
800-634-8978 or 503-248-9985
www.ata.org

Association of Late Deafened Adults
1131 Lake Street, #204
Oak Park, IL 60301
877-907-1738 (Voice/Fax)
(Continental United States only)
708-358-0135 (TTY)
www.alda.org

Cochlear Implant Education Center at the Clerc Center, Gallaudet University
800 Florida Avenue, NE
Washington, DC 20002-3695
www.clerccenter.gallaudet.edu/CIEC

Disability and Business Technical Assistance Centers
ADA Information Line
Toll-free telephone hotline: 800-949-4232 (Voice/TTY)

Disability Rights Education and Defense Fund
ADA Information Line
800-949-4232 (Voice/TTY)
www.dredf.org

Gallaudet University
800 Florida Avenue, NE
Washington, DC 20002-3695
202-651-5000 (Voice/TTY)
www.gallaudet.edu

Job Accommodation Network
800-526-7234 (Voice/TTY)
800-ADA-WORK (Voice/TTY)
www.jan.wvu.edu

National Association of the Deaf
814 Thayer Avenue
Silver Spring, MD 20910-4500
301-587-1788 (Voice)
301-587-1789 (TTY)
www.nad.org

National Institute on Deafness and Other Communication Disorders (NIDCD) Clearinghouse
1 Communication Avenue
Bethesda, MD 20892-3456
800-241-1044 (Voice)
800-241-1055 (TTY)
E-mail: nidcdinfo@nidcd.nih.gov

Registry of Interpreters for the Deaf
333 Commerce Street
Alexandria, VA 22314
703-838-0030 (Voice)
703-838-0459 (TTY)
703-838-0454 (Fax)
www.rid.org

Self Help for Hard of Hearing People, Inc.
7910 Woodmont Avenue, Suite 1200
Bethesda, MD 20814
301-657-2248 (Voice)
301-657-2249 (TTY)
www.shhh.org

TDI (Telecommunications Device for the Deaf)
8630 Fenton Street, Suite 604
Silver Spring, MD 20910-3803
301-589-3006 (TTY)
301-589-3797 (Fax)
301-589-3786 (Voice)
info@tdi-online.org or *www.tdi-online.org*

U.S. Department of Justice
Civil Rights Division
Disability Rights Section
POB 66738
Washington, DC 20035-6738
Toll-free ADA Information Line:
800-514-0301 (Voice)
800 514-0383 (TTY)
www.ada.gov

Vestibular Disorders Association
1015 NW 22nd Avenue, D-230
Portland, OR 97210-3079
503-229-7705
www.vestibular.org

APPENDIX II

Code of Ethics

Registry of Interpreters for the Deaf

The Registry of Interpreters for the Deaf, Inc. (RID) has set forth the following principles of ethical behavior to protect and guide interpreters and transliterators and hearing and deaf consumers. Underlying these principles is the desire to ensure for all the right to communicate.

This Code of Ethics applies to all members of the Registry of Interpreters for the Deaf, Inc. and to all certified nonmembers.

1. Interpreters/transliterators shall keep all assignment-related information strictly confidential.
2. Interpreters/transliterators shall render the message faithfully, always conveying the content and spirit of the speaker using language most readily understood by the person(s) whom they serve.
3. Interpreters/transliterators shall not counsel, advise, or interject personal opinions.
4. Interpreters/transliterators shall accept assignments using discretion with regard to skill, setting, and the consumers involved.
5. Interpreters/transliterators shall request compensation for services in a professional and judicious manner.
6. Interpreters/transliterators shall function in a manner appropriate to the situation.
7. Interpreters/transliterators shall strive to further knowledge and skills through participation in workshops, professional meetings, interaction with professional colleagues, and reading of current literature in the field.
8. Interpreters/transliterators, by virtue of membership or certification by the RID, Inc., shall strive to maintain high professional standards in compliance with the Code of Ethics.

6
Disabling Rheumatologic Conditions Affecting Women

M. E. Csuka

Arthritis is the most common chronic condition and cause of activity limitation in women (Table 6-1) (1–3). Data from the National Health Interview Survey from 1989–1991 estimate that 22.8 million (22.7%) women self-reported arthritis, and 4.6 million (4.6%) women reported arthritis as limiting their activity. Women with arthritis and rheumatic conditions account for more than 60% of hospital discharges, ambulatory care visits, and home health care visits (4). Arthritis and physical limitation is reported more commonly in women, regardless of age group studied (5).

To prescribe appropriate therapy for women with musculoskeletal complaints, differentiation between degenerative, inflammatory, and nonarticular soft-tissue conditions is essential. A history of prolonged morning stiffness, typically lasting more than 1 hour, is the hallmark of inflammatory arthritis. On physical examination objective findings of inflammation (swelling, erythema, warmth, and joint effusions) will confirm the history. Abnormal laboratory test results such as anemia, elevated sedimentation rate, and elevated C-reactive protein support the diagnosis of an inflammatory condition suggested by a careful history and physical examination. Some rheumatologic conditions have specific autoantibody markers. As a general rule, positive autoantibody tests are not helpful in the absence of a typical history and physical examination. The stiffness associated with degenerative joint disease occurs with inactivity. This phenomenon, termed *gelling,* is limited

TABLE 6-1. *Estimated average annual prevalence of self-reported chronic conditions and activity limitations among women aged ≥15 years, by condition—National Health Interview Survey (NHIS), United States, 1989–1991*

Condition	Overall no.[a]	No. with activity limitation[a]
Arthritis	22,755	4,597
Chronic sinusitis	17,511	80
Hypertension	15,720	1,875
Orthopedic deformity	14,536	3,689
"Hay fever," rhinitis	10,700	127
Hearing impairment	9,199	479
Ischemic heart disease	2,421	874
Other selected conditions[b]	11,825	2,356

[a]In thousands. To generate national estimates, NHIS rates were applied to the U.S. civilian, noninstitutionalized population.

[b]Diabetes, thyroid disorder, bladder disorder, cerebrovascular disease, breast neoplasm, and female reproductive malignancy.

(From Centers for Disease Control and Prevention (CDC). Prevalence and impact of arthritis among women—United States, 1989–1991. *MMWR* 1995;44:329–334, 517–518, with permission.)

to specific joints and is relieved with movement. Physical examination will localize the problem to a particular joint or pattern of joints. Fibromyalgia is the prototype of soft-tissue rheumatism. Although neither degenerative nor inflammatory, a history of prolonged morning stiffness may be elicited. On examination, however, there is no evidence of inflamed joints. Laboratory tests are normal in degenerative and soft-tissue rheumatism.

Osteoarthritis (OA) is the most common disabling condition affecting joints and is more prevalent in women. Other rheumatologic conditions such as rheumatoid arthritis (RA), systemic lupus erythematosus (SLE), systemic sclerosis (SSc), Sjögren's syndrome, and fibromyalgia are diagnosed two to ten times more frequently in women and carry even greater potential for disability. Onsets of rheumatic conditions are often insidious, making diagnosis difficult. Early diagnosis and treatment has the potential to prevent disability (6).

OSTEOARTHRITIS

OA, or degenerative joint disease, is a disease of synovial joints. The most common joints involved are the hand, foot, knee, hip, and spine. Loss of articular cartilage, loss of joint space, sclerosis of subchondral bone, subchondral bone cysts, and marginal osteophytes are features of the pathology. Its etiology is multifactorial, including genetic, developmental, metabolic, hormonal, and traumatic factors. Age is the most prominent risk factor for OA. Obesity also has been identified as a significant risk factor, particularly in women. Maintaining a healthy weight at an early age may reduce the risk of developing arthritis in later years, and reduction of weight can improve symptoms (7–15). Osteoporosis is inversely related to prevalence of OA and may relate to factors that cause bone sclerosis (16). Past or present users of postmenopausal estrogen therapy may have a lower incidence and less progression of knee OA (17). True benefit of estrogen replacement awaits a prospective study. Repetitive

stress on a normal joint has been associated with the development of OA, and occupations such as teaching and nursing that involve squatting or kneeling are associated with an increased risk for OA of the knee (18).

Pain localized to the involved joint and limitation of movement are the predominant symptoms of OA. In early disease, symptoms may be episodic and usually are related to activity and relieved with rest. Because cartilage is an aneural tissue, degeneration can progress with little symptomatology. Stretching of the periarticular ligaments or joint capsule, muscle spasm, subchondral microfractures, and patchy synovitis are sources of pain in OA. In early disease, physical findings may be limited to joint or periarticular tenderness on palpation and mild restricted joint motion. Crepitus, noninflammatory joint effusions, limitation of motion, and joint instability are found as the condition progresses. Radiographs may be normal when symptoms first occur, but over time joint space narrowing as a result of loss of articular cartilage, sclerosis of subchondral bone, and development of osteophytes become evident.

OA is not a single disease entity, and various subsets are recognized (Table 6-2). Involvement of the hand in OA is ten times more common in middle-aged women compared to men. It is recognized by bony enlargement of the distal interphalangeal (DIP) joints (Heberden's nodes), proximal interphalangeal (PIP) joints (Bouchard's nodes), and

TABLE 6-2. *Osteoarthritis clinical subsets*

Generalized OA
Heberden's and Bouchard's nodes
First carpometacarpal joint
Knee, hip, acromioclavicular joint
Inflammatory small joint OA (erosive OA)
Spontaneous osteonecrosis of the knee
Unifocal large joint OA
Multifocal large joint OA
Cervical and lumbar spondylosis
Lumbar spinal stenosis
Cervical spinal stenosis
Disseminated idiopathic skeletal hyperostosis (DISH)

OA, osteoarthritis.

the base of the thumb (first carpometacarpal complex). Hand involvement is often gradual and relatively painless. Patients may not present for evaluation until they have symptoms in a weightbearing joint such as the knee or hip. Progressive degeneration of the base of the thumb can be quite painful and interfere with activities that require gripping (19,20). One subset, erosive OA, is characterized by inflammatory findings of pain and swelling in the PIP and DIP joints with prominent nodule formation. This condition is more common in women and may begin in the premenopausal period (21).

There is no known cure for OA. Treatment is directed at alleviation of pain, maintenance of function, and prevention of joint instability. Patient education is as important as pharmacotherapy for maximizing a successful outcome (22). The positive impact of social support in improving pain and function was demonstrated when patients were contacted monthly by phone by trained nonmedical personnel to discuss issues of pain, medication compliance, drug toxicity, and barriers to attending follow-up clinic appointments (23).

Referral to physical therapy is helpful to establish a home exercise program to maintain muscle strength. The periarticular muscles are important for joint stabilization and for shock absorption. This is most noticeable in knee arthritis, where quadriceps atrophy is a common finding. Consequently, quadriceps strengthening is an important component of managing knee arthritis. Exercise programs have been found to decrease the need for analgesics (24–26). A combination of quadriceps strengthening and aerobic exercise has been found helpful for patients with OA of the knee (27). In addition to improving muscle strength, mobility, and coordination, improvement in pain and less disability were found in a study evaluating an exercise program for OA of the hip and knee (28). Exercise need not be strenuous or complicated. Additional benefit of quadriceps strengthening through a series of simple exercises that can be performed at home without specialized equipment can improve proprioception and perfor-

mance of activities of daily living (ADLs) (29). Because patients with lower-extremity arthritis often become sedentary, engaging in a low-impact, continuous-movement exercise program several times a week is important for reconditioning and maintaining cardiovascular health. This can be achieved through a variety of modalities, including fitness walking, participating in an aquatic exercise program, riding an exercise bicycle with low or no tension, or treadmill walking with no elevation, depending on the preference of the patient (30, 31).

Occupational therapy can offer guidance in principles of joint protection and energy conservation. Patients frequently resist the use of assistive devices. Proper use of a cane (i.e., in the contralateral hand) will unload an arthritic hip or knee joint, resulting in less pain and improved function. Wedged insoles may help correct abnormal biomechanics as a result of varus deformity of the knee (32).

Prescribing drug therapy is an important component of the comprehensive management of OA (Table 6-3) and is more effective when combined with nonpharmacologic treatment (33). Acetaminophen can provide relief for mild to moderate pain and in some studies is as effective as ibuprofen or naproxen when used in therapeutic doses. Dosage of acetaminophen should not exceed 4 g/day. A long-acting formulation allows dosing every 8 hours, which is beneficial for patients with night pain. Hepatotoxicity is rare if a dose of 4 g is not exceeded. Existing liver disease and chronic alcohol abuse are recognized clinical situations associated with increased risk for toxicity. Because acetaminophen commonly is present in combination analgesics and/or cold and sinus preparations, such dosing needs to be calculated into the total daily dose (34,35). Monitoring of the international normalized ratio is imperative if used in combination with warfarin (36). It is the safest analgesic for women with impaired renal function (37). Because of low cost and relatively low toxicity, acetaminophen is a good first choice for management of pain in OA. It also can be used on an as-needed basis with a non-

TABLE 6-3. *Management of osteoarthritis*

Nonpharmacologic	Pharmacologic	Surgical
Patient education	Oral analgesics 　Acetaminophen 　Tramadol 　Opioids	Arthroscopy
Psychosocial support	Antiinflammatory analgesics	Osteotomy
Physical/occupational therapy	Nonacetylated salicylate	Total joint replacement
Exercise	Nonselective NSAID 　COX-2 specific NSAID	
Weight reduction	Nutraceuticals 　Glucosamine sulfate 　Chondroitin sulfate Intraarticular 　Glucocorticosteroids 　Hyaluronan Topical 　Capsaicin	

COX, cyclooxygenase; NSAID, nonsteroidal antiinflammatory drug.

steroidal medication for additional pain relief if necessary (38,39).

Nonsteroidal antiinflammatory drugs (NSAIDs) are the most frequently prescribed class of drugs in the United States (Table 6-4). Studies have documented patient preference for these medications instead of acetaminophen for treatment of arthritis pain (40–42). Several of these drugs are available in low-dose, over-the-counter preparations (ibuprofen, naproxen, and ketoprofen). Their primary mode of action is to decrease the production of prostaglandin by inhibiting cyclooxygenase. Until recently, this inhibition was nonspecific, with inhibition of both constitutive prostaglandins responsible for maintenance of normal gastric mucosal barrier and inflammatory prostaglandins responsible for pain and inflammation. As a consequence, significant upper gastrointestinal (GI) toxicities, including gastric/duodenal ulceration, perforations, and death, have been reported. Before prescribing these agents patients should be evaluated for risk of GI toxicity (Table 6-5) (20,43).

TABLE 6-4. *Common nonsteroidal antiinflammatory drugs and typical doses used in osteoarthritis*

Medication	Typical dose
Ibuprofen	400–800 mg t.i.d./q.i.d.
Etodolac	200–400 mg b.i.d./t.i.d.
Ketoprofen	25–75 mg t.i.d./q.i.d.
Diclofenac	50–75 mg b.i.d./t.i.d.
Meclofenamate	50–100 mg t.i.d./q.i.d.
Nabumetone	1,000 mg q.d./b.i.d.
Naproxen	250–500 mg b.i.d.
Sulindac	150–200 mg b.i.d.
Oxaprozin	1,200 mg q.d.
Nonacetylated salicylates 　(Choline magnesium trisalicylate/salsaltate)	500–1,500 mg t.i.d.
Meloxicam[a]	7.5–15 mg q.d.
Celecoxib[b]	100 mg b.i.d. or 200 mg q.d.
Rofecoxib[b]	12.5–25 mg q.d.

[a]COX-2-selective in low dose.
[b]COX-2-specific at all doses.

TABLE 6-5. *Risk factors for upper gastrointestinal adverse events*

Age >65
Comorbid medical conditions
Use of oral glucocorticoids
History of peptic ulcer disease
History of upper gastrointestinal bleeding
Use of anticoagulants

(From American College of Rheumatology Subcommittee on Osteoarthritis Guidelines. Recommendations for the medical management of osteoarthritis of the hip and knee: 2000 update. *Arthritis Rheum* 2000;43:1905–1915, with permission.)

To prevent GI toxicity, concomitant use of gastroprotective agents such as misoprostol or a proton pump inhibitor has been recommended in the high-risk patient. It is important to remember that H_2 blockers have not been found to prevent ulcer development, although they can improve symptoms of dyspepsia, which may mask warning signs. Most GI ulcers are asymptomatic, so patients need to notify their medical care providers of a change in bowel habit and should be monitored for occult anemia (44).

Since 1999, cyclooxygenase 2 (COX-2)-specific inhibitors have been available with the potential of less GI toxicity. The COX-2-specific inhibitors are equivalent pain relievers when compared to traditional nonselective NSAIDs. In addition, COX-2-specific NSAIDs do not inhibit thromboxane production in platelets and therefore do not affect bleeding time or platelet aggregation. Therefore, as opposed to traditional NSAIDs, these drugs do not need to be discontinued prior to surgery and have a better safety profile for patients taking warfarin (45,46). Both traditional and COX-2-specific NSAIDs inhibit renal prostaglandins. As a consequence, fluid retention, hypertension, and renal failure may occur, particularly in the elderly. Renal insufficiency or clinical states of decreased intravascular volume (diuretic therapy, cirrhosis, and congestive heart failure) are conditions where there is an increased risk for NSAID-induced renal toxicity (47).

Although an effective analgesic, acetyl salicylic acid (ASA) is not recommended because of the need for multiple daily dosing and excessive GI risk. Unlike ASA, nonacetylated salicylates do not have antiplatelet effects nor do they impair renal function. When used in therapeutic doses salicylism may limit their usefulness, particularly in the elderly (48).

For patients with severe OA and in whom NSAIDs are contraindicated, opioid analgesics may be necessary. Tramadol is a centrally acting oral analgesic approved by the Food and Drug Administration (FDA) for treating moderate to severe pain. It has compared favorably to ibuprofen for management of OA pain and may be a useful adjunct for symptoms inadequately controlled with NSAIDs alone. As a synthetic opioid agonist, side effects include nausea, constipation, and drowsiness. It should not be used by women with epilepsy (49–51). For severe pain, more standard opiates may be necessary to relieve suffering and maintain function. Guidelines for use of opioids in the management of chronic, nonmalignant pain have been published (52). Use of opioids requires a close physician–patient relationship because of the risk of tolerance and dependence. Significant side effects include respiratory depression and constipation.

Topical therapy can be effective, particularly if only a single joint is causing pain, such as the first carpometacarpal joint of the hand or the knee. Capsaicin, a natural alkaloid derivative of capsicum, the hot pepper, depletes substance P, which is a signal protein for pain-sensitive C-fibers. A small amount is applied to the painful area four to five times per day. Patients may experience a slight burning when applied. Over time, as substance P is depleted from nerve endings, pain is lessened. Capsaicin needs to be applied regularly (not as needed) to be effective. Usually after 1 month of multiple applications, maintenance of twice a day can sustain benefit (53,54)

For management of acute painful flare associated with local inflammation and effusion, especially the knee, intraarticular glucocorticoids can be beneficial in conjunction with systemic therapy. Fluid that is aspirated should be sent for synovial analysis and culture (55). Newer intraarticular therapies have been developed, particularly for the patient unable to tolerate NSAIDs. There are two hyaluronate preparations (Hyalgan and Synvisc) approved for intraarticular injection. Both preparations require multiple weekly injections into the involved joint. The pain relief with hyaluronate injections is slower than with glucocorticoids but appears to last longer. This therapy is helpful, especially in patients intolerant of NSAIDs with localized disease. Currently, this treatment is approved by the FDA only for knee arthritis. Studies are planned to evaluate usefulness of this approach in the shoulder and hip (20,56).

Surgery is an option for patients who have become severely limited by pain and progressive impairment of ADLs with confirmatory radiographic joint damage. In younger patients, a tibial osteotomy is an option for pain relief of predominant medial compartment OA of the knee. Such intervention may delay the need for total joint replacement for years. In the appropriate patient total joint arthroplasty provides marked pain relief and functional improvement (57).

For reasons not entirely clear, women have worse pain and disability than men do prior to arthroplasty. One study suggested that women were more reluctant to undergo a surgical procedure because of concern of risks associated with the surgery and concerns about increasing their burden on the family. A survey performed in Canada found that women were less likely to discuss arthroplasty with their physicians, although they were more likely to seek treatment for arthritis. Compared with men, women had a higher prevalence of arthritis of the hip or knee, worse symptoms, and greater disability but were less likely to have undergone arthroplasty. In this study, women were equally willing to have surgery, but fewer women had discussed this treatment with their physicians (58,59).

Glucosamine sulfate and chondroitin sulfate are two dietary supplements (nutraceuticals) that have gained popularity as safe, nontoxic, and possibly effective treatments for OA. Although proposed beneficial regenerative effects on cartilage have not been proven, preliminary studies have shown these compounds to reduce pain and improve function in some patients with OA. The doses studied were 1,500 mg/day for glucosamine sulfate and 1,200 mg/day for chondroitin sulfate. The National Institutes of Health (NIH) is conducting a trial comparing these agents singly and in combination. Positive effects of reducing pain and stiffness generally are noted at 6–8 weeks (60,61).

RHEUMATOID ARTHRITIS

RA is the most common chronic polyarticular inflammatory disease in the United States, with an estimated 1% prevalence. Women are effected two to three times more often then men. By definition, RA symptoms of joint pain and swelling and morning stiffness lasting more than 1 hour have been present for at least 6 weeks. Usual onset is insidious over weeks to months. Signs and symptoms are unremitting without therapy.

Examination will confirm palpable, painful synovial swelling involving the wrists, metacarpalphalangeal, PIPs, and metatarsalphalangeal joints. Large joint involvement is associated with greater disability. Unlike OA, the thoracolumbar spine and the DIP joints are spared, although high cervical disease can result in neurologic impairment and death. Extraarticular manifestations include tenosynovitis, subcutaneous or periosteal nodules palpated at pressure points (typically along the proximal ulna or olecranon bursae), pulmonary disease, vasculitis, keratoconjunctivitis sicca, and peripheral neuropathy.

Rheumatoid factor (RF) is present in 85% of patients with established disease. A positive rheumatoid factor is not diagnostic of RA unless patients have objective findings of inflammation in a typical distribution of joints. Neither does a negative RF rule out the condition when history and physical findings are compatible. Radiographic changes include marginal erosions and joint space narrowing as a consequence of progressive synovitis.

The etiology is unknown, and although an infectious trigger has been postulated, no organism has been identified definitively. The association of severe disease when an individual possesses the HLA-DR4 haplotype suggests a genetic component (62).

TABLE 6-6. *Reproductive variables and rheumatoid arthritis*

Parity
  Nulliparous women have increased risk of developing RA
  A single live birth appears to permanently decrease risk of developing RA
Established RA
  Remission: symptoms improve in 75% of pregnancies
  Postpartum flare: worsening in first 6 weeks postpartum
  Maternal–fetal HLA mismatch predictive of clinical remission
New-onset RA
  Decreased risk for developing RA during pregnancy
  Increased risk for developing RA in first year postpartum
Oral contraceptives
  May decrease risk for developing RA
  No known treatment effect

HLA, human leukocyte antigen; RA, rheumatoid arthritis.
(From Dugowson CE. Rheumatoid arthritis. In: Goldman MB, Hatch MC, eds. *Women and health.* San Diego: Academic Press, 2000, with permission.)

Rheumatoid arthritis, unlike OA, commonly occurs in younger and middle-aged women. Hormonal and reproductive variables have been noted to affect the course of RA. Remission of symptoms with pregnancy were noted first in 1938. Association of reproductive variables and their relation to RA is presented in Table 6-6 (63).

Joint damage occurs early in most patients. Joint-space narrowing and erosions are noted in 50% of patients in the first 2 years. Half of young working patients will be disabled by 10 years. Even more alarming is decreased life expectancy of 7 years in men and 3 years in women (64,65). Five-year survival estimates for patients with severe functional disability were comparable to three-vessel coronary artery disease or with stage IV Hodgkin's disease (66,67).

Accurate diagnosis and determination of disease severity are important treatment principles. Morning stiffness, synovitis, fatigue, erythrocyte sedimentation rate, and functional limitations assess disease activity. The 1987 revised criteria for diagnosis of RA (Table 6-7) are use-

TABLE 6-7. *The 1987 revised classification of rheumatoid arthritis[a]*

Criterion	Definition
1. Morning stiffness	Morning stiffness in and around the joints, lasting at least 1 hour before maximal improvement.
2. Arthritis of three or more joint areas	At least three areas simultaneously have had soft-tissue swelling or fluid (not bony overgrowth alone) observed by a physician. The 14 possible areas are right or left PIP, MCP, wrist, elbow, knee, ankle, and MTP joints.
3. Arthritis of hand joints	At least one area swollen (as defined in 2.) in a wrist, MCP, or PIP joint.
4. Symmetric arthritis	Simultaneous involvement of the same joint areas (as defined in 2.) on both sides of the body (bilateral involvement of PIPs, MCPs, or MTPs is acceptable without absolute symmetry).
5. Rheumatoid nodules	Subcutaneous nodules, over bony prominences, or extensor surfaces, or in juxtaarticular regions, observed by a physician.
6. Serum rheumatoid factor	Demonstration of abnormal amounts of serum rheumatoid factor by any method for which the result has been positive in less than 5% of normal control subjects.
7. Radiographic changes	Radiographic changes typical of rheumatoid arthritis on posteroanterior hand and wrist radiographs, which must include erosions or unequivocal bony decalcification localized in or most marked adjacent to the involved joints (osteoarthritis changes alone do not qualify).

MCP, metacarpalphalangeal; MTP, metatarsalphalangeal; PIP, proximal interphalangeal.
[a]For classification purposes, a patient shall be said to have rheumatoid arthritis if he or she has satisfied at least four of these seven criteria. Criteria 1 through 4 must have been present for at least 6 weeks. Patients with two clinical diagnoses are not excluded. Designation as classic, definite, or probable rheumatoid arthritis is not to be made.
(From Arnett FC, Edworthy SM, Bloch DA, et al. The American Rheumatism Association 1987 revised criteria for the classification of rheumatoid arthritis. *Arthritis Rheum* 1988;31:315–324, with permission.)

ful in established disease when patients are evaluated for participation in studies, but may not be sensitive enough to diagnose early disease (68).

Importance of patient education cannot be overestimated. Initial exercise programs should emphasis range of motion with progression to conditioning and strengthening exercises as inflammation is controlled. Instruction in joint protection and use of splints, particularly for the wrists, may help improve symptoms and function. Nonsteroidal inflammatory medica-tions work quickly to improve symptoms, but have no effect on disease course. Low-dose prednisone may be necessary in severe disease initially while awaiting the effect of disease-modifying antirheumatic drugs (DMARDs). Alternatively, intraarticular injection of large joints with long-acting corticosteroids can provide significant relief without the long-term complications of oral prednisone.

Recognition of early morbidity has changed the approach to treatment. No longer should patients be asked to wait for the first occur-

TABLE 6-8. *Disease modifying antirheumatic drugs used to treat rheumatoid arthritis*

Drug	Usual dosing regimens	Common adverse effects	Rare, serious toxicities
Azathioprine	50–200 mg/d	Nausea, hepatic abnormalities	Leukopenia, thrombocytopenia, infection (e.g., herpes zoster), secondary neoplasia
Cyclosporine	2.5–4 mg/kg/d	Diarrhea, gingivitis, hypertension, increased hair growth, paresthesias	Renal insufficiency
D-penicillamine	500–1,000 g/d	Pruritic rash, oral ulcers Proteinuria, hematuria Dysgeusia (metallic taste)	Thrombocytopenia, neutropenia Hypersensitivity pneumonitis Polymyositis, SLE, myasthenia gravis
Etanercept	25 mg s.c. twice weekly	Cutaneous injection site reactions	Possible risk of sepsis; possible ANA, DNA seropositivity; ? malignancy
Gold salts			
Injectable gold	50 mg IM q week	Pruritic rash, oral ulcers Proteinuria	Thrombocytopenia Granulocytopenia, hypersensitivity pneumonitis
Oral	3 mg b.i.d.	Diarrhea	
Hydroxychloroquine	200–400 mg q.d (<6.9 mg/kg/d)	Nausea, diarrhea	Rash, pruritus, retinopathy, neuromyopathy
Infliximab	3 mg/kg IV q8wk	Headache, fever, dyspnea Hypertension	Possible risk of sepsis Possible ANA, DNA seropositivity; ? malignancy
Leflunomide	100 mg × 3 d then 20 mg q.d.	Nausea, diarrhea Alopecia	Hepatotoxicity (increased risk in combination with methotrexate)
Methotrexate	10–25 mg q/wk (PO or IM)	Nausea, diarrhea, headache, somnolence Increased liver enzymes	Oral ulcers, bone marrow suppression, hypersensitivity pneumonitis Hepatic fibrosis
Minocycline	100 mg b.i.d.	Photosensitivity, skin discoloration, gastrointestinal upset, drug-induced hepatitis, dizziness	Drug-induced SLE
Sulfasalazine	2 to 3 g/d	Nausea, abdominal pain, diarrhea	Hemolytic anemia, leukopenia
		Rash, increased hepatic enzymes	Thrombocytopenia
		Increased hepatic enzymes	Stevens-Johnson syndrome

ANA, antinuclear antibodies; SLE, systemic lupus erythematosus.

rence of joint erosions to begin taking potentially disease-modifying agents. A list of drugs now used to treat RA is summarized in Table 6-8. Choice of therapy depends on disease severity and individual patient risk factors. Over the past decade, more aggressive management includes beginning disease-modulating drugs early in the course; use of combination chemotherapy and the development of new biologic agents are becoming the standards of therapy (69,70).

Methotrexate has supplanted intramuscular gold as the "gold standard." Lack of true remission with monotherapy methotrexate has prompted the use of combination chemotherapy akin to cancer therapy (71). Increased understanding of the role of tumor necrosis factor (TNF)-α as a proinflammatory cytokine has lead to the development of biologic agents that block its effects. Two injectable drugs are available. Etanercept is a recombinant soluble human TNF receptor blocker administered by subcutaneous injection twice a week. Infliximab is a chimeric human/mouse anti-TNF monoclonal antibody administered intravenously in a maintenance dose every 8 weeks. Simultaneous dosing with methotrexate to prevent the development of antichimeric antibodies is recommended. Both biologic agents have unknown long-term risks with respect to malignancy. They are contraindicated in patients with serious infections. Because of cost ($10,000–$12,000 per patient per year), most insurance policies will not allow such treatment as first line, although recent studies have documented true disease-modifying properties by the demonstration of decreased occurrence of erosions. Recognition of the serious morbidity and mortality associated with RA has led to investigation of these drugs in early disease. In comparison to methotrexate, TNF receptor blockers have shown greater potential for retarding progression of joint damage in RA (72,73). Biologic therapy is a new frontier in the management of RA. A recombinant human interleukin-1 receptor antagonist (IL-1Ra; anakinra) also has shown radiographic regression of bone erosions and was approved by the FDA in 2002 (74). All DMARDs require frequent monitoring for side effects. Hopefully, the expense of new therapies will be outweighed by real benefits of improved function and decreased morbidity and mortality.

SYSTEMIC LUPUS ERYTHEMATOSUS

SLE is an acute and chronic inflammatory multisystem disease characterized by the production of antinuclear antibodies (ANA) and immune complexes that cause tissue injury. SLE has a peak incidence between the ages of 15 and 45, with an estimated female-to-male ratio of 12:1 (75). African-American women are diagnosed with SLE three to four times more frequently than white women and suffer disproportionate disability and mortality. It is not clear whether poorer prognosis is truly a factor of race as opposed to socioeconomic status (76).

As with most autoimmune disease, a specific cause is unknown. A genetic propensity to immunologic dysfunction may be triggered by environmental, infectious, or hormonal factors. Environmental factors reported to predispose to SLE include exposure to ultraviolet light, drug use, smoking, and stress (77). Although 90% of patients are female of childbearing age, cases can be diagnosed at any age and in either sex. Abnormalities of sex hormones, particularly estrogen metabolism, have been found in both male and female patients with SLE (78,79).

The American College of Rheumatology (ACR) criteria for diagnosis of SLE are presented in Table 6-9 (80). Additional signs and symptoms associated with SLE are Raynaud's phenomenon, alopecia (typically along the frontal hairline), fever, weight loss, and severe fatigue. These are not included in the diagnostic criteria because they are not specific to SLE. Diagnosis is generally not difficult in fulminant disease. However, milder cases may present more insidiously, and only over time does the full constellation of signs become manifest.

Laboratory tests are helpful in confirming diagnosis. Unexplained anemia, leukopenia,

TABLE 6-9. *The 1982 revised criteria for classification of systemic lupus erythematosus*[a]

Criterion	Definition
1. Malar rash	Fixed erythema, flat or raised, over the malar eminences, tending to spare the nasolabial folds
2. Discoid rash	Erythematous raised patches with adherent keratotic scaling and follicular plugging; atrophic scarring may occur in older lesions
3. Photosensitivity	Skin rash as a result of unusual reaction to sunlight, by patient history or physician observation
4. Oral ulcers	Oral or nasopharyngeal ulceration, usually painless, observed by physician
5. Arthritis	Nonerosive arthritis involving two or more peripheral joints, characterized by tenderness, swelling, or effusion
6. Serositis	a. Pleuritis—convincing history or pleuritic pain or rubbing heard by a physician or evidence or pleural effusion b. Pericarditis—documented by ECG or rub or evidence of pericardial effusion OR
7. Renal disorder	a. Persistent proteinuria greater than 0.5 g/d or greater than 3+ if quantitation not performed OR b. Cellular casts—may be red cell, hemoglobin, granular, tubular, or mixed
8. Neurologic disorder	a. Seizures—in the absence of offending drugs or known metabolic derangements (e.g., uremia, ketoacidosis, or electrolyte imbalance) OR b. Psychosis—in the absence of offending drugs or known metabolic derangements (e.g., uremia, ketoacidosis, or electrolyte imbalance)
9. Hematologic disorder	a. Hemolytic anemia—with reticulocytosis OR b. Leukopenia—less than 4,000/mm³ total on two or more occasions OR c. Lyphopenia—less than 1,500/mm³ on two or more occasions OR d. Thrombocytopenia—less than 100,000/mm³ in the absence of offending drugs
10. Immunologic disorder	a. Positive lupus erythematous cell preparation OR b. Anti-DNA: antibody to native DNA in abnormal titer OR c. Anti-Sm: presence of antibody to Sm nuclear antigen OR d. False-positive serologic test for syphilis known to be positive for at least 6 months and confirmed by *Treponema pallidum* immobilization or fluorescent treponemal antibody absorption test
11. Antinuclear antibody	An abnormal titer of antinuclear antibody to immunofluorescence or an equivalent assay at any point in time or in the absence of drugs known to be associated with "drug-induced lupus" syndrome

ECG, electrocardiogram.

[a]The proposed classification is based on 11 criteria. For the purpose of identifying patients in clinical studies, a person shall be said to have systemic lupus erythematosus if any four or more of the 11 criteria are present, serially or simultaneously, during any interval of observation.

(From Tan EM, Cohen AS, Fries JF, et al. The 1982 revised criteria for the classification of systemic lupus erythematosus. *Arthritis Rheum* 1982;25:1271–1277, with permission.)

and thrombocytopenia are clues to the diagnosis of SLE. A urinalysis should be performed at each evaluation to identify occult renal disease. A positive ANA is nearly 100% when performed by indirect immunofluorescence on HEp-2 cells (81,82). Although a sensitive test, it is not specific and denotes SLE only in the proper clinical setting. A more specific test is antibody to double-stranded DNA (dsDNA) by the FARR or Crithidiae assays. High titer dsDNA antibody and low complement levels are associated with renal disease and may fluctuate with disease activity (83). Anti-Smith (anti-Sm) is another autoantibody, which is specific for SLE and is present in 30% of patients. Other less-specific antibodies include anti-U1RNP, anti-Ro (SSA), and anti-La (SSB), which are found in other systemic rheumatic conditions (84).

As with RA, patient education is essential to successful management. Regular application of sunscreens and wearing protective clothing are helpful in avoiding ultraviolet light as a trigger of disease activation. Mild disease often can be managed with simple analgesics or NSAIDs. Topical glucocorticoids are useful for treatment of skin lesions. Antimalarial medications, including hydroxychloroquine, chloroquine, and quinacrine, are prescribed for management of constitutional symptoms, cutaneous disease, and musculoskeletal manifestations. Methotrexate is helpful for arthritis and skin manifestations. Serious organ involvement, including renal disease, neuropsychiatric disease, and systemic vasculitis, requires intensive immunosuppressive therapy. High-dose prednisone may be life saving, but prolonged use is complicated by secondary morbidity such as osteoporosis and cardiovascular disease. Immunosuppressive therapy, including cyclophosphamide, azathioprine, and cyclosporine A, are prescribed for serious organ involvement (85). Monthly intravenous cyclophosphamide is now standard therapy for serious renal involvement because it has been shown to preserve renal function and prevent the need for dialysis (86,87).

Mycophenolate mofetil, a reversible inhibitor of inosine monophosphate dehydrogenase, selectively inhibits lymphocyte activity. Commonly used in renal transplantation, it has been found useful in patients with SLE refractory to other therapy, particularly nephritis (88). One randomized controlled trial comparing mycophenolate mofetil to oral cyclophosphamide therapy showed comparative efficacy with less toxicity (89). An NIH trial is comparing this immunosuppressive to intravenous cyclophosphamide.

Immunoablative therapy with high-dose cyclophosphamide with and without autologous stem-cell transplantation has shown promise for severe life-threatening disease in preliminary studies (85). An NIH-sponsored trial is being conducted and hopefully will clarify the benefit of disease remission against death.

Reduced levels of androgens have been noted in women with active lupus. Hormonal manipulation has had some success. Autoimmune-mediated thrombocytopenia and autoimmune hemolytic anemia have been treated successfully with danazol, a synthetic attenuated androgen (90,91). Dehydroepiandrosterone (DHEA) has been useful in mild to moderate disease but not in severe disease (92,93). Doses of 200 mg/day were found to be helpful in reducing prednisone dose in one large study (94).

Animal studies have demonstrated an immunomodulatory role for prolactin. Antibody formation and cell-mediated immune responses were suppressed when serum prolactin levels were lowered artificially. Elevated prolactin levels have been noted in both male and female patients with SLE. Bromocriptine, a prolactin antagonist, has been found to be useful in combination with conventional therapy to reduce flares (95–98).

Renal and neuropsychiatric disease are the cause of the most serious morbidity. Since 1955 there has been an improvement of the 5-year survival rate from 55% to 90% (99). Earlier diagnosis, improved treatments, and diagnoses of milder cases are the most likely cause of better outcome. Mortality is still three times greater than the general population. Cause of death is attributed to serious organ involvement and complications of therapy, particularly infection. Complications of premature atherosclerosis are the leading cause of death in late disease (77,100).

Pregnancy and SLE exacerbation are controversial. Pregnancy during active disease is discouraged because of increased maternal and fetal mortality. In general lupus flares during pregnancy are not more serious than in the nonpregnant SLE population. A flare may occur at any time during the pregnancy or in the postpartum period. Careful monitoring during the pregnancy and in the postpartum period is imperative. Conception in the presence of active disease should be discouraged (101,102).

Obstetric complications, including an increased risk for preeclampsia, are more common in patients with SLE. Risk factors for preeclampsia include preexisting hypertension, nephritis, and the presence of antiphospholipid (aPL) antibodies. Negative fetal outcomes include increased occurrence of fetal wastage, prematurity, and intrauterine growth restriction (101).

Exogenous estrogen supplements in women with SLE remain controversial (103, 104). A study entitled "Safety of Estrogens in Lupus Erythematosus—National Assessment (SELENA)" was designed to clarify this issue (105). Estrogen-containing oral contraceptives and estrogen for postmenopausal hormone replacement should be used with caution in women with SLE, particularly if there are aPL antibodies. Estrogens are contraindicated if the patient has a known history of thrombosis. Depot progesterone is an alternative hormonal approach to contraception; side effects include irregular bleeding, bloating, and weight gain. Intrauterine contraceptive devices are associated with increased risk of infection. Mechanical barrier methods (condoms, diaphragms) are probably the safest choice, although they are not the most effective (101).

The aPL syndrome is found more commonly in women with SLE, although it may present without evidence of another connective tissue disorder (primary aPL syndrome, or PAPS). In the presence of antibodies to phospholipid protein complexes, patients are predisposed to recurrent arterial and venous thrombosis and thrombocytopenia. Mid-trimester abortion as a result of thrombosis and infarction of the placenta is a consequence. Other complications include stroke, peripheral gangrene, epilepsy, chorea, livedo reticularis, and (rarely) multisystem arterial occlusion (catastrophic antiphospholipid syndrome). An elevated partial thromboplastin time is a clue to the presence of aPL antibodies. Because of the presence of blocking antibodies (lupus anticoagulant) the clotting time does not correct when normal serum is added to the assay. Antibodies (immunoglobulin G [IgG] or immunoglobulin M [IgM]) to purified anticardiolipin can be tested by immunoassay. It long has been recognized that patients with SLE often demonstrate biologic false-positive serologic tests for syphilis. This is another example of antibody to phospholipid, although the clinical syndrome is less common when just this test is abnormal.

A 2% prevalence of aPL antibodies in the general population is estimated. Therefore, treatment without a recognized complication is not indicated. Risk of thrombosis is associated with high titer IgG anticardiolipin or aPL antibodies, particularly if the test for lupus anticoagulant is also positive (106,107). An immunoassay to detect anti-B_2-glycoprotein I is felt to more specific for the clinical syndrome and less likely to be associated with false-positive test results for syphilis (108).

In the setting of recurrent thrombosis, anticoagulation therapy is indicated. Women with a history of recurrent abortion and presence of aPL antibodies and/or lupus anticoagulant need close monitoring for both maternal and fetal complications. Low-dose aspirin and subcutaneous heparin are used to maintain pregnancy. High-dose intravenous immunoglobulin also has been used with some success, particularly when thrombocytopenia is a complication (109).

Neonatal lupus erythematosus (NLE) syndrome is a condition in newborns born of mothers with SSA/Ro antibody. The risk is 7% in mothers who are positive for SSA/Ro (101). Transient rash and primary congenital heart block are key features. Primary congenital complete heart block is a consequence of the transplacental passage of maternal antibody to the Ro antigen (SSA). In women known to possess this antibody, administration of low-dose prednisone during heart development may prevent this complication. An alternative approach is to administer maternal dexamethasone at the first sign of any fetal heart abnormality (101). Long-term follow-up of healthy mothers identified to have SSA antibodies as a result of bearing children with NLE frequently will develop a connective tissue disorder, such as SLE or Sjögren's syndrome (110).

SYSTEMIC SCLEROSIS

SSc (scleroderma) is a generalized disorder of connective tissue with characteristic skin findings of thickening and fibrosis and internal organ involvement. The most common presentation is in women between the ages of 30 and 60 years old with female-to-male ratios of 7 to 12:1. Although considered a rare disease, there are more estimated cases of SSc in the United States than multiple sclerosis or muscular dystrophy (111).

Etiology is unknown. One hypothesis implicates microchimerism, the low-level persistence of fetal progenitor cells in maternal blood for decades after childbirth. Support for this hypothesis comes from the predominance of women with SSc, the peak incidence after the childbearing years, and clinical manifestations similar to graft versus host disease. Although this is an intriguing theory, not all women with SSc exhibit this phenomenon, and microchimerism can be demonstrated in normal healthy women (112,113).

The disease currently is classified as either diffuse or limited based on skin involvement. Limited scleroderma (lcSSc) characteristically is more indolent, with skin thickening confined to the face and distal to the elbows and knees. The term CREST syndrome (*c*alcinosis, *R*aynaud's phenomenon, *e*sophageal dysmotility, *s*clerodactyly, and *t*elangiectasias) is no longer used because many patients with long-standing diffuse disease develop features of CREST over time (114). The 1980 criteria for diagnosis are presented in Table 6-10 (115).

TABLE 6-10. *Criteria for the classification of systemic sclerosis (scleroderma)*

A. Major criterion
   Proximal scleroderma: symmetric thickening, tightening, and induration of the skin of the fingers and the skin proximal to the metacarpophalangeal or metatarsophalangeal joints. The changes may affect the entire extremity, face, neck, and trunk (thorax and abdomen).
B. Minor criteria
   1. Sclerodactyly: previously indicated skin changes limited to the fingers.
   2. Digital pitting scars or loss of substance from the finger pad: depressed areas at tips of fingers or loss of digital pad tissue as a result of ischemia.
   3. Bibasilar pulmonary fibrosis: bilateral reticular pattern of linear or lineonodular densities most pronounced in basilar portions of the lungs on standard chest roentgenogram; may assume appearance of diffuse mottling or "honeycomb" lung. These changes should not be attributable to primary lung disease.

(From Preliminary criteria for the classification of systemic sclerosis (scleroderma). Subcommittee for Scleroderma Criteria of the American Rheumatism Association Diagnostic and Therapeutic Committee. *Arthritis Rheum* 1980;23:581–590, with permission.)

Patients with lcSSc may experience symptoms of Raynaud's phenomenon for many years prior to diagnosis. Major organ involvement other than esophageal dysmotility is uncommon. Ischemic digital ulcerations are a source of significant morbidity. Scleroderma renal crisis is rare in lcSSc. Mortality in lcSSc is usually secondary to pulmonary hypertension, which occurs in 10%–15% of patients with lcSSc. Anticentromere antibody, a serologic marker for lcSSc, is found in 70%–80% of patients with limited disease.

The diffuse form of the disease is characterized by rapid progression of skin thickening. Diffuse cutaneous scleroderma (dcSSc) is a much more aggressive disease. Onset of Raynaud's phenomenon usually follows within 1 year, with evidence of puffy or hidebound skin changes. Tendon friction rubs may be palpated and heard over extensor and flexor surfaces of joints. Renal disease, interstitial lung disease, diffuse GI involvement, and myocardial disease account for significant morbidity and mortality. Anti-Scl-70 (antitopisomerase) is a serologic marker for pulmonary interstitial disease and occurs in 30% of patients (116).

In contrast to RA and SLE, there are no disease-modifying agents. Penicillamine, once considered the "drug of choice," has not proved effective in a large multicenter trial comparing low- to high-dose regimens (117). Methotrexate was not shown to be effective in a double-blind, placebo-controlled trial (118). Relaxin, a hormone produced during pregnancy, can inhibit collagen production *in vitro*. Initial enthusiasm for recombinant relaxin therapy was not confirmed when this treatment was subjected to a large placebo-controlled trial (119). Interest in minocycline has been raised after report of improvement in six of 11 patients treated for 1 year in an open-label trial (120). Thalidomide has shown some promise in short-term studies (121). For management of severe multisystem disease, trials are being conducted to assess bone-marrow transplantation. Although there have been some successes, mortality has been high with this treatment (122). Because there is no "gold" standard for therapy, anecdotal reports are encouraging but are not a substitute for randomized control trials. Although the majority of patients with diffuse disease experience progression, reports of spontaneous resolution of skin thickening are not rare. Until a definitive therapy is identified, treatment of scleroderma remains largely symptomatic.

General management of Raynaud's phenomenon includes common-sense measures such as wearing gloves and avoiding undue exposure to cold temperatures, including air conditioning. Discontinuing smoking and other vasoconstrictor agents (e.g., caffeine) is obvious. Treatment with calcium channel blockers is prescribed for management of Raynaud's with variable success but may cause worsening of esophageal symptoms. A recent trial of losartan has been found to be more effective than nifedipine for management of Raynaud's (123). Digital sympathectomy is a useful surgical intervention to treat severe Raynaud's associated with ischemic digital ulceration (124).

Before the availability of angiotensin converting enzyme (ACE) inhibitors, scleroderma hypertensive renal crisis was the most common cause of death. Factors predictive of renal crisis include diffuse skin involvement, rapid progression of skin thickness, disease duration of less than 4 years, recent high-dose glucocorticoid use, new anemia, and new cardiac event (pericardial effusion/congestive heart failure). Early recognition of this complication and treatment with ACE inhibitors have been associated with less end-stage renal disease and/or death. Factors associated with early death or permanent dialysis include male sex, older age at onset, concomitant scleroderma heart disease, pretreatment creatinine of more than 3 mg/dl, and inability to control blood pressure within 72 hours (125–127). Occasionally rapidly progressive unexplained azotemia will occur in the presence of a normal blood pressure. The actual blood pressure value is higher than the patient's baseline. So-called normotensive renal crisis is associated with features of microangiopathic hemolytic anemia and thrombocytopenia (128).

Progressive interstitial lung disease is now the most common cause of death. High-resolution computerized tomography scan of the lung may help differentiate active inflammatory disease from end-stage fibrosis. Immunosuppression is not indicated once fibrosis is the primary pathology. Single lung transplants may be an option for patients without significant other organ damage (129,130). Open-label trials and retrospective studies have suggested some benefit for immunosuppression with cyclophosphamide if there is active alveolitis. A placebo-controlled trial evaluating daily oral cyclophosphamide is being conducted by the Scleroderma Clinical Trials Consortium. Management of secondary pulmonary hypertension is the same as primary pulmonary hypertension. Epoprostenol is approved for management of this complication (131).

Esophageal dysmotility is the most common manifestation of GI dysmotility. Management is symptomatic and aimed at preventing reflux. Measures such as elevation of the head of the bed and limiting food or fluid ingestion for several hours before bedtime are helpful. Proton pump inhibitors often are required in high doses. Prokinetic agents may be of some benefit in early disease but not helpful once fibrosis has replaced contractile smooth muscles. Long-term complications include strictures that may require dilation. Progressive dysmotility of both the small and large bowel is associated with both limited and diffuse disease. Poor nutritional intake and malabsorption may require hyperalimentation (132).

In contrast to SLE, pregnancy is not associated with any serious risk for mother or fetus. Premature birth and small full-term infants were more common in women with SSc when compared with healthy pregnant women. Complications of pregnancy were similar to a group of women with RA (133). Pregnancy is ill advised during early, rapidly progressive disease when there is a higher risk of renal crisis.

SJÖGREN'S SYNDROME

Primary Sjögren's syndrome is a systemic autoimmune disease characterized by xerostomia (dry mouth) and xerophthalmia (dry eye) and is primarily a disease of perimenopausal and postmenopausal women. After RA it is the second most common autoimmune disease, although it frequently is underdiagnosed in clinical practice. Extraarticular manifestations include arthralgia, myalgia, rash, interstitial pneumonitis, renal tubular acidosis, and vasculitis. Risk of developing lymphoma is reported to be 5%. When symptoms are present in a defined rheumatologic condition, the term secondary Sjögren's syndrome is used (134,135). Dyspareunia may be an early symptom preceding more typical complaints of dry eye or mouth (136). Fatigue and fibromyalgia are common and may be a consequence of interrupted sleep as a result of the need to drink followed by voiding as well as a consequence of systemic inflammatory pathways (137,138).

Because symptoms of sicca (dry eyes/ mouth) are common particularly in aging and secondary to common drug therapy, it is important to use objective criteria to make a definitive diagnosis. A Schirmer's test can be performed in the office to quantify absence of tearing (less than 5 mm wetting in 5 minutes). An ophthalmologist can confirm keratoconjunctivitis sicca by slit lamp examination using Rose bengal stain or Lissamine green. Criteria for histologic diagnosis have been established for minor salivary gland biopsy. ANA antibodies and RF commonly are found. Presence of SSA/anti-Ro and SSB/anti-La are more specific (139).

Unless systemic disease is present, treatment is primarily symptomatic. Preservative-free artificial tears are helpful for managing dry eye. Surgical occlusion of the inferior and/or superior punctate can decrease drainage of in a patient who still produces tears. Use of sugar-free gum or candy can help stimulate saliva production. Artificial saliva can be helpful for managing dry mouth, particularly at night or when talking. Muscarinic agonists may be prescribed to help stimulate saliva and tear production. Pilocarpine long has been shown to increase salivation. More recently, cevimeline, a derivative

of acetylcholine, has been approved for treatment of Sjögren's syndrome. None of these modalities has been shown to prevent dental caries. Attention to optimal oral hygiene and close consultation with a dentist is advised. Topical treatment of erythematous oral candidiasis is preferred because systemic administered antifungals do not reach the oral cavity in adequate concentration. Dissolution of vaginal preparations in the mouth is preferred over "oral" topical antifungal agents containing glucose and sucrose for flavoring, which increases the risk of dental caries in individuals with teeth (140,141).

FIBROMYALGIA

Fibromyalgia is a noninflammatory syndrome characterized by complaints of widespread musculoskeletal pain for at least 3 months in the absence of other conditions to account for the pain. The documentation of discrete tender points on physical examination is essential to making a diagnosis. Additional somatic complaints include fatigue, headaches, irritable bowel syndrome, subjective sensation of joint swelling, Raynaud's syndrome, and psychologic distress. The 1990 ACR criteria for the classification of fibromyalgia are presented in Table 6-11 (142).

More than 75% of patients report a nonrestorative sleep pattern. Alpha-wave intrusion during non–rapid eye movement sleep (stage 3 and 4) occurs with increased frequency in patients with fibromyalgia and may account for the subjective sensation of awakening unrefreshed as well as contributing to fatigue (143,144).

Fibromyalgia is associated with increased psychologic distress manifested by depression, somatization disorders, and anxiety. Increased rates of divorce, smoking, physical and sexual abuse, and alcohol or drug use has been reported (145). Women are affected eight times more frequently than men, and symptoms most commonly present in middle age. Prevalence is estimated to be 2% in the general population. An estimated 3.7 million people in the United States are estimated to be

TABLE 6-11. *American College of Rheumatology 1990 criteria for the classification of Fibromyalgia[a]*

1. History of widespread pain
   Definition. Pain is considered widespread when all of the following are present: pain in the left side of the body, pain in the right side of the body, pain above the waist, and pain below the waist. In addition, axial skeletal pain (cervical spine or anterior chest or thoracic spine or low back) must be present. In this definition, shoulder and buttock pain are considered as pain for each involved side. "Low back" pain is considered lower segment pain.
2. Pain in 11 of 18 tender point sites on digital palpation
   Definition. Pain, on digital palpation, must be present in at least 11 of the following 18 sites:
   Occiput: bilateral, at the suboccipital muscle insertions.
   Low cervical: bilateral, at the anterior aspects of the intertransverse spaces at C5–C7.
   Trapezius: bilateral, at the midpoint of the upper border.
   Supraspinatus: bilateral, at origins, above the scapula spine near the medial border.
   Second rib: bilateral, at the second costochondral junctions, just lateral to the junctions on upper surfaces.
   Lateral epicondyle: bilateral, 2 cm distal to the epicondyles.
   Gluteal: bilateral, in upper outer quadrants of buttocks in anterior fold of muscle.
   Greater trochanter: bilateral, posterior to the trochanteric prominence.
   Knee: bilateral, at the medial fat pad proximal to the joint line.
   Digital palpation should be performed with an approximate force of 4 kg.
   For a tender point to be considered "positive," the subject must state that the palpation was painful. "Tender" is not to be considered "painful."

[a]For classification purposes, patients will be said to have fibromyalgia if both criteria are satisfied. Widespread pain must have been present for at least 3 months. The presence of a second clinical disorder does not exclude the diagnosis of fibromyalgia.

(From Wolfe R, Smythe HA, Yunus MB, et al. The American College of Rheumatology 1990 Criteria for the classification of fibromyalgia: report of the multicenter criteria committee. *Arthritis Rheum* 1990;33: 160–172, with permission.)

affected (146). A specific etiology has not been defined. Structural or functional muscle abnormalities never have been found consistently. Changes in muscle are attributed to deconditioning (147).

Dysfunction of the hypothalamic–pituitary—adrenal axis has been studied, but consistent abnormalities have not been found. Treatment with glucocorticoids is not helpful. Serotonin is a neurotransmitter that modulates pain and stage 4 sleep. Abnormalities of serotonin and its precursor, tryptophan, have been reported in fibromyalgia. Large doses of tryptophan have not been helpful. Selective serotonin receptor inhibitors may be useful in treating associated depression but not the primary symptoms of fibromyalgia. Another neurotransmitter involved in pain pathways is substance P, and was found to be elevated in the cerebrospinal fluid of patients with fibromyalgia. Whether this finding is unique to fibromyalgia or present in other pain syndromes is not known. Evidence for hormonal modulation on pain and other symptoms of fibromyalgia are limited (145).

Although patients usually first are diagnosed in middle age, symptoms may have been present since childhood. The typical patient notes a gradual onset of diffuse musculoskeletal problems. Onset of symptoms traced to trauma (motor-vehicle accident, work injuries, surgery, "viral" illness) is more likely to cause patients to have limitations in daily activity, to be unemployed, or to receive disability payments. Patients may perceive emotional trauma as the cause of fibromyalgia. Overall, there is lack of consensus regarding trauma as a definite initiating event (145).

Misdiagnosis of fibromyalgia as RA or OA is common because the patient may present with complaints of joint pain and morning stiffness. Absence of signs of joint pathology and the presence of pain in typical tender points differentiates fibromyalgia from these conditions. SLE may be misdiagnosed in patients with Raynaud's phenomenon and low-titer ANA. Accurate diagnosis is important to avoid unnecessary therapy. It is important to note that fibromyalgia may be diagnosed concomitantly with another rheumatologic condition. Recognizing fibromyalgia as the cause of the patient's symptoms rather than the activity of the systemic disease will avoid unnecessary escalation of immunosuppressive therapy (148).

Laboratory tests are distinctly normal. Unnecessary diagnostic testing is to be avoided. Screening for occult hypothyroidism is reasonable given the common occurrence of this endocrine disorder, which may present with nonspecific musculoskeletal complaints. Detection of RF and ANA should be reserved for patients who have actual inflammatory disease. Positive tests have little significance when the diagnosis is fibromyalgia and contribute to anxiety and concern that a more serious condition is not being diagnosed.

The goal of therapy is to maintain function despite pain. When managing a patient with fibromyalgia, it is important that the treating physician relay with confidence the diagnosis as a real entity and not just a "wastebasket" diagnosis. Although the condition is chronic, it is not life threatening. The majority of patients are relieved to learn that they do not have a progressive, disabling condition. Treatment of concomitant depression and anxiety will allow patients to have a more active role in the treatment program. Identification of individuals factors associated with symptom flares allows patients to take an active role in therapy. Patients may need to change their type of employment. Emphasis on a healthy lifestyle, sleep hygiene, and practice of stress reduction are important factors to emphasize. Social interactions and employment are to be encouraged.

Pharmacotherapy of fibromyalgia in general has not proven to be of any long-lasting benefit, and side effects are frequently more troublesome. NSAIDs in general are little better than placebo. Because many patients are older than age 50, use of NSAIDs may be beneficial for treatment of associated symptoms of OA. Low-dose amitriptyline and cyclobenzaprine may be helpful for short-term use. A double-blind, placebo-controlled study showed no benefit after 6 months (149). Fluoxetine, a selective serotonin reuptake inhibitor, was found to be more effective in combination with low-dose amitriptyline than with either drug alone with respect to sleep and global well-being (150).

Aerobic exercise has been the only treatment modality to show any consistent improvement in symptoms of fibromyalgia. When an indoor bicycle aerobic exercise group was compared to a group assigned to stretching, pain threshold scores, patient and physician global assessment scores, and pain scores improved (151). Additional benefits of exercise include improvement in self-efficacy, a general sense of improved well-being, and improved quality of life (152). A study in 2001 compared a pool-based to a land-based aerobic exercise program. The pool-based group showed greater improvement on self-reported physical impairment and symptoms (pain, depression, and anxiety) as compared to the land-based exercise group (153). Local Arthritis Foundation chapters offer self-help courses for fibromyalgia and warm-water exercise programs in community pools.

Narcotic analgesics are generally not considered appropriate. Recent guidelines encourage use of these agents in nonmalignant pain syndromes (154). It is the rare patient who requires such therapy to function. In general, complaints of pain continue despite use of narcotics. Prescription use of narcotics needs to be monitored carefully to avoid abuse. Modest benefits were noted in a recent multicenter, randomized, placebo-controlled study evaluating tramadol (155).

Various adjunctive therapies have been tried. These include use of S-adenosyl-L-methionine (SAMe), biofeedback, hypnotherapy, acupuncture, and Cognitive Behavioral Treatment. No long-term benefits have been found. Positive treatment response may be hampered by the long duration of symptoms prior to entry into studies (143).

ANTIRHEUMATIC DRUGS AND PREGNANCY

When treating women of childbearing age, issues regarding reproductive function are a consideration. Women are advised not to become pregnant during active disease. However, disease course is variable and many patients may experience remissions, either through medical therapy or (rarely) spontaneously. Before initiating immunosuppressive or antiinflammatory therapy, the risks regarding effects on fertility, timing of conception, fetal development, and lactation should be discussed. The general principle of avoiding all drugs other than folate-enriched multivitamins prior to and during pregnancy is not always practical in the woman with a rheumatic disease. One goal of treatment is to restore function, which for many women includes the desire to become pregnant.

For ethical reasons, pregnant women are not included in drug trials to test toxicity. Studies of immunosuppressive and antiinflammatory drugs require that women agree not to become pregnant. Information regarding effects of drug therapy relies on animal studies and anecdotal case reports. Table 6-12 summarizes recommendations regarding re-productive function with respect to common immunosuppressive and antiinflammatory drugs used in the treatment of rheumatic disease (156).

Until recently glucocorticoids were considered the only "safe" treatment of rheumatic disease in pregnancy. Supplementation with calcium and vitamin D are recommended to help prevent the complication of glucocorticoid-induced osteoporosis. Chronic use requires stress dosing for emergency surgery, cesarean section, and prolonged labor and delivery.

NSAIDs generally are considered safe in early pregnancy, although studies in animals suggest that they may be associated with infertility related to blastocyst implantation. No harmful effects have been reported on early

TABLE 6-12. *Antirheumatic drugs and reproduction[a]*

Drug	FDA risk category[a]	Conception	Pregnancy	Breastfeeding
Aspirin	C (D, third T)	Compatible	d/c 6–8 wk before expected delivery	Compatible
NSAIDs[b]	B (C, high dose)	Compatible	d/c 6–8 wk before expected delivery	Compatible
Corticosteroids[c]	B	Compatible	IUGR	Compatible
Etanercept	B	?	Caution	?
Infliximab	B	?	Caution	?
Hydroxychloroquine	C	Compatible	Compatible	Compatible
Cyclosporin A	C	Compatible	IUGR	Contraindicated
Azathioprine	D	Compatible	IUGR	Contraindicated
Cyclophosphamide	D	Avoid	Avoid, first trimester	Contraindicated
Methotrexate	X	Contraindicated	Contraindicated	Contraindicated
Leflunomide	X	Contraindicated	Contraindicated	Contraindicated

d/c, discontinue; FDA, Food and Drug Administration; NSAID, nonsteroidal antiinflammatory drug; IUGR, intrauterine growth restriction.

[a] The FDA risk categories are (A) controlled studies in women fail to demonstrate a risk to the fetus in the first trimester (and there is no evidence of a risk in the later trimesters) and the possibility of fetal harm seems remote; (B) either animal reproduction studies have not demonstrated a fetal risk but there are no controlled studies in pregnant women, or animal reproduction studies have shown an adverse effect (other than a decrease in fertility) that was not confirmed in controlled studies in women in the first trimester (and there is no evidence of a risk in later trimesters); (C) either studies in animals have revealed adverse effects on the fetus (teratogenic or embryocidal or other) and there are no controlled studies in women, or studies in women and animals are not available. Drugs should be given only if the potential benefit justifies the potential risk to the fetus; (D) there is positive evidence of human fetal risk, but the benefits from use in pregnant women may be acceptable despite the risk (e.g., if the drug is needed in a life-threatening situation or for a serious disease for which safer drugs cannot be used or are ineffective); and (X) studies in animals and human beings have demonstrated fetal abnormalities or there is evidence of fetal risk based on human experience or both, and the risk of the use of the drug in pregnant women clearly outweighs any potential benefit. The drug is contraindicated in women who are or may become pregnant.

[b]Diclofenac, flurbiprofen, ibuprofen, indomethacin, ketoprofen, naproxen, piroxicam. (Diflunisal, etodolac, ketorolac, mefenamic acid, nabumetone, oxaprozin, oxyphenbutazone, phenylbutazone, and tolmetin are FDA risk categorized as C/D.)

[c]Prednisone and methylprednisolone.

fetal development. Except for low-dose aspirin, NSAIDs should be discontinued 6–8 weeks prior to delivery to avoid both maternal and fetal effects (157).

Sulfasalazine has shown no effect on early pregnancy in women taking this drug for management of inflammatory bowel disease. Because there is no reason to believe that women with RA are different in this respect, it should be considered as first-line therapy when treating a young woman with RA. Because hydroxychloroquine crosses the placenta, there is concern regarding accumulation in the fetal uveal tract. To date there are no reports of congenital malformations. Available data support the use of hydroxychloroquine during pregnancy, especially if cessation would risk a flare of disease. This is particularly true for women with SLE when a flare may be life threatening to both the mother and fetus. Gold compounds have a long history of use in RA and do not appear to impair fertility or cause neonatal malformations, although these compounds cross the placenta with deposition into the fetal liver and kidneys. Breastfeeding is discouraged because gold is excreted in breast milk. Most rheumatologists recommend discontinuing injections if patients become pregnant during therapy (158).

Based on data from the renal transplant experience, azathioprine is considered "relatively" safe by some rheumatologists. Informed consent is important because the FDA lists it as risk category D, although no definite teratogenicity has been documented. Use of azathioprine in pregnancy is reserved for women with severe life-threatening disease. Breastfeeding is not recommended. Data on cyclosporine A is also primarily from the renal transplant experience and is considered in a B risk category by the FDA.

Methotrexate is embryotoxic, and women are advised not to become pregnant until discontinuing the drug for 3 months before conception. As a folic acid antagonist, supplemental folate is imperative to prevent neural tube defects. Most of the adverse experience with methotrexate in human pregnancy is derived from high-dose chemotherapy or preg-

nancy termination (159). Data on toxicity with low-dose therapy used in RA is conflicting (160,161). Methotrexate is FDA risk category X and therefore is contraindicated.

Cyclophosphamide is a cytotoxic drug used for management of severe and life-threatening complications of rheumatic disease. Daily oral dosing is associated with a 70% rate of ovarian failure within the first year. Monthly intravenous dosing also can cause ovarian failure, particularly in women older than age 31 years (162). If possible, preservation of ovarian function by timing of monthly dosing, use of oral contraceptives, use of gonadotropin-releasing hormone antagonists, and/or cryopreservation of oocytes can be considered (163). Cyclophosphamide is teratogenic in early pregnancy but may be considered for life-threatening complications after the third trimester.

Newer therapies have no anecdotal cases to assess possible risk. The FDA has given leflunomide an X risk category based on animal data. Because of its prolonged half-life, a drug elimination protocol with cholestyramine 8 g tid for 11 days is recommended prior to contemplation of conception (164). Two other therapies for RA, etanercept and infliximab, both are risk category B for pregnancy. There are no data on fertility, carcinogenesis, or lactation effects. At this time it is prudent to advise patients to use contraception to avoid pregnancy while taking these medications (164,165).

DEPRESSION AND MUSCULOSKELETAL PAIN

The diagnosis of depression is more common in women; therefore it is not surprising that depression is a significant comorbid condition for women suffering functional disability and pain. Significant depression is detected in 49% of patients with chronic soft-tissue pain, 37% of patients with RA, and 33% with OA (167). Increased pain levels are noted in patients with depression and arthritis. Cognitive behavioral treatment, which includes relaxation techniques, coping skills, and cognitive restructuring, may help decrease affective stress and pain in patients with chronic arthritis (168).

EDUCATIONAL RESOURCES

The *Arthritis Sourcebook* by Earl J. Brewer, Jr, MD, and Kathy Cochran Angel is an excellent informational tool to help patients understand their rheumatic condition. Women and their health care providers can obtain reliable, up-to-date information from the American College of Rheumatology and the Arthritis Foundation Web sites (*www.rheumatology.org* and *www.arthritis.org*). Patients should no longer feel that there is nothing to be done but live with pain and progressive disability.

REFERENCES

1. Centers for Disease Control and Prevention (CDC). Prevalence and impact of arthritis among women—United States, 1989–1991. *MMWR* 1995;44:329–334, 517–518.
2. Callahan LF, Rao J, Boutaugh M. Arthritis and women's health: Prevalence, impact, and prevention. *Am J Prev Med* 1996;12:401–409.
3. Centers for Disease Control and Prevention. Arthritis prevalence and activity limitations—United States, 1990. *MMWR* 1994;43:433–438.
4. Centers for Disease Control and Prevention. Impact of arthritis and other rheumatic conditions on the healthcare system—United States, 1997. *MMWR* 1999;48:349–353.
5. National Center for Health Statistics. Health, United States, 1995. Public Health Service, Hyattsville, MD. Available at www.cdc.gov/nchswww/products/pubs/pubd/hus/hus.htm. Accessed July 8, 2003.
6. Buckwalter JA, Lappin DR. The disproportionate impact of chronic arthralgia and arthritis among women. *Clin Orthop* 2000;372:159–168.
7. Davis MA, Neuhaus JM, Ettinger WH, et al. Body fat distribution and osteoarthritis. *Am J Epidemiol* 1990;132:701–707.
8. Anderson JJ, Felson DT. Factors associated with osteoarthritis of the knee in the first National Health and Nutrition Examination Survey (HANES I). Evidence for an association with overweight, race, and physical demands of work. *Am J Epidemiol* 1988;128:179–189.
9. Hartz AJ, Fischer MF, Bril G, et al. The association of obesity with joint pain and osteoarthritis in the HANES data. *J Chronic Dis* 1986;39:311–319.
10. Hochberg MC, Lethbridge-Cejtku M, Scott WW Jr, et al. The association of body weight body fatness and body fat distribution with osteoarthritis of the knee: data from the Baltimore Longitudinal Study of Aging. *J Rheumatol* 1995;22:488–493.
11. Tepper S, Hochberg MC. Factors associated with hip osteoarthritis: data from the first National Health and Nutrition Examination Survey (NHANES I). *Am J Epidemiol* 1993;137:1081–1088.
12. Felson DT, Anderson JJ, Naimark A, et al. Obesity and knee osteoarthritis. The Framingham Study. *Ann Intern Med* 1988;109:18–24.
13. Carman WJ, Sowers M, Hawthorne VM, et al. Obesity as a risk factor for osteoarthritis of the hand and wrist: a prospective study. *Am J Epidemiol* 1994;139:129.
14. Felson D. Weight and osteoarthritis. *J Rheumatol* 1995;22(suppl 43):7–9.
15. Sahyoun NR, Hochberg MC, Helmick CG, et al. Body mass index, weight change and incidence of self-reported physician-diagnosed arthritis among women. *Am J Public Health* 1999;89:391–394.
16. DeQueker J, Mokassa L, Aerssens J. Bone density and osteoarthritis. *J Rheumatol* 1995;22(suppl 43):98–100.
17. Felson DT, Nevitt MC. Estrogen and osteoarthritis: how do we explain conflicting study results. *Prev Med* 1999;28:445–448, discussion 449–450.
18. Cooper C. Occupational activity and the risk of osteoarthritis. *J Rheumatol* 1995;22(suppl 43):10–12.
19. Holderbaum D, Haqqi TM, Moskowitz RW. Genetics and osteoarthritis: exposing the iceberg. *Arthritis Rheum* 1999;42;397–405.
20. American College of Rheumatology subcommittee on osteoarthritis guidelines. Recommendations for the medical management osteoarthritis of the hip and knee. *Arthritis Rheum* 2000;43:1905–1915.
21. Eirlich GE. Inflammatory osteoarthritis–I. The clinical syndrome. *J Chron Dis* 1972;25:317–328.
22. Superio-Cabuslay E, Ward MM, Lorig KR. Patient education interventions in osteoarthritis and rheumatoid arthritis: a meta-analytic comparison with nonsteroidal anti-inflammatory drug treatment. *Arthritis Care Res* 1996;9:292–301.
23. Weinberger M, Tierney WM, Cowper PA, et al. Cost-effectiveness of increased telephone contact for patients with osteoarthritis: a randomized, controlled trial. *Arthritis Rheum* 1993;36:243–246.
24. Slemenda C, Brandt KD, Heilman DK, et al. Quadriceps weakness and osteoarthritis of the knee. *Ann Intern Med* 1997;127:97–104.
25. Slemenda C, Heilman DK, Brandt KD, et al. Reduced quadriceps strength relative to body weight: a risk factor for knee osteoarthritis in women? *Arthritis Rheum* 1998;41:1951–1959.
26. Hurley MV. The role of muscle weakness in the pathogenesis of osteoarthritis. *Rheum Dis Clin North Am* 1999;25:283–298.
27. Ettinger WH Jr, Burns R, Messier SP, et al. A randomized trial comparing aerobic exercise and resistance exercise with a health education program in older adults with knee osteoarthritis: The Fitness Arthritis and Seniors Trial (FAST). *JAMA* 1997;277:25–31.
28. Van Baar ME, Dekker J, Oostendorp RAB, et al. The effectiveness of exercise therapy in patients with osteoarthritis of the hip or knee: a randomized clinical trial. *J Rheumatol* 1998;25:2432–2439.
29. Hurley MV, Scott DL. Improvements in quadriceps sensorimotor function and disability of patients with knee osteoarthritis following a clinically practicable exercise regime. *Br J Rheumatol* 1998;37:1181–1187.
30. Rogind H, Bibow-Nielsen B, Jensen B, et al. the effects of a physical training program on patients with

osteoarthritis of the knees. *Arch Phys Med Rehabil* 1998;79:1421–1427.

31. Jette AM, Lachman M, Giogetti MM, et al. Exercise—it's never too late: the Strong-for-Life Program. *Am J Public Health* 1999;89:66–72.

32. Keating EM, Faris PM, Ritter MA, et al. Use of lateral heel and sole wedges in the treatment of medial osteoarthritis of the knee. *Orthop Rev* 1993;22:921–924.

33. American Geriatrics Society Panel on Chronic Pain in Older Persons. The management of chronic pain in older persons. *J Am Geriatric Soc* 1998;46:635–651.

34. Schhiodt FV, Rochling FA, Casey DL, et al. Acetaminophen toxicity in an urban country hospital. *N Engl J Med* 1997;337:1112–1127.

35. Whitcomb DC, Block GD. Association of acetaminophen hepatotoxicity with fasting and ethanol use. *JAMA* 1994;273:1845–1850.

36. Hyleck EM, Heiman H, Skates SJ, et al. Acetaminophen and other risk factors for excessive warfarin anticoagulation. *JAMA* 1998;279:657-62.

37. Henrich WL, Agodaoa LE, Barret B, et al Analgesics and the kidney: summary and recommendations to the Scientific Advisory Board of the National Kidney Foundation from an Ad Hoc Committee of the National Kidney Foundation. *Am J Kidney Dis* 1996;27:162–165.

38. Bradley JD, Brandt KD, Katz BP, et al. Comparison of an antiinflammatory dose of ibuprofen, an analgesic dose of ibuprofen, and acetaminophen in the treatment of patients with osteoarthritis of the knee. *N Engl J Med* 1991;325:87–91.

39. Williams HJ, Ward JR, Egger MJ, et al. Comparison of naproxen and acetaminophen in a two-year study of treatment of osteoarthritis of the knee. *Arthritis Rheum* 1993;36:1196–1206.

40. Wolfe F, Zhao S, Lane N. Preference for nonsteroidal anti-inflammatory drugs over acetaminophen by rheumatic disease patients: a survey of 1,799 patients with osteoarthritis, rheumatoid arthritis, and fibromyalgia. *Arthritis Rheum* 2000;43:378–385.

41. Pincus T, Swearingen C, Cummins P, et al. Preference for nonsteroidal anti-inflammatory drugs versus acetaminophen and concomitant use of both types of drugs in patients with osteoarthritis. *J Rheumatol* 2000;27:1020–1027.

42. Pincus T, Koch GG, Sokka T, et al. A randomized, double-blind, crossover clinical trial of diclofenac plus misoprostol versus acetaminophen in patients with osteoarthritis of the hip or knee. *Arthritis Rheum* 2001;44:1587–1598.

43. Wolfe MM, Lichtenstein DR, Singh G. Gastrointestinal toxicity of nonsteroidal antiinflammatory drugs. *N Engl J Med* 1999;340:1888–1899.

44. Lanza FL. A guideline for the treatment and prevention of NSAID-induced ulcers. Members of the Ad Hoc Committee on Practice Parameters of the American College of Gastroenterology. *Am J Gastroenterol* 1998;93:2037–2046.

45. Silverstein FE, Faich G, Goldstein J, et al. Gastrointestinal toxicity with celecoxib vs nonsteroidal anti-inflammatory drugs for osteoarthritis and rheumatoid arthritis: the CLASS study. A randomized controlled trial. *JAMA* 2000;284:1247–1255.

46. Bombardier C, Laine L, Reicin A, et al. Comparison of upper gastrointestinal toxicity of rofecoxib and naproxen in patients with rheumatoid arthritis. *N Engl J Med* 2000;343:1520–1528.

47. Perazella MA, Eras J. Are selective COX-2 inhibitors nephrotoxic? *Am J Kidney Dis* 2000;35:937.

48. Furst DE. Are there differences among nonsteroidal anti-inflammatory drugs? Comparing acetylated salicylates, nonacetylated salicylates and nonacetylated nonsteroidal anti-inflammatory drugs. *Arthritis Rheum* 1994;37:1–9.

49. Anonymous. Drugs and pain. *Medical Letter* 1998;40:79–84.

50. Dalgin P. Comparison of tramadol and ibuprofen for the chronic pain of osteoarthritis (abstract). The TPS-OA Study Group. *Arthritis Rheum* 1997;40 (Suppl) 9:S86.

51. Roth SH. Efficacy and safety of tramadol HCl in breakthrough musculoskeletal pain attributed to osteoarthritis. *J Rheumatol* 1998;25:1358–1363.

52. American Academy of Pain Medicine and American Pain Society. The use of opioids for the treatment of chronic pain. Glenview, IL: American Academy of Pain Medicine and American Pain Society, 1997.

53. McCarthy GM, McCarty DJ. Effect of topical capsaicin in the treatment of painful osteoarthritis of the hands. *J Rheumatol* 1992;19:604–607.

54. Matucci-Cerinic M, McCarthy G, Lombardi G. Neurogenic influences in arthritis: potential modification by capsaicin. *J Rheumatol* 1995;22:1447–1449.

55. Creamer P. Intra-articular corticosteroid injections in osteoarthritis: do they work and if so, how? *Ann Rheum Dis* 1997;56:634–636.

56. Kirwan JR, Rankin E. Intra-articular therapy in osteoarthritis. *Baillieres Clin Rheumatol* 1997;11:769–794.

57. Dieppe P, Basler HD, Chard J, et al. Knee replacement surgery for osteoarthritis: effectiveness, practice variation, indications and possible determinants of utilization. *Rheumatol* 1999;38:73–83.

58. Karlson EW, Daltroy LH, Liang MH, et al. Gender differences in patient preferences may underlie differential utilization of elective surgery. *Am J Med* 1997;102:524–530

59. Hawker GA, Wright JG, Coyte PC, et al. Differences between men and women in the rate of use of hip and knee arthroplasty. *N Engl J Med* 2000;342:1016–1022.

60. McAlindon TF, LaValley MP, Gulin JP, et al. Glucosamine and chondroitin for treatment of osteoarthritis: a systematic quality assessment and meta-analysis. *JAMA* 2000;283:1469–1475.

61. Deal CL, Moskowitz RW. Nutraceuticals as therapeutic agents in osteoarthritis. *Rheum Dis Clin North Am* 1999;25:379–395.

62. van Zeben D, Hazes JMW, Zwiderman AH, et al. Association of HLA-DR4 with a more progressive disease course in patients with rheumatoid arthritis. Results of a followup study. *Arthritis Rheum* 1991;34:822–830.

63. Dugowson CE. Rheumatoid arthritis. In: Goldman MB, Hatch MC, eds. *Women and health.* San Diego: Academic Press, 2000.

64. Mitchell CM, Spitz PW, Young DY, et al. Survival, prognosis, and causes of death in rheumatoid arthritis. *Arthritis Rheum* 1986;29:706–714.

65. Wolfe F, Mitchell DM, Sibley JT, et al. The mortality of rheumatoid arthritis. *Arthritis Rheum* 1994;37:481–494.

66. Pincus T, Brooks BS, Callahan LF. Prediction of Long-term mortality in patients with rheumatoid arthritis according to simple questionnaire and joint count measures. *Ann Intern Med* 1994;120:26–34.

67. Pincus T, Callahan LF. What is the natural history of rheumatoid arthritis? *Rheum Dis Clin North Am* 1993; 19:123–151.

68. Arnett FC, Edworthy SM, Bloch DA, et al. The American Rheumatism Association 1987 revised criteria for the classification of rheumatoid arthritis. *Arthritis Rheum* 1988;31:315–324.

69. Pincus T. Aggressive treatment of early rheumatoid arthritis to prevent joint damage. *Bull Rheum Dis* 1998;46:2–8.

70. Kremer JM. Rational use of new and existing disease modifying agents in rheumatoid arthritis. *Ann Intern Med* 2001;134:695–796.

71. Pincus T, O'Dell JR, Kremer JM. Combination therapy with multiple disease-modifying anti-rheumatic drugs in rheumatoid arthritis: a preventive strategy. *Ann Intern Med* 1999;131:768–774.

72. Bathon JM, Martin RW, Fleischmann RM, et al. A comparison of etanercept and methotrexate in patients with early rheumatoid arthritis. *N Engl J Med* 2000;343:1586–1593.

73. Lipsky PE, van der Heijde DM, St. Clair EW, et al. Infliximab and methotrexate in the treatment of rheumatoid arthritis. *N Engl J Med* 2000;343:1594–1602.

74. Jiang Y, Genant HK, Watt I, et al. A multicenter, double-blind, dose-ranging, randomized, placebo-controlled study of recombinant human interleukin-1 receptor antagonist in patients with rheumatoid arthritis. *Arthritis Rheum* 2000;43:1001–1009.

75. McCarty DJ, Manzi S, Medsger TA, Jr., et al. Incidence of systemic lupus erythematosus. Race and gender differences. *Arthritis Rheum* 1995;38:1260–1270.

76. Gladman DD. Prognosis and treatment of systemic lupus erythematosus. *Curr Opin Rheumatol* 1996;8: 430–437.

77. Petri M. Hopkins Lupus Cohort. *Rheum Dis Clin North Am* 2000;26:199–213.

78. Hahn BH. An overview of the pathogenesis of systemic lupus erythematosus. In: Wallace DJ, Hahn BH, eds. *Dubois' lupus erythematosus*, 5th ed. Baltimore: Williams & Wilkins, 1997:69–75.

79. Cooper GS, Dooley MA, Treadwell EL, et al. Hormonal, environmental, and infectious risk factors for developing systemic lupus erythematosus. *Arthritis Rheum* 1998;41:1714–1724.

80. Tan EM, Cohen AS, Fries JF, et al. The 1982 revised criteria for the classification of systemic lupus erythematosus. *Arthritis Rheum* 1982;25:1271–1277.

81. Forslid J, Heigl Z, Jonsson J, et al. The prevalence of antinuclear antibodies in healthy young persons and adults comparing rat liver tissue sections with HEp-2 cells as antigen substrate. *Clin Exp Rheumatol* 1994;12:137–141.

82. Von Muhlen CA, Tan EM. Autoantibodies in the diagnosis of systemic rheumatic diseases. *Semin Arthritis Rheum* 1995;24:323–358.

83. Weinstein A, Bordwell B, Stone B, et al. Antibodies to native DNA and serum complement (C3) levels. Application to diagnosis and classification of systemic lupus erythematosus. *Am J Med* 1983;74:206–216.

84. Maddison PJ, Skinner RP, Vlachoyiannopoulos P, et al. Antibodies to nRNP, Sm, Ro(SSA) and La (SSB) detected by ELISA: their specificity and interrelationship in connective tissue disease sera. *Clin Exp Immunol* 1985;62:337–345.

85. Ruiz-Irastorza G, Khamashta MA, Castellino G, et al. Systemic lupus erythematosus. *Lancet* 2001;357: 1027–1032.

86. Gourley MF, Austin HA, Scott D, et al. Methylprednisolone and cyclophosphamide alone or in combination in patients with lupus nephritis: a randomized, controlled trial. *Ann Intern Med* 1996;125:549–557.

87. Austin HA III, Klippel JH, Balow JE, et al. Therapy of lupus nephritis. *N Engl J Med* 1986;314:614–619.

88. Glickich D, Acharya A. Mycophenolate mofetil for lupus nephritis refractory to intravenous cyclophosphamide. *Am J Kidney Dis* 1998;32:318–322.

89. Chan TM, Li FK, Tang CSO, et al. Efficacy of mycophenolate mofetil in patients with diffuse proliferative lupus nephritis. *N Engl J Med* 2000;343:1156–1162.

90. Ahn YS, Harrington WJ, Simon SR, et al. Danazol for the treatment of idiopathic thrombocytopenic purpura. *N Engl J Med* 1983;308:1396–1399.

91. Ahn YS, Harrington, Mylvaganam R, et al. Danazol therapy for autoimmune hemolytic anemia. *Ann Intern Med* 1985;102:298–301.

92. Van Vollenhoven RF, Engleman EG, McGuire JL. Dehydroepiandrosterone in systemic lupus erythematosus: Results of a double-blind placebo-controlled, randomized clinical trial. *Arthritis Rheum* 1995;38: 1826–1831.

93. Van Vollenhoven RF, Park JL, Genovese MC, et al. A double-blind, placebo-controlled clinical trial of dehydroepiandrosterone in severe systemic lupus erythematosus. *Lupus* 1999;8:181–187.

94. Petri M, Lahita R, McGuire J, et al. Results of the GL701 (DHEA) multicenter steroid-sparing SLE study. *Arthritis Rheum* 1997;40:S327 (abstr.)

95. Bernton EW, Meltzer MS, Holaday JW. Suppression of macrophage activation and T lymphocyte function in hypoprolactinemic mice. *Science* 1988;239:401–404.

96. McMurray R, Keisler D, Kanuckel K, et al. Prolactin influences autoimmune disease activity in the female B/W mouse. *J Immunol* 1991;147:3780–3787.

97. Pauzner R, Urowitz MB, Gladman DD, et al. Prolactin in systemic lupus erythematosus *J Rheumatol* 1994; 21:2064–2067.

98. Alvarez-Nemegyei J, Cobarrubias-Cobos A, Escalantc-Triay F, ct al. Bromocriptine in systemic lupus erythematosus: a double blind, randomized, placebo-controlled study. *Lupus* 1998;7:414–419.

99. Uramoto KM, Michet CJ, Thumboo J, et al. Trends in the incidence and mortality of systemic erythematosus, 1959-1992. *Arthritis Rheum* 1999;42:46–50.

100. Abu-Shaker M, Urowitz MD, Gladman DD, et al. Mortality studies in systemic lupus erythematosus: Results from a single center, I—cause of death. *J Rheumatol* 1995;22:1259–1264.

101. Mok CC, Wong RWS. Pregnancy in systemic lupus erythematosus. *Postgrad Med J* 2001;77:157–165.

102. Ramsey-Goldman R, Manzi S. Systemic lupus erythematosus. In: Goldman MB, Hatch MC, eds. *Women and health*. San Diego: Academic Press, 2000: 713–714.

103. Lahita RG. The role of sex hormones in systemic lu-

pus erythematosus. *Curr Opin Rheumatol* 1999;11: 352–356.

104. Buyon JP, Kalunian KC, Skovron ML, et al. Can women with systemic lupus erythematosus safely use exogenous estrogens? *J Clin Rheumatol* 1995;1: 205–212.

105. Petri M, Buyon J. Flares in the SELENA oral contraceptive trial (abstract). For the SELENA Group. *Arthritis Rheum* 1999;42:S265.

106. Harris EN. Anticardiolipin antibodies and autoimmune diseases. *Current Opin Rheum* 1989;1:215–220.

107. Silver RM, Porter TF, van Leeuween I, et al. Anticardiolipin antibodies: clinical consequences of low titers. *Obstet Gynecol* 1996;87:494–500.

108. Amengual O, Atsumi T, Khamashta MA, et al. Specificity of ELISA for antibody to beta 2-glycoprotein I in patients with antiphospholipid syndrome. *Br J Rheum* 1996;35:1239–1243.

109. Cowchock S. Prevention of fetal death in the antiphospholipid syndrome. *Lupus* 1996;5:467–472.

110. Waltuck J, Buyon JP. Autoantibody associated complete heart block: outcome in mothers and children. *Ann Intern Med* 1994;120:544–551.

111. Monsky S. Scleroderma: A case study of policy. In: Haseltine FP, Jacobson BG, eds. *Women's health research*. Washington, DC: American Psychiatric Press, 1997:285–300.

112. Miyashita Y, Ono M, Ono M, et al. Y chromosome microchimerism in rheumatic autoimmune disease. *Ann Rheum Dis* 2000;59:655–656.

113. Nelson JL. Microchimerism and scleroderma. *Curr Rheum Dis* 1999;1(1):15–21.

114. Wigley fibromyalgia. When is Scleroderma really scleroderma? *J Rheumatol* 2001;28:1471–1473.

115. Preliminary criteria for the classification of systemic sclerosis (scleroderma). Subcommittee for Scleroderma Criteria of the American Rheumatism Association Diagnostic and Therapeutic Criteria Committee. *Arthritis Rheum* 1980;23:581–590.

116. White B. Systemic sclerosis and related syndromes. In: Klippel JH, ed. *Primer on the rheumatic diseases,* 11th ed. Atlanta: Arthritis Foundation, 1997:263–266.

117. Clements PJ, Furst DE, Wong WK, et al. High-dose versus low-dose D-penicillamine in early diffuse systemic sclerosis: analysis of a two-year, double-blind, randomized, controlled clinical trial. *Arthritis Rheum* 1999;42:1194–1203.

118. Pope JE, Bellamy N, Seibold, et al. A randomized, controlled trial of methotrexate versus placebo in early diffuse scleroderma. *Arthritis Rheum* 2001;44: 1351–1358.

119. Seibold JR, Korn JH, Simms R, et al. Recombinant human relaxin in the treatment of scleroderma. A randomized, double-blind, placebo-controlled trial. *Ann Intern Med* 2000;132:871–879.

120. Le CH, Morales A, Trentham DE. Minocycline in early diffuse scleroderma. *Lancet* 1998;352(9142): 1755–1756.

121. Oliver ST. The Th1/Th2 paradigm in the pathogenesis of scleroderma and its modulation the thalidomide. *Curr Rheum Rep* 2000;2:486–491.

122. Viganego I, Nash R, Furst DE. Bone Marrow Transplantation in the treatment of systemic sclerosis. *Curr Rheum* 2000;2:492–500.

123. Dziadzio M, Denton CP, Smith R, et al. Losartan ther-

apy for Raynaud's phenomenon and scleroderma: clinical and biochemical findings in a fifteen-week, randomized, parallel-group, controlled trial. *Arthritis Rheum* 1999;52:2646–2655.

124. Yee AMI. Adventitial Stripping: a digit saving procedure in refractory Raynaud's phenomenon. *J Rheumatol* 1998;25:269–276.

125. Steen VD, Medsger RA Jr. Long-term outcomes of scleroderma renal crisis. *Ann Intern Med* 2000;133: 600–603.

126. Steen VD, Costantino JP, Shapiro AP, et al. Outcome of renal crisis in systemic sclerosis: relation to availability of angiotensin converting enzyme (ACE) inhibitors. *Ann Intern Med* 1990;113:352–357.

127. Steen VD. Scleroderma renal crisis. *Rheum Dis Clin North Am* 1996;22:861–878.

128. Helfrich DJ, Banner B, Steen, et al. Normotensive renal failure in systemic sclerosis. *Arthritis Rheum* 1989; 32:1128–1134.

129. Davas EM, Peppas C, Maragou M, et al. Intravenous cyclophosphamide pulse therapy for the treatment of lung disease associated with scleroderma. *Clin Rheumatol* 1999;18;455–461.

130. White B, Moore W, Wigley fibromyalgia, et al. Cyclophosphamide is associated with pulmonary function and survival benefit in patients with scleroderma and alveolitis. *Ann Intern Med* 2000;132:947–954.

131. Badesch DB, Tapson VF, McGoon MD, et al. Continuous intravenous epoprostenol for pulmonary hypertension due to the scleroderma spectrum of disease. *Ann Intern Med* 2000;132:425–434.

132. Weston S, Thumshirn M, Wiste J, et al. Clinical and upper gastrointestinal motility features in systemic sclerosis and related disorders. *Am J Gastroenterol* 1998;93:1085–1089.

133. Steen V, Medsger TM. Pregnancy. *Arthritis Rheum* 1999;42:763–768.

134. Talal N. What is Sjögren's syndrome and why it is important? *J Rheumatol* 2000;27(suppl):1–3.

135. Anaya J-M, Talal N. Sjögren's syndrome comes of age. *Semin Arthritis Rheum* 1999;28:355–359.

136. Mulherin DM, Sheeran TP, Kumararatne DS, et al. Sjögren's syndrome in women presenting with chronic dyspareunia. *Br J Obstet Gynaecol* 1997;104: 1019–1023.

137. Bonafede RP, Downey DC, Bennett RM. An association of fibromyalgia with primary Sjögren's syndrome: a prospective study of 72 patients. *J Rheumatol* 1995; 22:133–136.

138. Bennett R. Fibromyalgia, chronic fatigue syndrome, and myofascial pain. *Curr Opin Rheumatol* 1998;10: 95–103.

139. Fox R. Classification criteria for Sjögren's syndrome: current controversies in rheumatology. *Rheum Dis Clin North Am* 1994;20:391–407.

140. Daniels TE. Evaluation, differential diagnosis, and treatment of xerostomia. *J Rheumatol* 2000;27(suppl 61):6–10.

141. Fox RI, Michelson P. Approaches to the treatment of Sjögren's syndrome. *J Rheumatol* 2000;27(suppl 61): 1521.

142. Wolfe R, Smythe HA, Yunus MB, et al. The American College of Rheumatology 1990 criteria for the classification of fibromyalgia: report of the multicenter criteria committee. *Arthritis Rheum* 1990;33:160–172.

143. Levanthal LJ. Management of fibromyalgia. *Ann Intern Med* 1999;131:850–858.
144. Roizenblatt S, Moldofsky H, Benedito-Silva AA, et al. Alpha sleep characteristics in fibromyalgia. *Arthritis Rheum* 2001;44:222–230.
145. Hawley DJ, Wolfe F. Fibromyalgia. In: Goldman MB, MC Hatch MC, eds. *Women and health.* San Diego: Academic Press, 2000:1068–1083.
146. Wolfe F, Ross K, Anderson J, et al. The prevalence and characteristics of fibromyalgia in the general population. *Arthritis Rheum* 1995;38:19–28.
147. Simms RW. Fibromyalgia is not a muscular disorder. *Am J Med Sci* 1998;315:346–350.
148. Clauw DJ, Katz P. The overlap between fibromyalgia and inflammatory rheumatic diseases: when and why does it occur. *J Clin Rheumatol* 1995;1:335–341.
149. Carette S, Bell MJ, Reynolds WJ, et al. Comparison of amitriptyline, cyclobenzaprine, and placebo in the treatment of fibromyalgia. *Arthritis Rheum* 1994;37:32–40.
150. Goldenberg D, Mayskiy M, Mossey C, et al. A randomized, double-blind crossover trial of fluoxetine and amitriptyline in the treatment of fibromyalgia. *Arthritis Rheum* 1996;39:1852–1859.
151. McCain GA, Bell CA, Mai fibromyalgia, et al. A controlled study of the effects of a supervised cardiovascular fitness training program on the manifestations of fibromyalgia. *Arthritis Rheum* 1988;31:1135–1141.
152. Burckhardt CS, Mannerkorpi K, Hedenberg L, et al. A randomized, controlled clinical trial of education and physical training for women with fibromyalgia. *J Rheumatol* 1994;21:714–720.
153. Jentoft ES, Kvalvik AG, Mengshoel AM. Effects of pool-based and land-based aerobic exercise on women with fibromyalgia/chronic widespread musculoskeletal pain. *Arthritis Care Res* 2001;45:42–47.
154. The Federation of State Medical Boards of the United States, Inc. *Model Guidelines for the Use of Controlled Substances for the Treatment of Pain.* Adopted, May 2, 1998.
155. Russell IJ, Kamin M, Sager D, et al. Efficacy of Ultram™ (Tramadol HCL) treatment of fibromyalgia syndrome: Preliminary analysis of a multi-center, randomized, placebo-controlled study. *Arthritis Rheum* 1997;40(Suppl):S117.
156. Janssen NM, Genta MS. The effects of immunosuppressive and anti-inflammatory medications on fertility, pregnancy, and lactation. *Arch Intern Med* 2000;160:610–615.
157. Dawwood MY. Nonsteroidal anti-inflammatory drugs and reproduction. *Am J Obstet Gynecol* 1993;169: 1255–1265.
158. Briggs GG, Freman RK, Yaffe SJ. *Drugs in pregnancy and lactation,* 5th ed. Baltimore: Williams & Wilkins, 1998.
159. Hausknecht RU. Methotrexate and misoprostol to terminate early pregnancy. *N Engl J Med* 1995;333: 537–540.
160. Kozlowski RD, Steinbrunner JV, MacKenzie AH. Outcome of first-trimester exposure to low-dose methotrexate in eight patients with rheumatic disease. *Am J Med* 1980;88:589–592.
161. Buckley LM, Bullaboy CA, Leichtman L, et al. Multiple congenital anomalies associated with weekly low-dose methotrexate treatment of the mother. *Arthritis Rheum* 1997;40:971–973.
162. Boumpas DT, Austin HA, Vaughn EM, et al. Risk for sustained amenorrhea in patients with systemic lupus erythematosus receiving intermittent pulse cyclophosphamide therapy. *Ann Intern Med* 1993;119:366–369.
163. Slater CA, Liang MH, McCune JW, et al. Preserving ovarian function in patients receiving cyclophosphamide. *Lupus* 1999;8:3–10.
164. Leflunomide (package insert) Kansas City, MO: Hoescht Marion Roussel, 1998.
165. Enbrel (package insert). St. David's, PA: Wyeth-Ayerst Laboratories and Immunex Corp., 1998.
166. Remicaide (package insert). Malvern, PA: Centocor, Inc., 2000.
167. Bradley LA. *Primer on rheumatic disease.* Atlanta: Arthritis Foundation, 1997:413–415.
168. Huyser BA, Parker JC. Negative affect and pain in arthritis. *Rheum Dis Clin North Am* 1999;25:105–121.

7

Management of Urinary Incontinence in Women with Disabling Conditions

Matteo Balzarro and Rodney A. Appell

The management of urinary incontinence in women with disabling conditions is a problem that severely affects individuals, their families, and caregivers. It is true that all diseases create a state of psychologic, social, and physical disability; moreover, the matter of urinary incontinence treatment may be affected by other female pathologic entities. A simple example is use of estrogen for a voiding problem in a patient who has had breast cancer. In these situations, an individual case may become a management problem and become frustrating for the patient and the physician. However, in this chapter we have limited the definition of a disabling condition to an entity that creates a severe obstacle to performing activities of daily living. These are neuropathic entities, which have been described as upper– or lower–motor neuron disease. However, the attempt to correlate a clinical and/or urodynamic finding to an anatomic position of the lesion has failed, which makes these definitions improper (1). For this reason the evaluation now must be considered with respect to the urodynamic pattern as opposed to the specific entity.

PHYSIOLOGY OF THE LOWER URINARY TRACT

The urinary bladder is a reservoir with two purposes: the storage of urine and the evacuation of urine. To attain this, a perfect interaction between bladder, urethral internal and external sphincters, and pelvic musculature is required. This simplified concept of filling and emptying requires a very complex neurologic mechanism to permit constant sensory information from all of these anatomic structures to result in an appropriate motor action to be completed.

Learmonth (2) recognized the trigone of the bladder to be the origin of sensation related to overdistension of the bladder, such as pain or fullness. Other fibers gather sensory information related to the increase of the pressure in the bladder (3). Animal models have demonstrated the presence of an extensive plexus of nerves under the urothelium within the lamina propria as well as within the bulk of the overlying detrusor muscle (4).

The neurologic sensory and motor pathways that permit the necessary synergy are summarized in Fig. 7-1. Pressure-volume bladder sensations travel to the sacral cord by the afferent pelvic, hypogastric, and pudendal nerves. Here the majority of the fibers cross the midline and ascend to the micturition center in the pons. Other fibers activate the cortex to make the individual conscious of bladder fullness.

The majority of fibers from pelvic and pudendal nerves pass through the spinal cord and arrive at the pontine nuclei, whereas other fibers reach higher centers such as the cortex, cerebellum, extrapyramidal system, and brainstem (5). The neuronal connections between the pontine center and higher centers may help to explain the relation between micturition, the conscious idea of full bladder,

69

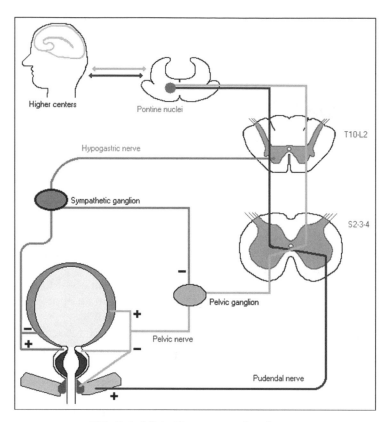

FIG. 7-1. Micturition neuronal pathways.

and emotions. This information established by micturition pontine nuclei and other higher centers then must synchronously input different structures. For example, to reach the pelvic floor muscles, neurologic impulses originating in the anterior horn cells at S_{2-4} then are transmitted via the *pudendal nerve*. To reach the bladder the impulses pass from Onuf's nucleus, also located in the anterior horn of the spinal cord, directly via the *pelvic nerve*. To reach the bladder neck, information is transmitted from the anterior horn of T_{10}-L_2 via the *hypogastric nerve*. Some fibers directly innervate the bladder neck and proximal urethral smooth muscle, whereas others project to the pelvic ganglion, where they have an inhibitory effect on parasympathetic nerve transmission (6,7).

Sacral parasympathetic (pelvic) nerves provide the major excitatory (motor) input to the bladder. However, simultaneous sphincter relaxation during micturition and sphincter contraction during the urinary storage phase also must take place. The precise role of sympathetic (hypogastric nerve) function has been postulated as protection from excess sensory information until a specific threshold is reached, meaning that bladder fullness is not detected until a certain minimum activity threshold has been reached (8).

FOUR MAIN URODYNAMIC PATTERNS OF VESICOURETHRAL DYSFUNCTION

Neurogenic voiding problems can be the result of dysfunction of the detrusor, sphincter, or a combination of both (9). The four main urodynamic patterns of neurogenic bladder are demonstrated in Fig. 7-2. In the case of *hyperreflexia of the detrusor combined with hyperreflexia (spasticity) of the*

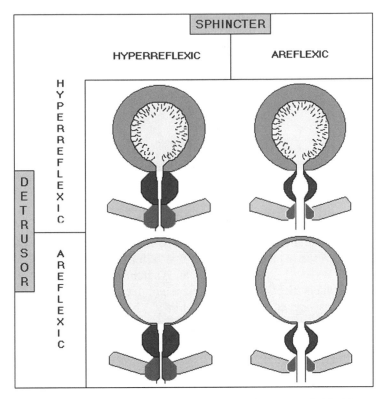

FIG. 7-2. Four main urodynamic patterns of neurogenic bladder.

sphincter, spontaneous reflex voiding is present. However, the presence of detrusor contractions and the concomitant sphincter spasticity make the micturition pathways unbalanced and uncontrolled, resulting in incontinence. *Areflexia of the detrusor combined with areflexia of the sphincter* is the pattern for the condition, which previously had been labeled "lower motor neuron lesion" and results in overflow incontinence. The presence of an areflexic sphincter may be the cause of stress urinary incontinence (SUI); this kind of incontinence can be combined with overflow incontinence caused by an areflexic bladder. *Areflexia of the detrusor combined with hyperreflexia (spasticity) of the sphincter* can be another cause of overflow incontinence. *Hyperreflexia of the detrusor combined with areflexia of the sphincter* can result in a combination of urge incontinence (UI) associated with SUI called mixed incontinence.

CAUSES AND ASSESSMENT

In the case of abnormal neural activity with respect to the bladder, there is a pathologic condition called neurogenic bladder. Several causes may produce abnormal neural transmission. Moreover, lesions may interfere with normal neural transmissions at different levels. The level and the extent of damage may display different clinical presentations, as listed in Table 7-1.

Cerebrovascular Accident

Cerebrovascular accident (CVA) is the third leading cause of death in the United States (10). The prevalence of CVA is 60/1,000 in individuals older than age 65 years and increases to 95/1,000 in patients older than 75 years (11). Animal models confirm that after induced cerebral infarction there is upregulation of excitatory pathways

TABLE 7-1. *Causes and level of lesions in neurogenic bladder*

At or above the brain	Spinal cord	Conus medullaris and cauda equina
Multiple sclerosis		Multiple sclerosis
Cerebral trauma		Spinal cord injury
Encephalitis		Myelitis
Dementia	Multiple sclerosis	Diabetes mellitus
Cerebrovascular disease	Spinal cord injury	Vitamin B_{12} deficiency
AIDS	Myelitis	Spina bifida
Brain tumor	Cervical spondylitis	Metastatic carcinoma
Parkinson's disease	Spinal cord infarction	Sacral agenesis
Shy-Drager syndrome	Spina bifida	Spinal stenosis
Cerebral palsy	Spinal cord tumor	Tabes dorsalis
Lyme disease		Disc disease
Hereditary spastic paraplegia		Herpes zoster

and downregulation of a tonic inhibitory activity resulting in a decrease in bladder capacity (12).

Detrusor hyperreflexia is the most common bladder dysfunction associated with CVA (13,14). The neurogenic bladder in patients who have had a CVA commonly is associated with irritative voiding symptoms of frequency, urgency, and UI. The mechanisms recognized as responsible for urinary incontinence in stroke victims are the deregulation of micturition pathways resulting in urge incontinence; incontinence associated with cognitive, functional, or language deficits; and concurrent neuropathy or medication that may cause bladder areflexia and resultant overflow incontinence (13). Goals in these patients are to reduce detrusor hyperreflexia and to preserve upper urinary tract function, which usually is accomplished with a combination of behavioral modification, pelvic floor exercise, and the judicious use of anticholinergic pharmacologic agents, such as tolterodine and oxybutynin.

Dementia

Incontinence is a hallmark of moderate or severe dementia and of early vascular dementia, but little is known about its inception in different types of dementing disease (15–17). Bladder and bowel incontinence frequently appears in the late stages of dementia, and loss of urine is an item included in the functional assessment of dementia (18–21). Loss of continence is associated with severe cognitive failure and the severity of the confusion in Alzheimer's disease, but usually precedes mental decline in patients affected by cortical Lewy body disease or patients with Alzheimer's disease with vascular lesions (16).

Urodynamic studies have demonstrated as many as 40% of patients have a normal bladder, whereas 38% demonstrate detrusor instability. Other findings include 16% of patients have SUI and 5% present with retention and associated overflow incontinence (22).

Successful management of neurogenic bladder dysfunction in patients with dementia is complicated by the fact that behavioral modification is affected by the degree of confusion; it must be remembered that anticholinergic drugs may increase confusion. Goals in these patients are to attain urinary continence and to preserve upper urinary tract function.

Parkinson's Disease

Parkinson's disease is a degenerative disorder of dopaminergic neurons of unknown cause resulting in a relative dopamine deficiency in the nigrostriatal pathway and cholinergic predominance in the corpus striatum. Several animal models have had varying results in an attempt to recognize the cause of bladder symptoms probably because anesthesia can affect the results of such studies. A recent study done in conscious, free-moving rats suggests that activating the dopamine D_1 receptors results in an inhibition of voiding reflex and that activating dopamine D_2 receptors stimulates micturition (23).

Detrusor hyperreflexia is a consequence of dopamine depletion of the substantia nigra, whereas hyporeflexia remains unexplained (24). Overactive bladder symptoms of frequency, urgency, and UI are associated with detrusor hyperreflexia and often are present in these patients (24,25). These symptoms can be exacerbated by decreases in general mobility and cognitive function. In addition, the heterogeneity and the progressive nature of the lesions of Parkinson's disease may explain the variations seen in detrusor tone and the consequent onset of symptoms.

Urodynamic assessment of a patient with Parkinson's disease may demonstrate a lower maximum cystometric capacity, detrusor hyperreflexia, and/or outflow obstruction (sphincter and/or pelvic floor) (26,27). Nevertheless, hypocontractility also may be observed (24). The urodynamic findings are not disease specific and also may be age related (28,29) with the primary finding of detrusor hyperreflexia with impaired contractility during the voiding phase—a very difficult problem to treat.

In patients affected by Parkinson's disease, the use of levodopa with the intent to restore the lack of dopamine neurotransmitter in the basal ganglia may or may not improve bladder function. Anticholinergic medications may cause acute retention in patients in the presence of outlet obstruction or those with impaired contractility and may exacerbate certain other parkinsonian symptoms. Elevated residual urines actually may require catheterization.

Shy-Drager Syndrome

Shy-Drager syndrome, also known as multiple system atrophy, creates damage in the basal ganglia positioned in the intermediolateral cell columns creating loss of both sympathetic and parasympathetic neurons. Onuf's nucleus also is attacked from the disease; the loss of these cells creates a deficit in the nor-mal pathways to the pelvic floor, intrinsic urethral sphincter, and anal sphincter.

Although this disease more frequently affects middle-aged males than females, early urinary symptoms in women are urgency and frequency. Postural drop of blood pressure on standing also is a strong indicator. Voiding dysfunction seems to be more common and is often an earlier manifestation than orthostatic hypotension (30). Although urinary disturbances are more frequent in Shy-Drager syndrome, it can be misdiagnosed as Parkinson's disease, especially when orthostatic hypotension and urinary symptoms are present in a patient with Parkinson's disease (31). However, 60% of the patients with Shy-Drager syndrome present with urinary problems before neurologic clinical evidence, whereas 94% of patients with Parkinson's disease have a neurologic diagnosis before the urogenital symptoms (32).

Evidence of a denervated pelvic floor and external urethral sphincter during electromyography is useful in making the diagnosis of Shy-Drager syndrome (32). Video-urodynamic investigation demonstrates open bladder neck, decreased bladder compliance, and incontinence caused by the associated rhabdosphincter incompetence.

Landry-Guillan-Barré Syndrome

Landry-Guillan-Barré syndrome is an acute symmetric peripheral polyneuropathy characterized by a demyelinating disorder as a result of an immune response. The syndrome presents with a typical weakness to the lower extremities that will progress to a motor paralysis. Urinary incontinence may occur as overflow from detrusor areflexia (33). Full recovery of detrusor function is possible, but prognosis is guarded and recovery may require months (34). Goals in these patients are to prevent upper urinary tract degeneration and urinary tract infections.

Spinal Cord Injury

The effects of spinal cord injury on the lower urinary tract depend on the level, duration, and completeness of the lesion. The lesions can be divided into suprasacral or infrasacral.

Suprasacral lesions disconnect the conus and sacral roots from the micturition center in the pons. For this reason, there is an isolation of the bladder from the neuronal impulses in the immediate posttraumatic period, which results in areflexia. Bladder overfilling and fecal impaction occur in the early months following injury. With an incomplete transection of the spinal cord, reflexes may return a few hours after injury. In humans, this spinal shock may last a few weeks to 6 months (35). The patient emerges from acute spinal shock with a gradual return to reflex activity. Bladder reflexes may be slower to recover than plantar, ankle jerk, and knee jerk (36). The return of reflex activity at the level of the pelvic floor is characterized by the presence of bulbocavernosus and anal skin reflexes. The presence of these reflexes confirms the integrity of the spinal reflex center for micturition located in the conus medullaris. Usually these patients lose control of the sphincteric mechanism, developing a *detrusor-sphincter-dyssynergia* (DSD). In other words, there is a lack of appropriate sphincter relaxation during detrusor contractions. Of the patients with

a suprasacral spinal cord injury, 70%–100% develop DSD (37,38). Several DSD classifications have been proposed (39,40). Otherwise, no significant association has been documented between the specific level of injury and DSD type showing no crucial clinical significance in any DSD classification (41).

Patients with a cord injury at T6 or higher often have a clinical condition called *autonomic dysreflexia*. In this pathologic condition stimuli such as bladder distension, fecal impaction, or visceral inflammation send inputs to the spinal cord below the level of the lesion. These inputs activate the sympathetic pathways inducing piloerection and sweating of the skin innervated by the efferent impulses below the level of the lesion. Additionally, arteriolar vasoconstriction results in dangerously high blood pressure. This rapid hypertension activates the baroreceptor reflex, thus stimulating the vagus nerve, which causes bradycardia (Fig. 7-3).

The protracted high pressure generated inside the bladder by this abnormal mechanism may cause hydronephrosis to develop. For this reason evaluation for the presence of vesicoureteral reflux and the level of renal function must be strictly controlled. Other complications related to suprasacral spinal cord

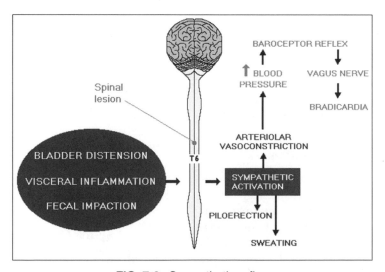

FIG. 7-3. Sympathetic reflex.

injury are elevated postvoid residual (PVR) urine, recurrent urinary tract infections, and bladder stones.

With *sacral and infrasacral lesions*, a complete damage to the sacral cord, or to the conus, creates a total neuronal disconnection and results in an acontractile bladder, which is unable to empty. Credé's maneuver has been proposed to empty the bladder. However, this procedure may induce a functional obstruction at the level of the striated external sphincter despite complete paralysis of the musculature of the pelvic floor and may not serve to improve bladder emptying; in fact, it may make it worse (9,42).

In spinal cord injury, varying urodynamic findings are possible. In case of a suprasacral lesion, the urodynamic pattern will change in relation to the completeness of the lesion and the time elapsing posttrauma. In the majority of the cases, both voluntary motor function as well as sensory activity are damaged. Initially the majority of the patients will have an areflexic bladder, which may change to a hyperreflexic bladder if the spinal lesion is above the spinal micturition center at S_{2-4}. DSD occurs if the lesion disconnects the pontine micturition center and the spinal micturition center; the lesion interrupting the data incoming from the pontine center maintains a permanent storage situation that is in conflict with detrusor contractions.

Congenital Cord Lesion

Congenital cord lesions are myelomeningocele, lumbosacral lipoma, dermoid cysts, and tethered cord syndrome. These classes of diseases are rare. Prenatal screening of alpha-fetoprotein has reduced the incidence of myelomeningocele, but it is still the most common congenital cord lesion. In general, the position of myelomeningocele has a correlation with the severity of the clinical manifestation and the seriousness of interrupting in the cord. Thoracolumbar and lumbar myelomeningoceles usually create a complete lesion, whereas lumbosacral and sacral myelomeningoceles usually result in an in-

complete lesion. Patients with cervical and upper thoracic lesions have a lower risk of voiding disorders and upper-tract deterioration (43). Urodynamic findings vary between a hyperreflexic detrusor with no sphincter weakness resulting in incontinence to an acontractile bladder with varying degrees of sphincter weakness also resulting in incontinence (44,45).

The aim for therapy in these patients principally is to achieve urinary continence and to prevent upper urinary tract damages (46). Additionally, these patients must have strict surveillance to prevent urinary tract infections or calculi.

Multiple Sclerosis

Multiple sclerosis (MS) is a pathologic demyelination in the white matter of the brain and spinal cord; the etiology is unknown. The clinical course of these patients is extremely variable and generally is characterized by progressing from a quiescent to a progressive phase. However, remission phases between the progressive phases are common. Duration of disease, older age at diagnosis, and the lack of motor or sensory function correlate well with the degree of urologic impairment (47).

More than 80% of patients with MS have symptoms of lower genitourinary tract dysfunction, and this increases to more than 96% with duration of disease beyond 10 years (48). Lower urinary tract problems so rarely are present in patients without pyramidal dysfunction that the degree of lower-extremity motor dysfunction seems to be the best predictor of bladder dysfunction (49).

Suprasacral plaques may explain detrusor hyperreflexia and therefore urge incontinence, just as demyelinization of the sacral cord/conus medullaris may explain hypocontractility and areflexia. DSD is highly correlated with cervical lesions (47). However, the exact correlation between plaque position and lower urinary tract dysfunction remains uncertain and debatable.

Genitourinary tract symptoms range from irritative symptoms, such as frequency and urgency, to incontinence and other voiding dysfunction, such as obstruction with urinary retention. DSD, when present, is correlated with stranguria and incomplete emptying. Male and female sexual dysfunctions are well reported and vary from a decreased sensation to fatigue and erectile and orgasmic dysfunction (50,51).

Urodynamic findings and bladder compliance may change in patients with MS. For this reason urodynamic evaluation should be repeated to confirm the appropriate management and to prevent complications (52).

Lumbar Disc Disease

In intervertebral disc prolapse (IDP) the most frequent compression is between L4-L5 and L5-S1 in the posterolateral spaces so as to not affect the majority of the cauda equina. If a migration of a posterolateral IDP happens, cauda equina compression is possible. Central disk prolapse is only 1%–15% of all IDP, and compression of cauda equina may result (53).

Using an animal model, Delamarter and colleagues (54) demonstrated how a 75% constriction of the cauda equina can evoke detrusor areflexia, increased bladder capacity, and overflow incontinence. These results make it more clear how IDP may interfere with stimuli *from the bladder*, which initiate micturition, as well as stimuli *to the bladder*, which are required for a detrusor contraction to occur. This creates a potential for overflow incontinence (55).

Voiding dysfunctions have been reported from 27% (56) to 92% (57) of patients with an IDP. The most frequent urinary symptoms are retention, compromised urinary flow, interrupted stream because of abnormal straining to void, and incontinence. Impaired sensation of filling is also a frequent manifestation. A large PVR, frequency, and urinary tract infections are other common clinical findings in these patients (58).

Urinary retention caused by bladder areflexia and associated with sphincter neuropathy is the most common urodynamic pattern

(58), and it also has been reported as a finding in the absence of neurologic signs (59). However, detrusor overactivity also has been identified in lower IDP, with the pathophysiology resulting from an irritation of the sacral roots, which may be accentuated by walking (60,61).

Treatment consists of correcting the cause of the problem, usually requiring laminectomy. Shapiro (62) reevaluated his patients with cauda equina syndrome secondary to IDP and noted the importance of the time period from the onset of symptoms to laminectomy. Detrusor recovery after central disk prolapse is not expected in all patients, and, in fact, after 24 months, up to 65% of patients still may have an areflexic bladder (63). In addition, the laminectomy itself also may result in damage to the sacral nerve roots (53). In patients with IDP the treatment goal is to obtain symptomatic relief by adequate bladder emptying without incontinence and preservation of upper-tract function. With adequate bladder compliance a trial of bethanechol chloride (50 mg four times daily) alone or with metoclopramide (5–10 mg up to four times daily) may help to give an adequate cholinergic stimulation. The therapy should not be protracted. If after 1 month no change is noted, therapy should be stopped (58).

Diabetes Mellitus

Making an epidemiologic quantification of lower urinary tract dysfunction in women with diabetes mellitus (DM) is difficult because the symptoms and presentation may mimic, or be masked by, other pathologies (64). Thus, a large number of women with diabetes, even when asymptomatic, on careful evaluation may be found to have bladder dysfunction.

There are several theories regarding the pathophysiology of diabetic neuropathy. However, derangements in the peripheral and autonomic nervous system may explain alterations in bladder function and a portion of the symptoms in these patients (64). Generally, the first symptom is impaired bladder sensation. Other urinary symptoms, also known as diabetic cystopathy, are infrequent voiding, reduced stream, hesitancy, the sensation of incomplete emptying, dribbling, and overflow incontinence (65). Other authors give more importance to symptoms such as nocturia more than twice a night (87%) and urinary frequency greater than every 2 hours (78%) (66). Moreover, these patients may develop urinary tract infections easily, which may be difficult to treat because of a high PVR and the reduced defensive barriers caused by DM.

Urodynamically, patients with DM have retarded sensations, increased cystometric capacity, decreased detrusor contractility, impaired uroflow, and increased PVR. Some patients present with detrusor areflexia, whereas others have detrusor instability (64). In people with diabetes, the aim of treatment is symptomatic relief, adequate bladder emptying, prevention of infections, control and maintenance of renal function, and (when necessary) continence.

ASSESSMENT

In assessing patients with neurogenic bladder, medical history and physical examination with a simple neurologic examination can be helpful in understanding the cause. Factors that may predispose to detrusor hyperreflexia in women—such as prior pelvic surgery, caffeine and tobacco intake, and poor estrogen status—must be considered. A micturition diary and PVR are indispensable in documenting the nature and severity of the clinical situation. Bulbocavernous reflex, catheter tug reflex, and an anocutaneous reflex can give information on the assessment of the sacral cord and pathways relating to nerves S_{2-4} (67).

Urodynamic evaluation permits identification of which one of the four possible patterns, previously described, is present. Furthermore, it has been proved how compliance can worsen progressively (66,68). Furthermore, different patients with the same disorder (e.g., MS) may present with differing clinical and urodynamic patterns (8,67,68).

MANAGEMENT

Management of urinary incontinence in women with these disabling conditions is complicated, and the psychologic impact on patients, their families, and caregivers also must be considered. However, individualizing the diagnosis by urodynamic findings will show the pattern promoted by the disease in that individual and help to direct the therapeutic regimen. The urodynamic patterns may change over time. For these reasons it is mandatory to have urodynamic follow-up.

There are several guidelines for the management of such patients (9,69). The correct management will preserve an independent lifestyle and social interactions. Table 7-2 lists

TABLE 7-2. *International Continence Society guidelines for the management of neurogenic bladder*

Detrusor pattern	Sphincter	Management
Hyperreflexia	Hyperreflexia	Intermittent catheterization Pharmacotherapy Electrotherapy Condom-catheters Triggered reflex voiding[a]
	Areflexia	Bladder relaxant agents Electrotherapy
Areflexia	Areflexia	Intermittent catheterization Bladder expression (Credé)[a]
	Hyperreflexia	Intermittent catheterization

[a]Recommended only if it is urodynamically safe.

the International Continence Society guidelines for the management of the four main patterns of neurogenic bladder (70).

As reported, hyperreflexia of the detrusor may be combined with an areflexia or a hyperreflexia of the sphincter. In both these clinical situations the first aim is to decrease detrusor contractility. However, in the presence of sphincter spasticity intermittent catheterization (IC) is considered the gold standard to empty the bladder (9,71).

In the case of areflexia of the detrusor associated with hyperreflexia or areflexia of the sphincter, the aim is to empty the bladder. In both these clinical situations IC is considered the treatment of choice. However, in the case of an areflexic sphincter bladder expression (Credé's maneuver) also has been proposed (9, 72).

Several medications are available to improve urinary incontinence and the related symptoms. Each kind of urinary incontinence has different causes; therefore, varying drugs have been proposed for the different types of incontinence (Table 7-3). However, the risk/benefit ratio is difficult to gauge precisely. To decrease detrusor contractility, new anticholinergic pharmacologic agents have been proposed. The excellent efficacy and safety profiles are comparable between extended release oxybutynin and tolterodine (73).

In all the different patterns of neurogenic bladder dysfunction, it is essential to prevent the complications related to neuropathic voiding dysfunction. Early diagnosis and proper management can prevent urologic complications. Hyperreflexia, decreased compliance, and fixed outlet resistance must be well controlled because of the high risk of impairment of upper urinary tract dysfunction. In these cases anticholinergic medications may be used, and in some cases it can be combined with self-catheterization. If this is unsuccessful, then surgical bladder augmentation may be necessary to achieve a sufficient bladder capacity and to reduce detrusor pressure to protect the upper urinary tract. General measures can improve urinary incontinence such as treating other medical conditions, discontinuing certain types of medications, regulating fluid intake, and reducing environmental barriers with varying forms of behavioral modification (when possible).

To conclude, multiple pathologies may cause urinary incontinence in women with disabling conditions. Each condition is related to a different pathophysiologic mechanism that is usually well detected by urodynamic studies. There is, in general, no single perfect management to suggest; each patient must be evaluated and treated on an individual basis, with respect to the urodynamic findings and the physically disabling condition. Choose reasonable management to accomplish the desired goals—normalizing bladder filling and emptying, preventing complications, and improving the quality of life of the patient.

TABLE 7-3. *Drugs related to the different kinds of incontinence*

Detrusor pattern	Effect	Drugs
Hyperreflexia	Anticholinergic agents	Oxybutynin
		Tolterodine
		Dicyclomine
		Propantheline
	Tricyclic antidepressants	Imipramine
		Doxepin
		Desipramine
		Nortriptyline
Areflexia	Parasympathomimetic	Bethanechol hydrochloride
Stress incontinence	α-adrenergic agonist agents	Ephedrine
		Pseudoephedrine
Enuresis	Antidiuretic hormone	Desmopressin
Hormonal deficiency	Estrogen therapy	Conjugated estrogens

REFERENCES

1. Kaplan SA, Chancellor MB, Blaivas JG. Bladder and sphincter behavior in patients with spinal cord lesions. *J Urol* 1991;146:113–117.
2. Learmonth J. A contribution to the neurophysiology of the urinary bladder in man. *Brain* 1931;54:147–176
3. Iggo A. Tension receptors in stomach and urinary bladder. *J Physiol* 1955;128:593–607.
4. Gabella G. The structural relations between nerve fibres and muscle cells in the urinary bladder of the rat. *J Neurocytol* 1995;24:159–187.
5. Morrison J. Bladder control: role of higher levels of the central nervous system. In: *The physiology of the lower urinary tract.* Berlin: Springer-Verlag, 1987;237–274
6. Daniel EE, Cowan W, Daniel VP. Structural bases for neural and myogenic control of human detrusor muscle. *Can J Physiol Pharmacol* 1983;61:1247–1273.
7. Dixon JG. Structure and innervation in the human. In: *The physiology of the lower urinary tract.* Berlin: Springer-Verlag, 1987;3–22
8. DeGroat WC, Booth AM. Physiology of the urinary bladder and urethra. *Ann Intern Med* 1980;92:312–315.
9. Abrams PK, Wein A. Incontinence. In: Abrams PK, Wein A, ed. *1st International Consultation on Incontinence.* Paris: World Health Organization 1998:778–779.
10. American Heart Association. *Heart and stroke facts: 1997 statistical supplement.* Dallas: AHA, 1998.
11. Walshe TM. Approach to cerebrovascular disease. In: *Manual of clinical problems in geriatric medicine.* Vol. 1. Boston: Little Brown & Co., 1985:326–330.
12. Yokoyama O, Yoshiyama M, Namiki M, et al. Role of the forebrain in bladder overactivity following cerebral infarction in the rat. *Exp Neurol* 2000;163: 469–476.
13. Gelber DA, Good DC, Laven LJ, et al. Causes of urinary incontinence after acute hemispheric stroke. *Stroke* 1993;24:378–382.
14. Khan Z, Starer P, Yang WC, et al. Analysis of voiding disorders in patients with cerebrovascular accidents. *Urology* 1990;35:265–270.
15. Ouslander JG, Palmer MH, Rovner BW, et al. Urinary incontinence in nursing homes: incidence, remission and associated factors. *J Am Geriatr Soc* 1993;41:1083–1089.
16. Del-Ser T, Munoz DG, Hachinski V. Temporal pattern of cognitive decline and incontinence is different in Alzheimer's disease and diffuse Lewy body disease. *Neurology* 1996;46:682–686.
17. Kotsoris H, Barclay LL, Kheyfets S, et al. Urinary and gait disturbances as markers for early multi-infarct dementia. *Stroke* 1987;18:138–141.
18. Blessed G, Tomlinson BE, Roth M. The association between quantitative measures of dementia and of senile change in the cerebral grey matter of elderly subjects. *Br J Psychiatry* 1968;114:797–811.
19. Reisberg B, Ferris SH, de Leon MJ, et al. The Global Deterioration Scale for assessment of primary degenerative dementia. *Am J Psychiatry* 1982;139:1136–1139.
20. Roman GC, Tatemichi TK, Erkinjuntti T, et al. Vascular dementia: diagnostic criteria for research studies. Report of the NINDS-AIREN International Workshop. *Neurology* 1993;43:250–260.
21. Chui HC, Victoroff JI, Margolin D, et al. Criteria for the diagnosis of ischemic vascular dementia proposed by the State of California Alzheimer's Disease Diagnostic and Treatment Centers. *Neurology* 1992;42:473–480.
22. Skelly J, Flint AJ. Urinary incontinence associated with dementia. *J Am Geriatr Soc* 1995;43:286–294.
23. Seki S, Igawa Y, Kaidoh K et al. Role of dopamine D1 and D2 receptors in the micturition reflex in conscious rats. *Neurourol Urodyn* 2001;20:105–113.
24. Aranda B, Cramer P. Effects of apomorphine and L-dopa on the parkinsonian bladder. *Neurourol Urodyn* 1993;12:203–209.
25. Pavlakis AJ, Siroky MB, Goldstein I, et al. Neurourologic findings in Parkinson's disease. *J Urol* 1983;129:80–83.
26. Berger Y, Blaivas JG, DeLaRocha ER, et al. Urodynamic findings in Parkinson's disease. *J Urol* 1987;138:836–838.
27. Fitzmaurice H, Fowler CJ, Rickards D, et al. Micturition disturbance in Parkinson's disease. *Br J Urol* 1985;57:652–656.
28. Castleden CM, Parker SG. Lower urinary tract dysfunction in Parkinson's disease: changes relate to age not disease. *Age Ageing* 1996;25:336.
29. Gray R, Stern G, Malone-Lee J. Lower urinary tract dysfunction in Parkinson's disease: changes relate to age and not disease. *Age Ageing* 1995;24:499–504.
30. Sakakibara R, Hattori T, Uchiyama T, et al. Urinary dysfunction and orthostatic hypotension in multiple system atrophy: which is the more common and earlier manifestation? *J Neurol Neurosurg Psychiatry* 2000;68:65–69.
31. Bonnet AM, Pichon J, Vidailhet M, et al. Urinary disturbances in striatonigral degeneration and Parkinson's disease: clinical and urodynamic aspects. *Mov Disord* 1997;12:509–513.
32. Chandiramani VA, Palace J, Fowler CJ. How to recognize patients with parkinsonism who should not have urological surgery. *Br J Urol* 1997;80:100–104.
33. Kogan BA, Solomon MH, Diokno AC. Urinary retention secondary to Landry-Guillain-Barre syndrome. *J Urol* 1981;126:643–644.
34. Nickell K, Boone TB. Peripheral neuropathy and peripheral nerve injury. *Urol Clin North Am* 1996;23:491–500.
35. Tanago RS. Neuropathic bladder disorder. In: *Smith's general urology.* Norwalk/San Mateo: Appleton & Lange, 1992:460.
36. Austin G. Recovery from spinal shock. In: *The spinal cord: basic aspects and surgical considerations.* Springfield, IL: Charles C Thomas, 1972:265.
37. Hackler RH. A 25-year prospective mortality study in the spinal cord injured patient: comparison with the long-term living paraplegic. *J Urol* 1977;117:486–488.
38. D.G. Thomas KJOF. Spinal cord injury. In: Mundy AR, Stephenson TP, Wein AJ. *Urodynamics: Principles, practice and application.* Edinburgh: Churchill Livingstone, 1994:345–358.
39. Blaivas JG, Sinha HP, Zayed AA, et al. Detrusor–external sphincter dyssynergia: a detailed electromyographic study. *J Urol* 1981;125:545–548.
40. Yalla SV, Blunt KJ, Fam BA, et al. Detrusor-urethral sphincter dyssynergia. *J Urol* 1977;118:1026–1029.
41. Weld KJ, Graney MJ, Dmochowski RR. Clinical significance of detrusor sphincter dyssynergia type in patients with post-traumatic spinal cord injury. *Urology* 2000;56:565–568.

42. Madersbacher H. The neuropathic urethra: urethrogram and pathophysiologic aspects. *Eur Urol* 1977;3: 321–332.

43. Perez LM, Wilbanks JT, Joseph DB, et al. Urological outcome of patients with cervical and upper thoracic myelomeningocele. *J Urol* 2000;164:962–964.

44. McGuire EJ, Woodside JR, Borden TA, et al. Prognostic value of urodynamic testing in myelodysplastic patients. *J Urol* 1981;126:205–209.

45. Mundy AR, Shah PJ, Borzyskowski M, et al. Sphincter behaviour in myelomeningocele. *Br J Urol* 1985;57: 647–651.

46. Persun ML, Ginsberg PC, Harmon JD, et al. Role of urologic evaluation in the adult spina bifida patient. *Urol Int* 1999;62:205–208.

47. Koldewijn EL, Hommes OR, Lemmens WA, et al. Relationship between lower urinary tract abnormalities and disease- related parameters in multiple sclerosis. *J Urol* 1995;154:169–173.

48. Litwiller SE, Frohman EM, Zimmern PE. Multiple sclerosis and the urologist. *J Urol* 1999;161:743–757.

49. Kurtzke JF. Rating neurologic impairment in multiple sclerosis: an expanded disability status scale (EDSS). *Neurology* 1983;33:1444–1452.

50. Valleroy ML, Kraft GH. Sexual dysfunction in multiple sclerosis. *Arch Phys Med Rehabil* 1984;65:125–128.

51. Minderhoud JM, Leemhuis JG, Kremer J, et al. Sexual disturbances arising from multiple sclerosis. *Acta Neurol Scand* 1984;70:299–306.

52. Ciancio SJ, Mutchnik SE, Rivera VM, et al. Urodynamic pattern changes in multiple sclerosis. *Urology* 2001;57:239–245.

53. O'Flynn KJ, Murphy R, Thomas DG. Neurogenic bladder dysfunction in lumbar intervertebral disc prolapse. *Br J Urol* 1992;69:38–40.

54. Delamarter RB, Bohlman HH, Bodner D, et al. Urologic function after experimental cauda equina compression. Cystometrograms versus cortical-evoked potentials. *Spine* 1990;15:864–870.

55. Goldman HB, Appell RA. Voiding dysfunction in women with lumbar disc prolapse. *Int Urogynecol J* 1999;10:134–138.

56. Bartolin Z, Gilja I, Bedalov G, et al. Bladder function in patients with lumbar intervertebral disk protrusion. *J Urol* 1998;159:969–971.

57. Rosomoff HL, Johnston JD, Gallo AE, et al. Cystometry as an adjunct in the evaluation of lumbar disc syndromes. *J Neurosurg* 1970;33:67–74.

58. Goldman HB, Appell RA. Voiding dysfunction in women with lumbar disc prolapse. *Int Urogynecol J* 1999;10:134–138.

59. Sylvester PA, McLoughlin J, Sibley GN, et al. Neuropathic urinary retention in the absence of neurological signs. *Postgrad Med J* 1995;71:747–748.

60. Yamanishi T, Yasuda K, Sakakibara R, et al. Detrusor overactivity and penile erection in patients with lower lumbar spine lesions. *Eur Urol* 1998;34:360–364.

61. Ando M, Nagamatsu H, Tanizawa A, et al. [Neurogenic bladder in patients with lumbar vertebral disorders]. *Nippon Hinyokika Gakkai Zasshi* 1990;81:1322–1329.

62. Shapiro S. Medical realities of cauda equina syndrome secondary to lumbar disc herniation. *Spine* 2000;25: 348–351.

63. Fanciullacci F, Sandri S, Politi P, et al. Clinical, urodynamic and neurophysiological findings in patients with neuropathic bladder due to a lumbar intervertebral disc protrusion. *Paraplegia* 1989;27:354–358.

64. Goldman HB, Appell RA. Voiding dysfunction in women with diabetes mellitus. *Int Urogynecol J Pelvic Floor Dysfunct* 1999;10:130–133.

65. Frimodt-Moller C. Diabetic cystopathy: epidemiology and related disorders. *Ann Intern Med* 1980;92:318–321.

66. Kaplan SA, Te AE, Blaivas JG. Urodynamic findings in patients with diabetic cystopathy. *J Urol* 1995;153: 342–344.

67. Comarr AE. Neurourology of spinal cord-injured patients. *Semin Urol* 1992;10:74–82.

68. Blaivas JG. Pathophysiology of lower urinary tract dysfunction. *Urol Clin N Amer* 1985;12:215–224.

69. *Urinary incontinence in adults: acute and chronic management.* Clinical Practice Guideline Number 2 (1996 Update). AHCPR Publication No. 96-0682: March 1996.

70. Watanabe T, Rivas DA, Chancellor MB. Urodynamics of spinal cord injury. *Urol Clin North Am* 1996;23: 459–473.

71. Weld KJ, Dmochowski RR. Effect of bladder management on urological complications in spinal cord injured patients. *J Urol* 2000;163:768–772.

72. Chang SM, Hou CL, Dong DQ, et al. Urologic status of 74 spinal cord injury patients from the 1976 Tangshan earthquake, and managed for over 20 years using the Crede maneuver. *Spinal Cord* 2000;38:552–554.

73. Appell RA. Recent clinical studies of new pharmacology agents and their efficacy in the treatment of incontinence. *Rev Urol* 2001;3(Suppl 1):S15–S18.

8

Management of Fecal Incontinence

Kirsten Bass Wilkins and Kirk A. Ludwig

Fecal incontinence is defined as the inability to control gas or stool. It can be a severely disabling condition, with an estimated 5% of the world's population affected. Because childbirth injury is the most common cause of fecal incontinence, it occurs in a female to male ratio of approximately 4:1 (1). As many as 50% of elderly women may be affected by incontinence (2), and in both men and women, fecal incontinence is one of the most common reasons for nursing home placement (3).

Defecation and the act of deferring defecation are complicated physiologic processes. Continence is dependent on many variables including stool consistency, small bowel and colon transit, rectal compliance, intact neural pathways, and an intact and functional pelvic floor. Ultimately, each of these variables functioning at a minimum level, combined with the integrated action of the internal and external anal sphincters, determine an individual's ability to defer defecation and maintain fecal continence. Although beyond the scope of this text, an understanding of how each of these physiologic variables affects continence is essential in treating patients with fecal incontinence. Only after each of these variables has been evaluated can the proper approach to an individual patient be formulated. Based on the patient's primary problem, nonoperative or operative therapy, or a combination of both, may be appropriate.

PHYSIOLOGY

As mentioned, the ability to defer defecation and maintain fecal continence relies on the complex coordination of many physiologic variables. Many of these variables and their perturbations are difficult to study, and the methods available for study in and of themselves cause change. There is much that is not fully understood. This should be kept in mind.

Rectal compliance is very important for continence (4–8). Rectal compliance refers to the ability of the rectum to fill (increase volume) without a significant increase in pressure (Fig. 8-1). Development and maintenance of normal rectal compliance are related to normal function of the anal sphincter complex (9). The rectum develops compliance when forced to fill as a result of the sphincters producing an outlet obstruction. Rectal compliance decreases in the face of poor sphincter function. If the sphincters gradually lose their ability to defer defecation in response to rectal distention, the rectum becomes less compliant, resulting in higher rectal pressure with lesser degrees of volume increase.

Sensation of rectal fullness is mediated through pelvic nerves (4,10). Although there are stretch receptors located in the muscle layer of the rectal wall (11), the rectum itself is not necessary for the urge to defecate (12). Patients who undergo proctectomy with either coloanal anastomosis or ileal pouch anal anastomosis still can sense the urge to defecate. This is because much of the urge comes from stimulation of stretch receptors in the puborectalis and pelvic floor muscles (13,14).

It cannot be emphasized too strongly that the anal sphincters are only part of the picture. Experience tells us that there are many

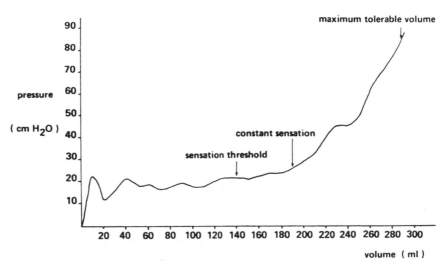

FIG. 8-1 This curve illustrates how volume in the rectum can increase significantly before pressure starts to rise. This type of curve can be produced in the anorectal physiology laboratory with the three specific volumes (volume of sensation threshold, volume of constant urge, and maximal tolerated volume) recorded. (From Hemond M, Bedard G, Bouchard H, et al. Step-by-step manometry: small balloon tube. In: Smith L, ed. *Practical guide to anorectal testing,* 2nd ed. New York: Igaku-Shoin Medical Publishers, Inc., 1995:130, with permission.)

women, in particular, with far less than anatomically perfect sphincters (usually as a result of childbirth) that maintain a normal level of continence based on the fact that they have good function of the colon, rectum, or both. There are others with poorly functioning colons or rectums that despite an anatomically normal anal sphincter will experience various degrees of fecal incontinence.

ETIOLOGY OF FECAL INCONTINENCE

Based on the multiple variables involved in maintaining fecal continence, it is not surprising that there are many potential causes of it. Etiologies of fecal incontinence may be grouped into several broad categories including altered stool consistency, overflow incontinence, inadequate rectal capacity or compliance, neurologic abnormalities, and sphincter defects (Table 8-1).

A number of disorders that result in the presentation of liquid stool to the rectum and anus may lead to incontinence. The anus has the difficult task of controlling gas, liquid stool, and solid stool. It is more difficult to maintain continence for liquid stool or gas than it is to maintain continence of solid stool. Irritable bowel syndrome, inflammatory bowel disease, malabsorption syndromes (including short gut syndrome), infectious diarrhea, laxative abuse, and other causes of diarrheal states frequently are associated with some degree of fecal incontinence. Fortunately, many of these conditions can be treated and continence can be improved with medical therapy directed at the underlying cause of diarrhea.

Related to altered stool consistency is overflow incontinence around a fecal impaction caused by chronic constipation. As a result of many factors, this is a common problem in elderly and hospitalized patients. Medications

TABLE 8-1. *Conditions associated with fecal incontinence*

I. Diarrheal states—altered stool consistency
    A. Inflammatory bowel disease
    B. Irritable bowel disease
    C. Infectious diarrhea
II. Inadequate reservoir capacity or compliance
    A. Inflammatory bowel disease
    B. Absent rectal reservoir
        (sphincter-preserving operation)
    C. Rectal ischemia
    D. Collagen vascular diseases (scleroderma)
    E. Rectal neoplasms
    F. Extrinsic rectal compression
III. Inadequate rectal sensation
    A. Neurologic conditions
        1. Dementia
        2. Cerebrovascular accidents
        3. *Tabes dorsalis*
        4. Multiple sclerosis
        5. Injuries
        6. Neoplasms
            a. Brain
            b. Spinal cord
            c. Cauda equina
    B. Overflow incontinence
        1. Fecal impaction
        2. Encopresis
        3. Psychotropic drugs
        4. Antimotility drugs
IV. Abnormal sphincter mechanism or pelvic floor
    A. Anatomic sphincter defects
        1. Traumatic
            a. Obstetric injury
            b. Anorectal surgery
        2. Neoplastic
            a. Inflammatory
    B. Pelvic floor degeneration
        1. Primary ("idiopathic" neurogenic
            incontinence)
        2. Secondary
            a. Injuries to spinal cord/cauda
                equina/pelvic floor nerves
            b. Diabetic neuropathy
    C. Congenital abnormalities
        1. Myelomeningocele
        2. Spina bifida
        3. Imperforate anus
    D. Miscellaneous
        1. Aging
        2. Rectal prolapse

often are implicated as a cause. Commonly associated with constipation are narcotics, psychotropic drugs, and antimotility agents. Diuretics, which can cause a chronic state of dehydration, also can contribute to constipation. Antihypertensive agents such as beta blockers and calcium channel blockers can slow transit by their effects on bowel wall

smooth muscle and therefore cause or contribute to constipation. In addition to medications, overall inactivity and confinement to a bed or wheelchair can contribute to constipation. Inability of bedridden patients to get up and answer the call to stool or having to repeatedly defer the call for long periods can lead to constipation and fecal impaction.

The mechanism of this overflow incontinence is as follows (14). As the proximal colon works against the impaction, liquid stool, under some amount of pressure, is generated above the impaction. With the rectum being full, the internal sphincter is reflexively open and the external sphincter eventually fatigues (or is unable to contract in the first place) and the patient leaks liquid stool around the impaction, producing paradoxic diarrhea with incontinence. This leakage of liquid stool is aggravated by the administration of oral laxatives, which only increase the amount of liquid stool reaching the rectum without relieving the obstruction. An attempt at disimpaction using enemas may be attempted, but frequently manual disimpaction is required to relieve obstruction. After the obstruction has been relieved, patients are managed best on a strict bowel regimen consisting of diet modification, elimination of constipating medications if possible, and the routine administration of stool softeners and enemas. Regular evacuation of the rectum is critical to avoiding this cause of fecal incontinence.

Inadequate rectal capacity or compliance can lead to fecal incontinence. Inflammatory bowel disease, pelvic irradiation, and collagen vascular diseases, such as scleroderma (15), all can lead to loss of rectal compliance as a result of fibrosis in the rectal wall. Large rectal neoplasms or extrinsic compression from neoplasms or inflammatory masses also may cause decreased rectal capacity.

An iatrogenic cause of fecal incontinence encountered more commonly today than in the past is that secondary to proctectomy and sphincter-saving operations for cancer and inflammatory bowel disease. This postoperative incontinence is in some part the result of lack of compliance in the neorectum. Over time the compliance of the neorectum improves, and this coincides with improvement in bowel function and continence. Diet modification and the use of medications to manipulate the stool consistency and colon transit time are helpful in minimizing bowel dysfunction and incontinence after proctectomy and reconstruction.

A large number of neurogenic abnormalities are associated with fecal incontinence. These neurogenic abnormalities may disturb continence by producing rectal sensory defects (patient cannot feel when the rectum is full), pelvic floor abnormalities (patient cannot sense rectal distention or cannot effectively assist evacuation), or a combination of both.

As mentioned previously, many elderly patients are disabled secondary to incontinence. Dementia resulting from Alzheimer's disease or multiinfarct dementia, among other causes, frequently is associated with fecal incontinence presumably from inadequate rectal sensation and poor control of the external sphincter. Rectal prolapse of varying degrees is not uncommon, especially in elderly females, and frequently is associated with fecal incontinence.

Diabetes mellitus is associated with severe anorectal dysfunction, presumably from autonomic neuropathy, in approximately 30% of patients (16,17). In both continent and incontinent patients with diabetes, resting internal anal sphincter tone can be reduced (18–20). Impaired rectal sensation also is present in patients with diabetes (21). Typically, patients with diabetes have the most difficulty with liquid stool incontinence.

Bowel dysfunction is a major problem for patients following spinal cord injury (22,23). Spinal cord injury causes changes in bowel motility, sphincter control, and overall motor dexterity, making bowel management a problem that can consume a tremendous amount of time for patients with spinal cord injury and/or their caregivers. In fact, many patients with spinal cord injury rank colorectal problems as more disabling than bladder and sexual dysfunction (24,25). Anorectal abnormalities associated with spinal cord injury include decreased or absent rectal sensation, increased

rectal contraction and anal relaxation in response to rectal distention, reduced resting internal anal sphincter tone, decreased external anal squeeze pressures, or paradoxic squeeze of the external anal sphincter with failure to relax in response to straining. Depending on the level and degree of spinal cord injury, diverse anorectal abnormalities may be present that lead to problems with fecal incontinence as well as bowel evacuation abnormalities. Related to spinal cord injuries is multiple sclerosis, a demyelinating disease of the central nervous system that affects young women. Spinal cord abnormalities from multiple sclerosis frequently are associated with bowel dysfunction, particularly as the disease progresses (26–28). Congenital abnormalities, including spina bifida and myelomeningocele, also often cause disabling bowel dysfunction resulting in fecal incontinence (29–33).

Pelvic floor denervation may present as a primary or a secondary problem that leads to problems with fecal incontinence. Secondary causes of pelvic floor denervation have been discussed earlier in this chapter and include etiologies such as spinal cord injury and diabetic neuropathy. Incontinence resulting from primary pelvic floor denervation commonly is referred to as idiopathic neurogenic incontinence (33). Here, the fecal incontinence results from denervation of the external anal sphincter and puborectalis muscle with no obvious neurologic disease (34–37). These patients are usually women, and many have had multiple vaginal deliveries. There is usually no direct evidence of an anatomic sphincter injury. Idiopathic incontinence may be associated with prolonged pudendal nerve terminal motor latency (PNTML) and consequent low resting and squeeze anal pressures. However, several studies have shown that a fair number of patients with idiopathic incontinence do not have prolonged PNTML. A normal PNTML is possible in this situation because much neurologic dysfunction can be present before this latency becomes prolonged. A normal latency does not mean completely normal neurologic function (38). A prolonged latency, however, does indicate significant neurologic damage. Other than, or in addition to, vaginal (single or multiple) delivery (39), factors that have been implicated in the development of idiopathic incontinence include chronic straining at defecation and descending perineum syndrome (40). Whether as a result of severe traction during childbirth or severe traction from longstanding constipation and straining, these conditions may result in a neuropathy from stretching forces exerted on the terminal portion of the pudendal nerve. This type of incontinence generally develops over a long period (41). Its development after childbirth may not be evident for years or decades after the injury. When the nerve damage results from chronic straining and constipation, the patient often notices gradually that minor, then increasing, degrees of fecal incontinence replace her problem with straining to stool.

Anatomic sphincter defects represent a very common cause of fecal incontinence. Sphincter damage following vaginal delivery is the most common cause of fecal incontinence in women (42,43). Factors associated with obstetric sphincter damage include forceps delivery, prolonged labor, primiparous delivery, birth weight of more than 4 kg, and third- and fourth-degree perineal lacerations or extensive episiotomy. Midline episiotomy more commonly is associated with sphincter injuries as compared to mediolateral episiotomy (44). Approximately 5% of vaginal deliveries are associated with third- or fourth-degree perineal tears. The obstetrician usually repairs these injuries shortly after delivery. Nonetheless, approximately 5% of these patients will experience moderate to major fecal incontinence during short-term follow-up (45,46). Endoanal ultrasound study of these patients reveals external sphincter damage in approximately 80%, internal sphincter damage in more than 50%, and disruption of the perineal body in more than 40% (47). Furthermore, pudendal nerve damage is present in a significant number of these patients, most likely a result of nerve compression and stretch during delivery (48). As previously mentioned, pudendal nerve damage can, and does, occur without evidence of anatomic sphincter defects, and the resulting

incontinence is referred to as idiopathic neurogenic incontinence.

Sphincter defects and fecal incontinence also are associated with anorectal surgery. Hemorrhoidectomy and lateral internal sphincterotomy are associated with a low, but real, incidence of long-term incontinence. Fecal incontinence is encountered more commonly in patients who have undergone surgery for anal fistulae. Anal fistula operations almost always divide a portion of both the internal and external anal sphincters. Depending on a number of factors, these operations can lead to varying degrees of fecal incontinence. Finally, congenital abnormalities such as imperforate anus often lead to lifetime problems with some degree of bowel dysfunction and fecal incontinence either secondary to the congenital abnormality itself or the surgery undertaken to correct the problem (49).

EVALUATION

The initial evaluation of the patient with fecal incontinence must include a thorough history focused on determining the etiology and severity of incontinence because these variables will lead to the selection of appropriate therapy. First, the physician must verify that fecal incontinence actually exists and that fecal or mucous soilage secondary to hemorrhoids, fistulae, or rectal prolapse is not the actual problem. After a history of true incontinence has been elicited, the frequency, duration, and severity (whether for flatus, liquid stool, or solid stool) of the problem are determined. A full medical history is obtained with emphasis on associated neurologic, endocrine, collagen vascular, and gastrointestinal diseases. Questions are asked regarding stool consistency (diarrhea). All medications are reviewed including usage of laxatives and enemas. All previous operations around the anus, rectum, colon, and small bowel should be documented carefully. In female patients, a careful obstetric history should be obtained focusing on the number of vaginal deliveries, the birthweight of children, the duration and difficulty of labor, the use of forceps, the severity of perineal lacerations, and the use of episiotomy. The exact onset of incontinence in relation to surgical procedures or obstetric events should be noted. The presence or absence of bladder dysfunction should be noted because bowel and bladder incontinence frequently occur together, often as a result of neurologic dysfunction.

An attempt should be made to broadly categorize the incontinence as passive or urge incontinence. Passive incontinence is characterized by the passage of feces without the patient being aware of it. This and nocturnal incontinence may indicate neurologic abnormalities and impaired rectal sensation or dysfunction of the internal anal sphincter. Urge incontinence, however, occurs with the patient being aware of the impending bowel movement but without the ability to prevent it. This commonly is observed with abnormalities of rectal compliance and dysfunction of the external sphincter complex.

The physical examination begins with a careful inspection of the anus and perineum. The presence or absence of soilage, scars, visible mucosa, a patulous anus, the loss of perineal body, and obvious muscle defects are noted. Next, perianal sensation and the anal wink reflex are assessed. Impairment of sensation suggests the presence of peripheral neuropathy or a more central lesion. The patient is asked to contract the sphincter, and lack of contraction on squeeze commands suggests neurogenic incontinence as well. The patient is asked to bear down and strain. Extensive perineal descent or the presence of rectal prolapse suggests severe pelvic floor weakness and possibly neurogenic impairment. Digital examination permits a gross determination of resting internal sphincter tone and external anal squeeze pressure. Obvious sphincter defects may be appreciated. The presence or absence of a rectocele is noted. Assessment of the function of the puborectalis muscle can be obtained by palpation in the upper, posterior anal canal. Contraction of the puborectalis and sphincter muscles during attempted squeeze normally pushes the palpating finger anteriorly. Proctoscopy routinely is obtained to rule out rectal neoplasm,

TABLE 8-2. *Severity of incontinence: functional groups*

Mild
   Occasional seepage and escape of flatus
   Continent for liquid and solid stool
   Rarely or never wears a pad
Moderate
   Frequently incontinent for flatus and occasionally
     for liquid stool
   Continent for solid stool
   Often wears a pad
Severe
   Frequently or permanently incontinent for both solid
     and liquid stool
   Symptoms severely restrict social involvement
   Always wears a pad

proctitis, or mucosal disease as a cause of symptoms. Evidence of internal rectal prolapse may be revealed on proctoscopy.

By the end of the initial interview and physical examination, the physician should be able to place the patient into a functional

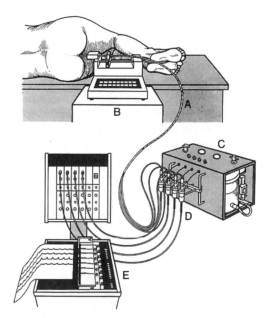

FIG. 8-2. The components and set-up for performing anorectal manometry. *A:* catheter, (*B*) withdrawal motor, (*C*) perfusion apparatus, (*D*) transducers, (*E*) multichannel recorder. (From Timmcke AE. Methodology and applications of water perfusion anal manometry. In: Smith L, ed. *Practical guide to anorectal testing,* 2nd ed. New York: Igaku-Shoin Medical Publishers, Inc., 1995:29, with permission.)

group of mild, moderate, or severe incontinence (50) (Table 8-2). The etiology of incontinence likely will be revealed, and based on the severity and etiology, plans for nonoperative or operative intervention are initiated. Initial therapy is usually medical and focuses on manipulation of stool consistency and frequency. Based on the severity of the fecal incontinence (51,52) and the presumed cause, physiologic and radiographic testing may be offered to assist in objectifying the etiology of the incontinence and therefore the treatment. Testing generally involves anal manometry, measurement of PNTML, and transrectal ultrasound to visualize the anatomy of the anal sphincter complex.

Anorectal manometry is the most commonly used method to assess anal sphincter function. Although various manometry systems are available, the most common use water perfusion through soft plastic multichannel catheters (Fig. 8-2). Manometry allows

measurement of anal resting tone, which reflects function of the internal anal sphincter, and squeeze pressure, which is a measure of external anal sphincter function. Isolated decreases in resting and/or squeeze pressures may indicate defects in the internal and external sphincter, respectively. Other variables measured include the functional length of the anal canal (high-pressure zone) and rectal compliance and sensation (by rectal balloon inflation).

The anal sphincters are innervated by the pudendal nerves. Proper function of at least one of these paired nerves is critical to the proper function of the anal sphincters. The PNTML is a measure of conduction velocity across the distal part of the nerve as it passes out of Alcock's canal at the ischial spine and crosses the ischioanal fossa to innervate the sphincters. This latency can be measured using a special electrode called the St. Mark's electrode (33) (Fig. 8-3). A prolonged latency

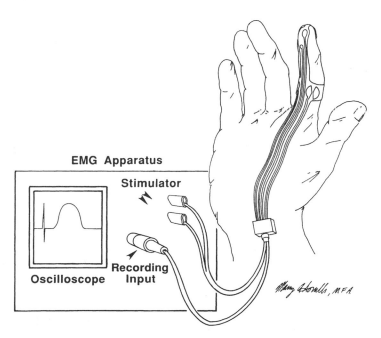

FIG. 8-3. The St. Mark's electrode used for testing the pudendal nerve terminal motor latency. The stimulating electrode at the tip of the finger is placed on the ischial spine at Alcock's canal, and the response of the external sphincter is recorded by the electrodes at the base of the finger. (From Fleshman JW. Determination of pudendal nerve terminal motor latency. In: Smith L, ed. *Practical guide to anorectal testing*, 2nd ed. New York: Igaku-Shoin Medical Publishers, Inc., 1995:225, with permission.)

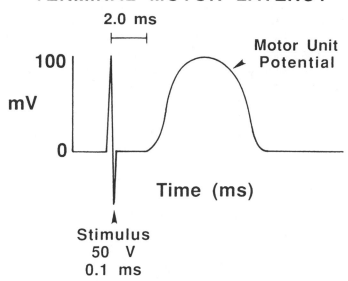

TERMINAL MOTOR LATENCY

FIG. 8-4. The pudendal nerve terminal motor latency as recorded on the electromyography apparatus. The latency is the time elapsed between stimulation and response of muscle. (From Fleshman JW. Determination of pudendal nerve terminal motor latency. In: Smith L, ed. *Practical guide to anorectal testing*, 2nd ed. New York: Igaku-Shoin Medical Publishers, Inc., 1995:224, with permission.)

is associated with injury and subsequent demyelination (Fig. 8-4). Because conduction along the fastest conducting fibers is measured, even in the presence of significant nerve injury, a normal PNTML may be recorded. Assessment of the neurologic status of the sphincter may be especially important in patients in whom sphincter repair is planned because several studies have revealed suboptimal outcomes after sphincter repair in patients with concomitant nerve injury (53–56).

In the past, formal sphincter electromyography (EMG) was used to map sphincter defects. It is no longer used routinely for this purpose. It is still useful in assessing the degree of active or chronic denervation and reinnervation. Today, most physicians rely on transrectal or endoanal ultrasonography or, to a much lesser degree, magnetic resonance imaging (MRI) techniques to define sphincter anatomy. These radiologic techniques have a number of advantages over EMG sphincter mapping. Unlike EMG, which can be quite

painful because of multiple needle passes, these techniques are, for the most part, pain free. Ultrasound can be performed in the office, and it is highly accurate in defining sphincter anatomy. Endoanal ultrasound is most useful in the preoperative evaluation in a patient in whom sphincter repair is planned. Currently, it is the test of choice for defining the anatomy of the internal and external anal sphincters. The accuracy of endoanal ultrasound for defining anatomic defects has been reported as 90%–95%. Endoanal MRI also has a reported accuracy of 90%–95% for defining sphincter defects, but the test is more expensive, is time consuming, and requires an experienced and interested radiologist (56).

TREATMENT

The treatment of fecal incontinence is guided in large part by the severity of the problem and by the etiology of the disorder. Generally speaking, patients with mild to moderate dysfunction and no evidence of an anatomic defect initially are managed with nonsurgical therapy including dietary modification, enforcement of a strict bowel regimen, and possible biofeedback therapy. Patients with an anatomic sphincter defect are usually candidates for surgical repair, most commonly an overlapping sphincteroplasty. For patients with a denervated sphincter or an anatomically absent sphincter, implantation of an artificial anal sphincter may be offered after they have failed conservative treatment or previous operative repair. In certain patients, fecal diversion may offer the best option for relief.

Patients with mild incontinence may require only medical measures to improve function (Table 8.3). These measures often include dietary modifications, which include the

TABLE 8-3. *Nonsurgical treatment of fecal incontinence*

Dietary manipulation (consider intolerance to lactose, sorbitol, fructose, and gluten-containing foods)
Avoiding diarrhea-causing food
  Caffeine, alcohol, fruit juice, prunes, figs, licorice, spicy or fatty foods, beans, broccoli, cauliflower, cabbage, green leafy vegetables
Constipating foods
  Cheese, yogurt, plain boiled rice, pasta, bananas, applesauce
Stool bulking agents
  High-fiber foods or fiber supplements, mild fluid restriction

Medications
Antidiarrheal agents
  Adsorbents and coating agents
    Kaopectate (Pharmacia & Upjohn, Peapack, NJ), bismuth subsalicylate, aluminum hydroxide
  Antimotility agents
    Codeine, paregoric, tincture of opium, loperamide (Imodium, McNeil Consumer Healthcare, Fort Washington, PA), diphenoxylate hydrochloride (Lomotil, Searle, Chicago, IL)
  Bile salt binders
    Cholestyramine (Questran, Apothecon, Princeton, NJ), colestipol (Colestid, Pharmacia & Upjohn, Peapack, NJ)

Bowel management
Scheduled defecation; dietary modification; stool-consistency and frequency-modifying medications; stimulated defecation using suppositories, enemas, or manual disimpaction

Biofeedback

avoidance of foods that induce diarrhea. At the same time, constipating foods, stool-bulking agents, and antidiarrheal medications may be administered to change stool consistency and frequency. Patients who have problems with rectal sensation or difficulties with complete rectal evacuation may benefit from the administration of "cleansing" enemas on a scheduled basis to keep the rectum empty and decrease the incidence of soilage. Medical management is associated with only moderate success, but because of its noninvasive nature, it is usually a reasonable initial approach.

Patients with spinal cord injuries can remain "continent" by following a strict bowel management program making use of scheduled evacuation stimulated by digitalization, suppositories, or enemas. A low-fiber diet combined with stool softeners and antidiarrheals, if needed, can be helpful.

An approach related to the maintenance of a strict bowel regimen is the creation of an antegrade colonic enema (ACE). Although originally designed for use in children, the ACE procedure has been modified and is used in adults with fecal incontinence (57,58). Most surgeons perform an orthotopic appendicocecostomy, carefully maintaining the appendiceal blood supply. Seromuscular cecal imbrication is performed to ensure a conduit that is continent of gas and stool. Fairly good results have been reported, especially in patients who have the ability to squeeze the external anal sphincter to some degree.

Another noninvasive alternative is biofeedback training (59). This treatment modality may be used in patients with fecal incontinence of various etiologies, but some degree of rectal sensation must be intact and the patient must be able to contract the external sphincter for biofeedback training to be successful. During biofeedback training, a manometric catheter with an attached rectal balloon is placed in the rectum. Patients are taught how to perceive small volumes of air in the rectal balloon and then contract the external sphincter in response to this rectal distention. A pressure-sensing device attached to the manometric catheter converts the pressure exerted by the patient to a visual or auditory signal, allowing the patient to monitor external anal sphincter contraction. This technique requires both a dedicated therapist and a patient willing to attend multiple sessions. In approximately 70%–80% of patients some degree of improvement is appreciated with biofeedback training (60,61).

Operative Sphincter Repair

In the patient with significant fecal incontinence and a sphincter defect, sphincteroplasty is the treatment of choice. Although patients with concomitant pudendal neuropathy also may be candidates for sphincter repair, superior results are reported in patients who have pure anatomic sphincter defects without associated neuropathy. Several techniques have been described for sphincter repair including direct apposition and overlapping anterior sphincteroplasty. Direct apposition of the internal and external sphincters most commonly is used for primary repair at the time of obstetric injury and is associated with moderate success. Most failed repairs following this technique have been attributed to suture line tension and subsequent separation.

In general, women with an anterior sphincter defect and fecal incontinence following delivery are best served by delayed repair after 3–6 months. During this time period, acute inflammation is allowed to resolve and firm, fibrous tissue develops at the divided ends of the sphincter. Incontinence is treated temporarily with diet modification, antidiarrheal medications, and a strict bowel regimen.

For elective repair of most sphincter defects, an overlapping sphincteroplasty is the treatment of choice. The majority of these repairs are performed on women to manage anterior defects that are a result of childbirth injury. The goal of overlapping sphincter repair is to restore the entire anterior sphincter, keeping in mind the continuity of the external anal sphincter and the levator muscles.

Of patients, 70%–90% experience moderate to excellent improvement following overlapping anterior sphincteroplasty. Young patients with no previous attempt at repair and intact pudendal nerves tend to experience the best results after repair. Recent studies point out that long-term results are not spectacular. Patients should be counseled accordingly (62).

Postanal Repair

As discussed previously, medical management is the mainstay of therapy when no sphincter defect is identified and the cause of incontinence is thought to be pudendal neuropathy. However, some operative interventions are available for the treatment of neurogenic incontinence. The postanal repair, as described by Parks and colleagues (63), was designed to address physiologic abnormalities associated with neurogenic incontinence including a short anal canal, a poor anorectal angle, and perineal descent with straining. Postanal repair does not alter basal anal pressures, but it may increase squeeze pressures and lengthen the anal canal. Posterior plication of the puborectalis theoretically restores the anorectal angle, but this has not been demonstrated. Success rates of approximately 70%–80% are reported immediately after repair, but sustained long-term benefit is not always attained (64). This operation rarely is performed in the United States.

Total pelvic floor repair deserves mention as one option for surgical repair. This operation consists of a combination of anterior sphincter repair with levatoroplasty and postanal repair (65,66). Potential candidates for this repair include patients with complex sphincter injuries at more than one site as well as pudendal neuropathy. Experience with this repair is limited, and the operation is not performed widely.

Neosphincter Options

Neosphincter construction may be appropriate in patients in whom previous operative attempts at repair have failed. The principle of anal sphincter substitution involves the use of biologic material or artificial mechanical devices to fashion a neosphincter around the nonfunctioning anal canal.

Bilateral gluteus maximus transposition (gluteoplasty) (67) and gracilis muscle transposition (graciloplasty) (68–70) have been used for neosphincter construction. Graciloplasty was used more commonly. Gracilis wrap has been used in patients who have failed attempts at sphincter repair and thus have a very thin and scarred perineum. Electrical stimulation has been added to graciloplasty (dynamic graciloplasty) in an attempt to convert fatigable, fast-twitch (Type II) muscle fibers to fatigue-resistant (Type I) muscle fibers. Good results have been reported with dynamic graciloplasty, with 70%–90% of the patients reporting improvement of continence after the procedure. Complications including infection and mechanical failure of the electrical stimulator have been reported. Some patients also report difficulties evacuating stool after the procedure. Currently, the stimulator is not available in the United States. This operation, therefore, rarely is performed today.

An implanted, artificial anal sphincter device also may be used to construct a neosphincter (71–73). The artificial sphincter device represents a modification of the artificial urinary sphincter that has been used successfully for many years. The device consists of three parts and is made of silastic material (Fig. 8-5). The first part is an inflatable cuff that is implanted around the anus. The second part is a control pump that is implanted in the labia in women and in the scrotum in men. When pumped, water is removed from the cuff, and the cuff is deflated. The water from the pump flows into the third part, a regulating balloon that is implanted in the space of Retzius. The cuff is deflated just prior to defecation. The cuff is automatically slowly reinflated with water, closing the anal canal after defecation. Just as with graciloplasty, complications include infection, device failure, and difficulties with stool evacuation. Only small numbers of patients have been treated using this technique. Initial and long-term results are encouraging, but the major problem, in-

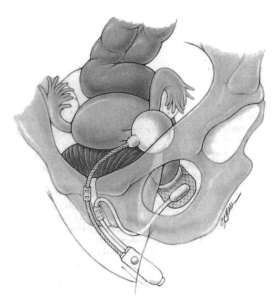

FIG. 8-5. The artificial bowel sphincter. The cuff is in place around the anus, the reservoir is in the retroperitoneal space anterior to the bladder, and the pump is in the labium. (From Aitola PT, Congilosi SM. Artificial anal sphincter: the current status. Congilosi S, ed. *Seminars in colon and rectal surgery*, Vol 12, No 2, Anal Incontinence. Philadelphia: WB Saunders Co., 2002: 116, with permission from Elsevier Science.)

fection of the prosthesis or erosion of the device necessitating removal, is not uncommon and complicates up to 33% of implantations.

Sacral Nerve Stimulation

Electrical stimulation of sacral nerve is a well-established treatment of urinary incontinence. This technique is being applied to and evaluated for the treatment of fecal incontinence (74,75). Patients first undergo a short trial period with direct stimulation of the S3 nerve root via the foramen. If significant improvement in reduction of incontinence episodes and symptoms occur, then the stimulation is stopped, and the patient is considered for implantation of a permanent stimulation device. It initially was thought that this stimulation worked by enhancing the ability of the external sphincter to generate a squeeze. Recent investigations suggest, however, that improvement may be the result of neuromodulation of sacral reflexes responsible for rectal sensitivity and contractility (76). Results at this point are promising, but more studies are needed.

Fecal Diversion

The final surgical option for patients with fecal incontinence refractory to medical and operative management is the creation of an end sigmoid colostomy. In most cases, this stoma can be created using laparoscopic techniques that minimize pain and length of hospital stay. Many will find that a well-constructed stoma is much more manageable than the constant disability associated with fecal incontinence.

REFERENCES

1. Drossman DA, Zhming L, Andruzzi E, et al. U.S. householder survey of functional gastrointestinal disorders. *Dig Dis Sci* 1993;38:1569–1580.
2. Van Nostrand JF, Zappolo A, Hing E, et al. *The national nursing home survey: 1977 summary for the United States* (DHEW Publication No. PHS 79-1794). Washington DC: U.S. Government Printing Office, Statistics-Series 13-No. 43, 1979.
3. Lahr CJ. Evaluation and treatment of incontinence. *Pract Gastroenterol* 1988;12:27-35.
4. Goligher JC, Hughes ES. Sensibility of the rectum and colon. *Lancet* 1951;122:599–609.
5. Ihre T. Studies on anal function in continent and incontinent patients. *Scand J Gastroenterol* 1974;9(Suppl 25):1–64.
6. Varma JS, Smith AN, Busuttil A. Correlation of clinical and manometric abnormalities of rectal function following chronic radiation injury. *Br J Surg* 1985;72: 875–878.
7. Beart RW, Dozois RR, Wolff BG, et al. Mechanisms of rectal continence. *Am J Surg* 1985;149:31–34.
8. Pedersen IK, Hint K, Olsen J Christiansen J, et al. Anorectal function after low anterior resection for carcinoma. *Ann Surg* 1986;204:133–135.
9. Rasmussen OO, Christensen B, Sorensen M, et al. The value of rectal compliance in the assessment of patients with fecal incontinence. *Dis Colon Rectum* 1990;33: 650–653.
10. Frenckner B, Euler CV. Influence of pudendal nerve block on the function of the anal sphincters. *Gut* 1975;16:482–489.
11. Parks AG, Porter NH, Melzak J. Experimental study of the reflex mechanism controlling the muscles of the pelvic floor. *Dis Colon Rectum* 1962;5:407–414.
12. Lane RH, Parks AG. Function of the anal sphincters following colo-anal anastomosis. *Br J Surg* 1977;64: 596–599.
13. Scarli AF, Kiesewetter WB. Defecation and continence. *Dis Colon Rectum* 1970;13:81–107.
14. Read NW, Abouzekry L. Why do patients with faecal impaction have faecal incontinence. *Gut* 1986;27:283–287.
15. Trezza M, Krogh K, Egekvist H, et al. Bowel problems in patients with systemic sclerosis. *Scand J Gastroenterol* 1999;34:409–413.
16. Epanomeritakis E, Koutsoumbi P, Tsiaoussis I, et al. Impairment of anorectal function in diabetes mellitus parallels duration of disease. *Dis Colon Rectum* 1999;42: 1394–1400.
17. Feldman M, Schiller L. Disorders of the gastrointestinal motility associated with diabetes mellitus. *Ann Intern Med* 1983;98:378–384.
18. Erckenbrecht JF, Winter HJ, Cimir I, et al. Fecal incontinence in diabetes mellitus: Is it correlated to autonomic or peripheral neuropathy? *Z Gastroenterol* 26; 1988:731–736.
19. Schiller RL, Santa Ana CA, Schmulen AC, et al. Pathogenesis of fecal incontinence in diabetes mellitus. Evidence of internal anal sphincter dysfunction. *N Engl J Med* 1982;307:1666–1671.
20. Sun WM, Katsinelos P, Horowitz M, et al. Disturbances in anorectal function in patients with diabetes mellitus and faecal incontinence. *Eur J Gastroenterol Hepatol* 1996;8:1007–1012.
21. Aitchison M, Fisher BM, Carter K, et al. Impaired anal sensation and early diabetic faecal incontinence. *Diabet Med* 1991;8:960–963.
22. Lynch AC, Wong C, Anthony A, et al. Bowel dysfunction following spinal cord injury: a description of bowel function in a spinal cord-injured population and comparison with age and gender matched controls. *Spinal Cord* 2000;38:717–723.
23. Lynch AC, Anthony A, Dobbs BR, et al. Anorectal physiology following spinal cord injury. *Spinal Cord* 2000;38:573–580.
24. Levi R, Hultling C, Nash MS, et al. The Stockholm spinal cord injury study: Medical problems in a regional SCI population. *Paraplegia* 1995;33:308–315.
25. De Looze D, Van Laere N, De Muynck M, et al. Constipation and other chronic gastrointestinal problems in spinal cord injury patients. *Spinal Cord* 1998;36:63–66.
26. Hinds JP, Eidelman BH, Wald A. Prevalence of bowel dysfunction in multiple sclerosis. *Gastroenterol* 1990; 98:1538–1542.
27. Norbendo AM, Anderson JR, Anderson JT. Disturbances of anorectal function in multiple sclerosis. *J Neurol* 1996,243.445–451.
28. Caruana ET, Wald A, Hinds JP, et al. Anorectal sensory and motor function in neurogenic fecal incontinence. *Gastroenterol* 1991;100:465–470.
29. Shepherd K, Hickstein R, Shepherd R. Neurogenic fecal incontinence in children with spina bifida: Rectosphincteric responses and evaluation of physiologic rationale for management including biofeedback conditioning. *Aust Pediatr J* 1983;19:97–99.
30. King JC, Currie DM, Wright E. Bowel training in spina bifida: Importance of education, patient compliance, age, and anal reflexes. *Arch Phys Med Rehabil* 1994;75: 243–247.
31. Pappo I, Meyer S, Winter S, et al. Treatment of fecal incontinence in children with spina bifida by biofeedback and behavioral modification. *Z Kinderchir* 1988;43 (Suppl II);36–37.

32. Ponticelli A, Iacobelli BD, Silveri M, et al. Colorectal dysfunction and faecal incontinence in children with spina bifida. *Br J Urol* 1998;31(Suppl 3):117–119.

33. Kiff ES, Swash M. Slowed conduction in the pudendal nerves in idiopathic (neurogenic) faecal incontinence. *Br J Surg* 1984;71:614–616.

34. Dhaenens G, Emblem R, Ganes T. Fibre density in idiopathic ano-rectal incontinence. *Electromyogr Clin Neurophysiol* 1995;35:285–290.

35. Neill ME, Swash M. Increased motor unit fibre density in the external anal sphincter muscle in ano-rectal incontinence: a single fibre EMG study. *J Neurol Neurosurg Psychiatry* 1980;43:343–347.

36. Parks AG, Swash M. Denervation of the anal sphincter causing idiopathic ano-rectal incontinence. *J R Coll Surg Edinb* 1979;24:94–96.

37. Parks AG, Swash M, Urich H. Sphincter denervation in ano-rectal incontinence and rectal prolapse. *Gut* 1977; 18:656–665.

38. Osterberg A, Graf W, Edebol Eeg-Olofsson K, et al. Results of neurophysiologic evaluation in fecal incontinence. *Dis Colon Rectum* 2000;43:1256–1261.

39. Snooks SJ, Setchell M, Swash M, et al. Injury to the innervation of the pelvic floor sphincter musculature in childbirth. *Lancet* 1984:546–550.

40. Jones PN, Lubowski DZ, Swash M, et al. Relation between perineal descent and pudendal nerve damage in idiopathic faecal incontinence. *Int J Colorectal Dis* 1987;2:93–95.

41. Rasmussen OO, Christiansen J, Tetzschner T, et al. Pudendal nerve function in idiopathic fecal incontinence. *Dis Colon Rectum* 2000;43;633–636.

42. Madoff RD, Williams JG, Caushaj PF. Fecal incontinence. *N Engl J Med* 1992;326:1002–1007.

43. Kamm MA. Obstetric damage and faecal incontinence. *Lancet* 1994;344:730–733.

44. Thacker SB, Banta DH. Benefits and risks of episiotomy: an interpretive review of the English language literature, 1860-1980. *Obstet Gynecol Survey* 1983;38: 322–338.

45. Legino LJ, Woods MP, Rayburn WF, et al. Third and fourth degree perineal tears: experience at a university hospital. *J Reprod Med* 1988;33:423–426.

46. Go PM, Dunselman GA. Anatomical and functional results of surgical repair after total perineal rupture at delivery. *Surg Gynecol Obstet* 1988;166:121–124.

47. Sultan AH, Kamm MA, Hudson CN, et al. Third degree obstetric anal sphincter tears: risk factors and outcome of primary repair. *BMJ* 1994;308:887–891.

48. Sangwan YP, Coller JA, Barret RC, et al. Unilateral pudendal neuropathy: impact on outcome of anal sphincter repair. *Dis Colon Rectum* 1996;39:686–689.

49. Pena A, Guardino K, Tovilla JM, et al. Bowel management for fecal incontinence in patients with anorectal malformations. *J Pediatr Surg* 1998;33:133–137.

50. Jorge M, Wexner S. Etiology and management of fecal incontinence. *Dis Colon Rectum* 1993;36:77–97.

51. Rockwood TH, Church JM, Fleshman JW, et al. Fecal incontinence quality of life scale: quality of life instrument for patients with fecal incontinence. *Dis Colon Rectum* 2000;43:9–17.

52. Hull TL, Floruta C, Piedmonte M. Preliminary results of an outcome tool used for evaluation of surgical treatment for fecal incontinence. *Dis Colon Rectum* 2001; 44:799–805.

53. Laurberg S, Swash M, Henry MM. Delayed external sphincter repair for obstetric tear. *Br J Surg* 1988;75: 786–788.

54. Wexner SD, Marchetti F, Jagelman DG. The role of sphincteroplasty for fecal incontinence reevaluated: a prospective physiologic and functional review. *Dis Colon Rectum* 1991;34:22–30.

55. Gilliland R, Altomare DF, Moreira H, et al. Pudendal neuropathy is predictive of failure following anterior overlapping sphincteroplasty. *Dis Colon Rectum* 1998; 41:1516–1522.

56. Stoker J, Halligan S, Bartram CI. Pelvic floor imaging. *Radiology* 2001;218:621-41.

57. Teichman JMH, Harris JM, Currie DM, et al. Malone antegrade continence enema for adults with neurogenic bowel disease. *J Urol* 1998;160:1278—1281.

58. Williams NS. Surgery of anorectal incontinence. *Lancet* 1999;353(Suppl 1):31–32.

59. Ryn A, Morren GL, Hallbook O, et al. Long-term results of electromyographic biofeedback training for fecal incontinence. *Dis Colon Rectum* 2000;43: 1262–1266.

60. Keck JO, Staniunas RJ, Coller JA, et al. Biofeedback training is useful in fecal incontinence but disappointing in constipation. *Dis Colon Rectum* 1994;37: 1271–1276.

61. Guillemot F, Bouche B, Gower RC, et al. Biofeedback for the treatment of fecal incontinence. Long-term clinical results. *Dis Colon Rectum* 1995;38:393–397.

62. Malouf AJ, Norton CS, Engel AF, et al. Long-term results of overlapping anterior anal-sphincter repair for obstetric trauma. *Lancet* 2000;355:260–265.

63. Parks AG, Porter NH, Hardcastle J. The syndrome of descending perineum. Proceedings of the Royal Society of Medicine 1966;59:477–482.

64. Setti Carraro P, Kamm MA, Nicholls RJ. Long-term results of postanal repair for neurogenic faecal incontinence. *Br J Surg* 1994;81:140–144.

65. Browning GGP, Henry MM, Motson RW. Combined sphincter repair and postanal repair for the treatment of complicated injuries to the anal sphincters. *Ann R Coll Surg Engl* 1988;70:324–328.

66. Pinho M, Ortiz J, Oya J, et al. Total pelvic floor repair for treatment of neuropathic fecal incontinence. *Am J Surg* 1992;163:340–343.

67. Devesa JM, Madrid JM, Gallego BR, et al. Bilateral gluteoplasty for fecal incontinence. *Dis Colon Rectum* 1997;40:883–888.

68. Baeten CG, Geerdes BP, Adang EM, et al. Anal dynamic graciloplasty in the treatment of intractable fecal incontinence. *N Engl J Med* 1995;332:1600–1605.

69. Baeten CG, Bailey HR, Bakka A, et al. Safety and efficacy of dynamic graciloplasty for fecal incontinence: report of a prospective, multicenter trial. *Dis Colon Rectum* 2000;43:743–751.

70. Niriella DA, Deen KI. Neosphincters in the management of faecal incontinence. *Br J Surg* 2000;87: 1617–1628.

71. Christiansen J, Rasmussen OO, Lindorff-Larsen K. Long-term results of artificial anal sphincter implantation for severe anal incontinence. *Ann Surg* 1999;230: 45–48.

72. Wong WD, Jensen LL, Bartolo DCC, et al. Artificial anal sphincter. *Dis Colon Rectum* 1996;39:1345–1351.

73. Devesa JM, Rey A, Hervas PL, et al. Artificial anal

sphincter: Complications and functional results of a large personal series. *Dis Colon Rectum* 2002;45: 1154–1163.

74. Matzel KE, Stadelmaier U, Hohenfellner M, et al. Electrical stimulation of sacral spinal nerves for treatment of faecal incontinence. *Lancet* 1995;346:1124–1127.

75. Malouf AJ, Vaizey CJ, Nicholls RJ, et al. Permanent sacral nerve stimulation for fecal incontinence. *Ann Surg* 2000;232:143–148.

76. Vaizey CJ, Kamm MS, Turner IC, et al. Effects of short term sacral nerve stimulation on anal and rectal function in patients with anal incontinence. *Gut* 1999;44:407–412.

9

General Health Concerns and the Physical Examination

Sandra L. Welner and Bliss Temple

An underlying theme that pervades the medical model of disability is that only a person who is physically agile and neurologically intact can be considered healthy (1). This inaccurately categorizes almost 30 million women with disabilities in the United States as being in poor health. Consequently, rather than having access to primary and preventive health care, the tendency may be for them to receive treatment only from specialists or on an emergency basis. Acknowledgment of the potential for wellness and tailored primary prevention can minimize the need for this stopgap care (2). A better approach to promoting wellness is to recognize that health issues may differ depending on the woman and her disability and to tailor preventive care strategies to each individual. The ultimate objective of health maintenance programs for women who are disabled is to maximize independence and well-being while minimizing deterioration and intercurrent illnesses (3,4).

The delivery of health care to women is multifaceted. When physical disabilities are added to the equation, there are yet more dimensions to consider. It is important to acknowledge that all women are similar, although physical challenges and medical conditions may affect some aspects of the care they require. Specifically, health care practitioners should realize that women with disabilities experience all of the health concerns that nondisabled women do in the areas of reproductive health, mental health, nutrition and weight management, cancer screen-

ing, cardiac screening, and so on. These issues may interact with disability issues in ways that are unique to each individual, but the disability does not take them away. Viewing health care for women with disabilities in this context emphasizes similarities between these individuals and other women without ignoring the differences that must be taken into account when delivering comprehensive services to women with challenging medical conditions.

Information and communication are key to providing good primary and preventive health care. Practitioners need to be able to gather relevant information from the professional literature, medical records, and the woman herself. Synthesizing this information and designing an individualized health care program can be challenging; often there will be no "roadmap" to follow. It is very important to involve patients in this process. They often will be far more knowledgeable about their disabilities than most health care practitioners. Good communication facilitates the design of effective individualized health care programs and effective patient education as well as being its own reward.

This chapter surveys the general issues that arise in providing primary and preventive care for women with disabilities in an outpatient setting, provides practical suggestions for addressing them, then briefly discusses issues particular to several disability groups. It is hoped that it will help you offer high-quality care that can maximize your disabled patients' independence and well-being over the course of their lives.

PHYSICAL ACCESS

Patients with physical disabilities have the right to expect a certain level of physical access to any "public accommodation," which includes doctors' offices. Beyond the question of rights, however, you certainly will be able to provide better care in an accessible facility, as well as enable your patients who are disabled to be more comfortable and autonomous.

When considering access overall, it is often useful to think of a hypothetic wheelchair user arriving at the building's parking lot, and imagine her path of travel from the lot to the entrance, from the lobby to your office (through elevators, waiting room, reception desk, examination room, bathroom, access to equipment, etc.), and out again. This exercise then could be repeated for another hypothetic patient using a walker or crutches and again for one with blindness.

It is worth noting that if you are leasing space in a medical building, the building owner/management has some access obligations under the law. If remodeling or retrofits are needed, you might consider trying to get the owner to share the expense. If the access problems exist in the path of travel to your office, the owner is obligated to provide that for you if it can be reasonably accomplished. Issues to consider in determining what is reasonable are the age of the building and the cost of any retrofits. If extensive remodeling is done for any reason, then there is a legal mandate to make the remodel accessible. More information on physical access mandated by law is in Chapter 3.

Parking

Access begins outside the building, in the parking lot (if there is one). Parking lots should have at least one handicap accessible parking space. Depending on the size of the lot, an additional accessible space should be added for every 50 regular spaces. There are readily available specifications for these spaces in handbooks for builders and architects. If the lot is extensive, there should be signage that clearly indicates where to find the accessible parking areas.

Often, the accessible parking spaces are placed very near the entrance; for many persons who are disabled, the easiest and shortest path to your office will be greatly appreciated. There is an obligation to create a safe and accessible path of travel from the parking spaces to the entrance of the building. "Safe" usually means that disabled pedestrians do not need to walk in the same roadway that cars are using to get in and out of the lot. If there is no way to avoid the roadway, then a clear path should be marked using crosshatched markings on the pavement. This is both to indicate the path and to alert drivers to a crosswalk.

Entrance

An accessible entrance is one a wheelchair user can use to get into the building without encountering curbs or steps. If necessary, a ramp can be used to create an alternative path for wheelchair users. There should be clearly visible signs indicating the accessible entrance, if there are multiple entrances. (If all of the entrances are accessible, then signage isn't necessary.)

Ramps are required to be at least 12″ to 1″–that is, 12 inches for every inch of elevation. If necessary, a ramp can be "wrapped," meaning that it has switchbacks rather than one very long, straight ramp. Specifications for both ramps and stairs—which have specific requirements for the height of a riser and for stair banisters—are readily available.

At least a portion of the path must be nonslip, meaning that the surface itself is not slippery or that nonslip strips are applied on top of a slippery surface. There also should be changes in pavement texture (usually ridges in the cement) to indicate the beginning and ending of stairs or ramps to individuals who are blind or visually impaired.

Doors

All doors used by patients need to be wide enough for a wheelchair to get through, minimally 30″ but preferably 32″ or 36″ when this is possible. Employees or possible future employees who use wheelchairs also should be a consideration when thinking about doorway access.

In many older buildings, there are sets of two narrow doors at the building entrance. If only one leaf of the set of these older doors is opened, the space is not wide enough for a wheelchair to pass through. There are two ways to solve this problem. Some choose to remove the two doors and replace them with one wider door and a strip of glass next to the wider door. Another option is to put in an automatic (powered) door opener, which will open both of the narrow doors at the same time.

Powered doors are not required at an otherwise accessible entrance. However, if it is an entrance that gets a lot of traffic, powered doors are an excellent idea. Powered doors *are* required if the path of travel immediately outside the door is sloped, such that a person in a manual wheelchair can't stop to open the door without rolling backward or forward.

The threshold(s) should be flush, or nearly so, with the floor on either side. There are inexpensive adapters that can be placed over thresholds that are high to smooth out the path for a wheelchair user.

"Lever hardware" should be installed on all doors used by the public. This refers to the type of doorknobs that are not actually knobs but rectangular handles that can be operated with a closed fist.

Lobby (Building and/or Individual Office)

How a lobby should be laid out depends entirely on the size of the space and how much traffic it gets. The most important aspect of a large lobby is the signage indicating where an office is, and, if necessary, where there are accessible restrooms.

When designing and positioning a building directory, you should think about the following:

- Using letters big enough for patients with vision impairments to see
- Avoiding having a reflective covering encasing the directory
- Indicating accessible restrooms with the blue wheelchair symbol
- Placing the directory at a height and angle that can be read by someone using a wheelchair

If there are chairs for use while waiting, they should not block any door or pedestrian pathway. There should be an area within the waiting area where someone in a wheelchair could park their chair without blocking pedestrian pathways or access to the other chairs in the waiting area. It is preferable for wheelchair "parking spaces" to be at a conversational distance from where able-bodied companions will sit and to feel like an extension of the existing seating. When positioning furniture, plants, or decorations, keep in mind leaving enough free floor space for maneuvering a wheelchair.

Telephones

In any building that provides a pay phone for visitors, there should be an accessible phone for visitors with disabilities. There are specific and detailed specifications available for these accessible phones. It is not necessary to have a TDD (telecommunications device for the deaf also known as a teletypewriter or TTY) in every location where there are pay phones, but there should be clear signage as to where the TDD is located if one is available.

Elevators

There are extremely detailed code requirements for elevators, which include size of buttons, Braille signage, height of the buttons, visible and sound indicators for floors, support railings inside of the cab, size of cab, and so on. These are readily available.

The main thing to watch out for on a day-to-day basis is that no plants, trash receptacles, or furniture block access to call buttons and elevator doors. Remember that even low obstacles can prevent wheelchair users from getting close enough to reach the buttons.

Reception

The reception desk or counter should have at least a portion at wheelchair-user height—the height that works best for the most number of people is 32″, which is the middle of the Americans with Disabilities Act's regulated counter heights. If the counter edge extends at least 18 inches beyond the lower support, it will enable many wheelchair users to pull up under the counter and interact with the receptionist eye to eye. This is a tremendous indication of respect for the patient using a wheelchair.

If a patient needs to fill out forms or sign anything and the counter does not work for them, they should be offered a clipboard. Some patients may need assistance in filling out forms. If they do, it should be given in a way that is respectful and mindful of the patients' privacy.

Inner Office

There should be a clear path of travel from the reception room to an accessible examin-ing room. This means that equipment should not be stored in the hallway if it blocks the hallway—there should be at least 36″ of clear space.

There should be enough space in the examination room that patients using wheelchairs can turn around, maneuver themselves into a good position to transfer to the examination table, and park themselves in an appropriate position for a conversation with the health care practitioner. There should be clear space in front of any assessment equipment, so that a wheelchair could pull up close enough to use it. It is common for a woman using a wheelchair to have never been weighed. To ensure comprehensive health assessments, a platform scale should be available (5). Also, having a height-adjustable examination table (see Fig. 9-1) is critical to performing a comprehensive health evaluation on patients who cannot climb onto a high table, as well as offering the practitioner more options for examining all patients.

BATHROOMS

Any public restroom in the building ideally should have an accessible option for wheelchair users. However, in older buildings it is not necessary to make all of the bathrooms

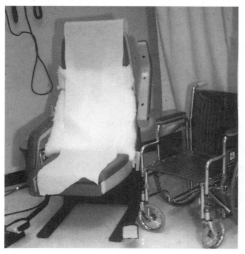
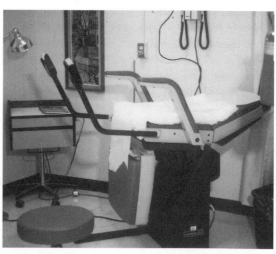

A

B

FIG. 9-1. Universally accessible examination table. (From Welner SL, inventor; Hausman Industries, assignee, US patent # 5507050, 1996, with permission.)

accessible. There does need to be at least one accessible restroom. It is extremely important that there be clear signage indicating the location of that restroom.

The specifications for accessible bathrooms are readily available. Among the accommodations in an accessible bathroom are larger stalls, bars beside and/or behind the toilet, space for wheelchair users to pull underneath sinks, lever-type faucet handles, and lowered paper towel dispensers. One important but often overlooked modification you should make is to insulate the pipes underneath sinks, which prevents wheelchair users from burning themselves on hot water pipes.

If you must retrofit your building, there is more than one way to achieve accessibility. In a large bathroom with multiple stalls, two small stalls may be remodeled into one accessible stall. Alternatively, if there are two small bathrooms, one for men and one for women, these could be remodeled into one larger unisex bathroom that is wheelchair accessible. Creative reconfiguration of space often can help you come up with a feasible, affordable solution.

Non–public use bathrooms do not need to be made accessible as a "public accommodation." Bathrooms for employees, however, also should provide an accessible option.

SCHEDULING, INTAKE FORMS, AND EDUCATIONAL MATERIALS

Paratransit is a door-to-door transportation service provided for people with disabilities who cannot use other means of public transportation. Although this service can be valuable, it is not always reliable. Public transportation also can provide unexpected surprises if elevators or lifts are broken or a vehicle already is carrying its full load of passengers in wheelchairs. Therefore, some women with disabilities who are not able to drive may not be in full control of whether they arrive on time for medical appointments. This may be disruptive to the office staff as well as frustrating for the woman. Whenever

possible, it is helpful to be more lenient with cancellation and late-arrival policies to accommodate women with these issues.

Women with hearing or speech impairments may have other scheduling concerns. Ideally, each office should have a TDD. Otherwise, women may need to use a telephone relay service when calling to schedule an appointment. Receptionists should become familiar with using a TDD or relay service to communicate with patients. For more information on TDD (TTY) and relay service, see Chapter 5.

Women with dexterity or visual impairments may have difficulty filling out medical forms. An office staff member may need to act as a scribe for these women. Employees who work at the reception counter should be trained to offer assistance in a professional and casual manner. "Do you need any help with that?" is much better than "Oh, let me do that for you!" or "Why haven't you filled out those forms yet?" To protect confidentiality, if personal information must be exchanged orally it is important to do it in a private space where others cannot overhear the exchange (6). When possible, it may be useful to mail forms to a woman in advance of her appointment.

Education about general and specific health concerns helps make a woman a partner in her medical care. Depending on the nature of the disability, alternative formats of this education may be required. If you keep educational materials such as posters or pamphlets in your waiting area, you should make copies available in Braille, in large print, and/or on audiotape for women with visual impairments. Remember that they may not even know that such materials exist unless you offer them. It is helpful when possible to have materials that are simple, colorful, and highly visual for women with cognitive impairments and those who are not fluent in written English.

It should be recognized that the woman who is hearing impaired may not have access to a comprehensive array of public health promotion sources because many of these are provided via radio and television. Therefore women with hearing impairments should be supplied with health information materials to supplement what is otherwise not available to them (7).

COMMUNICATION AND ATTITUDES ABOUT DISABILITY

It is critical to view each woman as a whole person—not just as her disability. Learning to respect each patient as a person will help you provide better care. Listening to her will help you understand her disability within the broader context of her health concerns.

It is important to acknowledge that patients who are disabled are susceptible to any and all health problems seen in able-bodied individuals. When treating patients who are disabled, clinicians need to strike a balance between learning enough about the patient's disability to understand how it affects her health and also focusing on broader health issues common to all patients and the specific symptoms or concerns revealed in the course of a particular visit.

When possible, it may be helpful to obtain a medical history of a woman with a disability before her visit. In this way, the practitioner can gain some basic knowledge about the disability and other concerns before she arrives. This will facilitate communication and also show the patient that she was important enough to the clinician that an effort was made to gain a better understanding of her diagnosis. To foster a stronger clinician–patient relationship, it is important for the practitioner to listen to and learn from the patient about her particular disability. She is most likely very knowledgeable about her situation, and learning from her not only educates the provider but also lets her know that her contribution to the medical interaction is valued.

Patients with complex medical conditions are usually very familiar with many issues pertaining to their health, and clinicians can benefit greatly by listening to them. Patients' input is not only valuable, it is critical, and patients with disabilities welcome open-minded practitioners who are willing to learn and listen as well as prescribe and treat. Patients can provide a wealth of information and detail about their disabilities, which educates the provider about their conditions and assists her in appropriately tailoring medical care. When the patient's expertise is not acknowledged and used, valuable time may be wasted and important symptoms may be missed. This causes frustration for both patient and practitioner, potentially delays diagnosis of serious conditions, and results in adverse health consequences.

It is not uncommon for women with disabilities to be accompanied by a family member, attendant, interpreter, or service animal. It is important to focus attention on the patient who has come for care or advice. After all, it is her appointment. Questioning her assistant, interpreter, or family member about her medical problems is unlikely to provide the practitioner with as much valuable personal information as talking with the woman herself. Furthermore, it sends a signal that the practitioner does not respect the woman's knowledge of her own situation or her need to have her own concerns addressed by her health care provider. Asking personal questions of those accompanying the patient, especially if her input is not sought, can be embarrassing and negating. The patient is the most reliable source of information and she should be questioned directly about her symptoms and concerns. (Of course, women who are unable to communicate or understand questions will not be able to answer for themselves, so in these exceptional cases practitioners will need to rely on family members or assistants. Even in cases like these, however, it is important to maintain a focus on the patient.)

When a woman is accompanied by a family member or attendant, you should offer her the option of having her appointment with or without the presence of these companions. She may prefer to have their physical and/or emotional support during the examination. However, in some cases women may be more able to bring up concerns without their presence. It is especially important to give women an opportunity to see you alone in cases where there may be abuse, when adolescents or young-adult women may want to discuss issues of sexuality and contraception, and/or when companions seem to have difficulty allowing the woman to speak for herself.

It is a good start but not enough for physicians and other practitioners to be sensitized to attitudes and communication issues when dealing with patients who are disabled. Staff training is essential to ensure that the entire health care team's interactions with a patient will be positive. If the staff has had limited interaction with people who are disabled, they may harbor misconceptions about the capabilities and intelligence of people with physical challenges. It is ideal for this training to be done by articulate people with disabilities who can educate and enlighten office personnel about sensitive ways in which their physical and other needs can be met. This may be especially critical for staff interacting with those who have speech impediments and cognitive dysfunctions.

THE EXAMINATION

History and Screening

In performing the examination, the practitioner should ask questions that are thorough and comprehensive. These questions should address general health, women's health, and disability-related issues. Remember that women with disabilities may have any or all of the health concerns that your nondisabled patients have. Do not, for instance, make the assumption that a disabled teenager is not sexually active or that an older woman with a physical disability is not at risk for cancer.

It is especially important with women who are disabled to make sure that you have a comprehensive list of the drugs they take regularly. It is common for women who are disabled to take several medications prescribed by different specialists. The general or woman's health care practitioner is often the only person monitoring all of her medications in relation to each other.

Many women who are disabled receive inadequate dental care. You should inquire about dental health and be ready to provide a referral to an accessible dental health provider if appropriate.

Osteoporosis and vaccines for pneumonia and influenza are particular preventive health issues you may want to address with some patients who are disabled. Women who are sedentary may develop osteoporosis at younger ages than their counterparts whose bones are subjected to load-bearing exercise. It may be useful to counsel patients who are disabled about obtaining adequate levels of calcium and vitamin D, obtaining bone scans, and/or considering drug therapy for osteoporosis as early as adolescence. Pneumonia vaccines are recommended for people older than 65 years of age; the vaccine also may be a good idea for younger patients with compromised lung function (such as quadriplegics with reduced lung capacity and difficulty coughing) and/or chronic illnesses and/or who live in long-term care facilities. Flu vaccines are recommended for people older than 50 years of age; they also should be received by those with chronic illnesses and/or who live in long-term care facilities.

The American College of Obstetricians and Gynecologists has established guidelines for appropriate routine counseling and screening for gynecologic health concerns of women in particular age groups. These guidelines should be followed in women with disabilities as well (8). You also should do screenings for colon cancer, melanomas, diabetes, hypercholesterolemia, and hypertension that are appropriate for the patient's age and risk factors.

Physical Examination

The physical examination may be affected by the woman's disability. This varies within disability groups and also may vary among patients in the same group.

It is helpful to orient a woman who is visually impaired to the examination room so that she is familiar with her surroundings. Statements such as, "Just go right down that hall into that room," or "The exam table is right over there," can be confusing. Try to be as specific as possible when giving directions. It is especially important that she knows where her clothing has been placed so that she may retrieve it after the examination is complete. Statements such as, "Your clothing has been hung on a hook behind the door, which is about two feet to your left," are more helpful than "Don't worry. Your clothes are right over here." For more information on examining the woman who is blind or visually impaired, see Chapter 4.

A person who is hearing impaired who is not able to respond to verbal instructions will need visual cues to help her work with a practitioner before and during the exam (6,7). It is important to ensure that she can see you during the examination. If an interpreter is present for the examination, the participants should be positioned so that the patient can see both the interpreter and the health care provider clearly; the health care provider should be focused on the patient rather than the interpreter. For more information on examination of the hearing impaired, see Chapter 5.

Physiatric disabilities include spinal cord injury, spina bifida, cerebral palsy, and muscular dystrophy, to name a few. These disorders are characterized by joint movement restrictions and increased spasticity. These mobility restrictions and pain syndromes may affect comfortable positioning when performing the examination. See Chapters 21 and 27 for more information. When wheelchair users will need to be examined on the examination table, they should be asked about transfer techniques that have worked for them in the past because they are most familiar with their own capabilities.

The initial part of the examination should be done in a seated position. Tables with an elevated backrest are ideal for this purpose. Palpation of the thyroid as well as auscultation of heart and lungs can be done in this position. Careful attention should be focused on the clinical breast examination because many women with extremity contractures and dex-

terity limitations may be unable to do an adequate self-examination. The observant practitioner should note these difficulties and develop a more complete breast health plan for them. Using a training video that has been produced for this purpose or with direct clinician involvement, a woman can be taught self-examination techniques that she can do on her own or with a trained companion. Otherwise, she could come to the provider for more frequent clinical examinations.

Assessment of the abdomen may be compromised by the presence of urinary or colonic drainage devices. Because the pelvic examination may involve exerting pressure on bowel or bladder structures, patients with neurogenic dysfunction should come to the physical examination after bowel and bladder have been evacuated to avoid embarrassing accidents and time-consuming clean-up (9). Even with this precaution, bowel and bladder accidents still may occur. To minimize inconvenience to the staff and assist in more expeditious disposal of soiled material, it is beneficial to place a water-resistant pad on the lower part of the table. This can be removed or changed during the examination as needed to keep the perineum clean.

To assist in appropriate positioning for the pelvic examination, placing a cloth sheet on the table under the woman will enable her to be moved down the table without requiring her physical assistance. (It may be easiest to do this before she transfers to the table.) Make sure to inform each woman when you need to reposition her, ask her permission to move her around, and let her know what you are planning to do before you do it. This is very important not only because it is respectful and sensitive to the woman's feelings, but also because it will prevent triggering spasticity in some patients. For women with rigid spasticity in their hip joints, discomfort may be intensified during positioning adjustments required for the physical examination. Small doses of anxiolytic or analgesic medication may be helpful in such patients, enabling them to tolerate the examination more successfully. Leg-adjusting movements may generate reflex spasticity. Quick and forceful movements on a spastic extremity can trigger increased rigidity and make it more difficult to adjust leg positioning. Gentle, slow movements of the patients' lower extremities are most effective.

Bootleg holders are ideal for positioning patients with weak legs (see Fig. 9-2) because they can eliminate the necessity for extra personnel to hold legs in position during the examination. Because these "boots" can be individually adjusted, they are especially helpful for women whose function and range of motion in one leg may differ from that of the other. Knee crutches (obstetric stirrups) may work well for some women, too. Disabilities where impaired leg control is often prominent include cerebral palsy, cerebral vascular accident (CVA), spinal cord injury, spina bifida, and multiple sclerosis.

The patient's positioning during the gynecologic exam depends on her particular physical limitations. Several positions have been found to work well for women with varying disabilities and levels of hip, knee, and back flexibility.

1. Diamond-shaped position. Knees set wide apart with the soles of the feet pressed together.

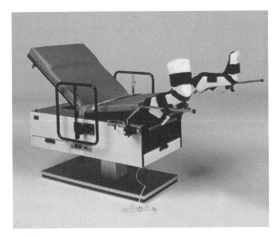

FIG. 9-2. Examination table with bootleg holders.

2. Knee-chest position. Legs bent and to one side, with the top knee drawn toward the patient's chest.
3. M-shaped position. Knees set wide apart with the soles of the feet pressed against the table.
4. V-shaped position. With knees straight, legs are held as far apart as possible.
5. OB stirrups position. Knees held in stirrups.[1]

Of course, variations may be necessary depending on the individual. The woman who is disabled and the health care practitioner should work together to discover what works.

In some of these positions, especially the V-shaped and diamond-shaped positions, the woman's pelvis may be tilted at an angle that makes it hard to visualize her cervix. Putting a rolled-up blanket or foam wedge under her buttocks may help, as may inserting the speculum upside down.

It is important to inspect the skin of women who use wheelchairs and/or have impaired circulation to check for skin breakdown or areas of redness. Inspection of the perineum should be especially meticulous, not only to identify skin breakdown but also to note the very common finding of perineal vulvovaginitis. Especially in women who use wheelchairs, excess buildup of moisture in the perineum is common. This can predispose to monilial vulvitis or vulvovaginitis. The woman's health clinician should perform a thorough examination, including inspection of the perineum, to uncover signs of abuse such as cigarette burns or cuts if they are present. Because some sexual abuse may not be apparent, it is important that all women be checked for sexually transmitted diseases. See Chapter 11.

Care should be taken to avoid discomfort during the examination. A cold speculum can trigger involuntary muscle movements even

---

[1]For further information, please refer to Ferreyra S, Hughes K. *Table manners*. San Francisco/Alameda: Planned Parenthood, 1982.

in able-bodied individuals; this reaction may be accentuated in women with neurologic or orthopedic disabilities. For nulliparous or elderly women, using a small speculum and applying lidocaine gel to the perineum may help reduce some of the pain felt when stretching the labia during speculum insertion while opening the blades. Because of the risk of autonomic dysreflexia, lidocaine gel also is recommended for examining women who are quadriplegic and have spinal cord injuries.

It may be necessary to examine women with certain disabilities in bed rather than in the ideal setting of a medical office. This may be the case for nursing home patients or women who are hospitalized for acute or chronic problems who develop gynecologic symptoms that need to be evaluated. The key to examining the patient in bed is to achieve as much elevation of the pelvis as possible to allow the clinician easy access to the perineum for insertion of the speculum. This is best achieved by making a thick blanket roll and threading it under the hips and buttocks of the patient. This arrangement is far more comfortable for the patient than the traditional upside-down bedpan. In these cases, because of the orientation of the pelvis in relation to the speculum, the cervix is best visualized with the speculum inverted. A number of positions are possible with the blanket roll elevation of the pelvis, including the diamond-shaped position (heels together, knees apart), the M-shaped position (knees on either end of the bed, feet touching sides of bed), and the V-shaped position (with both legs spread away from midline) (10). Modifications of these positions can be tried depending on the physical limitation of the individual patient.

When it is not possible to insert a speculum and specimens need to be obtained, the examiner can insert a gloved finger into the vagina, identify the cervical os, and introduce specimen-collection devices along the track of the pointing finger. Although accuracy of specimens collected in this way may not be ideal, sometimes it is the only way that these can be obtained.

SPECIAL CONCERNS FOR EXAMINATIONS OF WOMEN WITH COMMON DISABILITIES

Spinal Cord Injury

The main concerns in examining women with a spinal cord injury are the risks of triggering involuntary movements, excess spasticity, or even autonomic dysreflexia. Speculum selection usually is determined on the basis of parity; however, in women with certain types of spinal cord injury, such as cauda equina lesions, vaginal muscle tone may be so lax that a very large speculum will be needed to visualize the cervix (11). It has been noted that the application of lidocaine gel to insensate perineal structures can result in the reduction of spasticity through unknown neurologic pathways (12). This gel can be applied directly to the perineum as well as to the outer sides of the speculum blades. The pressure of the upper blades on the urinary tract system and lower blades on the lower bowel can result in the involuntary oozing of urine and feces during the speculum examination. Bowel and bladder emptying before the visit should minimize the likelihood of this occurrence.

In certain types of spinal cord injury, such as in women who have lesions that are above the splanchnic sympathetic nervous system chain (thoracic level 6–10), reaction to painful or uncomfortable stimuli may be translated into activation of the sympathetic nervous system (13). Patients usually will give a history that they have had symptoms of autonomic dysreflexia with urinary tract infections, fecal impaction, and other triggers, so that the staff will be alerted and prepared for this possibility. In such patients, digital rectal examination should be avoided because of the likelihood of triggering dysreflexia (9). Alternatively, cards that test for fecal occult blood can be given to the patient to take home.

For patients who have high spinal cord injuries, blood pressure monitoring throughout the examination will alert the staff to this impending complication. Reactions can vary from mild to severe and can be initiated by numerous sources, including the pelvic examination. A full bladder or constipation also could be triggers. Signs of this reaction include facial flushing; irregular heartbeat; shortness of breath; increased muscle spasticity; and, of greatest concern, labile hypertension to a severe degree. If this reaction develops during the pelvic examination, all procedures should stop, the speculum should be removed, clothing should be loosened, and the head of the table should be elevated. Rapid-acting, short duration antihypertensive medications such as nifedipine (Procardia) at a recommended dosage of 10 mg can be administered sublingually or chewed and swallowed (14). It will be helpful to have a physiatrist or anesthesiologist on hand for patients who have a history of developing autonomic dysreflexia. For further information on autonomic dysreflexia see Chapter 15.

Many women with spinal cord injury have the combination of difficulty with perineal care, excessive moisture in the perineal region as a result of bladder leaking and/or positioning, and reduced perineal sensation. For this reason, it is especially important to check them for skin breakdown and/or infections.

Be aware that in patients who are quadriplegic, impaired hand function may make breast self-examination difficult or impossible. Therefore, clinical breast examination and/or training companions or personal care attendants to do breast exams is key for these patients.

Spina Bifida

Women with spina bifida usually have health issues regarding perineal care. An especially careful examination of the perineum will help find areas of skin breakdown or infection. Most women with spina bifida have neurogenic bowel and bladder. As in women with spinal cord injury, it may be helpful to ask these patients to empty their bladder and bowels before performing the examination.

Be aware that many women with spina bifida have latex allergies. Latex gloves therefore should not be used to examine these pa-

tients (15). There have been case reports of anaphylactic shock in women with spina bifida after exposure to latex products. Fortunately, safe alternatives exist. Plastic or polyurethane examination gloves should be kept on hand for examining all women with spina bifida as well as any woman with known or suspected latex allergy.

Occasionally, surgical diversion devices or scarring from procedures to manage bowel and bladder incontinence will be palpated in the abdomen (16) or apex of the vaginal vault (17) during the bimanual examination. To clarify these issues, it might be helpful to communicate with the urologist so as to better interpret these physical findings. Because some women with spina bifida have absent pelvic sensation and leg control, perineal care and lower-extremity positioning issues may need to be taken into consideration.

Cerebral Palsy

Physical examination of women with cerebral palsy is made most challenging because of the presence of excess spasticity and joint contractures. It is not uncommon for lower-extremity joints to be rigidly flexed (spastic paraplegia). Women with this type of cerebral palsy usually are wheelchair users, and issues pertaining to perineal care are similar to those previously discussed. Because of the rigid spasticity often seen within these patients, alternative examination positions that will accommodate totally flexed lower extremities are most effective. Examples of these include variations of the knee–chest position (with knees up or to the side) or side-lying knee–chest with one knee abducted.

You will need to enlist the help of each patient in finding an examination position that will work given her particular limitations. To avoid excess spasticity during positioning, all adjustments should be made very slowly, giving the woman adequate warning before moving her.

Hand function is impaired in many women with cerebral palsy. If a woman's breast self-examination capabilities are limited, clinical breast examination is especially important.

Poliomyelitis

Women with poliomyelitis present unique issues during the physical examination. In addition to fatigue, which is a prominent feature of those with polio, muscle weakness and atrophy are also common findings (18). Pain may occur, usually associated with joint contractures resultant from disuse (19). All these physical sequelae of the postpolio syndrome need to be taken into account when performing physical examination on such patients. Because of weakness, patients may need assistance transferring onto an examination table. They may need to be assisted to sit upright for the examination of the upper body including auscultation of heart and lungs. Elevating backrests on the examination table can facilitate this process. Pulmonary function is a significant concern in some of these patients because weakness can affect diaphragmatic muscles and increase the risk for respiratory infections.

Because hand function may be affected in some women with postpolio syndrome, breast self-examination capabilities may be limited, in which case clinical breast examination is especially critical. Because shoulder contractures may be present, creative positioning may be required to palpate the axillary region during the clinical breast examination to ensure thorough assessment and to minimize discomfort.

Patients may not be able to voluntarily position extremities into stirrups or hold them in place for the pelvic examination. A number of factors can contribute to this, including weakness and limited range of motion because of contractures. As a result, the patient may need to be assisted and positioned on the examination table. It is important to recognize that although there may be significant mobility restrictions, patients with postpolio syndrome have completely intact pelvic sensation. Care should be taken to minimize discomfort during speculum insertion and bimanual examination.

Multiple Sclerosis

Multiple sclerosis is a neurologic disorder that has variable manifestations. The affected parts of the body are not consistent from one woman to another and may vary in the same woman over time.

In some women, range of motion in upper extremities may be affected, compromising breast care. Special attention to clinical breast examinations should be considered.

In wheelchair users, issues pertaining to perineal care are similar to those affecting women with other impairments. Pain, excess muscle tone, spasticity, and balance problems of neurologic origin are common in these patients (20). This may affect the woman's ability to transfer to the table or position her legs and hold them in place during the pelvic examination.

Some of these patients have difficulty with bowel and bladder control and should be counseled on addressing these issues prior to their visit. Although pelvic sensation may be affected in some women with multiple sclerosis, in others this is intact even when incontinence is present. Minimizing discomfort during the pelvic examination is important to decrease the likelihood of triggering increased spasticity (21).

Cerebral Vascular Accident

Women with CVA frequently have many other medical problems. The added burden of decreased physical functioning often will result in less frequent visits to the woman's health care provider for gynecologic evaluation. Certainly any time preventive health care is neglected, complications such as malignancies can progress to a much more advanced stage than they otherwise would.

Those who have experienced a CVA that left them with significant physical limitations are likely to avoid routine women's health screening, unless or until pain or bleeding develops. Involvement of the multidisciplinary team of neurologists, physiatrists, cardiologists, internists, and the like should give a number of different practitioners the opportunity to recognize the need for this important health assessment and provide referrals and encouragement.

Rheumatoid Arthritis/Osteoarthritis

Arthritic conditions are extremely common. Some are of autoimmune origin, such as rheumatoid arthritis, and others result from age-related degenerative conditions. Rheumatologic and arthritic disorders manifest as muscle aches, joint pain, and restrictions in range of motion (see also Chapter 6). Often, there is a permanent destruction of cartilage and joints with resulting chronic arthritic pain and stiffness.

The physical examination for women with rheumatologic and arthritic conditions is achieved most easily using a low examination table with supportive boots. Because range of motion in upper extremities may be compromised, breast self-examination is an issue for focused attention. Limitations in knee flexion and hip abduction may make it difficult for the woman to position her legs for the pelvic examination. Unlike woman with spasticity, the main limitations in these patients are joint pain, stiffness, and restricted movements. Therefore, the examination position for each patient may need to be individualized depending on her specific areas of discomfort.

It might be helpful for patients with arthritis to take nonsteroidal antiinflammatory agents prior to the examination, if this has been cleared with the rheumatologist or other provider. In women with acute hip or pelvic fractures, it is preferable when possible to defer the pelvic examination until the acute pain has diminished and healing is progressing. If the severity of the gynecologic problem does not permit this, the intact hip and knee joints may be flexed and abducted while stabilizing the painful joints. In this way, access to the pelvis may be achieved without excessive discomfort.

Developmental Disabilities

Women who are cognitively impaired may require special interventions for health main-

tenance (9). Pictures of the female anatomy and doll models can help inform these women about their needs.

Deafness

Women with hearing impairments need to be approached when the practitioner is ready for them because they may not be able to hear their name being called. Sign language interpreters should be available to assist in the sharing of medical information between patient and practitioner (8). Practitioners should remember to address their questions and comments to the patient rather than her interpreter and to maintain as much visual contact as possible throughout the examination. It is *extremely* preferable that the interpreter not be a family member because medical information may not be shared as freely when relatives are involved in the exchange. For more information about working with patients who are deaf or hearing impaired, see Chapter 5.

REFERENCES

1. Fiduccia BW, ed. *Multiplying choices: improving access to reproductive health services for women with disabilities.* Oakland: Berkeley Planning Associates, 1997.
2. Thomas DC. Primary care for people with disabilities. *Mount Sinai J Med* 1999;66:188–191.
3. Nosek M. The John Stanley Coulter lecture. Overcoming the odds: the healthcare of women with physical disabilities in the United States. *Arch Phys Med Rehabil* 2000;81(2):135–138.
4. Veltman A, Stewart DE, Gaétan S, et al. Perceptions of primary healthcare services among people with physical disabilities—Part 1: Access Issues MedGenMed, April 6, 2001. Full text available on-line through Entrez-PubMed.
5. Welner S. Screening issues in gynecologic malignancies for women with disabilities: critical considerations. *J Women's Health* 1998;7:281–285.
6. Faye E. Living with low vision: what you can do to help patients cope. *Postgrad Med* 1998;103:167–170, 175–178.
7. Weber RD. Hearing impaired patients: legal obligation to treat and pay for interpreters. *Mich Med* 1999;98:10.
8. American College of Obstetricians and Gynecologists. Primary care review for the obstetrician-gynecologist: primary and preventive care. Washington, DC: ACOG, 1997.
9. Welner SL, Foley CC, Nosek MA, et al. Practical considerations in the performance of physical examinations on women with disabilities. *Obstet Gynecol Surv* 1999; 54(7):457–462.

10. Ferreyra S, Hughes K. *Table manners*. San Francisco/Alameda: Planned Parenthood, 1982.
11. Light JK, Beric A, Petronic I. Detrusor function with lesions of the cauda equina with special emphasis on the bladder neck. *J Urol* 1993;17:24–28.
12. Colachis SC 3d. Autonomic hyperreflexia with spinal cord injury. *J Am Paraplegia Soc* 1992;15:171–186.
13. Welner SL. STIs in women with disabilities: diagnosis, treatment, and prevention: a review. *J Sexually Transmitted Diseases* May 2000:272–277.
14. Donaldson J. Neurologic emergencies in pregnancy. *Obstet Gynecol Clin North Am* 1991;18:199–212.
15. Niggemann B, Buck D, Michael T, et al. Latex allergy in spina bifida: at the turning point? *J Allergy Clin Immunol* 2000 Dec;106(6):1201.
16. Christiansen J. Advances in the surgical management of anal incontinence. *Baillieres Clin Gastroentrol* 1992;6:43–57.
17. Mann WJ, Jones DE. Pregnancy complicated by maternal neural tube defect and an ileal conduit: a case report. *J Reprod Med* 1976;17:339–341.
18. Grimby G, Jonsson AL. Disability in poliomyelitis sequelae. *Phys Ther* 1994;74(5):415–424.
19. Shah A, Asirvatham R. Hypertension after surgical release for flexion contractures of the knee. *J Bone Joint Surg Br* 1994;76(2):274–277.
20. Goodin DS. Survey of multiple sclerosis in northern California. Northern California MS Study Group. *Mult Scler* 1999;5(2):78–88.
21. Hulter BM, Lundberg PO. Sexual function in women with advanced multiple sclerosis. *J Neurol Neurosurg Psychiatry* 1995;59(1):83–86.

10

Contraceptive Choices for Women with Disabilities

Eleanor A. Drey and Philip D. Darney

Half of all pregnancies in the United States are unintended or mistimed, and about half of these end in abortion (1). If an unintended pregnancy poses a health risk and potential personal crisis in the life of any woman, pregnancy's dangers and difficulties can be more extreme for a woman with disabilities. All too often, women with disabilities or chronic medical conditions are not offered adequate contraceptive counseling as part of their routine preventive health care. This delay in the start of a contraceptive method until a pelvic exam can be performed may place a woman at unnecessary risk of unintended pregnancy (2,3). Women with disabilities who confront barriers to access should be prescribed hormonal contraception while arrangements are made for later examination.

METHODS AND THEIR SPECIAL CONSIDERATIONS

Although women with disabilities face special challenges, many of the initial approaches to contraceptive counseling remain the same as for patients who are not disabled. We will review counseling considerations that are relevant for the most commonly available methods, highlighting those related to disabilities before discussing each disability individually (see also refs. 4 nd 5). Contraceptive failure rates in the first year are summarized in Table 10-1. For any method that requires consistent use, the failure rate, or probability of pregnancy, is higher with typical than perfect use and often is highest in the first year. Using two methods at once can lower the risk of pregnancy still further.

METHOD BY METHOD

Hormonal Contraception

Oral Contraceptive Pills

The most effective oral contraceptive pills combine estrogen to control bleeding and a progestin to inhibit ovulation. In general, oral contraceptives are well tolerated, have low failure rates in compliant patients, and have numerous noncontraceptive benefits (Table 10-1). In women with disabilities, most medical concerns about combined oral contraception (COC) focus on the estrogen component of the pill. Many of the original precautions were based on risks observed with pills containing 50–100 µg of ethinyl estradiol or mestranol; however, risks are greatly reduced or eliminated with lower dose formulations. Other hormonal delivery methods with similar mechanisms and medical considerations include the vaginal ring (Nuvaring), the contraceptive patch (Ortho Evra), and the once-monthly combined injectable (Lunelle).

The increased risk of venous thromboembolism (VTE) remains the greatest concern; the World Health Organization (WHO) found a threefold to fourfold increased risk associated with even low-dose COCs (6,7). Because of these concerns, women with disabilities already thought to have an increased risk of VTE generally are encouraged either to avoid COC use altogether or to use progestin-only methods, reserving COCs if the benefits of use are evaluated by the practitioner to outweigh the VTE risks (Table 10-2).

TABLE 10-1. *Failure rates, noncontraceptive benefits, dangers, and side effects of the most frequently used contraceptive methods*

Method	Lowest expected (typical) failure rates during the first year of use	Noncontraceptive benefits	Adverse effects	Side effects
Combined pill (similar considerations in other delivery methods, such as the patch, ring, and combined E2/MPA injectable)	0.1 (7.6)%	Decreases menstrual blood loss, pain, cycle irregularities, and PMS. Protects against PID requiring hospitalization, some cancers (ovarian, endometrial, possibly colon), some benign tumors (leiomyomata, benign breast masses, and fibrocystic disease), and possibly ovarian cysts. Decreases iron-deficiency anemia. Reduces acne and hirsutism. Protects against loss of bone mass. Decreases ectopic pregnancy incidence.	Cardiovascular complications (stroke, heart attack, blood clots, high blood pressure), depression, hepatic adenomas, possible increased risk of breast and cervical cancers.	Nausea, breast tenderness, headaches, dizziness, spotting, chloasma
Progestin-only pill	0.5 (somewhat higher than combined oral contraceptives)	Decreases menstrual blood loss, pain, and PMS. Decreased breast tenderness.	May fail if taken even 3 hr late.	Breakthrough bleeding with no overall change in average . menstrual blood loss, acne, functional ovarian follicular cysts
Emergency contraception pills	Less than 2% per act of intercourse, or 75% decreased risk	None known	None known for progestin-only regimen	Nausea, vomiting, delayed menses
IUD—levonorgestrel (Mirena)	0.1 (0.1)	Dramatically decreases menstrual blood loss (about 90%) and pain	PID following insertion, uterine perforation	Initial irregular bleeding or spotting, abdominal pain or cramping, back pain, breast tenderness, headache, mood changes, nausea
IUD—copper T 380A	0.6 (0.8)	None known	PID following insertion, uterine perforation, anemia	Menstrual cramping, spotting, increased bleeding
Implant	0.05 (0.2)	May decrease menstrual cramps, pain, and blood loss	Infection at implant site, complicated removals, depression	Irregular menstrual bleeding, more frequent follicular cysts, infrequent weight gain, mood changes and headache, tenderness at site, hair loss, weight gain
Combined injectable (Lunelle)	0.1 (0.2)	See combined pill benefits (supposition based on insufficient data)	See combined pill dangers (supposition based on insufficient data)	See combined pill side effects

Method	Failure rate (perfect [typical])	Noncontraceptive benefits	Risks	Disadvantages
Progestin-only injectable (Depo-Provera, or DMPA)	0.3 (3.1)	Decreased frequency of seizures in women with epilepsy, decreased frequency of sickle cell crises, decreased endometrial cancer, increased volume of breast milk in lactating women	Allergic reactions, pathologic weight gain, decreased bone mineral density, possible depression	Irregular menstrual bleeding, including prolonged or frequent bleeding; weight gain; headaches; adverse effects on lipids
Female sterilization	0.05 (0.05)	Reduces risk of ovarian cancer and may protect against PID	Infection; anesthetic complications; if pregnancy occurs afterwards, high risk it will be ectopic	Pain at surgical site, psychologic reactions, subsequent regret that the procedure was performed
Male sterilization	0.1 (0.15)	None known	Infection; anesthetic complications	Pain at surgical site, psychologic reactions, regret
Barriers: diaphragm, cap, sponge	Diaphragm + spermicides 6.0 (12.1) Cervical cap 9.0–20 (20–40)	Provides modest protection against some STDs	Vaginal and urinary tract infections, toxic shock syndrome	Pelvic pressure, vaginal irritation, vaginal discharge if left in too long, allergy
Male condom	3.0 (13.9)	Protects against STDs, including HIV; delays premature ejaculation	Anaphylactic reaction to latex	Decreased sensation, allergy to latex, loss of spontaneity
Female condom	5.0 (21.0)	Protects against STDs	None known	Aesthetically unappealing and awkward to use for some
Spermicides	6.0 (25.7)	Provides modest protection against some STDs	Vaginal and urinary tract infections	Vaginal irritation, allergy
Abstinence	—	Prevents infections, including HIV	None known	Psychologic effects
Lactational amenorrhea method (LAM)	0.5–1.5 (perfect use for 6 mo)	Provides excellent nutrition for infants younger than 6 mo old	Increased risk of HIV transmission to infant if mother is HIV+	Mastitis from staphylococcal infection

DMPA, depot medroxyprogesterone acetate; HIV, human immunodeficiency virus; IUD, intrauterine device; MPA, medroxyprogesterone acetate; PID, pelvic inflammatory disease; PMS, premenstrual syndrome; STD, sexually transmitted disease.

(From Hatcher RA, Trussell J, Stewart F, et al. *Contraceptive technology.* New York: Ardent Media, 1998:216–235, with permission.)

TABLE 10-2. *World Health Organization medical eligibility criteria for starting contraceptive methods*

WHO categories for temporary methods:
WHO I **Can use** the method. No restriction on use.
WHO 2 **Can use** the method. Advantages generally outweigh theoretic or proven risks. Careful follow-up may be required.
WHO 3 **Should not use** the method unless clinician makes clinical judgment that the patient can safely use it. **Theoretic or proven risks usually outweigh the advantages** of method. Severity of the condition and availability, practicality, and acceptability of alternative methods should be considered. Method of last choice, with careful follow-up required.
WHO 4 **Should not use** the method. Condition represents an unacceptable health risk if method is used.

The four categories can be simplified into two categories:

WHO category	With clinical judgment	With limited clinical judgment
1	Use the method in any circumstances	Use the method
2	Generally use the method	
3	Use of the method not usually recommended unless other, more appropriate methods are not available or acceptable	Do not use the method
4	Method not to be used	

Boxes that are divided refer to initiation, followed by continuation. For example, initiating an IUD in a woman with endometrial cancer is category 4, whereas continuing it is category 2.

	COC	Comb. inject.	POP	DMPA NET-EN	LNG implants	Cu-IUD	LNG-IUD
PERSONAL CHARACTERISTICS AND REPRODUCTIVE HISTORY							
Pregnancy	NA	NA	NA	NA	NA	4	4
Age	<40 = 1	<40 = 1	<18 = 1	<18 = 2	<18 = 1	<20 = 2	<20 = 2
	>40 = 2	>40 = 2	18–45 = 1	18–45 = 1	18–45 = 1	>20 = 1	>20 = 1
			>45 = 1	>45 = 2	>45 = 1		
Parity							
Nulliparous	1	1	1	1	1	2	2
Parous	1	1	1	1	1	1	1
BREASTFEEDING							
<6 wk postpartum	4	4	3	3	3		
6 wk to <6 mo (primarily breastfeeding)	3	3	1	1	1		
>6 mo postpartum	2	2	1	1	1		
Postpartum (not breastfeeding)							
<21 d	3	3	1	1	1		
>21 d	1	1	1	1	1		
Postpartum (breastfeeding or not, including postcesarean section)							
<48 hr						2	3
>48 hr to <4 wk						3	3
>4 wk						1	1a
Puerperal sepsis						4	4

TABLE 10-2. *(Continued)*

	COC	Comb. inject.	POP	DMPA NET-EN	LNG implants	Cu-IUD	LNG-IUD
POSTABORTION							
First trimester	1	1	1	1	1	1	1
Second trimester	1	1	1	1	1	2	2
Immediate postseptic abortion	1	1	1	1	1	4	4
Past ectopic pregnancy	1	1	2	1	1	1	1
Past pelvic surgery (including cesarean section)	1	1	1	1	1	1	1
Smoking							
Age <35	2	2	1	1	1	1	1
Age >35							
<15 cigarettes/d	3	2	1	1	1	1	1
>15 cigarettes/d	4	3	1	1	1	1	1
Obesity>30 kg/m^2 BMI	2	2	1	2	2	1	2
ANATOMIC ABNORMALITY							
Distorts uterine cavity						4	4
Does not distort uterine cavity						2	2
Blood pressure unmeasured	NA	NA	NA	NA	NA	NA	NA
CARDIOVASCULAR DISEASE							
Multiple risk factors for CAD (e.g., older age, smoking, diabetes, HTN)	3 or 4	3 or 4	2	3	2	1	2
HYPERTENSION							
History of hypertension where blood pressure CANNOT be evaluated	3	3	2	2	2	1	2
Adequately controlled hypertension, where blood pressure CAN be evaluated	3	3	1	2	1	1	1

TABLE 10-2. *(Continued)*

	COC	Comb. inject.	POP	DMPA NET-EN	LNG implants	Cu-IUD	LNG-IUD
Systolic 140–159 or diastolic 90–99	3	3	1	2	1	1	1
Systolic >160 or diastolic >100	4	4	2	3	2	1	2
Vascular disease	4	4	2	3	2	1	2
History of high BP in pregnancy (where current BP is measurable and normal)	2	2	1	1	1	1	1
Deep venous thrombosis/Pulmonary embolism							
History of DVT/PE	4	4	2	2	2	1	2
Current DVT/PE	4	4	3	3	3	1	3
Family history (first-degree relatives)	2	2	1	1	1	1	1
MAJOR SURGERY							
With prolonged immobilization	4	4	2	2	2	1	2
Without prolonged immobilization	2	2	1	1	1	1	1
Minor surgery without immobilization	1	1	1	1	1	1	1
SUPERFICIAL VENOUS THROMBOSIS							
Varicose veins	1	1	1	1	1	1	1
Superficial thrombophlebitis	2	2	1	1	1	1	1
Ischemic heart disease current and past	4	4	2 / 3	3	2 / 3	1	2 / 3
Stroke (history of cerebrovascular accident)	4	4	2 / 3	3	2 / 3	1	2
Known hyperlipidemia	2 or 3 (b)	2 or 3 (b)	2	2	2	1	2
VASCULAR HEART DISEASE							
Uncomplicated	2	2	1	1	1	1	1
Complicated (pulmonary hypertension, atrial fibrillation, h/o SBE)	4	4	1	1	1	2	2

TABLE 10-2. *(Continued)*

	COC		Comb. inject.		POP		DMPA NET-EN		LNG implants		Cu-IUD		LNG-IUD	
NEUROLOGIC CONDITIONS														
Headaches														
Nonmigrainous (mild or severe)	1	2	1	2	1	1	1	1	1	1	1		1	1
Migraine without focal neurologic symptoms														
Age <35	2	3	2	3	1	2	2	2	2	2	1		2	2
Age >35	3	4	3	4	1	2	2	2	2	2	1		2	2
Migraine with focal symptoms (at any age)	4	4	4	4	2	3	2	3	2	3	1		2	3
Epilepsy	1		1		1		1		1		1		1	
REPRODUCTIVE TRACT INFECTIONS AND DISORDERS														
Benign ovarian tumors (including cysts)	1		1		1		1		1		1		1	
VAGINAL BLEEDING PATTERNS														
Irregular pattern without heavy bleeding	1		1		2		2		2		1		1	2
Prolonged or heavy bleeding (regular or irregular)	1		1		2		2		2		2		1	2
UNEXPLAINED VAGINAL BLEEDING														
Before evaluation	2		2		2		3		3		4	2	4	2
Endometriosis	1		1		1		1		1		2		1	
Severe menstrual cramps	1		1		1		1		1		2		1	
TROPHOBLASTIC DISEASE														
Benign gestational trophoblastic disease	1		1		1		1		1		3		3	
Malignant gestational trophoblastic disease	1		1		1		1		1		4		4	
Cervical ectropion	1		1		1		1		1		1		1	
Cervical intraepithelial neoplasia	2		2		1		2		2		1		2	

TABLE 10-2. *(Continued)*

	COC	Comb. inject.	POP	DMPA NET-EN	LNG implants	Cu-IUD		LNG-IUD	
Cervical cancer (awaiting treatment)	2	2	1	2	2	4	2	4	2
BREAST DISEASE									
Undiagnosed mass	2	2	2	2	2	1		2	
Benign breast disease	1	1	1	1	1	1		1	
Family history of breast cancer	1	1	1	1	1	1		1	
Current breast cancer	4	4	4	4	4	1		4	
Past breast cancer and no evidence of current disease for 5 yr	3	3	3	3	3	1		3	
Endometrial cancer	1	1	1	1	1	4	2	4	2
Ovarian cancer	1	1	1	1	1	3	2	3	2
UTERINE FIBROIDS									
Without distortion of uterine cavity	1	1	1	1	1	2		2	
With distortion of uterine cavity	1	1	1	1	1	4		4	
Pelvic inflammatory disease									
Past PID (assuming no current risk factors of STDs)									
With subsequent pregnancy	1	1	1	1	1	1	1	1	1
Without subsequent pregnancy	1	1	1	1	1	2	2	2	2
PID—current or within last 3 mo	1	1	1	1	1	4	3	4	3
SEXUALLY TRANSMITTED DISEASES									
Current or within 3 mo (incl. purulent cervicitis)	1	1	1	1	1	4		4	
Vaginitis without purulent cervicitis	1	1	1	1	1	2		2	

TABLE 10-2. *(Continued)*

	COC	Comb. inject.	POP	DMPA NET-EN	LNG implants	Cu-IUD	LNG-IUD
Increased risk of STDs (e.g., multiple partners or partner with multiple partners)	1	1	1	1	1	3	3
HIV/AIDS							
High-risk of HIV	1	1	1	1	1	3	3
HIV-positive	1	1	1	1	1	3	3
AIDS	1	1	1	1	1	3	3
OTHER INFECTIONS							
Schistosomiasis							
Uncomplicated	1	1	1	1	1	1	1
Fibrosis of the liver	1	1	1	1	1	1	1
Tuberculosis							
Nonpelvic	1	1	1	1	1	1	1
Known pelvic	1	1	1	1	1	4 3	4 3
Malaria	1	1	1	1	1	1	1
ENDOCRINE CONDITIONS							
Diabetes							
History of gestational disease	1	1	1	1	1	1	1
Nonvascular disease							
Noninsulin dependent	2	2	2	2	2	1	2
Insulin dependent	2	2	2	2	2	1	2
Nephropathy/ retinopathy/ neuropathy	3 or 4	3 or 4	2	3	2	1	2
Other vascular disease or diabetes of >20 yr duration	3 or 4	3 or 4	2	3	2	1	2
Thyroid							
Simple goiter	1	1	1	1	1	1	1
Hyperthyroid	1	1	1	1	1	1	1
Hypothyroid	1	1	1	1	1	1	1

TABLE 10-2. *(Continued)*

	COC	Comb. inject.	POP	DMPA NET-EN	LNG implants	Cu-IUD	LNG-IUD
GASTROINTESTINAL CONDITIONS							
Gallbladder disease							
Symptomatic							
Treated by cholecystectomy	2	2	2	2	2	1	2
Medically treated	3	2	2	2	2	1	2
Current	3	2	2	2	2	1	2
Asymptomatic	2	2	2	2	2	1	2
Past COC-related	3	2	2	2	2	1	2
HISTORY OF CHOLESTASIS							
Pregnancy-related	2	2	1	1	1	1	1
VIRAL HEPATITIS							
Active	4	3 or 4	3	3	3	1	3
Carrier	1	1	1	1	1	1	1
CIRRHOSIS							
Mild (compensated)	3	2	2	2	2	1	2
Severe (decompensated)	4	3	3	3	3	1	3
LIVER TUMORS							
Benign (adenoma)	4	3	3	3	3	1	3
Malignant (hepatoma)	4	3 or 4	3	3	3	1	3
ANEMIAS							
Thalassemia	1	1	1	1	1	2	1
Sickle cell disease	2	2	1	1	1	2	1
Iron-deficiency anemia	1	1	1	1	1	2	1
DRUG INTERACTIONS							
Commonly used drugs that affect liver enzymes							
Certain antibiotics (rifampin and griseofulvin)	3	3	3	2	3	1	1
Certain anticonvulsants (phenytoin, carbamazepine, barbiturates, primidone)	3	3	3	2	3	1	1

TABLE 10-2. *(Continued)*

	COC	Comb. inject.	POP	DMPA NET-EN	LNG implants	Cu-IUD	LNG-IUD
Other antibiotics (excluding rifampin and griseofulvin)	1	1	1	1	1	1	1

AIDS, acquired immunodeficiency syndrome; BMI, body mass index; BP, blood pressure; CAD, coronary artery disease; COC, combined oral contraception; Comb. inject., combined injectable; Cu, copper; DMPA, depot-medroxyprogesterone acetate; DVT, deep venous thrombosis; HIV, human immunodeficiency virus; h/o, history of; HTN, hypertension; IUD, intrauterine device; LNG, levonorgestrel; NA, not applicable; PE, pulmonary embolism; PID, pelvic inflammatory disease; POP, progestin-only pills; SBE, subacute bacterial endocarditis; STD, sexually transmitted disease; WHO, World Health Organization.

Notes

A If the woman is breastfeeding, the LNG-IUD becomes a category 3 until 6 wk postpartum.

B Depending on severity of disease.

C Barrier methods, especially condoms, always are recommended for prevention of STD/HIV/PID.

Adapted from WHO Medical Eligibility Criteria, 2001 (87).

COCs provide numerous noncontraceptive health benefits that can be useful in patient management (Table 10-1). For example, continuous administration of COCs may be useful in women for whom menses may cause problems, such as with dysmenorrhea, hygiene, or menstrually related seizures or migraines. COCs are marketed as Seasonale™, specifically for prolonged use, providing four pill-free intervals a year.

Other pill packs can be used the same way. The primary disadvantage is intermenstrual bleeding.

Progestin-only contraceptive pills (POPs) prevent conception by combining several mechanisms, including suppressing ovulation in some cycles, thickening cervical mucus, and altering the endometrium and tubal ciliary function. POPs must be taken at the same time each day because the hormone usually is eliminated within 24 hours, with their protection diminishing after 20 hours. As a result POPs have higher typical failure rates than COCs. POPs do not appear to be associated with an increased risk of VTE (8). Most women with disabilities can use POPs (Table 10-2). Anticipatory guidance about the frequent side effect of scant, irregular bleeding can decrease concern and dissatisfaction with the method.

Combined Injectables

The most widely available, monthly injectable combination of estrogen and progestin contains 25 mg of depot-medroxyprogesterone acetate (DMPA; Depo-Provera) and 5 mg of estradiol cypionate (Lunelle). Although as effective as Depo-Provera, because of the inclusion of estrogen, it is associated with less menstrual irregularity or amenorrhea (9–13). Generally, combined injectables have the same medical considerations as COCs. The peak levels of estradiol are lower than the midcycle preovulatory surge. These physiologic levels are unlikely to cause cardiovascular side effects. However, because of the estrogen, combined injectables are relatively contraindicated in women with a personal or close family history of idiopathic VTE.

Depot-Medroxyprogesterone Acetate

DMPA is administered as 150 mg of microcrystals intended to be injected in the gluteal or deltoid muscle every 3 months. Because it is not a "sustained-release" system, its mechanism relies on high serum levels of progestins to attain its contraceptive effects (inhibiting ovulation, thickening the cervical mucus, and altering the endometrium). The most common problem is the change in menstrual bleeding, which decreases progressively with reinjection, progressing to amenorrhea after 5 years in 80% of users (14). Other common problems are breast tenderness and weight gain in some patients. The significance of bone density loss seen in some DMPA studies is uncertain because the evidence is mixed; however, it appears unlikely that permanent bone loss occurs sufficiently to increase osteoporosis later in life for most patients (15). Evidence linking DMPA to depression also is mixed (16,17). DMPA's noncontraceptive benefits that are useful in women with disabilities include causing amenorrhea, raising the seizure threshold, and decreasing the frequency of sickle cell crises.

Subdermal Implants

Subdermal implants provide long-acting, reversible, and extremely effective contraception with sustained release of low-dose progestins. They include Norplant, Jadelle, and Implanon. Implants prevent conception by suppressing ovulation and thickening cervical mucus (18). Implant contraceptives have few absolute contraindications—only active thrombophlebitis or thromboembolic disease and acute liver disease (Table 10-2). A controlled cohort study including 78,323 women-years of observation showed no significant excess risk of serious morbidity in Norplant users with two exceptions: increased incidence of gallbladder disease (rate ratio, or RR, 1.52; 95% confidence interval, or CI, 1.02, 2.27) and hypertension and borderline hypertension (RR 1.81, 95% CI 1.12, 2.92) (19).

Intrauterine Contraceptive Devices

The two types of intrauterine contraceptive devices (IUCDs or IUDs) have distinct advantages and disadvantages. Given their unparalleled ease of use, high efficacy, and strong user satisfaction, IUDs are remarkably underused in the United States. IUDs are recommended for women in monogamous relationships or who consistently use condoms for protection against sexually transmitted diseases (STDs), including human immunodeficiency virus (HIV). Because of the cost, most providers prefer IUD users to be interested in at least 2 years of contraception.

By producing a spermicidal intrauterine environment, the copper-containing IUD (CuT 380A) provides excellent contraception for at least 10 years. However, it is not recommended for women with menorrhagia, anemia, or dysmenorrhea because on average, users have more menstrual blood loss and cramps. The copper IUD has few other medical contraindications: principally, concerns about a possible increased failure or pelvic inflammatory disease rate (PID) in the immunosuppressed (20) and the rare concern of Wilson's disease or a copper allergy.

The levonorgestrel intrauterine device (LNG IUD) system relies on local hormonal effects to thin the endometrial lining and thicken the cervical mucus. It is the most effective form of contraception currently available; it is even more effective than sterilization. The LNG IUD (marketed as Mirena) offers at least 7 years of protection and has noncontraceptive health benefits that may be especially helpful in women with disabilities. Unlike the copper IUD, LNG IUD users have markedly less menstrual flow and cramps. After an initial 3–6 months of increased number of days of bleeding and spotting (although with a decreased average overall blood loss) (21,22), most women become amenorrheic or have only minimal bleeding 1–2 days each month. This can be a boon for women with anemia (such as anemia of chronic disease or sickle cell disease) or menorrhagia or women with menstrual hygiene difficulties. This IUD is an effective treatment for menorrhagia and dysmenorrhea (23). Because one of the contraceptive actions of LNG is that it makes cervical mucus more viscous, the LNG IUD may decrease the risk of STDs (24, 25). Because it is a progestin-only method with local action and relatively limited systemic effects, it may be appropriate for women in whom estrogen-containing methods are contraindicated or less effective, such as COCs for women with epilepsy or women with cardiovascular or thrombogenic risks.

Female Sterilization

Female sterilization, most commonly tubal ligation either by minilaparotomy or laparoscopy, provides highly effective permanent contraception with few contraindications. Special considerations in women with disabilities include anesthesia risks and issues of informed consent. Successful reversal is uncommon, and other reversible forms of contraception are equally effective. Therefore, thorough counseling is critical to help patients avoid regret.

Male Sterilization

All too often vasectomy is not discussed when counseling women with disabilities, although it may be the best choice for a couple desiring no more children. Vasectomy is notable for having a lower failure rate, lower costs, and fewer complications than female sterilization. It requires only local anesthesia and has few risks. For example, there is no evidence that vasectomy is associated with heart or prostate disease. The main concern is post-procedure regret. For example, the partner of a woman who is chronically ill with a poor long-term prognosis may want to consider the possibility of outliving his partner before choosing this method. Success in reversing vasectomy is related to the length of time since the operation—the sooner reanastomosis is attempted, the greater the chance of reestablishing fertility.

Barrier Methods

Condoms, Diaphragms, and Cervical Caps

Barrier methods prevent conception by physically preventing sperm from entering the uterus. They provide approximately a 50% reduction in STDs and PID (26–28), but only the condom has been proven to prevent HIV infection. Barrier methods rarely are associated with even minor side effects (usually allergies); however, couples must use them consistently and correctly to achieve acceptable efficacy.

Spermicides

Spermicides are chemical barriers made of two components: a spermicidal chemical and a delivery base. They can be used alone or with another contraceptive method. Efficacy varies greatly. Although they provide some protection against infection, condoms are a more effective form of infection prevention if that is the primary objective of the user. Spermicides have no serious side effects or problems, with allergy being the only rare, minor problem.

Emergency Contraception

Any woman whose primary contraceptive method requires compliance should be educated about and have ready access to emergency contraception methods that can prevent conception *after* intercourse. The most commonly used method is hormonal (also called postcoital contraception or the "morning after" pill), which consists of either two doses of COCs or of levonorgestrel (LNG). In either regimen, the first dose is to be taken as soon as possible and ideally within 72 hours after unprotected intercourse, with the second dose taken 12 hours later. Some studies suggest continued effectiveness of this method up to 5 days and that one dose is nearly as effective as two (29). Mifepristone (10 mg) also may be used as emergency contraception up to 5 days after intercourse. The copper-containing IUD may be used as an emergency contraceptive with even greater effectiveness than oral methods up to 5 days after unprotected intercourse.

Hormonal emergency contraception has no significant medical contraindications, with WHO concluding that there are no contraindications to either COC or LNG-only emergency contraception pills, and the American College of Obstetricians and Gynecologists advising that progestin-only methods are preferable in women with a history of idiopathic thrombosis (30,31). The only absolute contraindication is pregnancy because hormonal emergency contraception is ineffective if a woman is already pregnant. However, neither method has any proven teratogenicity, so if a woman already is pregnant, an ineffective dose is not of great concern. In women with disabilities or chronic medical conditions, the only group for whom LNG-ECP would be contraindicated is women who cannot follow the directions.

Because of its greater efficacy and fewer side effects, the 0.75-mg LNG-only emergency contraception regimen (available in the United States as Plan B, Women's Capital Corporation) is preferable to those containing estrogen. Compared with the COC regimen, LNG-only pills were 60% more effective (32). The only advantage of a combined regimen is that a woman already may have packs of pills at home that she can use. However, advance provision of either a prescription for Plan B or, better yet, the pills themselves obviates that advantage. Because of its safety, efficacy, and lack of teratogenicity, emergency contraception pills ought to be available over the counter in the United States, as it is in Europe (33).

CONTRACEPTIVE CONSIDERATIONS FOR SPECIFIC DISABILITIES

Physical Disabilities

Clinicians often give the reproductive needs of the physically disabled a low priority because of the misguided assumption that the disabled are not sexually active. This problem is exacerbated when physical access to family planning clinics is limited. To illustrate this, a U.S. study showed that few women with paralysis, impaired motor function, or physical deformities were offered contraception (34). However, another U.S. study found that disabled adolescents had the same patterns of

sexual activity as their nondisabled peers (35). Clearly, contraceptive counseling is an important part of health care for the physically disabled and a part of providers' responsibility to acknowledge the full lives and health needs of people who are disabled.

Contraceptive recommendations often will depend on underlying medical conditions and will vary with the quality of circulation to the extremities, coagulation abnormalities, physical sensation impairment, dexterity, possible drug interactions, and problems with menstrual hygiene (36). Difficulties with immobilization or limited dexterity affect contraceptive choice, but many reliable options are available.

The primary concern about COCs is the risk of thromboembolism, the sequelae of which could be aggravated if a woman has impaired sensation in the lower extremities and therefore does not detect thrombophlebitis. Although data are limited, women with impaired circulation, a history of stroke, or immobile extremities generally are advised to avoid COCs (37). Thus this recommendation may affect women with cerebral palsy, spinal cord injury, poliomyelitis, and muscular dystrophy and some women with rheumatoid arthritis (38).

Impaired mobility may pose the risk of lower extremity venous stasis, which may cause hesitation about using estrogen-containing methods. However, progestin-only hormonal methods (LNG IUD, POPs, DMPA, LNG implants) remain an option because they are not associated with VTE. The main concern about DMPA in women with paralysis is their increased risk for osteoporosis. Long-term use of DMPA has been associated with decreased bone density in some women, particularly in adolescents (39,40), although the effect is thought to be reversible. Neither Norplant nor the LNG IUD has been associated with this risk.

The amenorrhea that DMPA or the LNG IUD frequently achieves may be a welcome side effect in women who lack the dexterity to use tampons or menstrual pads. However, because of irregular bleeding, both methods initially may exacerbate hygiene difficulties, which may be a complaint with hormonal implants as well. Although implants are a good option, their insertion or removal may be more difficult in women with upper extremity contractures or spasticity if positioning is difficult.

IUDs, with their high efficacy and relative ease of use, may be an excellent choice. In women with disabilities, IUDs require some additional considerations. Some providers worry that a woman with limited sensation in her pelvis, such as with multiple sclerosis or spinal cord dysfunction, may not recognize symptoms of infection or of ectopic pregnancy. However, in monogamous women, evidence has shown that virtually all of the small risk of PID occurs within 20 days of insertion (41). Preinsertion screening for risk factors and cultures for gonorrhea and chlamydia and careful follow-up, including postinsertion examination, should minimize this risk. Although some authors have expressed concern that sensory impairment could make IUDs dangerous (42), with the extremely low rate of infectious complications in low-risk IUD users (43) and no data to support their concern, this must be viewed as a hypothetic risk. In women who experience adductor spasms of the thighs, such as some with severe scoliosis, cerebral palsy, or multiple sclerosis, insertion may be difficult (44). If a woman has limited mobility, her partner may need to assist with palpating the strings monthly to check for expulsion. Unlike the LNG IUD, which dramatically decreases menstrual bleeding, copper-containing IUDs tend to increase it. If this leads to anemia, women with respiratory compromise, such as with poliomyelitis, may want to discontinue its use.

Clinicians should encourage women who are physically disabled at risk for STDs to use barrier methods. This is especially important in women with decreased pelvic sensation who may not recognize PID symptoms. Women found to have STDs also should be screened for sexual abuse, which can be an unrecognized problem. An able-bodied partner can assist with condom use. Women may lack the dexterity needed to use other barrier methods, such as the diaphragm or cervical cap. Practitioners can assess any physical limitations to proper use by having the patient demonstrate placement of the barrier method during the visit.

Women expressing interest in permanent sterilization should be screened carefully to ensure that they are aware of all temporary methods and that they are not being pressured into a permanent method. Vasectomy also should be offered as an option to decrease their surgical risk.

Mental Disabilities and Psychiatric Illnesses

Choosing an optimal form of contraception can be particularly difficult for women challenged by mental illness, mental retardation, substance abuse, or a combination of these problems. The unstable lives of many of these patients not only make an ongoing clinical relationship more unlikely but also increase the risks and stress associated with an undesired pregnancy. For example, women with a history of psychiatric disorders are at increased risk for postpartum depression or psychosis, as well as the risk of losing custody of their children. At the same time, women suffering from mental retardation, anxiety, depression, or thought disorganization may be unable to use some types of contraception reliably.

A U.S. study demonstrated the magnitude of the risks for the severely mentally ill. Although about half of the 178 study patients had been recently sexually active, more than half never had used condoms. For those about whom data were available, nearly half had multiple partners, a third had used drugs during sex, and a third had traded sex for drugs or something else they needed (45).

A small study of female adolescents who were mentally retarded showed decreasing levels of sexual activity with increasing levels of retardation, with a high rate of abuse and incest and a high pregnancy rate (46). Mildly disabled women may be at an increased risk of abuse (47). Profoundly mentally retarded women are rarely sexually active by choice.

Successful contraceptive counseling depends on the patient's level of understanding and trust in her provider. For the provider, the counseling is made more difficult by frequent noncompliance, poor access to follow-up care, and the patient's possibly heightened fears of side effects or complications (48). Paramount considerations about these women include the type of disability and her level of functioning, the setting in which she lives, and her ability to understand the consequences of her contraceptive choices. Also important is the risk that pregnancy will exacerbate her mental disturbance, her level of sexual activity, her risk for abuse, her ability to comply with a contraceptive regimen, and her capacity to consent to a permanent contraceptive method. To optimize compliance, contraceptive counseling for women who are mentally disabled is most successful when it is reinforced over time with consistent follow-up, when it is discussed using concrete educational materials (such as models or the devices themselves), and when it involves the partner and mental health agency staff (36).

Mentally handicapped or behaviorally disordered patients who are in long-term treatment programs generally have better contraceptive compliance. For example, someone who already receives depot haloperidol or fluphenazine or who is enrolled in a methadone maintenance program may be well served by DMPA or a monthly combined injectable contraceptive. Other outpatients may benefit from implants or DMPA, although bleeding irregularities may be of concern to them (49).

Clinicians must know the legal criteria for informed consent when considering the appropriateness of long-term or permanent contraception, such as implants, IUDs, or sterilization. The ethics of sterilization of the mentally handicapped is controversial. For example, some ethicists contend that if an impaired mother were to get pregnant but inevitably would lose custody of that child, sterilization is not wrong. Others conclude

that one primarily must consider the genetic etiology of the retardation as well as parenting potential in making an ethical decision (50,51).

OC use may require close supervision and review of interactions with other medications, such as antiseizure medications. However, motivated or well-supervised women may benefit from decreased menstrual bleeding, especially if pills are used continuously. DMPA has a similar benefit, although one can expect increased menstrual irregularity, which is less problematic in combined injectables, such as Lunelle™. Some women view monthly menstrual cycles as a sign of health (52) and therefore may be distressed by cycle alterations. For the mentally ill, as for the mentally handicapped, the amount of supervision needed to ensure reliable pill-taking is often most critical. OCs are most successful in women whose lives are more structured, whereas women whose lives are disorganized, with such additional challenges as homelessness or substance use, are unlikely to be well protected by them.

A concern about hormonal methods for the mentally ill is whether they will increase the woman's symptoms. In considering steroidal preparations, clinicians should review the patient's other medications. COCs increase the concentrations of some benzodiazepines and therefore may not be ideal. However, patients who take phenothiazines or tricyclic antidepressants may benefit from COCs. Because these drugs can lower the levels of estrogen or progesterone, COCs may alleviate symptoms of hormone deficiency, such as vaginal dryness. Most antiseizure medications may accelerate steroid metabolism, which may lead to breakthrough bleeding, possible increased risk of contraceptive failure, and the need for a higher dose pill, which may increase the risk of thromboembolism.

The irregular bleeding associated with DMPA or hormonal implants may make women anxious. There is little evidence that Norplant or DMPA cause mood disorders (16,53), but many providers are cautious about long-term progestin methods that cannot be easily removed or stopped. We predict that this problem will not be a concern with the LNG IUD, in which systemic hormone levels are low, having largely a local effect. Some studies have suggested that COCs may lessen the severity of schizophrenic symptoms (54).

IUDs have not been recommended for women who are mentally handicapped because of concerns that they may not be able to report if they are having a complication that causes pain. For mentally ill women who may be at high risk for STDs, IUDs also may not be recommended, especially if the patient is at high risk at the time of insertion. Except after insertion, a LNG IUD may be associated with decreased infection risks because it causes thickening of the cervical mucus (25,55).

Mentally ill and retarded patients are at risk for STDs, as well as pregnancy. Some studies have shown sexual activity among the mentally ill, including those in institutions, to be higher than among the unaffected population (56–58). Therefore, in addition to determining an appropriate contraceptive method, clinicians should encourage use of a barrier method. However, for contraception, barrier methods are usually unreliable in the mentally disabled population, unless motivation, dexterity, and understanding are high. Progestin-only methods or the LNG IUD may be useful for their effect in thickening the cervical mucus and offering some protection against STDs if barriers are not used.

Cardiovascular Disorders

Women with thrombophlebitis, thromboembolic disorders, coronary artery disease, myocardial infarction, and cerebrovascular disease should avoid COCs (59). COCs have been associated with an increased risk of myocardial infarction and stroke. However, much of the risk is confined to hypertensive users who smoke, and the risk is modified by age. The risk increases with age as cardiovascular risk factors become more prevalent, including hypertension, diabetes, thromboembolic disease, and a sedentary lifestyle.

Among 100,000 COC users younger than age 45 years, the pill accounts for about 1.5 deaths per year (60). When considering COCs in women with angina, for example, additive risk factors are important. Because progestin-only contraceptives have not been associated with serious cardiovascular effects (61), progestin implants, POPs, DMPA, and LNG-containing IUDs are generally good choices. Barrier methods are safe, as are copper-containing IUDs, which only have the consideration of monitoring increased blood loss to avoid the additional risk that anemia could pose.

Sickle Cell Disease

Women with sickle cell disease greatly benefit from effective contraception because of the maternal and fetal risks of pregnancy (62,63). It is fortunate that some of the most effective methods are beneficial in management of the disease. Progestin-based methods that decrease menstrual blood loss can be useful and have been shown to be safe (64,65), which leads one to conclude that the LNG IUD may especially benefit these patients. DMPA in particular is associated with both decreased sickling and improved anemia (65,66). The use of COCs is a less desirable choice primarily because of theoretic concerns about estrogens causing increased sickling, thrombosis, and tissue infarction, but observational studies have not demonstrated increased risks of COCs in women with sickle cell disease (67–69). For women who are unwilling to consider other effective methods, the possible risks of COCs must be balanced against the known and substantial risks of pregnancy. POPs and the combined injectables have not been studied in women with sickle cell anemia. A small study showed no adverse health effect of Norplant (64); however, with lower progestin blood levels, one might not expect the benefits seen with DMPA. According to WHO guidelines, the benefits of copper IUDs may outweigh the risks, including the increased blood loss. If sterilization is desired and the partner is willing, vasectomy is a safer method than tubal ligation because vasectomy is faster, is simpler, and does not use general anesthesia. Patients should use condoms to prevent STDs in addition to using another effective method for contraception.

Neurologic Disorders

Epilepsy/Seizure Disorders

Epilepsy can complicate pregnancy not only by the maternal and fetal dangers of seizures but also by the teratogenic effects of many of the most frequently used antiseizure medications. DMPA has been strongly recommended for patients with epilepsy because it may reduce seizures; DMPA's high blood levels of progestin both ensures its efficacy and has been associated with decreased seizure frequency (70).

However, both COCs and progestin-only OCs have drawbacks. Although COCs are not believed to increase seizure frequency, by inducing hepatic enzymes many of the neuroleptics reduce the efficacy of COCs and progestin implants (71). Such drugs include phenytoin, carbamazepine, phenobarbital, and paramethadione but *not* valproate or benzodiazepines. If a woman wants to use COCs most effectively, she could change to valproate for seizure control. A less desirable option because of thromboembolic risk is to use an OC with at least 35 μg ethinyl estradiol and consider switching to a 50 μg pill for spotting that lasts longer than 3 months, which may indicate decreased effectiveness, although there is no direct evidence for this. At the same time, because estrogen can alter the metabolism of anticonvulsant medications, after starting COCs, blood levels should be checked and doses should be adjusted as needed (72).

For excellent and safe temporary contraception, either the copper- or levonorgestrel-containing IUD is a good choice. Barrier methods also may be adequate for women committed to using them consistently. With perioperative precautions, sterilization also is

an option for women desiring permanent contraception.

Multiple Sclerosis

Little data exist about the influence of OCs on multiple sclerosis. Cohort studies have not shown an elevated risk of multiple sclerosis from prior, current, or previous use of OCs (73,74). Other evidence suggests that estrogens may stabilize some symptoms of multiple sclerosis (75,76). Even less evidence guides practice about other contraceptive options.

Stroke

Not all of the numerous causes of stroke in women of childbearing age preclude the use of COCs. However, with a history of thrombotic stroke or other thromboembolic events or in women with such hypercoagulable states as factor V Leiden or protein C or S deficiency, contraceptive agents containing estrogens should be avoided. POPs also are relatively contraindicated primarily because of a concern about arterial thrombosis, although this risk is less than with COCs. Copper-containing IUDs are safe, as are barrier methods, and DMPA and LNG IUDs also may be considered.

Disabling Rheumatologic Conditions

Systemic Lupus Erythematosus

Case reports have shown that oral contraceptive use can exacerbate systemic lupus erythematosus (SLE). Lupus-associated vascular disease is a contraindication for estrogen-containing oral contraceptives, as are high levels of antiphospholipid antibodies and active nephritis (77,78). Progestin-only methods are a recommended alternative (79). In women with stable or inactive disease and without renal involvement or antiphospholipid antibodies, low-dose COCs may be considered (80). In these patients, noncontraceptive benefits may include decreased menstrually related flares with continuous use, decreased menstrual irregularity, and possibly decreased risk of osteoporosis (80). A National Institutes of Health-funded, ongoing, randomized, controlled clinical trial of OCs and hormone replacement therapy (HRT) in women with SLE should provide better guidance about OC and HRT use in SLE. POPs have not been associated with an increase in SLE flares (79). Progestin implants and IUDs are good choices. A controlled cohort of 16,021 women did not show an association between Norplant or copper-containing IUDs and arthropathies and related disorders (including SLE and rheumatoid arthritis) (19). Copper-containing IUDs are not associated with excessive bleeding or pelvic infection in patients with SLE, but the same study did not discuss the effect of steroids or immunosuppression (81).

Rheumatoid Arthritis

Although initial epidemiologic studies suggested a protective association between oral contraceptives and rheumatoid arthritis, later data have been mixed (82). The majority of 18 studies found some protective effect (83). Some studies suggest long-term COC use may protect women particularly against severe forms of rheumatoid arthritis (84,85). There is little information to guide recommendations about other contraceptive methods.

CONCLUSION

Any attempt to describe contraceptive choices for such a diverse group of women is destined to overgeneralize. Ultimately, each patient must be evaluated and treated on the basis of her individual needs and preferences. It is hoped that the information contained in this chapter provides some useful guidelines for doing so.

When considering contraception for women with disabilities, it is tempting to concentrate on the small risks of contraceptive methods, usually impossible to quantify,

rather than the greater risks of an unintended pregnancy. Careful assessment of a woman's contraceptive preferences must be weighed against a clinician's concerns about balancing her risks with each method's efficacy and noncontraceptive benefits.

USEFUL WEB SITES FOR INFORMATION ON CONTRACEPTION

Alan Guttmacher Institute: *www.agi-usa.org/index.html*
American College of Obstetricians and Gynecologists: *www.acog.org*
Association of Reproductive Health Professionals: *www.arhp.org*
Cochrane Library: *www.cochranelibrary.com*
CONRAD Program: *www.conrad.org*
The Emergency Contraception Web site: *www.not-2-late.com*
Family Health International: *www.fhi.org*
Healthy People 2010: *www.healthypeople.gov*
JAMA and Archives: Women's Contraception: *http://pubs.ama_assn.org/cgi/collection/*
Managing Contraception: *www.managingcontraception.com*
MEDLINE/PubMed: *www.ncbi.nlm.nih.gov/PubMed/*
ReproLine (Reproductive Health Online): *www.reproline.jhu.edu*
World Health Organization Medical Eligibility Criteria *www.who.int/reproductive-health/publications/RHR_00_2_medical_eligibility_criteria_second_edition*

REFERENCES

1. Abma JC, Chandra A, Mosher WD, et al. Fertility, family planning, and women's health: new data from the 1995 National Survey of Family Growth. *Vital Health Stat* 1997;19:1–114.
2. Stewart FH, Harper CC, Ellertson CE, et al. Clinical breast and pelvic examination requirements for hormonal contraception: current practice vs evidence. *JAMA* 2001;285(17):2232–2239.
3. Sawaya GF, Harper C, Balistreri E, et al. Cervical neoplasia risk in women provided hormonal contraception without a Pap smear. *Contraception* 2001;63:57–60.
4. Jones KP, Wild RA. Contraception for patients with psychiatric or medical disorders. *Am J Obstet Gynecol* 1994;170(Pt 2):1575–1580.
5. Trussell J, Leveque JA, Koenig JD, et al. The economic value of contraception: a comparison of 15 methods. *Am J Public Health* 1995;85:494–503.
6. Effect of different progestagens in low oestrogen oral contraceptives on venous thromboembolic disease. World Health Organization Collaborative Study of Cardiovascular Disease and Steroid Hormone Contraception. *Lancet* 1995;346(8990):1582–1588.
7. Venous thromboembolic disease and combined oral contraceptives: results of international multicentre case-control study. World Health Organization Collaborative Study of Cardiovascular Disease and Steroid Hormone Contraception. *Lancet* 1995;346(8990):1575–1582.

8. Cardiovascular disease and use of oral and injectable progestogen-only contraceptives and combined injectable contraceptives: results of an International, Multicenter, Case-Control Study. World Health Organization Collaborative Study of Cardiovascular Disease and Steroid Hormone Contraception. *Contraception* 1998; 57(5):315–324.

9. Kaunitz AM, Garceau RJ, Cromie MA. Comparative safety, efficacy, and cycle control of Lunelle™ monthly contraceptive injection (medroxyprogesterone acetate and estradiol cypionate injectable suspension): assessment of return of ovulation after three monthly injections in surgically sterile women. *Contraception* 1999; 60:179.

10. Hall P, Bahamondes L, Diaz J, et al. Introductory study of the once-a-month, injectable contraceptive Cyclofem in Brazil, Chile, Columbia, and Peru. *Contraception* 1997;56(6):353–359.

11. Garza-Flores J, Morales del Olmo A, Fuziwara JL, et al. Introduction of Cyclofem® once-a-month injectable contraceptive in Mexico. *Contraception* 1998;58(1): 7–12.

12. Cuong DT, Huong M. Comparative phase III clinical trial of two injectable contraceptive preparations, depotmedroxyprogesterone acetate and Cyclofem® in Vietnamese women. *Contraception* 1996;543:169–179.

13. A multicentred phase III comparative study of two hormonal contraceptive preparations given once-a-month by intramuscular injection. II. The comparison of bleeding patterns. World Health Organization Task Force on Long-Acting Systemic Agents for Fertility Regulation. *Contraception* 1989;40(5):531–551.

14. Gardner JM, Mishell DR Jr. Analysis of bleeding patterns and resumption of fertility following discontinuation of a long-acting injectable contraception. *Fertil Steril* 1970;21(4):286–291.

15. Speroff L, Darney PD. *A clinical guide for contraception*. Philadelphia: Lippincott Williams & Wilkins, 2001:207–209.

16. Westhoff C, Truman C, Kalmuss D, et al. Depressive symptoms and Depo-Provera®. *Contraception* 1998;57 (4):237–240.

17. Sangi-Haghpeykar H, Poindexter A, Bateman L, et al. Experiences of injectable contraceptive users in an urban setting. *Obstet Gynecol* 1996;88:227–233.

18. Roy S, Mishell DR Jr, Robertson D, et al. Long-term reversible contraception with levonorgestrel-releasing silastic rods. *Am J Obstet Gynecol* 1984;148:1006–1013.

19. Meirik O, Farley TMM, Sivin I. Safety and efficacy of levonorgestrel implant, intrauterine device and sterilization. *Obstet Gynecol* 2001;97(4):539–547.

20. Zerner J, Doil KL, Drewry J, et al. Intrauterine contraceptive device failures in renal transplant patients. *J Reprod Med* 1981;26(2):99–102.

21. Sivin I, Stern J, Coutinho E, et al. Prolonged intrauterine contraception: a seven-year randomized study of the levonorgestrel 20 mcg/day (LNg 20) and the Copper T380 AgIUDS. *Contraception* 1991;44(5):473–480.

22. Sivin I, Stern J. Health during prolonged use of levonorgestrel 20 micrograms/d and the Copper TCu 380Ag intrauterine contraceptive devices: a multicenter study. International Committee for Contraception Research (ICCR). *Fertil Steril* 1994;61(1):70–77.

23. Crosignani PG, Vercellini P, Mosconi P, et al. Levonorgestrel-releasing intrauterine device versus hysteroscopic endometrial resection in the treatment of dysfunctional uterine bleeding. *Obstet Gynecol* 1997;90 (2):257–263.

24. Andersson K, Odlind V, Rybo G. Levonorgestrel-releasing and copper-releasing (Nova T) IUDs during five years of use: a randomized comparative trial. *Contraception* 1994;49(1):56–72.

25. Toivonen J, Luukkainen T, Allonen H. Protective effect of intrauterine release of levonorgestrel on pelvic infection: three years' comparative experience of levonorgestrel- and copper-releasing intrauterine devices. *Obstet Gynecol* 1991;77(2):261–264.

26. Rosenberg MJ, Davidson AJ, Chen JH, et al. Barrier contraceptives and sexually transmitted diseases in women: a comparison of female-dependent methods and condoms. *Am J Public Health* 1992;82(5):669–674.

27. Feldblum PJ, Morrison CS, Roddy RE, et al. The effectiveness of barrier methods of contraception in preventing the spread of HIV. *AIDS* 1995;9(Suppl A):S85–93.

28. Cates W Jr, Stone K. Family planning, sexually transmitted diseases and contraceptive choice: a literature update: Part I. *Fam Plann Perspect* 1992;24(2):75–84.

29. Rodrigues I, Grou F, Joly J. Effectiveness of emergency contraceptive pills between 72 and 120 hours after unprotected sexual intercourse. *Am J Obstet Gynecol* 2001;184(4):531–537.

30. ACOG Practice Bulletin 25. 2001

31. WHO Family Planning and Population. Emergency contraception: a guide for service delivery. WHO: Geneva, 1998.

32. Randomised controlled trial of levonorgestrel versus the Yuzpe regimen of combined oral contraceptives for emergency contraception. Task Force on Postovulatory Methods of Fertility Regulation. *Lancet* 1998;352 (9126):428–433.

33. Grimes DA, Raymond EG, Scott Jones B. Emergency contraception over-the-counter: the medical and legal imperatives. *Obstet Gynecol* 2001;98(1):151–155.

34. Beckman CR, Gittler M, Barzansky BM, et al. Gynecologic health care of women with disabilities. *Obstet Gynecol* 1989;74(1):75–79.

35. Suris JC, Resnick MD, Cassuto N, et al. Sexual behavior of adolescents with chronic disease and disability. *J Adol Health* 1996;19(2):124–131.

36. Leavesley G, Porter J. Sexuality, fertility and contraception in disability. *Contraception* 1982;26(4):417–441.

37. Haefner HK, Elkins TE. Contraceptive management for female adolescents with mental retardation and handicapping disabilities. *Curr Opin Obstet Gynecol* 1991; 3(6):820–824.

38. Best K. Disabled have many needs for contraception. *Network* 1999;19(2):16–18.

39. Cundy TJ, Cornish H, Roberts H, et al. Spinal bone density in women using depot medroxyprogesterone contraception. *Obstet Gynecol* 1998;92(4):569–573.

40. Cundy T, Evans M, Roberts H, et al. Bone density in women receiving depot medroxyprogesterone acetate for contraception. *BMJ* 1991;303(6793):13–16.

41. Farley MM, Rosenberg MJ, Rowe PJ, et al. Intrauterine devices and pelvic inflammatory disease: an international perspective. *Lancet* 1992;339:785–788.

42. Charlifue SW, Gerhart KA, Menter RR, et al. Sexual issues of women with spinal cord injuries. *Paraplegia* 1992;30(3):192–199.

43. Hubacher D, Lara-Ricalde R, Taylor DJ, et al. Use of copper intrauterine devices and the risk of tubal infertility among nulligravid women. *New Engl J Med* 2001; 345(8):561–567.

44. Neinstein L. Contraception in women with special medical needs. *Compr Ther* 1998;24(5):238.

45. McKinnon K, Cournos F, Sugden R, et al. The relative contributions of psychiatric symptoms and aids knowledge to HIV risk behaviors among people with severe mental illness. *J Clin Psychiatry* 1996;57(11):506–513.

46. Chamberlain A, Rauh J, Passer A, et al. Issues in fertility control for mentally retarded female adolescents: I. Sexual activity, sexual abuse, and contraception. *Pediatrics* 1984;73(4):445–450.

47. McCormack B. Sexual abuse and learning disabilities. *BMJ* 1991;303(6795):143–144.

48. Vu KK, Zacur HA. Contraception in women with intercurrent disease. *Curr Opin Obstet Gynecol* 1994;6(6): 547–551.

49. Hankoff LD, Darney PD. Contraceptive choices for behaviorally disordered women. *Am J Obstet Gynecol* 1993;168(6 Pt 2):1986–1989.

50. Duncan SL. Ethical problems in advising contraception and sterilization. *Practitioner* 1979;223(1334): 237–242.

51. Denekens JP, Nys H, Stuer H. Sterilisation of incompetent mentally handicapped persons: a model for decision making. *J Med Ethics* 1999;25(3):237–241.

52. Elkins TE, Gafford LS, Wilks CS, et al. A model clinic approach to the reproductive health concerns of the mentally handicapped. *Obstet Gynecol* 1986;68(2): 185–188.

53. Westhoff C, Truman C, Kalmuss D, et al. Depressive symptoms and Norplant® contraceptive implants. *Contraception* 1998;57(4):241–245.

54. Kulkarni J, de Castella A, Smith D, et al. A clinical trial of the effects of estrogen in acutely psychotic women. *Schizophr Res* 1996;20(3):247–252.

55. Baveja R, Bichille LK, Coyaji KJ, et al. Randomized clinical trial with intrauterine devices (levonorgestrel intrauterine device [Lng], CuT 380ag, CuT 220c and CuT 200b). A 36-month study. Indian Council of Medical Research Task Force on IUD. *Contraception* 1989; 39(1):37–52.

56. Abernethy V. Sexual knowledge, attitudes, and practices of young female psychiatric patients. *Arch Gen Psychiatry* 1974;30(2):180–182.

57. Abraham SF, Bendit N, Mason C, et al. The psychosexual histories of young women with bulimia. *Aust N Z J Psychiatry* 1985;19(1):72–76.

58. Akhtar S, Crocker E, Dickey N, et al. Overt sexual behavior among psychiatric inpatients. *Dis Nerv Sys* 1997;38(5):359–361.

59. Sullivan JM, Lobo RA. Considerations for contraception in women with cardiovascular disorders. *Am J Obstet Gynecol* 1993;168(6S):2006–2011.

60. Harlap S, Kost K, Forrest JD. Preventing pregnancy, protecting health: a new look at birth control choices in the United States. New York: The Alan Guttmacher Institute, 1991.

61. McCann MF, Potter LS. Progestin-only oral contraception: a comprehensive review. *Contraception* 1994;50: S1–S195.

62. Sun PM, Wilburn W, Raynor BD, et al. Sickle cell disease in pregnancy: twenty years of experience at Grady Memorial Hospital, Atlanta, Georgia. *Am J Obstet Gynecol* 2001;184(6):1127–1130.

63. Smith JA, Espeland M, Bellevue R, et al. Pregnancy in sickle cell disease: experience of the Cooperative Study of Sickle Cell Disease. *Obstet Gynecol* 1996;87: 199–204.

64. Ladipo OA, Falusi AG, Feldblum PJ, et al. Norplant® use by women with sickle cell disease. *Int J Gynaecol Obstet* 1993;41(1):85–87.

65. DeCeular K, Gruber C, Hayes R, et al. Medroxyprogesterone acetate and homozygous sickle-cell disease. *Lancet* 1982;2(8292):229–231.

66. de Abood M, de Castillo Z, Guerrero F, et al. Effect of Depo-Provera® or Microgynon® on the painful crises of sickle-cell anemia patients. *Contraception* 1997;56 (5):313–316.

67. Blumenstein BA, Douglas MB, Hall WD. Blood Pressure changes and oral contraceptive use: a study of 2676 black women in the southeastern United States. *Am J Epidemiol* 1980;112(4):539–552.

68. Lutcher CL, Harris P, Henderson PA, et al. A lack of morbidity from oral contraception in women with sickle cell anemia. *Clin Res* 1981;29:863A.

69. Lutcher CL, Milner PF. Contraceptive-induced vascular occlusive events in sickle cell disorders—fact or fiction? *Clin Res* 1986;34:217A.

70. Mattson RH, Cramer JA, Caldwell BV, et al. Treatment of seizures with medroxyprogesterone acetate: preliminary report. *Neurology* 1984;34:1255–1258.

71. Odlind V, Olsson SE. Enhanced metabolism of levonorgestrel during phenytoin treatment in a woman with Norplant® implants. *Contraception* 1986;33(3): 257–261.

72. Neinstein L. Contraception in women with special medical needs. *Compr Ther* 1998;24(5):229–250.

73. Thorogood M, Hannaford PC. The influence of oral contraceptives on the risk of multiple sclerosis. *Br J Obstet Gynaecol* 1998;105(12):1296–1299.

74. Villard-Mackintosh L, Vessey MP. Oral contraceptives and reproductive factors in multiple sclerosis incidence. *Contraception* 1993;47(2):161–168.

75. Zordrager A, De Keyser J. Menstrually related worsening of symptoms in multiple sclerosis. *J Neurol Sci* 1997;149(1):95–97.

76. Sandyk R. Estrogen's impact on cognitive functions in multiple sclerosis. *Int J Neurosci* 1996;86(1–2):23–31.

77. Julkunen HA. Oral contraceptives in systemic lupus erythematosus: side-effects and influence on the activity of SLE. *Scand J Rheumatol* 1991;20(6):427–433.

78. Jungers P, Dougados M, Pelissier C, et al. Influence of oral contraceptive therapy on the activity of systemic lupus erythematosus. *Arthritis Rheum* 1982;25(6):618–623.

79. Mintz G, Guttierez G, Deleze M, et al. Contraception with progestagens in systemic lupus erythematosus. *Contraception* 1984;30(1):29–38.

80. Petri M, Robinson C. Oral contraceptives and systemic lupus erythematosus. *Arthritis Rheum* 1997;40(5): 797–803.

81. Julkunen HA, Kaaja R, Friman C. Contraceptive practice in women with systemic lupus erythematosus. *Br J Rheumatol* 1993;32(3):227–230.

82. Vessey MP, Villard-Mackintosh L, Yeates D. Oral contraceptives, cigarette smoking and other factors in relation to arthritis. *Contraception* 1987;35(5):457–464.

83. Brennan P, Bankhead C, Silman AJ. Oral contraceptives

and rheumatoid arthritis: results from a primary care-based incident case-control study. *Semin Arthritis Rheumatol* 1997;26(6):817–823.

84. Spector TD, Hochberg MC. The protective effect of the oral contraceptive pill on rheumatoid arthritis: an overview of the analytic epidemiological studies using meta-analysis. *J Clin Epidemiol* 1990;43:1221–1230.

85. Jorgensen C, Picot MC, Bologna C, et al. Oral contraception, parity, breast feeding, and severity of rheumatoid arthritis. *Ann Rheum Dis* 1996;55(2):25–37.

86. Hatcher RA, Trussell J, Stewart F, et al. *Contraceptive technology.* New York: Ardent Media, 1998:216, 235.

87. *www.who.int/reproductive-health/publications/RHR_00_2_medical_eligibility_criteria_second_edition*

11

Genital Infections—Diagnostic and Therapeutic Challenges

Sandra L. Welner

INTRODUCTION

Sexually transmitted diseases (STDs) are common in the United States. Indeed, the most recent statistics from the Centers for Disease Control and Prevention indicate that more than 65 million people in the United States are living with an incurable STD. It is estimated that there are 15 million new cases of STDs per year, half of which are lifelong infections (1). The incidence of STDs is increasing in the United States (2). Prevalence of STDs can vary with geographic location, socioeconomic status, and comorbidities.

Women with disabilities represent 10% of the female population of the United States, which is between 28 and 30 million individuals. Therefore, issues regarding diagnosis and treatment of STDs are relevant to the health care needs of women with different types of impairments. There are few data on the prevalence of STDs in women with disabilities. One nationwide survey of 506 women with disabilities disclosed that 22% have been diagnosed with an STD in the past year, which was similar to that seen in the 434 women in the control group, who had an STD rate of 24% (3). The National Health Interview Survey is collecting more complete data on these issues, but they are not yet available.

This chapter will discuss incidence, symptoms, diagnostic tests, and treatments of common STDs. It also will address specific points of interest related to unique concerns for management of STDs in women with disabilities.

VAGINAL INFECTIONS

Bacterial Vaginosis

Bacterial vaginosis (BV), the most common vaginal infection, is a clinical syndrome that results from the replacement of the normal H_2O_2-producing *Lactobacillus* in the vagina with high concentrations of anaerobic bacteria (4). Although BV is not considered an STD, its presence has been linked with pelvic inflammatory disease (PID) (5), cystitis (6), and pregnancy complications (7). According to the CDC, studies suggest that the prevalence of this infection varies among different members of ethnic and racial populations; among pregnant women, up to 6% of Asians, 9% of whites, 16% of Hispanics, and 23% of African Americans are infected with BV (8). BV, although quite prevalent, is asymptomatic in 50% of infected cases. Symptoms, if they are present, include thin, grayish-beige discharge with a strong fishy odor. This odor is thought to be linked to the presence of certain amine-producing anaerobic bacteria, such as putrescine and cadaverine (9).

The presence of BV infection can be documented by three of the four following criteria (10):

1. A thin, homogenous discharge that is not flocculent or curdlike
2. Vaginal pH of greater than 4.5
3. Clue cells on saline wet mount
4. A fishlike odor when 10% KOH (potassium hydroxide) is added to the discharge

Treatment of asymptomatic BV is controversial. Frequent recurrences of this infection often are noted even after treatment. Because of the change in vaginal pH and link to cystitis, treatment of infected asymptomatic women who have neurogenic bladders might be beneficial.

The choice of antimicrobial agent should take into consideration the women's physical limitations. Intravaginal preparations, such as clindamycin cream and metronidazole gel (4), may be difficult to use for women with dexterity limitations. However, because the oral agents (clindamycin tablets and metronidazole capsules) are not available in liquid formulations, vaginal preparations may be useful alternatives for those with dysphagia. Additionally, in rare cases, metronidazole may be associated with the development of abnormal neurologic findings such as numbness and paresthesia. Use of this agent in women with central nervous system diseases is not advisable (11).

Yeast Infection

Yeast infections are the second most common vaginal infection and are very prevalent in women who use wheelchairs. Increases in the temperature and moisture level of the external genitalia appear to predispose women to candidal infections and reinfection and to delay the response to treatment (9). Yeast infections may be caused by a number of organisms, most commonly *Candida albicans*. It is thought that a reservoir of *C. albicans* exists in the gastrointestinal tract (9).

Symptoms of yeast infection are vaginal itching and sometimes burning, especially during urination. Those with paralysis may not detect this discomfort; however, skin irritation can develop not only inside the vagina but also on the perineum and upper inner thighs. In severe infections thick, white, curd-like discharge may develop at the opening of the vagina.

Diagnosing yeast infections can be done with a microscopic evaluation of vaginal discharge and are confirmed with culture. The sensitivity of microscopic detection of yeast infection can range from 50% to 90% (9), whereas cultures can have a sensitivity of 94% (12). Cultures are usually not necessary unless poor response to standard antifungal medications is encountered. In these cases, cultures can provide useful antifungal sensitivity information as well as rule out other sources of the infection.

Four alternative treatment regimens are available for yeast infections: intravaginal creams at 3- to 7-day dosing; single-dose butoconazole 2% cream (13); intravaginal suppositories at 1-, 3-, and 7-day regimens; or oral agents, such as fluconazole. Two main drug categories of antifungal medications are available: the nystatins and the imadazols.

Simplified dosing regimens are clearly most suitable for women with physical disabilities. Cream preparations are good choices because they can be applied topically on the perineum or inserted intravaginally. Topical application of antifungal creams combined with low-dose cortical steroids is especially useful when treating perineal, vulvar, and upper-inner-thigh irritations from yeast infection. After the irritation has subsided with successful treatment, topical antifungal powder can be applied to combat moisture and provide prophylactic antifungal protection (14). Unfortunately, cream preparations usually use a plunger system, which may be difficult for a woman with dexterity limitations to use. In these cases, suppositories would be preferable. One-day dose suppositories to treat yeast infections are available. Because their efficacy may be slightly less than longer dosing regimens, they may not be suitable for the treatment of recurring yeast infections in this population.

Fluconazole, an oral agent, should be reserved for women who are not able to use vaginal preparations. Its use has been associated with a number of undesirable side effects. One study comparing side-effect profiles of oral fluconazole to vaginal preparations demonstrated that 26% of patients had undesirable side effects when using fluconazole, whereas only 16% had such side effects from vaginal preparations (15). Additionally, frequent use of fluconazole can give rise to resistant strains of yeast (16); therefore, oral fluconazole should not be used as a first-line agent to treat routine vulvovaginal candidiasis.

Furthermore, it has been noted that drug interactions can occur in women using antifungal agents in the imadazol category. Azols have been shown to reduce the catabolism of the following drugs: antihistamines, warfarin, cyclosporin (prescribed for rheumatoid arthritis), digoxin, lovastatin, methylprednisolone, phenytoin, and nortriptyline (17). Many of these agents commonly are prescribed to women with disabilities. Concomitant administration of azol antifungals with these pharmaceuticals could result in higher drug levels and may require dosing-regimen modifications. Women taking medications in the previously mentioned categories who have a yeast infection should be prescribed antifungal medications from the nystatin class to avoid harmful interactions.

SEXUALLY TRANSMITTED DISEASES

Trichomoniasis

Trichomoniasis, the most common curable STD with approximately 5 million new cases per year, is caused by the flagellated protozoa *Trichomonas vaginalis*. Many women have several signs and symptoms of *Trichomonas* infection, which usually appear within 5 to 28 days after exposure. Trichomoniasis is associated with a frothy, yellow–green vaginal discharge with a strong odor. The infection also can cause discomfort during intercourse and urination and can cause itching in the female genital tract. In rare cases, lower abdominal pain may occur. Those with pelvic sensory impairments may note only nonspecific signs such as malaise and increased spasticity, but they still could recognize the strong odor and know to seek attention.

Sensitivities for detection of trichomonas using a saline-mounted microscopic evaluation range from 56% to 86%. Monoclonal antibody staining to diagnose trichomonas can detect this infection accurately at a rate of 86%. To improve accuracy in detection, repeat or combination test can be used. For example, wet mount combined with culture increases accuracy detection 60% to 90%. Repeating a Pap test suggesting trichomoniasis can increase detection from 56% to 86%.

The mainstay of treatment for trichomoniasis is metronidazole, with a single-day dosing of 2 g; this regimen usually eradicates 97% of infections. Because this high dose may be poorly tolerated in some individuals, with most common side effects being gastrointestinal disturbance and metallic taste, lower dosing regimens also can be used over a 7-day period. Also, see earlier comment on use of metronidazole in women with neurologic disabilities. In rare cases trichomonas infection is resistant to metronidazole. New agents are being tested to provide further options for such patients. These include tinadazole, secnidazole, and paromomycin cream (18,19,20).

Gonorrhea

Gonorrhea is an STD caused by gram-negative diplococci. It has declined in prevalence but may be undergoing a resurgence as a result of treatment-resistant strains of the organism (21). It is reported that approximately 650,000 cases of gonorrhea occur per year in the United States (4).

In the early stages, gonorrhea frequently is asymptomatic; however, if it remains untreated, pelvic pain, vaginal discharge, dysuria, dyspareunia, dysfunctional uterine bleeding, pelvic adhesions, and even bacteremia can develop (22). Diagnostic dilemmas can arise because some of these findings commonly are seen in women with disabilities. For example, dysuria can mimic urinary tract infections, which are very common in this population. Dysfunctional uterine bleeding also is seen with many disabling conditions, especially those that have an autoimmune basis. Sensory impairment may mask the symptoms of pelvic pain. Because of these confusing confounders, gonorrhea may not be treated promptly, leading to increased risk for disseminated gonococcal infection. If this occurs, the resultant malaise and arthralgias could be confused with the women's underlying disability, further delaying treatment.

With 85% to 95% accuracy, cervical cultures are the most reliable indicator for gonorrhea. (23,24). The accuracy of cervical cultures can be affected by specimen handling; therefore other diagnostic techniques have been developed. These include DNA probes and enzyme immunoassays (EIA). These tests vary in their reliability; they are most accurate in populations with a high STD prevalence. It should be noted that there may be false-positive results related to bacterial overgrowth in the vagina when using enzyme-based assays. This finding has been noted in the screening of asymptomatic women and will be of special importance in women with disabilities who frequently have gram-negative bacterial colonization of the perineum (25).

There are many single-dose treatments for gonorrhea, including cefixime, ceftriaxone, ciprofloxacin, and ofloxacin. Cure rates range from 97% to 99% with these regimens. Of these, cefixime comes in liquid formulation, which is suitable for women with dysphagia.

Chlamydia

Chlamydia is an obligate intracellular parasite that contains both DNA and RNA (26). It is the most commonly reported infectious disease in the United States, with an estimated 3 million new cases per year (27).

The majority (75%) of women infected with chlamydia are asymptomatic (28). In some disabilities, such as spinal cord injury, spina bifida, and multiple sclerosis, pelvic sensory impairment may limit self-diagnosis in cases that otherwise would be experienced as pelvic pain and dysuria. Women with spinal cord injury, especially those with lesions above T6, may note activation of the autonomic nervous system as response to pelvic pain, with increased blood pressure, flushing, and spasticity being the most common complaints (Table 11-1). In these cases, a special line of questioning looking for symptoms of autonomic activation may be more beneficial than inquiring about pelvic discomfort.

The gold standard for the diagnosis of chlamydia is the culture; however, special medium and handling of the specimen must be performed to ensure an accurate result. Because this may be cumbersome, alternative diagnostic modalities may be more suitable. These include EIA (sensitivity of 70% to 90%) (29), DNA probe (sensitivity of 60% to 75%) (30), and polymerase chain reaction (PCR; sensitivity of 60% to 75%) (31). Perineal overgrowth with gram-negative bacteria could result in false-positive enzyme-based chlamydia assays (32). In high-prevalence

TABLE 11-1. *Autonomic dysreflexia*

Etiology	Painful stimulation from visceral organs results in activation of the autonomic nervous system
Manifestations	Autonomic nervous system activity results in diffuse muscle spasms commonly seen in the lower extremities
Target vessels	Affects aorta, large blood vessels in brain
Target muscles	Visceral smooth muscle
Symptoms and findings	Headache, labile hypertension, autonomic nervous activity resulting in sweating and piloerection above the level of the lesion, vagus nerve—mediated cardiac arrhythmias, pupillary dilatation
Potential gynecologic triggers	Severe menstrual cramps, ruptured ovarian cyst, UTIs or blocked catheter, severe constipation or fecal impaction, STDs
Potential surgical triggers	Ectopic pregnancy, appendicitis
Treatment	Identify and remove causative factors, speculum kinked catheter, semisupine positioning, rapid-acting antihypertensive agents
Worst scenario if mismanaged	Seizures, intracranial hemorrhage, coma
Risk of death	Significant

STDs, sexually transmitted diseases; UTIs, urinary tract infections.

TABLE 11-2. *Disability-friendly treatment regimens for sexually transmitted diseases*

Disease	Simplified oral	Liquid[a]
Chlamydia	Azithromycin (1 tablet four times daily)	Azithromycin and doxycycline
Gonorrhea	Cefixime, ciprofloxacin (1 tablet daily)	Cefixime
HSV	Famciclovir (1 tablet three times a day)	Acyclovir
HIV	—	Zidovudine and lamivudine

HIV, human immunodeficiency virus; HSV, herpes simplex virus.
(From *Physicians' Desk Reference*, 55th edition. Montvale, NJ: Medical Economics Company, Inc., 2001, with permission.)

populations, sensitivity for detection of chlamydia can be greater than 95%.

The most suitable antibiotic to treat chlamydia infection in women with disabilities is azithromycin because it is effective in a 1-day dosing regimen and is also available in liquid form. One study showed that azithromycin had a cure rate of 98% (33). Other agents to treat chlamydia are available (Table 11-2).

Syphilis

Syphilis is an STD caused by the bacteria *Treponema pallidum* and can present diagnostic challenges (34). In the year 2000, there were nearly 530 cases of the disease reported in the United States (35).

After exposure, the latency period can range from 10 to 90 days, with an average of 21 days (35). Symptoms of syphilis vary depending on the stage of the disease.

Primary syphilis reflects the first exposure to the microorganism. Symptoms are variable. The most common manifestation of this infection is a solitary chancre, or single, painless, firm ulcer with raised edges, present at the site of initial exposure (22,36). In as many as 40% of cases, multiple lesions appear (22). The skin lesions of primary syphilis resolve spontaneously without treatment in 1 to 8 weeks (22,35,36). Attendants of women with sensory deficits may note skin lesions while assisting with personal hygiene, but they may disregard their observations when these lesions disappear spontaneously.

Serologic tests are used to detect antibodies to *Treponema pallidum*. The most common screening test is the VDRL (Venereal Disease Research Laboratory), which can be confirmed with the FTA (fluorescent treponemal antibody-absorption). There may be subgroups of women with disabilities who may exhibit false-positive VDRLs. These include those with collagen vascular diseases, such as rheumatoid arthritis and lupus (37,38). The sensitivity of VDRL in predicting the presence of syphilis is 62% to 76% (37) and that of FTA is 84% in primary syphilis (37). At the early stages, serology may be negative because an antibody response takes 1 to 2 weeks to develop; therefore false reassurance of negative findings can lead to delay in treatment (22,37).

Treatment of primary syphilis is fairly straightforward. One injection of 2.4 million units of penicillin-G can affect a cure rate of 95% (39). Even so, it is important to confirm efficacy of treatment by checking for a fourfold decline in serologic titers at 3, 6, and 12 months (39).

Secondary syphilis develops about 6 weeks after primary syphilis if the infection has not been treated (36). Symptoms of secondary syphilis can be variable, ranging from a nonpruritic rash to fever, sore throat, myalgia, headache, fatigue, weight loss, and lymphadenopathy (35). This constellation of symptoms can be confusing in women with special medical problems. In certain disabilities myalgias, elevated temperature, enlarged lymph nodes, and skin rashes are not uncommon. These symptoms could be attributed falsely to rheumatologic or other disorders or to drug eruptions from one of the many medications taken by these women (40) (Table 11-3).

TABLE 11-3. *Diagnostic dilemmas in neurosyphilis*

	AIDS	MS	Syphilis
Visual impairment	Yes	Yes	Yes
Cognitive impairment	Yes	Yes	Yes
Spasticity	Yes	Yes	Yes
Balance spasticity	Yes	Yes	Yes
Gait disturbance	Yes	Yes	Yes
Pain	Yes	Yes	Yes
Paresthesias	Yes	Yes	Yes
Bowel/bladder dysfunction	Yes	Yes	Yes
Fatigue	Yes	Yes	No

AIDS, acquired immunodeficiency syndrome; MS, multiple sclerosis.

Confirming the diagnosis of secondary syphilis is straightforward. If this disease is considered in the differential diagnosis of symptoms, serologic tests approach 100% accuracy in detecting syphilis.

Treatment and follow-up of secondary syphilis resembles that for primary syphilis, with one injection of 2.4 million units achieving an eradication efficacy of 95% (39). If no treatment is given in secondary syphilis, symptoms will resolve spontaneously, usually within 3 to 12 weeks (36). The latent phase of syphilis then begins. The latent phase is defined as a stage of infection where no visible symptoms of syphilis are evident and in some cases serologic titers can decrease (37,39). Approximately two-thirds of untreated patients will remain in the latent stage for the remainder of their lives (39). Because progression of the disease can have such serious ramifications, it is important to identify those individuals who are in the latent phase and to treat them. Unfortunately during the latent phase serologic titers do not always remain elevated. Indeed, in 25% of people titers can decrease (37). Serologic test sensitivity averages only 70% (37). Although these serologic assays will decline, FTA always will remain positive, with a sensitivity of 97% (39). Treatment of women in the latent phase of syphilis involves therapy with penicillin G, 2.4 million units once per week for 3 weeks (4). Women with infections of unknown duration should be considered to be in latent phase and should

be treated accordingly. Women with disabilities who have transportation problems may have difficulty complying with these weekly injections, and every effort must be made by the medical team to assist her in completing this therapeutic course.

Of those infected with syphilis, 30% develop tertiary syphilis if untreated (39). There are three main types of tertiary syphilis: cardiovascular, gummatous, and neurosyphilis. Of the three types of tertiary syphilis, neurosyphilis can occur in approximately 10% to 30% of infected patients (39,41). Neurosyphilis is defined as an advanced tertiary syphilitic infection affecting the nervous system, with positive evidence of syphilis in the spinal fluid (39,42). Symptoms of neurosyphilis can be extremely variable, including one or any combination of the following: headaches, memory loss, apathy, seizures, visual or auditory changes, cranial nerve palsies, dementia, paralysis, shooting pains, impaired muscle coordination, and loss of pain sensitivity (35,36,39). These symptoms may be confused with manifestations of disabilities, such as multiple sclerosis (see Table 11-3).

Suspicion of neurosyphilis can be confirmed with evidence of elevated protein, pleocytosis, and reactivity in the VDRL test in the cerebral spinal fluid (37). Treatment is with intravenous crystalline penicillin G for 10 to 14 days, intramuscular penicillin G with oral probenecid, or 2.4 million units of penicillin G weekly for three doses. Efficacy of treatment (i.e., decrease in serologic titers and normalization of cerebral spinal fluid findings) can be as high as 90% (43). However, this is dependent on appropriate follow-up. Treatment regimens may be cumbersome, especially for women with disabilities who have difficulty arranging transportation to medical appointments (43). Unfortunately, even if therapies are successful neurosyphilis can result in permanent damage to the central and peripheral nervous system (35).

Pelvic Inflammatory Disease

The prevalence of PID has not been well characterized. PID denotes a polymicrobial infection, where bacteria have ascended through the endometrial cavity into the pelvis. Symptoms of PID range from discomfort to high fever; evidence of infection, such as elevated white blood cell count and increased sedimentation rate, often are present. This disorder must be treated aggressively because serious long-term sequelae can arise from delayed therapy. These include a significantly increased risk for chronic pelvic pain, pelvic adhesions, and ectopic pregnancy. Unfortunately, barriers in accessing medical care and pelvic sensory impairment may lead to a greater likelihood that PID would occur in a woman with a disability, although no data are yet available to confirm this.

Herpes Simplex Virus

Herpes simplex virus (HSV) is a common viral infection. There are three main forms of HSV infection: primary, recurrent, and chronic. It is estimated that 1 million people contract the virus each year (44). As many as 60% of infected individuals are asymptomatic (38). Even when the infection is asymptomatic, the virus still can be shed and the disease can be contracted by others (45). Symptoms of HSV are variable. Appearance of lesions may be delayed for 3 to 7 days after exposure (46). Because of blunted symptomatology in those with sensory impairments and delay in the appearance of lesions, association between prior sexual activity and HSV may not be made automatically. Usually primary herpes is more symptomatic and extremely painful, with ulcers and blisters at the site of initial contact.

Sensory impairment may compromise the capacity of women with disabilities to accurately detect this infection. In women who have impaired pelvic sensation resulting from a spinal cord injury, the presence of infectious vesicles and ulcers could stimulate increased spasticity in lower extremities. Perineal skin, which may be more sensitive to breakdown in these patients, may confuse the women and her caregiver about the nature of the ulcer. Therefore the diagnosis of a decubitus ulcer may be

assumed without testing for HSV. Additionally, healing of active blisters in perineal ulcerations may be a challenge for those who are wheelchair users because they will be unable to be mobile during the recovery phase of the infection. It may be necessary to use special procedures, such as heat lamps and other approaches, to accelerate healing of these lesions.

Recurrent HSV infection can occur in as many as 90% of patients (46). These recurrences often are preceded by a prodrome, which in able-bodied women can consist of tingling or burning at the site of the previous outbreak. Women with disabilities who have had previous herpes infections may respond differently to the symptoms of the prodrome of reactivation; they may have nonspecific symptoms such as flushing, sweating, increased muscle spasticity, malaise, elevated temperature, and other flulike symptoms (47).

Topical acyclovir may be beneficial in some cases to reduce symptoms and hasten healing (48). Patients with spinal cord injury may benefit from topical application of lidocaine gel to the ulcerated lesions because this may decrease spasticity (49). Such patients also may develop autonomic dysreflexia when faced with an outbreak of genital herpes. Timing topical applications may be challenging because these antiviral medications usually are applied six times per day (50). It may be difficult to schedule a time where lidocaine gel could be applied to improve dysreflexic symptoms without interfering with topical antiviral treatments, especially in cases where the women empties her bladder with intermittent self-catheterization. An indwelling full catheter may need to be inserted temporarily in severe cases. It also should be noted that women with autoimmune disorders who may be taking immunosuppressive agents may develop more severe symptomatic outbreaks of HSV (51).

Herpes cultures are considered the gold standard for diagnoses. Cultures taken from vesicles have the highest yield of accuracy, with assays of these sites detecting the presence of HSV in 93% of cases (52). However, there are drawbacks to viral culture methods.

They are time-consuming and technically demanding and have a low sensitivity in asymptomatic patients (52). These drawbacks have stimulated the development of newer methods to detect HSV infection. The most common ones include EIA and PCR. Some EIA methods successfully may detect up to 98% of infection (53), whereas PCR has been reported in some studies to detect 100% of infections (54). However, these methods also have limitations. PCR and EIA react with nonviable virus particles and can overestimate the risk of infection (52).

Treatment of HSV can be cumbersome for any woman and especially for those with disabilities. Of all agents used to treat this infection only acyclovir is available in liquid form for those with dysphasia (see Table 11-2). Although previous regimens for primary HSV required frequent dosing and prolonged administration, new medications such as valacyclovir are available. This antiviral agent can be administered 1 g twice a day for 7 to 10 days (4), whereas earlier regimens with acyclovir required 200 mg five times a day for 7 to 10 days (36).

Treatment of recurrent episodes can help decrease the duration of symptom flares. These approaches use similar medications to those used to treat primary herpes, although the dosing schedule may be simpler, with most regimens calling for two doses per day for 5 days.

For women who have frequent recurrences, defined as greater than six per year, chronic suppressive therapy may be in order. This therapy consists of 1,000 mg of oral valacyclovir once a day.

Human Papillomavirus

Human papillomavirus (HPV) is a viral infection that affects the tissues in the external female genitalia (36). Approximately 5.5 million new cases of HPV are reported each year (55). Of people with HPV, 70% remain asymptomatic (36).

There are roughly 80 genotypes of HPV (56). Some, but not all, of these are onco-genic. Depending on the viral type different symptoms may develop. Viral types that are less oncogenic are associated more commonly with external genital condyloma, which can present as cauliflowerlike growths with large or pruritic lesions. These may or may not be associated with some vaginal discharge. Manifestations of HPV can develop in the perineal region as well.

It has been widely accepted that cervical dysplasia is an STD and results from HPV infection. Women with disabilities may harbor an increased risk for the development of more aggressive outbreaks of overt HPV infection if they are being treated with immunosuppressive agents. In these cases not only can HPV be more symptomatic, but progression to cervical cancer can occur more readily.

Diagnosing HPV usually is done with colposcopically directed biopsies performed to confirm Pap test results suggesting HPV infection and/or cervical dysplasia. Discrepancies of cytologic screening practices between women with and without disabilities can be as high as 15%, with screening rates for women without disabilities reaching 74% and screening rates for women who are disabled reaching only 59% (57). It has been reported that one of the major obstacles to regular screening for women with functional limitations is a lack of the availability of low accessible examination tables (see Fig. 9-1 in Chapter 9). Positioning for Pap tests, and even more so for colposcopy, may be challenging for women with lower-extremity contractures or limitations in range of motion. Therefore, some women may avoid procedures that would detect the presence of HPV and dysplasia. New techniques are available through which secretions from the cervix can be collected on a swab or tampon and analyzed for the presence of HPV. These methods can detect the presence of HPV in up to 80% of cases (58) and may be easier to collect for women who have access barriers to screening. Specific correlations between the presence of HPV and cervical dysplasia are still under study. Currently these modalities are used as a complement to the standard Pap test, and further investigation is needed to evaluate the effectiveness of this screening method.

Treatment of external HPV can vary based on the location of the infection. On the vaginal area interferon injections can be highly effective, with results achieving a resolution rate of 80% (59). Other effective methods include laser therapy (cure rate of 89%) (60) and cryotherapy (resolution rate of 62%) (61). Less effective methods include trichloroacetic acid, at 65%, and podophyllin (25% cure rate) (62,63).

Because genital HPV recurs frequently, self-administered treatments have become available, allowing the patients to administer their own therapy on an as-needed basis. For some women with disabilities this may not be a practical option. Women who have poor finger dexterity or hand–eye coordination may have difficulty applying the medication to the affected area to eradicate external evidence of the infection. In some cases, the agents can be caustic to the skin and result in burns or ulcerations. This is especially a problem for women whose perineal sensation is impaired because they may not be able to detect a skin reaction to the newly acquired medication. Some treatments are less painful and may be preferable.

Hepatitis B

Hepatitis B virus (HBV) infects approximately 200,000 individuals in the United States per year (64). It is highly infectious, with sexual contact accounting for approximately 50% of new HBV cases (4,65); the other 50% is related to intravenous drug use, blood transfusions, and vertical transmission. Of individuals exposed to HBV, 5% contract the disease per exposure (66). Disabilities related to trauma may have required emergency blood transfusions, which could have resulted in hepatitis B exposure. The risk of HBV infection through transfusion is one out of 63,000 units (63), which is improving as a result of careful screening of banked blood.

This viral infection may vary in its effects on those who contract this disease. Of those

exposed to hepatitis B, 25% develop acute symptomatology, whereas the other 75% remain relatively asymptomatic (64) but still show evidence of exposure to the virus through serologic tests (67). Also, 10% will become chronic HBV carriers (64,67), and of these 25% to 30% will develop disease leading to morbidity and mortality (64). The causes of morbidity include cirrhosis and liver dysfunction, and mortality can result from hepatocellular carcinoma or liver failure (64).

Symptoms of hepatis B infection can vary. The most common ones reported include fatigue, abdominal pain, anorexia, nausea, and vomiting (67). There are a number of classic findings linked with those infected with HBV. These include jaundice; dark, tea-colored urine; and clay-colored stools (65).

The principal screening test for detecting current HBV infection is the identification of HBsAg (hepatitis B surface antigen). Enzyme immunoassays for detecting HBsAg have a reported sensitivity greater than 98% (68).

Treatment of acute HBV infection is usually supportive and directed at symptom relief. Maintenance of good nutrition may be especially challenging as a result of nausea and vomiting. Foods should be selected from a low-protein diet to minimize additional stress on the liver (69). If acute infection improves and a chronic carrier state is identified, alpha-2b interferon can be used. It is successful in eradicating 40% of chronic HBV infections (4).

Some women with disabilities acquired from trauma may have been substance abusers, which could have contributed to trauma-related injuries, such as brain and spinal cord injury. Such patients premorbidly may have been in high-risk groups for hepatitis B infection but never have been tested or treated for this disease. If during acute or follow-up rehabilitation they are found to be serologically negative for hepatitis, vaccination should be encouraged. Simpler dosing regimens, consisting of one vaccination with a booster 6 months later (69), are currently available. It is most desirable to administer the first dose of vaccination early on in the rehabilitation process and track such patients during follow-up outpatient rehabilitation to ensure that they repeat their second dose of vaccine.

Hepatitis C

Hepatitis C (HCV) is a viral disease that is estimated to infect 36,000 people each year in the United States (70). HCV can be transmitted through a variety of routes, although the primary one is intravenous drug use, which accounts for 80% of cases (71). Blood transfusion, sexual contact with an infected partner, and vertical transmission are infrequent causes of HCV transmission. Exact figures regarding the prevalence of these factors are not readily available. One exception to this premise are those who received transfusions before 1992, when screening for HCV had not been performed on blood prior to transfusion (70). Therefore women who became disabled from trauma and required transfusions in the early 1990s should be screened for HCV.

The majority (75%) of those infected with HCV are asymptomatic (64,70). In those that are symptomatic, complaints are similar to those seen in HBV in some respects, such as jaundice, fatigue, and gastrointestinal problems; the long-term sequelae of liver failure and hepatocellular carcinoma also are similar to those seen in HBV (72). However, there are also significant differences (Table 11-4).

TABLE 11-4. *Symptoms and findings common to hepatitis C and autoimmune disease*

Symptoms
  Joint pain
  Muscle aches
  Fatigue
  Elevated temperature
  Xerostomia
  Xerophthalmia
  Fibromyalgia
  Cutaneous vasculitis

Findings
  Renal dysfunction
  Cryoglobulinemia
  Anticardiolipin antibodies (thrombosis) +
    rheumatoid factor
  Autoantibodies

HCV can manifest as a diffuse autoimmune syndrome with arthritic and vascular changes, including autoimmune thyroid disease, membranoproliferative glomerulonephritis, sporadic porphyria cutanea tarda, and autoimmune hepatitis (73). Many disabling conditions, especially those that are immunologically based, can share manifestations of myalgias, low-grade fever, arthralgias, and other nonspecific complaints. Those with underlying disabilities, which are associated with these symptom complexes, may be unaware that these complaints may be infectious in origin and not at all related to the disability. Because of this confusion, prompt diagnosis may be delayed.

Diagnosis of HCV is quite accurate. New tests using antibody detection methods yield rapid and accurate results of approximately 98% (74).

Standard therapy protocols for HCV include ribavirin and interferon-alpha 2b, which has a treatment efficacy of 10% to 40% (70,75). Dosing regimens may be cumbersome and may pose significant obstacles for those with disabilities because multiple medications are to be taken at different times during the day for extended periods. Standard dosing regimens for ribavirin and interferon-alpha 2b usually include taking 3 million units, three times a week, for 24 weeks (72).

Human Immunodeficiency Virus

As of the year 2000, 150,000 people in the United States were infected with human immunodeficiency virus (HIV) (76). Women account for an increasing percentage of all acquired immunodeficiency syndrome (AIDS) cases, from 6.7% in 1986 to 18% in 1999 (77). The distribution of AIDS cases among women by means of acquisition was 50% through intravenous drug use, 34% through heterosexual transmission, 8% through transfusion, and 7% undetermined (78). The estimated risk posed by each sexual contact is 0.05% for male to female transmission (79).

The symptoms of HIV infection are variable (see Table 11-3). Some of the manifestations of HIV infection mimic findings of immunologic or rheumatologic conditions. They may include any or all of the following: fever, sweats, malaise, fatigue, myalgias, arthralgias, generalized lymphadenopathy, and thrombocytopenia (79). Macular erythematous skin eruptions could be mistaken for a skin reaction to one of the many medications taken by women with disabilities. Other nonspecific symptoms, such as diarrhea, headaches, and sore throat (79), may be interpreted as a viral infection or a gastrointestinal disorder and also confuse the diagnosis.

The most common test used to detect HIV infection is an EIA (4). This test is approximately 99% sensitive and specific (79). However, the findings may be less accurate in patients who are multiparous, those with recent influenza or HBV vaccines, patients with autoimmune antibodies, or those with a history of multiple blood transfusions (79). The incidence of false-positive results in the general population is extremely low, although data are not known for women with disabilities (80). Women who screen positive with the EIA require a confirmatory evaluation, using a Western blot or immunofluorescence assay, to verify the diagnosis (4).

Treatment of HIV infection depends on the nature of the exposure. Compliance may be physically difficult because of the necessity to take multiple medications and frequent dosing schedules. This may be complicated further if the woman has been exposed to HIV as a result of sexual abuse from a partner/caretaker who now may need to be responsible for helping her take these medications. The recommended regimen for HIV prophylaxis is composed of three antiviral agents (81). Pharmacists need to be involved to ensure that the medications the woman requires for her disability do not interact with regimens essential for HIV prophylaxis. Liquid forms of zidovudine and lamivudine are available for those with dysphagia (82,83).

The focus of the clinicians who are caring for the pregnant woman with a disability frequently is her disabling condition; thus she may not be screened for HIV. Established protocols have demonstrated effectiveness in decreasing vertical transmission of HIV infection. Neonatal zidovudine elixir should be administered for at least 6 weeks postpartum (82). The mother with dexterity difficulties may need some assistance administering this medication to her newborn.

Women who are infected with HIV should be treated with antiviral agents to delay progression of disease and prevent secondary complications. One of these complications includes cervical dysplasia and cervical cancer, which can develop at a higher rate in women who are infected with HIV (84). Women with disabilities who may receive less frequent Pap tests may be more likely to be underdiagnosed for cervical dysplasia. Thus, the added increased link between HIV infection and aggressive progression of cervical dysplasia may be even more critical in this population (85).

Compliance with complicated medication regimens can be a serious issue for women with disabilities. Suppressive and treatment regimens for HIV infection must be continued on a long-term basis. Thus, the maze of multiple medications and interactions can be dizzying for anybody and even more so for women who have preexisting debilitating medical conditions. The side effects from some of the antiviral agents may be poorly tolerated, especially those that may exacerbate the woman's underlying fatigue, myalgia, and neuropathy. When treating women who are disabled and have renal dysfunction with antiretroviral agents, clinicians should be especially careful with indinavir because it may be linked with increased risk for the development of nephrolithiasis and even renal failure (86). Treatments, therefore, need to be individualized.

REFERENCES

1. Centers for Disease Control and Prevention. *Tracking the hidden epidemics: trends in STDs in the United States.* Atlanta: CDC, 2000.
2. Seltzer VL, Pearse WH. *Women's primary health care: office practice and procedures,* 2nd ed. New York: McGraw-Hill, 2000:138.
3. Findings on reproductive health and access to health care. Baylor College of Medicine. The Center for Re-

search on Women with Disabilities. Department of Physical Medicine and Rehabilitation. 20 June 1995.

4. 1998 guidelines for treatment of sexually transmitted diseases. Centers for Disease Control and Prevention. *MMWR Recomm Rep* 1998 Jan 23;47(RR-1):1–111.

5. Paavonen J, Teisola K, Heinonen PK. Microbiological and histopathological findings in acute pelvic inflammatory disease. *Br J Obstet Gynaecol* 1987;94:454.

6. Stamm WE, Hoote TM, Johnson JR, et al. Urinary tract infections: From pathogens to treatment. *J Infect Dis* 1989;155:400.

7. Martius J, Eschenbach DA. The role of bacterial vaginosis as a cause of amniotic fluid infection, chorioamnionitis, prematurity: a review. *Arch Gynecol Obstet* 1990;274:1.

8. Centers for Disease Control and Prevention. Division of Sexually Transmitted Diseases. Bacterial vaginosis. Available at http://www.cdc.gov/nchstp/dstd/Fact_Sheets/FactsBV.htm. Accessed March 28, 2000.

9. Meltzer RM. Vulvovaginitis. In: Sciarra JJ. *Gynecology and Obstetrics,* Vol 1. Philadelphia: Lippincott Williams & Wilkins, 2001.

10. Amsel R, Totten PA, Spiegel CA, et al. Nonspecific vaginitis: Diagnostic criteria and microbial and epidemiological associations. *Am J Med* 1983;44:14.

11. *Physicians' Desk Reference 2001.* Product Information. Searle: Flagyl375, 2001:3002.

12. Cibley LJ, Baldwin D. Diagnosing candidiasis. A new, cost effective technique. *J Reprod Med* 1998;11: 925–928.

13. Reuters Health Information 2000. FDA Approves KV Pharmaceuticals' Gynazole-1 Cream. Available at http://www.womenshealth.mescape.com/reuters/prof/2 000/06.13.htm. Accessed June 19, 2000.

14. Welner SW. Sexually transmitted infections in women with disabilities. *Sex Transm Dis* 2000 May;27(5): 272–277.

15. *Physicians' Desk Reference 2001.* Product Information. Pfizer: Diflucan, 2001:2487.

16. National Association of Managed Care Physicians. Vulvovaginitis: a practice protocol for managed care physicians. *Roundtable Highlights* 1996;1:8–12.

17. Albengres E, Le Louet H, Tillement JP. Systemic antifungal agents. Drug interactions of clinical significance. *Drug Saf* 1998;18(2):83–97.

18. Nyirjesy P. Managing resistant trichomonas vaginitis. *Curr Infect Dis Rep* 1999;1(4):389–392.

19. Gillis JC, Wiseman LR. Secnidazole. *Drugs* 1996;51 (4):621–638.

20. Aschenbach DA. Infection vaginitis. In: Sciarra JJ. *Gynecology and Obstetrics* Vol 1. Philadelphia: Lippincott Williams & Wilkins, 2001.

21. Centers for Disease Control and Prevention. *STD Surveillance National Profile 1999. Gonorrhea.* Atlanta: CDC, 1999:15.

22. Watts DH. Gonorrhea and syphilis in pregnancy. In: Sciarra JJ. *Gynecology and Obstetrics* Vol 3. Philadelphia: Lippincott Williams & Wilkins, 2001.

23. Goh BT, Varia KB, Ayliffe PF, et al. Diagnosis of gonorrhea by gram-stained smears and cultures in men and women: role of the urethral smear. *Sex Transm Dis* 1985;12:135–139.

24. Romanowski B, Harris JRW, Wood H, et al. Improved diagnosis of gonorrhea in women. *Sex Transm Dis* 1986;13:93–96.

25. Stamm WE, Cole B, Fennell C, et al. Antigen detection for the diagnosis of gonorrhea. *J Clin Microbiol* 1984; 19:399–403.

26. Eschenbach DA. *Chlamydia trachomatis* and genital mycoplasmas. In: Sciarra JJ. *Gynecology and Obstetrics,* Vol 3. Philadelphia: Lippincott Williams & Wilkins, 2001.

27. Cates W Jr. Estimates of the incidence and prevalence of sexually transmitted diseases in the United States. American Social Health Association Panel. *Sex Transm Dis* 1999;26(4 Suppl):S2–7.

28. Centers for Disease Control and Prevention. Division of Sexually Transmitted Diseases. Tracking the Hidden Epidemics 2000. Trends in STDs in the United States. Trends by disease. Chlamydia. Available at http://www. cdc.gov/nchstp/od/news/RevBrochure1pdfChlamydia.h tm . Accessed August 12, 2001.

29. Centers for Disease Control and Prevention. Recommendations for the prevention and management of Chlamydia trachomatis infections, 1993. *MMWR* 1993; 42(RR-12):1–39.

30. Blanding J, Hirsch L, Stranton N, et al. Comparison of the Clearview chlamydia, the PACE 2 assay, and culture for the detection of Chlamydia trachomatis from cervical specimens in a low-prevalence population. *J Clin Microbiol* 1993;31:1622–1625.

31. Bauwens JE, Clark AM, Stamm WE. Diagnosis of Chlamydia trachomatis endocervical infections by a commercial polymerase chain reaction assay. *J Clin Microbiol* 1993;31:3023-3027

32. Demaio J, Boyd RS, Resni R, et al. False-positive Chlamydiazyme results during urine sediment analysis due to bacterial urinary tract infections. *J Clin Microbiol* 1999;29:1436–1438.

33. Micoud M, Pepin LF. Azithromycin and genital infections. *Pathol Biol* 1995;43(6):542–546.

34. Centers for Disease Control and Prevention. Division of Sexually Transmitted Diseases. Treponema pallidum. Available at http://www.cdc.gov/od/ohs/biosfty/bmbl4/ bmbl4s7a.htm#Agent:%20Treponema%20pallidum. Accessed August 6, 2001.

35. Centers for Disease Control and Prevention. Division of Sexually Transmitted Diseases. Syphilis elimination: history in the making. Available at http://www.cdc. gov/nchstp/dstd/Fact_Sheets/Syphilis_Facts.htm. Accessed February 7, 2001.

36. Seltzer VL, Pearse WH. *Women's primary health care: office practice and procedures,* 2nd ed. New York: McGraw-Hill, 2000:236.

37. American Medical Association. Sexually Transmitted Disease Information Center. Available at *http://www. ama-assn.org/special/std/treatmnt/guide/cps/syph/ syph3.htm.* Accessed August 6, 2001.

38. Libman H. Sexually transmitted diseases. In: Carr PL, Freund KM, Somani S, eds. *The medical care of women.* Philadelphia: WB Saunders Company, 1995: 468.

39. Sutton MY, Wasserheit JN. Syphilis. In: Sciarra JJ. *Gynecology and Obstetrics,* Vol 1. Philadelphia: Lippincott Williams & Wilkins, 2001.

40. Fioravanti A, Montemerani M, Scola C, et al. Fever of unknown origin in rheumatology. *Recenti Prog Med* 1998;89:30–36.

41. Lee CT, Cheong WK, Thirumoorthy T, et al. Evaluation of cerebrospinal fluid in asymptomatic late syphilis. *Ann Acad Med Singapore* 1989;18(6):684–686.

42. On-line Medical Dictionary: neurosyphilis. Available at http://cancerweb.ncl.ac.uk/cgi-bin/omd?query=neurosyphilis. Accessed July 6, 2003.

43. Greco H, Toles A. Genital tract infections. In: Wallis LA. *Textbook of women's health*. Philadelphia: Lippincott-Raven, 1998;76:618.

44. Centers for Disease Control and Prevention. Division of Sexually Transmitted Diseases. Genital herpes. Available at http://www.cdc.gov/nchstp/dstd/Fact_Sheets/facts_Genital_Herpes.htm. Accessed August 6, 2001.

45. Esmann J. The many challenges of facial herpes simplex virus infection. *J Antimicrob Chemother* 2001;47 (Suppl T1):17–27.

46. Boggess KA, Eschenbach DA. Herpes, varicella, and rubella. In: Sciarra JJ. *Gynecology and Obstetrics,* Vol 3. Philadelphia: Lippincott Williams & Wilkins, 2001.

47. Baker DA. Herpes. In: Sciarra JJ. *Gynecology and Obstetrics,* Vol 1. Philadelphia: Lippincott Williams & Wilkins, 2001.

48. Laerum E, Gabrielsen BO, Halsos A, et al. Acyclovir creme in recurrent herpes genitalis. *Tidsskr Nor Laegeforen* 1989;109(7–8):847–849.

49. Colachis SC. Autonomic hyperreflexia with spinal cord injury. *J Am Paraplegia Soc* 1992;15:171–186.

50. *Physicians' Desk Reference 2001*. Product Information. Glaxo Wellcome: Zovirax, 2001:1512.

51. Hudnall SD, Rady PL, Tyring SK, et al. Hydrocortisone activation of human herpesvirus 8 viral DNA replication and gene expression in vitro. *Transplantation* 1999;67(5):648–652.

52. American Medical Association. Sexually Transmitted Disease Information Center. Available at http://www.ama-assn.org/special/std/treatmnt/guide/cps/herpes/herpes3.htm. Accessed August 6, 2001.

53. Martins TB, Woolstenhulme RD, Jaskowski TD, et al. Comparison of four enzyme immunoassays with a western blot assay for the determination of type-specific antibodies to herpes simplex virus. *Am J Clin Pathol* 2001;115(2):272–277.

54. Puthavathana P, Horthongkham N, Roongpisuthipong A, et al. Comparison between virus isolation method, Papanicolaou stain, immunoperoxidase stain and polymerase chain reaction in the diagnosis of genital herpes. *Asian Pac J Allergy Immunol* 1998;16(4):177–183.

55. Centers for Disease Control and Prevention. National Center for Infectious Diseases. Genital HPV infection fact sheet. Available at http://www.cdc.gov/nchstp/dstd/Fact_Sheets/FactsHPV.htm. Accessed February 7, 2001.

56. Matsukura T, Sugase M. Relationships between 80 human papillomavirus genotypes and different graces of cervical intraepithelial neoplasia: associations and causality. *Virology* 2001;283(1):139–147.

57. Center for Cost and Financing Studies, Agency for Healthcare Research and Quality. Medical Expenditure Panel Survey Household Component, 1996 (Round 1).

58. Harper DM, Hildesheim A, Cobb JL, et al. Collection devices for human papillomavirus. *J Fam Pract* 1999;48 (7);531–535.

59. Penna C, Fallani MG, Gordigiani R, et al. Intralesional beta-interferon treatment of cervical intraepithelial neoplasia associated with human papillomavirus infection. *Tumori* 1994;80(2):146–150.

60. Schneider A, Grubert T, Kirchmayr R, et al. Efficacy trial of topically administered interferon gamma-1 beta gel in comparison to laser treatment in cervical intraepithelial neoplasia. *Arch Gynecol Obstet* 1995;256(2): 75–83.

61. Mohanty KC, Lowe JW. Cryotherapy in the management of histologically diagnosed subclinical human papilloma virus (HPV) infection of the cervix. *Br J Clin Pract* 1990;44(12):574–577.

62. *Physicians' Desk Reference 2001*. Product Information. Neutraceutics: Condylox, 2001:2249.

63. Menendez Velazquez JF, Gonzalez Sanchez JL, Rodriguez de Santiago JD, et al. The treatment of cervical human Papillomavirus (HPV) infection with trichloroacetic acid. *Ginecol Obstet Mex* 1993;61: 48–51.

64. Silverman NS. Hepatitis virus infections during pregnancy. In: Sciarra JJ. *Gynecology and Obstetrics,* Vol 3. Philadelphia: Lippincott Williams & Wilkins, 2001.

65. Jackson Gastroenterology. Hepatitis B. Available at http://www.gicare.com/pated/ecdlv41.htm. Accessed May 1, 2001.

66. Unspeakable. Sexually Transmitted Diseases. Hepatitis B—the facts. Available at http://www.unspeakable.com/facts/hepatit.html. Accessed May 1, 2001.

67. Centers for Disease Control and Prevention. National Center for Infectious Diseases. Viral hepatitis B—fact sheet. Available at http://www.cdc.gov/ncidod/diseases/hepatitis/b/fact.htm. Accessed February 7, 2001.

68. Hu JF, Cheng Z, Chisari FV, et al. Repression of hepatitis B virus (HBV) transgene and HBV-induced liver injury by low protein diet. *Oncogene* 1997;15(23): 2795–2801.

69. Marsano LS, West DJ, Chang I, et al. A two-dose hepatitis B vaccine regimen: proof of priming and memory responses in young adults. *Vaccine* 1998;16(6):624–629.

70. Centers for Disease Control and Prevention. National Center for Infectious Diseases. Viral hepatitis C—fact sheet. Available at http://www.cdc.gov/ncidod/diseases/hepatitis/c/fact.htm. Accessed February 7, 2001.

71. Pradat P, Trepo C. HCV: epidemiology, modes of transmission and prevention of spread. *Baillieres Best Pract Res Clin Gastroenterol* 2000,14(2).201–210.

72. Seltzer VL, Pearse WH. *Women's primary health care: office practice and procedures,* 2nd ed. New York: McGraw-Hill, 2000:775.

73. Obermayer-Straub P, Manns MP. Hepatitis C and D, retroviruses and autoimmune manifestations. *J Autoimmun* 2001;16(3):275–285.

74. Buti M, Cotrina M, Chan H, et al. Rapid method for the detection of anti-HCV antibodies in patients with chronic hepatitis C. *Rev Esp Enferm Dig* 2000;92(3):140–146.

75. Kallinowski B, Liehr H, Moeller B, et al. Combination therapy with interferon-alpha 2b and ribavirin for the treatment of relapse patients and non-responders with chronic HCV infection. *Z Gastroenterol* 2001;39(3): 199–204, 206.

76. Centers for Disease Control and Prevention. HIV/AIDS Surveillance Report, 2000;12(No. 2). Available at http://www.cdc.gov/hiv/stats/hasr1202.htm. Accessed September 28, 2001.

77. Hader SL, Smith DK, Moore JS, et al. HIV infection in women in the United States: status at the Millennium. *JAMA* 2001;285(9):1186–1192.

78. Watts DH. Human immunodeficiency virus in obstetrics. In: Sciarra JJ. *Gynecology and Obstetrics,* Vol 3. Philadelphia: Lippincott Williams & Wilkins, 2001.

79. Apodaca CC, Maslow AS. Acquired immunodeficiency

syndrome in gynecology. In: Sciarra JJ. *Gynecology and Obstetrics,* Vol 1. Philadelphia: Lippincott Williams & Wilkins, 2001.

80. Mylonakis E, Paliou M, Lally M, et al. Laboratory testing for infection with the human immunodeficiency virus: established and novel approaches. *Am J Med* 2000;109(7):568–576.

81. Puro V, Ippolito G. Issues on antiretroviral post exposure combination prophylaxis. *J Biol Regul Homeost Agents* 1997 Jan–Jun;11(102):11–19.

82. *Physicians' Desk Reference,* 52nd ed. Montvale, NJ: Medical Economics Company, Inc., 1998:1167.

83. *Physicians' Desk Reference,*52nd ed. Montvale, NJ: Medical Economics Company, Inc., 1998:1150.

84. Fowler MG, Melnick SL, Mathieson BJ. Women and HIV. *Obstet Gynecol Clin North Am* 1997 Dec;24(4): 704–729.

85. U.S. Department of Health and Human Services. *Healthy People 2000: national health promotion and disease prevention objectives.* Washington: Public Health Service, 1997.

86. Witte M, Tobon A, Gruenfelder J, et al. Anuria and acute renal failure resulting from indinavir sulfate induced nephrolithiasis. *J Urol* 1998;159(2):498–499.

12

Chronic Neurologic Diseases and Disabling Conditions in Pregnancy

Ahmet A. Baschat and Carl P. Weiner

INTRODUCTION

Improved care for patients with a wide range of chronic debilitating illnesses has increased survival and the quality of life. Such illnesses do not preclude either a reproductive function or family life. Consequently, health care professionals increasingly will find themselves challenged by the obstetric care of women with chronic neurologic illnesses and other debilitating diseases. Neurologic manifestations may develop during pregnancy, or pregestational neurologic disorders may affect the management of the current pregnancy. Chronic debilitating illnesses and their secondary complications may be modified further by pregnancy. Antepartum, intrapartum, and postpartum care therefore focuses on management of the underlying disease and prevention or early detection of complications. The pregnant patient with a chronic debilitating illness typically requires a team that includes the primary physician, obstetrician, anesthesiologist, neurologist, and rehabilitation specialist. Complications may require additional care by appropriate subspecialists. Clinicians from each of these disciplines need to be aware of management issues pertinent to pregnancy if they are to institute early, appropriate treatment or referral.

Pregnancies ideally should be planned to allow preconceptual counseling. This includes issues concerning the interaction between the underlying disease and pregnancy and availability of prenatal diagnosis for inheritable disorders. A formal assessment of neurologic, renal, urologic, and pulmonary status may be appropriate prior to pregnancy. This allows planning of care with early consultation of subspecialists if necessary.

SPINAL CORD INJURY

As of 1995, more than 40,000 women were diagnosed with spinal cord injury in the United States (1). Injury is most frequent in teenagers and young adults, with an average age of injury of 29 years. Life expectancy after spinal cord injury has improved significantly, approximating 30 to 40 years from the time of injury. Thus, the majority of women with spinal cord injury are in their reproductive years (2). There are no controlled trials, but there are sufficient numbers of publications confirming the relative safety of pregnancy in women with spinal cord injury (2).

Discussing the care of the patient with spinal cord injury illustrates principles pertinent to other chronic neurologic illnesses. Neurologic disease may lead to secondary involvement of other organ systems. The disease progression and specific manifestations of the neurologic illness may be altered in pregnancy.

Antepartum Management

Physiologic changes in the urinary tract of pregnant women predisposes to ureteric atony, urinary stasis, and vesicoureteric reflux and therefore alters the risk profile in patients with asymptomatic bacteriuria (3). Pregnant women are at increased risk for the development of symptomatic *urinary tract infection* and/or *pyelonephritis* in the presence of pre-existing asymptomatic bacteriuria (2,3). In addition, urinary tract infection in pregnancy carries a higher risk of maternal sepsis, adult respiratory distress syndrome (2,4), and preterm delivery (5); the latter may be mediated by inflammatory cytokines (6).

Spinal cord injury can result in detrusor atony with subsequent bladder overdistention, large postvoid residuals, and vesicoureteric reflux and is associated with increased risk for urinary tract infection and nephrolithiasis in nonpregnant women (7,8). Loss of voluntary control with bladder and ureteric hypotonia may necessitate intermittent self-catheterization or placement of a chronic indwelling catheter, which contributes to the development of bacteriuria and chronic urinary tract infection (8). Furthermore, recurrent pyelonephritis may result in normocytic normochromic anemia and gradual loss of renal function eventually necessitating dialysis (9).

A primary goal of bladder management of patients with spinal cord injury and other disabilities associated with bladder dysfunction, such as spina bifida (10), is to achieve adequate bladder drainage, low-pressure urine storage, and low-pressure voiding to prevent urinary tract infections, bladder wall damage as a result of overdistention, and stone disease (11). The optimal management of bacteriuria in pregnant women with neurogenic bladder dysfunction cannot be determined from the available data (2,7). It is unclear whether frequent urine cultures are superior to prophylactic urinary antiseptics and/or antibiotics. Home dipstick testing may be of value for early detection of asymptomatic bacteriuria (8). Prior to prescription of antibiotics it is paramount to ensure good local hygiene and adequate bladder drainage. It generally is accepted that women with a prior history of pyelonephritis should have frequent urine cultures and prophylactic antibiotics should be considered. It seems reasonable to extend this practice to women with spinal injuries. Pa-

tients at particular high risk (self-catheterization, chronic indwelling catheters) may require urinary antiseptics (methyl mandelic acid), gentamycin bladder washings, or chronic suppression therapy with nitrofurantoin. Standard antibiotic therapy for urinary tract infection includes amoxicillin and trimethoprim/sulfamethoxazole, which provide cure rates greater than 80% in pregnant women without associated neurogenic bladder disease (12). Trimethoprim/sulfamethoxazole is contraindicated in late gestation because sulfonamides cross the placenta and can lead to neonatal kernicterus (13). For nonpregnant patients a 7- to 14-day course of antibiotic therapy has been recommended for symptomatic bacteriuria (8), and it seems reasonable to adopt this approach in pregnancy.

Increasing patient weight and decreasing mobility with advancing gestational age increases the risk of *decubitus ulcer* formation in patients with chronic spinal cord injury and other immobilizing diseases. Anemia during pregnancy is an additional risk factor for the development of decubiti (2,14). Ulcers typically develop over the sacrum and on the heels. Apart from the danger of secondary infection with bacteremia and sepsis, the development of decubitus ulcers may create a nutritionally catabolic state (2,14). The associated negative nitrogen balance can lead to intrauterine fetal growth restriction. Meticulous physiotherapy, skin care, and skin hygiene are essential for the prevention of decubitus ulcer formation during pregnancy. High-risk areas should be examined at each antenatal visit. Wound healing of skin ulcers is promoted by the correction of any coexisting anemia or hypoproteinemia.

There are no studies linking the degree of *anemia* with outcome of pregnancy in patients with spinal cord injury. The reported incidence of anemia during pregnancy in women with spinal cord injury ranges from 30% to 98% (2,14–17). Iron deficiency is the usual cause, although patients taking antiseizure medications including phenobarbital, phenytoin, or primidone also may have a folate deficiency (18). These medications commonly are used by women with epilepsy or head injury. Infected skin ulcers or pyelonephritis themselves may cause anemia of chronic disease. Iron supplementation therapy is generally sufficient. Patients invariably become constipated; thus stool softeners are recommended (14). Meals should be served at regular times to maintain a bowel routine. Blood transfusion has been advocated if the hemoglobin levels decline to less than 11 g/dl because severe anemia may predispose to decubitus ulcer formation.

Any neurologic disease affecting innervation of respiratory muscles may compromise *pulmonary function*. Women who have spinal cord injury, especially high thoracic or low cervical spine lesions, are predisposed to impaired respiratory function. Respiratory support should be available at delivery for these patients. Lesions at T10 or above may result in impairment of the cough reflex and render patients more susceptible to lower respiratory tract infections. Because pregnancy is associated with an increased arterioalveolar gradient and decreased functional residual capacity (19), serial pulmonary function testing should be performed in patients with cervical spinal cord lesions or other neurologic illnesses with impact on respiratory function, such as spinal muscular atrophy and poliomyelitis, to assess whether the enlarging uterus is causing further compromise of respiratory function. A decrease in the vital capacity below 13 to 15 mL/kg body weight may necessitate mechanical ventilation (19). Furthermore, the respiratory work required for a prolonged labor eventually may necessitate mechanical ventilation in patients with compensated respiratory function at rest (2). Physiotherapy and training of accessory muscles of respiration including the clavicular portion of the pectoralis may improve mechanical respiratory function (20).

Spinal cord injury and pregnancy individually are associated with an increased risk of *venous thrombosis* (14). Despite these associations, however, there are relatively few cases of deep venous thrombosis or pulmonary embolus reported in pregnant women with spinal cord injury (21). The risk of thrombosis seems to be related to the degree of immobility. Thus prophylactic anticoagulation cannot be recommended universally. It seems reasonable to start prophylactic heparin therapy for patients at high risk for thrombosis. These risk factors include previous deep venous thrombosis and/or pulmonary embolus, coexisting deficiency of inhibitors of coagulation (antithrombin III, protein C, protein S deficiencies), as well as decreased ambulation as a result of high lesions. Conventional and low molecular weight heparin both can be administered safely for prophylaxis in pregnancy. There seems to be no appreciable difference in the incidence of osteoporosis between both heparins (22). The long half-life of low molecular weight heparins offers the advantage of once-daily dosage; however, there have been reports of hematoma after epidural anesthesia in patients taking enoxaparin, which may be related to the higher dosage used in the United States (23). Because epidural anesthesia is such an integral part of labor management in women with spinal cord injury, we favor conventional heparin therapy near term because the shorter half-life allows more flexible dosage.

Patients should be assessed for risk factors of *unattended and/or preterm delivery* and the development of autonomic hyperreflexia (see later in this chapter). In patients with high spinal cord lesions (above the level of T6), the cervix should be examined weekly after 28 weeks of gestation (2,14,15). Hospitalization is recommended when cervical dilatation and effacement are apparent, especially in patients at increased risk for autonomic hyperreflexia. Patients with spinal cord lesions may be unable to recognize the onset of labor and are thus at increased risk for unattended delivery (2,14,15). Patients should be instructed to palpate the uterus to detect contractions at home. The rate of preterm delivery may be increased slightly from the expected 5% to 10% to about 18% in women with spinal cord injury (14). Previous injury or secondary contractures may distort pelvic anatomy. Clinical computed tomography or open magnetic res-

TABLE 12-1. *Medications commonly used by pregnant women with disabilities*

Medication	Information
Ampicillin	No fetotoxicity noted; use is acceptable
Nitrofurantoin	No fetotoxicity noted; use is acceptable
Propantheline bromide	No evidence of malformations; use is acceptable
Sulfonamide antibiotics	Use near term may result in neonatal hyperbilirubinemia
Baclofen	No studies in pregnancy available; avoid use if possible; intrathecal forms appear to be more acceptable
Dentrolene	No information available; avoid use if possible
Diazepam	Possible cleft palate after first-trimester exposure; neonatal complications include floppy infant and drug withdrawal; avoid all but brief low-dose use during second trimester
Corticosteroids	Safe in pregnancy; steroid boost in labor

onance imaging (MRI) pelvimetry may be necessary to assess the need for abdominal delivery (24). Common medications used by pregnant women with disabilities are listed in Table 12-1.

Intrapartum Management of the Woman with Spinal Cord Injury

Although there are no controlled trials, there is a sufficient number of publications confirming the relative safety of pregnancy in women with spinal cord injury (2,25). The fertility and miscarriage rate in women with spinal cord injury is the same as in the general population (16). A large number of nervous system tumors have been reported in pregnancy and may present during pregnancy, with symptoms consistent with spinal cord dysfunction (26). The features and management of these patients is similar in many ways to that of women with spinal cord injury. The majority of women with spinal cord injury are in their reproductive years (27). Most paraplegic women perceive labor, but their subjective experience may differ from able-bodied women. The level of the spinal cord lesion determines the patient's ability to detect labor (15–17,25). Labor pains may be perceived as intermittent gas or may present as signs or symptoms of autonomic hyperreflexia (15–17,25). Pain stimuli during the first stage of labor arise primarily from uterine contractions and cervical dilation. These stimuli are conveyed via afferent nerve impulses entering the spinal cord at T10–L1. In the late first and

second stage of labor, perineal stretch produces pain impulses conveyed via the pudendal nerves entering the spinal cord at S2–S4. Lesions below T11, T12, or L1 (uterine sensory afferents) allow the sensation of labor pains and thus enable the patient to perceive the onset of labor. Patients with lesions of the cauda equina have relaxation of perineal muscles and may not perceive perineal pain stimuli. Lesions in the midthoracic region (T5,6–T10) result in painless labor (19,28). Subjective perception of contractions reported by parturients range from total lack of sensation to a feeling of indigestion and aggravation of spasticity, flexor spasms, and clonus (15–17). Patients can detect the onset of labor by these nonspecific clues or by abdominal self-palpation of the uterus. Lesions above T5,6 are associated with painful labor and a high incidence of autonomic hyperreflexia (29).

In general, care of the patient is according to standard obstetric practice. Many pregnant women with spinal cord injuries can deliver safely at secondary-level community hospitals. Transfer to a tertiary care facility is indicated when there is a high risk for autonomic hyperreflexia, impaired respiratory function, or preterm delivery. Patients with lesions above T6 may require arterial and central venous pressure lines and continuous cardiac monitoring during labor (15–17).

During labor, the staff must be attentive to the danger of pressure ulcers and injuries. The woman's position should be changed frequently. She needs to be covered adequately because thermoregulation is deficient below the level of the spinal cord lesion (16,17). Temperature checks should be done more often in patients with high lesions. Delivery may be in a side-lying position if leg abduction is impaired, limiting ability to attain a lithotomy position. Frequent bladder emptying is necessary to prevent overdistention and remove one potential stimulus for autonomic hyperreflexia. It may be prudent to shorten the second stage of labor by using midforceps or vacuum, especially if there is evidence of autonomic hyperreflexia.

Identifiable stimuli in patients at high risk for autonomic hyperreflexia should be avoided. Vaginal examinations, Foley catheter placement, or rectal manipulation should be kept to an absolute minimum and preceded by the application of anesthetic jelly. Fetal heart rate monitor belts should be applied loosely. Epidural anesthesia is the best measure to prevent autonomic hyperreflexia. However, the level of epidural anesthesia may be more difficult to control and monitor in patients with spinal cord injury and typically produces a nonselective motor, sensory, and sympathetic blockade when enough anesthetic is given to control autonomic hyperreflexia. Although epidural administration of the opioid analgesic meperidine (Demerol) can provide adequate pain relief in labor, it does not provide a conduction block for prevention of autonomic hyperreflexia. It is our practice to administer empirically high enough doses of local anesthetic to block the patellar reflex (L2–3). This should provide adequate conduction blockade to the level of T10 to ablate the most serious effects of autonomic hyperreflexia. Excess sympathetic blockade results in vasomotor instability, which may be complicated by severe hypotension, bradycardia, and even asystole (25). Because cesarean section is associated with excess visceral stimulation, repeat dosage of local anesthetic may be required.

Acute Spinal Cord Injury

The first goal of the management of acute spinal cord injury is to stabilize the mother, using positioning and fluid management to maintain uteroplacental perfusion during neurogenic shock. The typical signs of hypovolemia—tachycardia and cold clammy skin—are obscured by the disease. Management of hemodynamic status requires invasive monitoring. During initial stabilization, viability and the condition of the fetus must be assessed. Despite the cushioning effect of amniotic fluid, maternal injury may result in fetal trauma. Fetal skull and long bone fractures have been reported (2). Fetal death can result either from placental abruption or the transient hypotension associated with neurogenic shock (30). Long-term pressor support with dopamine and/or dobutamine may be necessary. Fetal monitoring provides a means to assess uteroplacental perfusion and, indirectly, the maternal hemodynamic status. To minimize further injury to the spinal cord by unstable spinal fractures, surgical stabilization may be performed in individual cases (31). If this is attempted, the orthosis must provide sufficient space for uterine growth and the patient should be maintained in lateral tilt to optimize uterine perfusion.

The route of delivery depends on the individual circumstances. If the lesion is above T10, there may be no need for anesthesia if a cesarean section is indicated. Dopamine and dobutamine, particularly when used concurrently, are associated with uterine atony because their sympathomimetic effects potentiate each other (32). In patients in whom regular contractions are desired for vaginal delivery, phenylephrine may be used for pressor support without uterine relaxation (33).

Pregnant women with spinal cord injury require special attention to obstetric and medical disorders that may be exacerbated during pregnancy. The most serious complication of spinal cord injury is the development of autonomic hyperreflexia. The higher the level of the spinal cord lesion, the higher the risk for complications requiring close attention.

Autonomic hyperreflexia is the most lethal complication of spinal cord injury. It results from a disordered neurologic mass response to noxious stimuli occurring below the level of spinal cord injury. Symptoms occur when afferent somatic or sensory impulses ascend along the spinothalamic tracts or the posterior columns and initiate reflexes that are not modulated or inhibited by higher centers. The level of damage is characteristically above T7 (10); up to 85% of women with spinal cord lesions above T6 may experience autonomic hyperreflexia (19).

The clinical signs range from irritability to marked hypertension, headache, bradycardia, cardiac dysrhythmias, diaphoresis, flushing, and piloerection. Hypertension is mediated by peripheral and splanchnic vasoconstriction and commonly reaches levels of 200/150 mm Hg (27). It may mimic preeclampsia, and case fatalities occur (28). Headache, intracranial hemorrhage, coma, and ultimately death are all possible complications (Table 12-2). Intense reflex-mediated vagal stimulation of the aortic arch and carotid sinus baroreceptor stimulation result in the cardiac rhythm disturbances. Dysrhythmias include a prolonged PR interval, second-degree atrioventricular block, multiple ventricular premature beats, and bigeminy. Prostaglandin E_2 concentration increases during such episodes and may contribute to the headache. The unopposed increase of autonomic tone triggers catecholamine release, causing diaphoresis and piloerection in dermatomes above the cord lesion (28).

Autonomic hyperreflexia may be triggered by stimuli of varying severity, ranging from changing a urinary catheter to the pain of uterine contractions. Susceptibility of a patient to autonomic hyperreflexia may be heralded by adductor spasms occurring late in pregnancy. Adductor spasms also occur with high lesions; approximately 60% of such patients develop autonomic hyperreflexia during labor. Although the autonomic hyperreflexia most commonly is observed at the onset of labor, it also has been described antepartum, intrapartum, and postpartum. During labor, the signs and symptoms usually improve between contractions, helping to distinguish it from preeclampsia. The hypertension associated with autonomic hyperreflexia builds rapidly with uterine contractions and decreases between them. In contrast, persistent hypertension is consistent with preeclampsia (28). Other pointers towards preeclampsia are the presence of pro-

TABLE 12-2. *Autonomic hyperreflexia versus preeclampsia*

	Autonomic hyperreflexia	Preeclampsia
Etiology	Painful stimuli from visceral organs result in activation of the autonomic nervous system	Idiopathic—possible immunologic link
Manifestations	Proteinuria occasionally trace, central nervous system activity results in diffuse muscle spasms commonly seen in the lower extremities	Edema, proteinuria, hyperactive reflexes
Target vessels	Affects aorta, large blood vessels in brain	Affects small blood vessels in brain, eyes, kidneys, liver
Target muscles	Visceral smooth muscle	Skeletal muscles
Symptoms and findings	Headache, labile hypertension, autonomic nervous activity resulting in sweating and piloerection above the level of the lesion, vagus nerve–mediated cardiac arrhythmias, nasal stuffiness, facial flushing, pupillary dilatation	Headache, steady hypertension
Hypertensive manifestations best treated with...	Conduction anesthesia	Magnesium sulfate
Worst scenario if mismanaged	Seizures, intracranial hemorrhage, coma	Kidney failure, blindness, seizures, stroke
Risk of death	Significant	Rare

teinuria and edema and/or laboratory evidence of end-organ involvement, including elevated liver and renal function tests or an elevated uric acid level. Epidural anesthesia is the most effective approach to management of autonomic hyperreflexia because it is both prophylactic and therapeutic.

Patients at risk for autonomic hyperreflexia should deliver in a unit equipped for continuous intraarterial blood pressure and cardiac rhythm recording. If antihypertensive medication is necessary, agents with short onset and duration of action (e.g., nitroglycerin, nitroprusside, labetalol) are preferred to prevent prolonged periods of hypotension. However, nitroprusside should be given only for short periods because its prolonged use may be associated with accumulation of cyanide in the fetus (34). Nitrates may be poorly tolerated because they cause headache and may exacerbate preexisting headache of autonomic hyperreflexia (35). Sublingual nifedipine does not have these adverse effects and therefore may be tolerated better. It is safe in pregnancy (36) and has been used in the treatment and prophylaxis of autonomic hyperreflexia (37). Postpartum triggers that may provoke an attack of autonomic hyperreflexia include urinary bladder distention and painful stimuli from the perineum. Women with spinal cord injury can and do have successful pregnancies providing that prenatal, intrapartum, and postpartum issues are addressed competently.

Postpartum Management

Overdistention of the bladder postpartum may trigger autonomic hyperreflexia and must be avoided. Breastfeeding is recommended. No decrease in the letdown reflex has been reported (16,17,21,25). The quadriceps muscle may become dysreflexic during breastfeeding.

MULTIPLE SCLEROSIS

Multiple sclerosis (MS) is the most common acquired demyelinating disease in women during their reproductive years (38).

Uncomplicated MS has no effect on fertility, pregnancy, duration of labor, or delivery (39). The rates for spontaneous abortion, congenital malformations, or stillbirths are not increased. Pregnancy does not appear to have any causative relationship with MS (40). Pregnancy may suppress disease activity, as evidenced by increasing remission rates with advancing gestational age perhaps because of the immunosuppressive effect of pregnancy. Relapses tend to occur in the first trimester and become increasingly uncommon in the second and third trimesters. The risk increases again in the postpartum period. The highest relapse rate occurs during the first 3 months postpartum (39). In addition, pregnancy may have a protective effect on long-term disease progression (41).

No consistent changes in individual immunosuppressive factors of pregnancy correlate with the decreased exacerbation rate in the third trimester and the increased relapse rate in the puerperium (39). Some patients paradoxically experience worsening of the disease in pregnancy in the absence of any predictive marker.

The decision to become pregnant should be based predominantly on the degree of disability. In a 1983 study, 30% of women who were severely affected by MS were not able to care for their child adequately after delivery (41). Fortunately, adaptive parenting strategies have been developed, enabling effective parenting even in the face of such potentially insurmountable obstacles (see Chapter 14). Yet, the course of MS is unpredictable and only 30% of patients will be affected severely after 10 years (42). Nonessential medications and immunosuppressant drugs should be discontinued before becoming pregnant (Table 12-3).

Prenatal course usually is not affected by MS (43). Anemia should be avoided by early institution of oral iron supplementation. Prophylactic urinary antibiotics may be necessary for chronic bacteriuria associated with neurogenic bladder (see section on bladder management in spinal cord injury). The gravid uterus may worsen symptoms of MS secondary to mechanical effects on bladder

TABLE 12-3. *Medications used by pregnant women with multiple sclerosis*

Medication	Information
Interferon β-1B	Category C; animal studies using high dose, no teratogenesis but possible increased risk of fetal loss; no human studies; avoid in pregnancy
Copolymer-1	Category B; no controlled human studies, no evidence of adverse effects at high doses in animal studies
Corticosteroids	Safe in pregnancy; steroid boost in labor

and bowel function. If MS symptoms worsen, a short course of steroids may be used. Patients who received daily doses of 10 to 20 mg of prednisone for prolonged periods should receive a stress dose corticosteroid during labor (44,45).

Only patients with either myelopathy or spasticity require special provisions during labor. Spasticity may increase or fluctuate as a result of increased visceral stimuli from bowel, bladder, and uterine contractions (38). Epidural anesthesia is effective in preventing spasticity (46). Baclofen and diazepam are effective, and the former has been used intrathecally to treat spasticity in quadriplegic patients in labor (47). Diazepam carries the risk of neonatal depression, which can be reversed with flumazenil, a benzodiazepine antagonist. Patients with myelopathy may not feel the onset of labor and/or may have problems with expulsion. The patient's inability to push the baby out and increased rate of maternal exhaustion results in a slightly higher operative vaginal delivery rate.

Baclofen is classified as class C, but it is considered safe during breastfeeding by the American Academy of Pediatrics (48). Breastfeeding is encouraged because it has not been shown to increase the relapse rate (49). The intravenous administration of immunoglobulin postpartum has been shown to prevent relapse within the first 6 months of delivery (50) (see Chapter 14).

NEUROMUSCULAR DISEASE

Myasthenia gravis (MG) is an autoimmune disorder resulting from immunoglobulin G (IgG) antibody-mediated destruction of postsynaptic neuromuscular acetylcholine receptors. It occurs in 2 to 10 patients per 100,000 and is twice as common in women (38). The onset is in the second and third decade (38,51). Classically, myasthenia presents as progressive fatigability, diplopia, and speech and swallowing difficulty. The initial complaint is often diplopia, which progresses to generalized weakness in a 1 to 2 year period (38,51). Neck flexors, deltoids, and wrist extensors particularly are affected. Of patients, 75% have coexisting thymus lymph follicle hyperplasia (38). Diagnosis is made by demonstration of the autoantibody, or the Tensilon test. Patients with myasthenia are susceptible to neuromuscular blocking agents, sedatives, and narcotic analgesics (38,51,52). Furthermore, magnesium salts, beta blockers, and aminoglycoside antibiotics may exacerbate myasthenia and also are contraindicated (51–53).

Pregnancy has an inconsistent effect on myasthenia. The exacerbation rate is reported to be 41% antepartum and 29% postpartum with a maternal mortality rate of 40 per 1,000 (51). The IgG autoantibody may cross the placenta and can result in fetal myasthenic syndrome and occasionally fetal arthrogryposis, presumably from decreased movement (51). Primary concerns of management of the pregnant patient with myasthenia are early detection of progressive weakness; treatment of intercurrent infection, which may exacerbate the disease; and fetal monitoring.

Medical treatment does not differ in pregnancy; the treatment of choice is cholinesterase inhibitors (e.g., pyridostigmine), which increase the concentration of acetylcholine at the motor endplate (38). Enhanced renal clearance in pregnancy may necessitate increase of the dosage of pyridostigmine by 15- to 30-mg increments as pregnancy advances (52). Overdosage with cholinesterase inhibitors may result in a cholinergic crisis with paradoxic muscle weakness and gastrointestinal symptoms. Acute exacerbations of myasthenia related to increased antibody production show an 80% remission rate to steroid therapy (52). Mostly prednisone dosages of 60 to 80 mg/day with a taper over several months are favored. Concomitant azathioprine appears safe in pregnancy and may allow lower steroid dosage (49). Plasmapheresis also has been used successfully for myasthenic crisis in pregnancy (54). Pre-pregnancy thymectomy may decrease the relapse rate of myasthenia (38) and may be considered in patients with more generalized disease (55).

Patients should be seen every 2 weeks during the first trimester and weekly in the second and third trimesters (51,52). Intercurrent infections may exacerbate myasthenia and require prompt treatment. Because magnesium salts are contraindicated, preterm labor can be treated with sympathomimetics. However, some patients with MG have an associated cardiomyopathy, which may increase the risks of sympathomimetic therapy (51,52). Patients with MG may have involvement of respiratory muscles and therefore impaired respiratory function prior to pregnancy. Thus, in patients with generalized or advancing MG in pregnancy, respiratory function testing should be performed. Furthermore, all patients should be seen in consultation with an anesthetist (51,53).

MG involves voluntary muscle and therefore does not result in altered uterine contraction pattern (38). The course of the first stage of labor is not altered. Voluntary muscle fatigue and poor expulsive effort may require instrumental delivery at the end of the second stage of labor (51). Neostigmine may be administered intrapartum to counteract weakness. The dosage can be calculated from the predelivery pyridostigmine dosage (120 mg of pyridostigmine equals approximately 1 mg of neostigmine) (51,52). Vaginal delivery is desirable in patients with MG. Cesarean section under general anesthesia is poorly tolerated by patients with MG (51,53). Prolonged postoperative respiratory muscle paralysis re-sults in decreased clearance of secretions. Concomitant use of narcotic analgesics equally worsens myasthenia. For these principal reasons, epidural anesthesia is the analgesia of choice (51,52).

Transient weakness, presenting as hypotonia, and feeding and respiratory difficulty occur in 10% to 20% of neonates of mothers with myasthenia; the symptoms characteristically last for 24 hours, persisting up to 3 days in exceptions (51,52). Breastfeeding is not contraindicated in mothers with MG, including those who are taking azathioprine.

Myotonic Dystrophy

Myotonic dystrophy is a distal myopathy inherited in an autosomal dominant pattern (38). Prenatal diagnosis is possible for the gene defect, which is localized to the centromeric portion of chromosome 19 (38,56). Exacerbations of myotonia occur in pregnancy and are particularly common in the third trimester (57,58). Myotonic dystrophy is associated with a high miscarriage, preterm delivery, and neonatal mortality rate (57). Uterine involvement results in dysfunctional myometrium (59).

Patients are encouraged to maintain a high level of activity during pregnancy to prevent deterioration of myotonia (57,58). An electrocardiogram should be performed to assess the cardiac conduction (38). Myocardial involvement with myotonia resulting in maternal cardiac failure has been reported (60). Pulmonary function testing should be performed to assess the extent of respiratory muscle involvement (38,57,58). Because prenatal diagnosis is available, this option should be discussed with the parents (59). Fetal involvement may result in abnormal fetal movement patterns (61) and polyhydramnios, which carries a high risk of intrauterine fetal death and increases the likelihood of preterm labor (57). Hydramnios may be treated with amnioreduction and/or indomethacin (62). Regular cervical examinations should be performed during antenatal visits to detect premature cervical dilatation (57,58).

In addition to rapid preterm labor, myotonic involvement of uterine muscle may result in uterine inertia (59). Uterine muscle still is responsive to oxytocin (58). However, fatigue and muscular weakness may necessitate instrumental vaginal delivery. As a result of uterine muscle inertia, atony is common, and therefore the third stage should be managed with oxytocin (57,59). Vaginal delivery is preferred in patients with myotonic dystrophy. The patient should receive epidural analgesia if a cesarean section is performed because neuromuscular blocking agents result in prolonged muscular weakness (38,57,58).

Connective Tissue Disorders

Connective tissue disorders may present as a neurologic disorder through direct involvement of neural tissue by granulomas or antibodies (38). Vasculitis and antibodies can produce occlusive infarction of various organ systems, including the peripheral and central nervous systems. Because connective tissue disorders primarily afflict young women, any neurologic manifestation may occur during pregnancy and the initial presentation of such diseases may be predominantly by neurologic symptoms. There is no increased risk for neurologic manifestations during pregnancy (63). However, progression of the underlying disease is highly variable and assessment needs to be individualized (63,64). Pregnant patients with connective tissue disorders always should be considered high risk, and the onset of a neurologic symptom should prompt an urgent referral (63,64).

The association of neurologic dysfunction in pregnant women with connective tissue diseases is far more common with systemic lupus erythematosus (SLE) than in any other connective tissue disease (65). Classic associations with SLE include uteroplacental dysfunction resulting in an increased incidence of intrauterine growth restriction, fetal wastage, preeclampsia, and placental abruption (64,65). Common neurologic manifestations of SLE include seizures, occlusive stroke, and central nervous system hemorrhage. Less

common findings include peripheral neuropathies and myelopathy (64). The antiphospholipid syndrome may occur in association with SLE or in isolation. It also can present mimicking preeclampsia, eclampsia, or occlusive cerebrovascular disease (65,66).

Rheumatoid arthritis (RA) results in a deforming arthritis that rarely may be associated with neurologic disease due to rheumatoid nodules, which may develop in the central nervous system and spinal cord (38). In approximately 70% of pregnancies, RA improves, mainly in the first trimester (67). Flares tend to occur postpartum, invariably by 3 to 4 months after delivery (67).

Scleroderma can present as Raynaud's phenomenon, esophageal dysfunction, skin atrophy, and pulmonary/renal failure (38). *Sjögren's syndrome* is characterized by keratoconjunctivitis sicca and xerostomia and frequently is associated with other connective tissue diseases (38). *Mixed connective tissue disease* is a multisystem disorder with features overlapping with SLE, scleroderma, and *polymyositis* (38). Neurologic involvement of these three diseases is mild and usually restricted to neuropathies and carpal tunnel syndrome (38,66,67). Trigeminal sensory neuropathy with neuralgia and motor and sensory peripheral neuropathies occur (38). No adverse outcomes have been reported for mother and child. Whereas disease activity in Sjögren's syndrome and mixed connective tissue disease usually is unaltered in pregnancy, acceleration of scleroderma by pregnancy has been reported (68).

Systemic vasculitides such as *periarteritis nodosa* (PAN) may produce neurologic symptoms as part of multiorgan involvement by affecting the blood supply to nervous tissue (38). The most common type of neurologic impairment is a mononeuritis multiplex (38). The disability depends on the nerve involved and the extent of functional loss. Another presenting feature of PAN in pregnancy may be preeclampsia or even eclampsia, which may be a result of involvement of the placental vascular bed (69).

The management of patients with neurologic manifestations of connective tissue disease depends on the disability and activity of the underlying disease. Suppression of disease activity by corticosteroids is mandatory. Multisystem involvement may require treatment with cyclophosphamide and/or dialysis. If the doses of prednisone exceed 10 to 20 mg daily for a prolonged period, a stress dose of corticosteroid should have been given classically during labor. Recent evidence suggests that hypothalamic–-pituitary–adrenal function may be far less compromised even after bursts of steroid therapy (44,45). Therefore, peripartal coverage with steroids may be overused. Definitive recommendations on the use of "stress dose" steroids during delivery in patients treated with corticosteroids has not shown to be beneficial. If "stress dose" steroids are to be used during labor, intravenous Solu-Medrol, 100 mg every 6 hours, is an accepted regimen (44,45).

MOVEMENT DISORDERS

Chorea gravidarum is a generic term for chorea starting during pregnancy and includes a variety of diseases such as Sydenham's chorea (i.e., rheumatic), SLE, and neuroleptic-induced chorea (70–72). Less common but specifically treatable causes include hyperthyroidism, Wilson's disease, vascular diseases (hypercoagulability of pregnancy, valvular heart disease, congenital cerebrovascular disease), meningovascular syphilis, anticonvulsants, theophylline, lithium, tricyclic antidepressants, lead, amphetamine, and cocaine intoxication (71). Huntington's disease, neuroacanthosis, and adult-onset Tay-Sachs disease do not have specific treatments but are important to diagnose for prognostic and genetic counseling considerations (71). There are no controlled trials on exacerbation and complications of chorea gravidarum in pregnancy. There does not seem to be any adverse affect on pregnancy, fetus, or delivery (72,73).

The diagnostic workup is the same as applied for chorea occurring at any other time in life. A detailed family history is important. If the clinical examination and serologic workup are not diagnostic, an MRI should be performed to rule out caudate atrophy secondary to Huntington's disease, neuroacanthosis, striatal damage of Wilson's disease, or forms of small arterial disease such as SLE (38,72,73).

Chorea gravidarum usually can be managed nonpharmacologically (71). Treatment of the underlying disease is important. Drug treatment should be reserved for women whose chorea is so violent that their own health or fetal well-being are endangered by factors such as malnutrition, dehydration, insomnia, or injury (71,72). The drug of choice in pregnancy is probably haloperidol (74).

The most common presentation is an acute dystonic reaction to dopamine-blocking drugs, such as metoclopramide, that are given for nausea in pregnancy. Idiopathic torsion dystonia is far less common, and most cases begin before the childbearing years (71). This form of dystonia may have its onset in pregnancy and may improve or worsen. Dopa-responsive dystonia is similar in natural history to the idiopathic form but is exquisitely responsive to levodopa and/or carbidopa. Both are considered safe in pregnancy (49,71).

The treatment of idiopathic torsion dystonia and idiopathic focal dystonias of early adulthood typically includes an oral anticholinergic agent or locally injected botulinum, a toxin. Oral medications should be tapered and discontinued whenever possible prior to conception. Baclofen and diazepam may be given during pregnancy (49,71) (See Table 12-1).

Wilson's disease is an autosomal recessive defect of copper metabolism that can produce nearly any basal ganglia sign (38). Pregnancy may occur before the appearance of neurologic signs (75). A manifestation of untreated Wilson's disease in pregnancy may be the deposition of copper in the placenta and fetus (76). Penicillamine, a copper-chelating agent, is the treatment of choice (75,77). Unfortunately, penicillamine also inhibits collagen synthesis and may cause laxity of the connective tissue, resulting in neonatal inguinal hernia and reversible (after 2 months) cutis laxa (77). There also may be poor wound healing, hyperflexible joints, and vascular fragility. It has been suggested that a decrease in the daily dose from 1,000 mg to 250 mg will have significantly less effect on collagen synthesis to facilitate wound healing (71,77). Pregnancy itself does not appear to have any effect on Wilson's disease. Pregnancy and estrogens increase the serum ceruloplasmin levels and may produce a false-positive result for the screening assay (75,77).

Friedreich's ataxia is an autosomal recessive disease inherited by a gene located on chromosome 9, and prenatal diagnosis is possible (78). Gait unsteadiness begins between 5 to 20 years and then is followed by upper-extremity ataxia and dysarthria (38). Tremor is a minor feature, and patients are areflexic with loss of vibration and position sense (38). Pes cavum and scoliosis are common, and there may be progressive cardiomyopathy (38). Management in pregnancy focuses on symptomatic relief (79,80). Care should be taken to avoid magnesium salts, which may result in profound motor weakness (79).

CONCLUSION

Improved care for patients with a variety of chronic disabling diseases has increased the overall survival and quality of life. Therefore, becoming pregnant has become a reality for many of these patients, which may prove to be a challenge for the obstetrician. Pregnancy appears safe for the majority of women with chronic debilitating neurologic disease. To help make pregnancy a positive experience for everyone involved, a multidisciplinary approach is essential. This is of particular importance because many diseases may have secondary complications with which the obstetrician is unfamiliar. For this reason we recommend interdisciplinary management including the primary care physician, obstetrician, anesthesiologist, neurologist, rehabilitation specialist, and appropriate subspecialists. This approach has maximized the relative safety of pregnancy for women with chronic neurologic and other disabling conditions.

REFERENCES

1. Molnar GE. Cerebral palsy. In: Molnar GE, ed. *Pediatric rehabilitation.* Baltimore: Williams & Wilkins, 1985:481–533.
2. Baker ER, Cardenas DD: Pregnancy in spinal cord injured women. *Arch Phys Med Rehabil* 1996;77; 501–507.
3. Patterson TF, Andriole VT. Detection significance and therapy of bacteriuria in pregnancy. Update in the managed health care era. *Infect Dis Clin North Am* 1997;11; 593–608.
4. Towers CV, Kaminskas CM, Garite TJ, et al. Pulmonary injury associated with antepartum pyelonephritis: can patients at risk be identified? *Am J Obstet Gynecol* 1991;164:974–978.
5. Naeye RL. Causes of the excessive rates of perinatal mortality and prematurity in pregnancies complicated by maternal urinary-tract infections. *N Engl J Med* 1979;300:819–823.
6. Gomez R, Romero R, Edwin SS, et al. Pathogenesis of preterm labor and preterm premature rupture of membranes associated with intraamniotic infection. *Infect Dis Clin North Am* 1997;11:135–176.
7. Stover SL, Lloyd LK, Waites KB, et al. Urinary tract infection in spinal cord injury. *Arch Phys Med Rehabil* 1989;70;47–54.
8. The prevention and management of urinary tract infections among people with spinal cord injuries. National Institute on Disability and Rehabilitation Research Consensus Statement. January 27–29, 1992. *J Am Paraplegia Soc* 1992;15:194–204.
9. Vaziri ND, Mirahmadi MK, Barton CH, et al. Clinicopathological characteristics of dialysis patients with spinal cord injury. *J Am* Paraplegia Soc 1983;6:3–6.
10. Yamazaki Y, Yago R, Toma H, et al. Pregnancy after augmentation cytoplasty. A case report. *Nippon Hinyokika Gakkai Zasshi* 1997 Jun;88(6):632–635.
11. Perkash I. Long-term urologic management of the patient with spinal cord injury. *Urol Clin North Am* 20: 423-34, 1993.
12. Vercaigne LM, Zhanel GG. Recommended treatment for urinary tract infection in pregnancy. *Ann Pharmacother* 1994;28:248–251.
13. *Physician's Desk Reference.* 52nd ed. Montvale, NJ: Medical Economics Company, Inc., 1998:2438–2439.
14. Feyi-Waboso PA. An audit of five years experience of pregnancy in spinal cord damaged women. A regional unit's experience and review of the literature. *Paraplegia* 1992;30;631–635.
15. Nygaard I, Bartscht KD, Cole S. Sexuality and reproduction in spinal cord injured women. *Obstet Gynecol Surv* 1990;45;727–732.
16. Ohry A, Peleg D, Goldman J. Sexual function pregnancy and delivery in spinal cord injured women. *Gynecol Obstet Invest* 1988;9:281–286.
17. Hughes SJ, Short DJ, Usherwood M, et al. Management of the pregnant women with spinal cord injuries. *Br J Obstet Gynaecol* 1983;62;59–63.
18. Ono H, Sakamoto A, Eguchi T, et al. Plasma total homocysteine concentrations in epileptic patients taking anticonvulsants. *Metabolism* 1997 Aug;46(8):959–962.
19. Desmond J. Paraplegia: problems confronting the anaesthesiologist. *Can Anaesth Soc J* 1970;17:435–451.
20. De Troyer A, Estenne M, Heilporn A. Mechanism of ac-

tive expiration in tetraplegic subjects. *N Engl J Med* 1986;314:740–744.

21. Paonessa K, Fernard R. Spinal cord injury and pregnancy. *Spine* 1991;16;596–598.

22. Hunt BJ, Doughty HA, Majumdar G, et al. Thromboprophylaxis with low molecular weight heparin (Fragmin) in high risk pregnancies. *Thromb Haemost* 1997; 77:39–43.

23. Hynson JB, Katz JA, Bueff UH. Epidural hematoma associated with enoxaparin. *Anesth Analg* 1996;82: 1072–1075.

24. Sporri S, Hanggi W, Braghetti A, et al. Pelvimetry by magnetic resonance imaging as diagnostic tool to evaluate dystocia. *Obstet Gynecol* 1997;89:902–908.

25. Greenspoon JS, Paul RH. *Paraplegia* and quadriplegia: Special considerations during pregnancy and labor and delivery. *Am J Obstet Gynecol* 1986;155;738–741.

26. Donaldson JO. *Neurology of pregnancy.* Philadelphia: WB Saunders, 1978:12.

27. Stover SL. *Spinal cord injury: The facts and figures.* National SCI Data base. Birmingham: University of Alabama, 1986:1–40.

28. Young BK, Katz M, Klein S. Pregnancy after spinal cord injury: Altered maternal and fetal response to labor. *Obstet Gynecol* 1983;62;59–63.

29. Verduyn WH. Pregnancy and delivery in tetraplegic women. *J Spinal Cord Med* 1997;20:371–374.

30. Gilson GJ, Miller AC, Clevenger FW, et al. Acute spinal cord injury and neurogenic shock in pregnancy. *Obstet Gynecol Surv* 1995;50:556–564.

31. Bravo P, Labarta C, Alcaraz MA, et al. Outcome after vertebral fractures with neurological lesion treated either surgically or conservatively in Spain. *Paraplegia* 1993;31:358–366.

32. Brown L, Erdmann E. Concentration-response curves of positive inotropic agents before and after ouabain pretreatment. *Cardiovasc Res* 1985 May;19:288–298.

33. McGrath JM, Chestnut DH, Vincent RD, et al. Ephedrine remains the vasopressor of choice for treatment of hypotension during ritodrine infusion and epidural anesthesia. *Anesthesiology* 1994;80: 1073–1081.

34. Naulty J, Cefalo RC, Lewis PE. Fetal toxicity of nitroprusside in the pregnant ewe. *Am J Obstet Gynecol* 1981;139:708–711.

35. Olesen J, Thomsen LL, Lassen LH, et al. The nitric oxide hypothesis of migraine and other vascular headaches. *Cephalgia* 1995;15:94–100.

36. Gallery ED, Gyory AZ. Sublingual nifedipine in human pregnancy. *Aust N Z J Med* 1997;27:538–542.

37. Dykstra DD, Sidi AA, Anderson LC. The effect of nifedipine on cystoscopy-induced autonomic hyperreflexia in patients with high spinal cord injuries. *J Urol* 1987;138:1155–1157.

38. Berkow R, Fletcher AJ, eds. Neurologic disorders. In: *Merck manual,* 16th edition. Rahway, NJ: Merck & Co., 1992;1380–1526.

39. Davis RK, Maslow AS. Multiple sclerosis and pregnancy: A review. *Obstet Gynecol Surv* 1992;47; 290–296.

40. Abramsky O. Pregnancy and multiple sclerosis. *Ann Neurol* 1994;36;S38–S41.

41. Poser S, Poser W. Multiple sclerosis and gestation. *Neurology* 1983;33;1422–1432.

42. Verdru P, Theys P, D'Hooghe MB, et al. Pregnancy and multiple sclerosis: the influence on long term disability. *Clin Neurol Neurosurg* 1994;96:38–41.

43. Damek DM, Shuster EA. Pregnancy and multiple sclerosis. *Mayo Clin Proc* 1997 Oct;72(10):977–989.

44. Salem M, Tainsh RE Jr, Bromberg J, et al. Perioperative glucocorticoid coverage. A reassessment 42 years after emergence of a problem. *Ann Surg* 1994;219:416–425.

45. Glowniak JV, Loriaux DL. A double-blind study of perioperative steroid requirements in secondary adrenal insufficiency. *Surgery* 1997;121:123–129.

46. Salvador M, Redin J, de Carlos J, et al. Multiple sclerosis and obstetric epidural analgesia. *Rev Esp Anestesiol Reanim* 1997;44:33–35.

47. Delhaas EM, Verhagen J. Pregnancy in a quadriplegic patient treated with continuous intrathecal baclofen infusion to manage her severe spasticity. Case report. *Paraplegia* 1992;30:527–528.

48. Nelson LM, Franklin GM, Jones MC. Risk of multiple sclerosis exacerbation during pregnancy and breast feeding. *JAMA* 1988;259:3441–3443.

49. Briggs GG, Freeman RK, Jaffe SJ, eds. *Drugs in pregnancy and lactation,* 4th ed. Baltimore: Williams & Wilkins, 1994.

50. Achiron A, Rotstein Z, Noy S, et al. Intravenous immunoglobulin treatment in the prevention of childbirth-associated acute exacerbations in multiple sclerosis: a pilot study. *J Neurol* 1996;243:25–28.

51. Plauche WC. Myasthenia gravis in mothers and their newborns. *Clin Obstet Gynecol* 1991;34:82–99.

52. Finley JC, Pascuzzi RM. Rational therapy of myasthenia gravis. *Semin Neurol* 1990;10:70–82.

53. Lucot JP, Dufour P, Vinatier D, et al. Myasthenia in pregnancy. Two case reports. *J Gynecol Obstet Biol Reprod* 1996;25:179–185.

54. Levine SE, Keesey JC. Successful plasmapheresis for fulminant myasthenia gravis during pregnancy. *Arch Neurol* 1986;43:197–198.

55. Eden RD, Gall SA. Myasthenia gravis and pregnancy: a reappraisal of thymectomy. *Obstet Gynecol* 1983;62: 328–333.

56. Sermon K, Lissens W, Joris H, et al. Clinical application of preimplantation diagnosis for myotonic dystrophy. *Prenat Diagn* 1997;17:925–932.

57. Shore RN, MacLachlan TB. Pregnancy with myotonic dystrophy: course, complications and management. *Obstet Gynecol* 1971;38:448–454.

58. Nazir MA, Dillon WP, McPherson EW. Myotonic dystrophy in pregnancy. Prenatal, neonatal and maternal considerations. *J Reprod Med* 1984;29:168–172.

59. Webb D, Muir I, Faulkner J, et al. Myotonia dystrophica: obstetric complications. *Am J Obstet Gynecol* 1978; 132:265–270.

60. Fall LH, Young WW, Power JA, et al. Severe congestive heart failure and cardiomyopathy as a complication of myotonic dystrophy in pregnancy. *Obstet Gynecol* 1990;76:481–485.

61. Ito T, Tanikawa M, Miura H, et al. The movements of fetuses with congenital myotonic dystrophy in utero. *J Perinat Med* 1996;24:277–282.

62. Cabrol D, Jannet D, Pannier E. Treatment of symptomatic polyhydramnios with indomethacin. *Eur J Obstet Gynecol Reprod Biol* 1996;66:11–15.

63. Futrell N, Millikan C. Neurologic disorders of pregnancy. Connective tissue disorders. *Neurol Clin* 1994; 12:527–539.

64. Martinez-Rueda JO, Arce Salinas CA, Kraus A, et al. Factors associated with fetal losses in severe systemic lupus erythematosus. *Lupus* 1996;5:113–119.
65. Gatenby PA. Neurological and obstetric manifestations of the antiphospholipid syndrome. *Lupus* 1996;5:170–172.
66. Vyse T, Luxon LM, Walport MJ. Audiovestibular manifestations of the antiphospholipid syndrome. *J Laryngol Otol* 1994;108:57–59.
67. Nelson JL, Ostensen M. Pregnancy and rheumatoid arthritis. *Rheum Dis Clin North Am* 1997;23:195–212.
68. Steen VD. Scleroderma and pregnancy. *Rheum Dis Clin North Am* 1997;23:133–147.
69. Aya AG, Hoffet M, Mangin R, et al. Severe preeclampsia superimposed on polyarteritis nodosa. *Am J Obstet Gynecol* 1996;174:1659–1660.
70. Cervera R, Asherson RA, Font J, et al. Chorea in the antiphospholipid syndrome. Clinical, radiologic, and immunologic characteristics of 50 patients from our clinics and the recent literature. *Medicine* 1997;76:203–212.
71. Golbe LI. Pregnancy and movement disorders. *Neurol Clin* 1994;12:497–508.
72. Lubbe WF, Walker EB. Chorea gravidarum associated with circulating lupus anticoagulant: successful outcome of pregnancy with prednisone and aspirin therapy. Case report. *Br J Obstet Gynaecol* 1983;90:487–490.
73. Dike GL. Chorea gravidarum: a case report and review. *Md Med J* 1997;46:436–439.
74. Donaldson JO. Control of chorea gravidarum with haloperidol. *Obstet Gynecol* 1982;59:381–382.
75. Nunns D, Hawthorne B, Goulding P, et al. Wilson's disease in pregnancy. *Eur J Obstet Gynecol Reprod Biol* 1995;62:141–143.
76. Oga M, Matsui N, Anai T, et al. Copper disposition of the fetus and placenta in a patient with untreated Wilson's disease. *Am J Obstet Gynecol* 1993;169:196–198.
77. Berghella V, Steele D, Spector T, et al. Successful pregnancy in a neurologically impaired woman with Wilson's disease. *Am J Obstet Gynecol* 1997;176:712–714.
78. Monros E, Smeyers P, Ramos MA, et al. Prenatal diagnosis of Friedreich ataxia: improved accuracy by using new genetic flanking markers. *Prenat Diagn* 1995;15:551–554.
79. Bruner JP, Yeast JD. Pregnancy associated with Friedreich ataxia. *Obstet Gynecol* 1990;76:976–977.
80. MacKenzie WE. Pregnancy in women with Friedreich's ataxia. *Br Med J* 1986;293:308.

13

Obstetric Anesthesia

Ferne B. Sevarino

INTRODUCTION

It is the position of both the American Society of Anesthesiology and the American College of Obstetricians and Gynecologists that labor analgesia should be provided to any parturient who requests it (1). A woman with coexisting medical problems may be limited in her options or encouraged toward certain options based on her (and her baby's) overall condition. For women undergoing surgical delivery, anesthetic choices may be limited by maternal coexisting conditions and fetal status. This chapter first will review labor analgesia and discuss choices for surgical anesthesia. Then anesthetic implications of coexisting medical conditions and disabilities will be discussed.

LABOR ANALGESIA

Preparation for birth begins with childbirth education. Being prepared and informed about the birth process will help all patients have a positive labor experience.

Most patients, especially primigravida and/or high-risk parturients, will need or want some type of labor analgesia. Choices include intravenous (IV) or intramuscular (IM) analgesics, spinal analgesia, epidural analgesia, or a combination of these. In most institutions in the United States, spinal and epidural analgesia is administered by anesthesiologists at the patient's and obstetrician's request. American Society of Anesthesiologists guidelines (2) require that an obstetric practitioner examine the patient and that a physician with obstetric surgical privileges be readily available when the analgesia is provided. IM or IV analgesia can be ordered by and administered without the presence of the obstetric practitioner.

Pain during parturition varies in origin and intensity as labor progresses. During the first stage of labor, uterine contractions and cervical effacement cause pain transmitted through afferent fibers traveling through the tenth thoracic to the first lumbar nerves. During the second stage of labor, pain from the distension of the vagina, vulva, and perineum is transmitted through the second to the fourth sacral nerve. As labor progresses, the frequency and severity of contractions also increases; thus both intensity and site of analgesia vary as labor advances.

The ideal labor analgesic should provide complete pain relief with no maternal or fetal adverse effects. That analgesic also should not affect the course of labor or the outcome of the labor. This goal has proved elusive, mostly because of the nature of labor and its associated pain. As described earlier, labor pain is intermittent; the intensity, quality, and location of the pain change as labor progresses. Like all pain, the amount of pain experienced varies widely among women (3,4). The obvious benefit of labor analgesia is relief of maternal pain and anxiety. The risk is that all analgesia is associated with a potentially undesirable effect on the fetus or mother. Systemic opioids cause nausea, vomiting, and sedation in the mother; sedation in the infant; and often inadequate pain relief. Paracervical block relieves only the pain of the first stage of labor and has the risk of direct fetal injection. Regional analgesia—epidural and/or spinal—is the most efficacious analgesia but may be associated with an impact on the course of labor or may be contraindicated in patients with coexisting disease. The use of regional analgesia in patients with coexisting disease may, in some circumstances, be beneficial to the patient and her medical condition. For example, the patient who is paraplegic or quadriplegic needs regional blockade to prevent autonomic hyperreflexia (AH), and the patient with significant cardiac disease will experience less cardiovascular instability with regional analgesia in labor. Later sections of this chapter will discuss the use of regional analgesia in patients with specific medical conditions.

Parenteral Analgesia

Parenteral opioids frequently are used for analgesia in early labor and in institutions where obstetric anesthesia care is not available. It is also the analgesic choice for patients who have medical contraindications to regional analgesia. Disadvantages of parenteral analgesia include maternal sedation, pruritus, nausea, neonatal respiratory depression, and inadequate maternal pain relief.

Patients may receive IM or IV doses of opioid or may be provided with IV patient-controlled analgesia as ordered by their obstetric practitioner. Table 13-1 lists opioids commonly used for parenteral analgesia.

Regional Analgesia

Regional analgesia for labor can be administered subarachnoid, epidurally, or as a combined spinal epidural (CSE) technique. Indication for regional analgesia is primarily maternal request. Contraindication to regional analgesia is maternal refusal, coagulopathy, severe hypovolemia, and infection over the site of needle placement. Relative contraindications must be viewed in the context of risk or benefit to the patient.

Prior to the administration of regional analgesia the patient must be examined by a practitioner privileged in obstetrics and fetal well-being. An obstetrician must be readily available, and a preanesthetic assessment by the anesthesiologist must be performed. All patients must have an IV catheter inserted and must be monitored with an automated blood pressure cuff and heart rate monitor (2). Co-existing disease may warrant additional monitoring.

Epidural Analgesia

Lumbar epidural analgesia provides effective pain relief for all stages of labor and, if needed, can be extended into the postpartum period or for cesarean delivery. An epidural catheter is placed, and medication is administered intermittently or by continuous infusion. The indication for epidural analgesia is pri-

TABLE 13-1. *Opioids commonly used for parenteral analgesia*

| Opioid | Traditional dosing | | Patient-controlled analgesia |
	Dosage	Interval	
Morphine	10 mg IM	2–3 hr	1 mg q 6 min with CI 1 mg/hr
	2–4 mg IV	1–2 hr	
Hydromorphone	1–2 mg IM	2–3 hr	0.1 mg q 6 min with CI 0.1 mg/hr
	0.2–0.4 mg IV	1–2 hr	
Meperidine	25–50 mg IV	2–3 hr	5–10 mg q 6 min
	50–100 mg IM	2–4 hr	4-hr limit of 200–300 mg
Fentanyl	50–100 µg IV	½–1 hr	25–50 µg IVq 4–6 min with 5–10 µg/hr CI
	25–50 µg IV	1 hr	
Butorphanol	1–2 mg IV/IM	q 4 hr	N/A
Nalbuphine	10 mg IV/IM	q 4 hr	N/A

CI, continuous infusion; IM, intramuscularly; IV, intravenously.

TABLE 13-2. *Protocol for ambulatory epidural*

Bed rest for >30 min for maternal and fetal monitoring
Before ambulation fetal heart rate should be within
  normal limits
Allow only if patient has normal motor function
Ambulation in the labor and delivery suite with an
  escort

marily maternal request. Early and continuous use of epidural analgesia is indicated in maternal preexisting conditions, as discussed later in this chapter.

After the epidural catheter is placed and its function is confirmed, the patient is made comfortable with a "loading dose" of medication and then a continuous infusion of a local anesthetic/opioid solution is begun. Continuous infusion of dilute local anesthetic solutions throughout the course of labor provides consistent, albeit not complete, pain relief for the parturient and is recommended for labor analgesia. The coadministration of epidural opioids with local anesthetic allows one to significantly and effectively dilute the local anesthetic administered in the infusions and decrease the total dose of local anesthetic administered. This effectively will eliminate or decrease motor weakness, minimizing the incidence of malposition and also allowing the parturient to ambulate if she chooses (5,6). Parturients who wish to ambulate should be assessed for adequate motor function and proprioception. The parturient must be accompanied at all times, and maternal and fetal assessment still must be performed in the

standard for the institution (Table 13-2). Ambulation has been shown to neither help nor hinder the progress of labor (7); however, the absence of motor block and the *ability to ambulate* improve patient satisfaction (8).

Table 13-3 provides a list of effective local anesthetic/opioid combinations. All opioid use may be associated with pruritus, which can be treated effectively with small doses of IV naloxone (40 to 80 g). These dilute solutions will provide effective, although not complete, analgesia throughout labor. Patients should expect to feel pressure and perhaps a sensation of cramping. If forceps are to be used, the epidural analgesia may need to be "densened" with the additional administration of a small dose of local anesthetic (Table 13-4). In patients with certain medical conditions, a denser local anesthetic block may be indicated for labor, and the medications administered would be modified to accommodate this need.

Combined Spinal Epidural

The technique of CSE may provide additional advantage in some patients. Intrathecal opioids provide adequate analgesia in the first stage of labor (9) and, when combined with the placement of an epidural catheter, will allow continuing analgesia with the "activation" of epidural analgesia later in the course of labor (8). This technique is especially valuable when used in parturients who are either in very early labor—less than 4-cm dilata-

TABLE 13-3. *Epidural infusions for labor analgesia*

Loading dose	Local anesthetic concentration	Opioid concentration
Bupivacaine 0.125% *or* Ropivacaine 0.1% with Hydromorphone 10 µg/mL Volume: 10 mL	Bupivacaine 0.0625%–0.05% *or* Ropivacaine 0.1%–0.2%	Hydromorphone 3 µg/mL
Bupivacaine 0.125% *or* Ropivacaine 0.1% with Fentanyl 5 µg/mL Volume: 10 mL	Bupivacaine 0.125%–0.0625% *or* Ropivacaine 0.1%–0.2%	Fentanyl 2 µg/mL
Bupivacaine 0.125% *or* Ropivacaine 0.1% with Sufentanil 1 µg/mL Volume: 10 mL	Bupivacaine 0.125%–0.0625% *or* Ropivacaine 0.1%–0.2%	Sufentanil 0.2 µg/mL

TABLE 13-4. *Supplement of analgesia for stage II labor*

Bupivacaine 8–10 mL of 0.25% solution
Ropivacaine 8–10 mL of a 0.2% solution
Lidocaine 8–10 mL of a 2% solution
2-chlorprocaine 8–10 mL of a 3% solution

tion—or in advanced labor. Those needing analgesia in early labor benefit from the almost-complete analgesia of a small dose of intrathecal opioid for approximately 2 hours without the need to administer any local anesthetic. In late labor an intrathecal dose of opioid provides almost instantaneous analgesia, again without motor blockade. Epidural analgesia can be instituted immediately, following testing of the catheter, with a dilute local anesthetic/opioid combination. Table 13-5 lists commonly used intrathecal opioids for this technique.

Intrathecal Analgesia

In some circumstances, labor analgesia may be provided with intrathecal administration alone, without the placement of an epidural catheter for CSE. Table 13-4 lists medications used for intrathecal analgesia. The disadvantage to this technique is that the duration of analgesia is limited to the duration of the medication administered through the spinal needle. Some indications for this technique include a patient's inability to cooperate with the longer procedure of epidural or CSE placement and borderline coagulation status where the benefit of analgesia with a small-gauge spinal needle outweighs the risk of bleeding. Other indications for this analgesic choice may be discussed by the anesthesiolo-

gist at the time of consultation for labor analgesia.

To summarize, labor analgesia with epidural or CSE provides profound analgesia. Epidural analgesia is initiated with small doses of local anesthetics and maintained with infusion of dilute local anesthetic/opioid solutions. Parturients in early or very late stages of labor may benefit from CSE. The occasional parturient may receive intrathecal analgesia alone. Parturients receiving epidural analgesia or CSE as described here may be ambulatory.

ANESTHESIA FOR CESAREAN DELIVERY

Publications cautioning against vaginal birth after cesarean (10) and expressing concern about neonatal outcome following vaginal breech deliveries (11,12) coupled with rising obstetric malpractice rates have lead to an increasing cesarean delivery rate. In many institutions, more than 25% of deliveries are by cesarean. It is therefore imperative that patients understand the anesthetic choices for cesarean delivery.

Regional Anesthesia for Cesarean Delivery

Regional anesthesia (spinal or epidural) now accounts for approximately 84% of all anesthetics for cesarean delivery (13). Regional anesthesia allows for an awake mother and avoidance of general anesthesia and the associated complications of failed or difficult intubation, hypoxemia, and aspiration. Similar to regional analgesia for labor, there are few absolute contraindications to regional anesthesia for cesarean delivery: patient re-

TABLE 13-5. *Intrathecal opioids for labor*

Opioid	Dose for CSE	Dose for IT analgesia
Sufentanil	2–5 µg in 1 cc NS	5–10 µg with bupivacaine 1.5 mg in a total volume of 1 cc NS
Fentanyl	10–15 µg in 1 cc NS	25–50 µg with bupivacaine 1.5 mg in a total volume of 1 cc NS
Meperidine	10 mg in 1 cc NS	10 mg in 1 cc NS

CSE, combined spinal epidural; IT, intrathecal; NS, normal saline.

TABLE 13-6. *Spinal anesthesia for cesarian delivery*

Local anesthetic	Dose (mg)	With opioid	Dosage
0.75% bupivacaine/8.25% glucose	12.5–15	Fentanyl *or*	50 µg
		Sufentanil *or*	5–10 µg
		Meperidine	10 mg
0.5% bupivacaine (not FDA approved)	15	Fentanyl *or*	50 µg
		Sufentanil *or*	5–10 µg
		Meperidine	10 mg

fusal, coagulopathy, severe maternal hemodynamic instability, technical problems, sepsis, and some maternal neurologic and cardiac disorders.

Complications of regional anesthesia include hypotension, high spinal, failed block, postdural puncture headache, and nausea and vomiting. Hypotension, nausea, and vomiting can be minimized by adequate IV prehydration and treatment with vasopressors and/or antiemetics. Failed blocks occur in approximately 1% to 5% of regional anesthetics for cesarean delivery (14); the block can be repeated, or general anesthesia can be induced. Treatment of a high spinal is supportive. Postdural puncture headache occurs in 1% to 5% of patients and is treated with hydration, caffeine, and, if needed, epidural blood patches. Incidence of postdural puncture headaches can be decreased to approximately 1% with the use of small-gauge, pencil-point needles (15).

Spinal anesthesia rapidly provides surgical anesthesia, with a low failure rate and a small drug exposure. Similar to its use for labor analgesia, its disadvantage is a limited duration of action. It also is associated with a higher incidence of hypotension and nausea and vomiting than epidural anesthesia, probably because of the rapid onset of a sympa-

thectomy. Epidural anesthesia can be used for a longer operation because the catheter allows for repeated dosing if needed. The ability to slowly titrate the desired dermatomal level results in less hypotension, which may make this a better choice in patients with hypertension and cardiac disease.

Tables 13-6 and 13-7 list medications for spinal and epidural anesthesia, respectively. Opioid is added to the solutions to improve intraoperative anesthesia and to provide some postoperative analgesia.

General Anesthesia for Cesarean Delivery

General anesthesia is used in approximately 16% of cesarean deliveries. General anesthesia is indicated when regional anesthesia is contraindicated or has failed. It is also appropriate in cases of extreme fetal distress, where it is felt to be most expeditious in achieving surgical anesthesia. Risks of general anesthesia primarily are related to airway problems: failed or difficult intubation and aspiration. Intraoperative recall also may occur. The degree of neonatal depression mirrors the duration of general anesthesia. One-minute Apgar scores are lower; 5-minute Apgar scores are no different than in infants of mothers undergoing regional anesthesia.

TABLE 13-7. *Epidural anesthesia for cesarean delivery*

Local anesthetic	Dosage range (mg)
Lidocaine 1.5%–2% (with or without epinephrine with or without alkalinization)	400–500
Bupivacaine 0.5%	100–125
Ropivacaine 0.5%	100–125
2-chloroprocaine 3%	600–750

The requirements for induction agents in the pregnant patient are decreased by 30% to 40% when compared to nonpregnant patients. Thiopental is the agent used most commonly. Its long safety record speaks for itself. Ketamine, etomidate, and propofol are also acceptable agents. Ketamine is the agent of choice for patients with hypovolemia or asthma; etomidate is useful in patients with cardiac disease. Succinylcholine is used for tracheal intubation; if further relaxation is needed, a short- or intermediate-acting nondepolarizing agent is used. Volatile anesthetic gases are used for maintenance of general anesthesia.

SPECIFIC CONSIDERATION FOR MEDICAL CONDITIONS IN THE PARTURIENT

The disabled parturient may have certain preexisting conditions that limit her choices for labor analgesia or anesthesia for cesarean delivery. This section will discuss common disabilities and their associated "special" consideration. If a patient has special issues, early discussion among all of her physicians allows for the formulation of a labor and delivery plan based on the severity of her disease.

Cystic Fibrosis

The wide range of cardiorespiratory and/or endocrine problems associated with cystic fibrosis must be considered in the delivery plan of a patient with this disease. Assisted vaginal delivery will minimize cardiorespiratory demands and avoid pneumothorax associated with vigorous Valsalva maneuvers. If vaginal delivery is assisted, epidural or spinal analgesia is needed. If cesarean delivery becomes the route of delivery, general anesthesia is well tolerated by most patients, with the use of invasive monitoring if surgery is indicated for deteriorating maternal cardiorespiratory status. Epidural anesthesia for cesarean delivery is also safe, providing the patient is able to lie flat for surgery and tolerate a high anesthetic level (16).

Cardiac Disease

The etiology of cardiac disease in pregnancy has changed over the last 20 to 30 years. There has been a significant decline in rheumatic heart disease. Now more women with congenital heart disease are surviving to reproductive age, and more women in their reproductive years are older and at risk for coronary artery disease. The risk to the mother with congenital heart disease depends on the structural abnormality and the functional impairment. The risk to the parturient with coronary artery disease depends on exercise tolerance and the extent of left ventricular dysfunction.

The danger for a pregnant patient with heart disease is the inability of the heart to meet the cardiac demands imposed by the physiologic changes of pregnancy, labor, and delivery. With aggressive care many women deliver healthy babies without complication. However, despite that same aggressive care, cardiac disease can lead to significant morbidity or mortality.

Pregnant women with known heart disease require management by a team including an obstetrician, anesthesiologist, intensivist, cardiologist, and pediatrician or neonatologist. Patients who fall into the American Heart Association (AHA) Class I or II (17) will remain asymptomatic during pregnancy and also will tolerate labor and delivery well. Patients in Class IV tolerate pregnancy poorly, often decompensating early in pregnancy as blood volume and cardiac output gradually increase to the point where their hearts can no longer meet the physiologic demands. Patients in AHA Class III usually do well through the 32nd week of pregnancy, when they may develop signs of heart failure as cardiac output peaks at 50% above baseline. If a patient with Class I, II, or III disease has an uncomplicated pregnancy and delivery, decompensation still may occur in the first 48 hours postpartum when blood volume and cardiac output continue to rise. Thus, even a cardiac patient who experiences no complications throughout pregnancy and parturition should be moni-

TABLE 13-8. *Anesthetic implications of structural cardiac lesions*

Structural pathology	Anesthetic goals	Intervention
Mitral stenosis	Maintain sinus rhythm	Early labor epidural with dilute solution
	Avoid tachycardia	Maintain epidural or other venodilator into postpartum period
	Avoid rapid ↓ SVR	Avoid ephedrine
	Prevent ↑ central blood volume	Avoid/use caution with spinal anesthesia for operative delivery
Aortic stenosis	Maintain sinus rhythm	Early labor epidural with gradual titration of level
	Avoid bradycardia	Early epidural also allows avoidance of GA (and tachycardia/hypertension associated with intubation)
	Avoid sudden changes to SVR	Avoid/use caution with spinal anesthesia for operative delivery
Idiopathic hypertrophic subaortic stenosis (IHSS)	Maintain SVR	Spinal/epidural relatively contraindicated because may ↓ SVR
	Avoid tachycardia	Avoid ephedrine use

GA, general anesthesia; SVR, systemic vascular resistance.

tored in an intensive care unit (ICU) setting for the first 2 days postpartum. If a patient needs aggressive interventions during her pregnancy and delivery, these also should continue at least 48 hours postpartum.

Specific to anesthetic management of the cardiac patient may be the use of anticoagulation, the need for invasive monitoring, and/or the timing of analgesia in the laboring patient. A patient using low molecular weight heparin (LMWH) should be converted to regular heparin at least 12 to 24 hours prior to anticipated delivery because regional anesthesia is contraindicated with LMWH (18). Table 13-8 summarizes anesthetic considerations for common structural heart lesions.

The patient with coronary artery disease can have a stress-free labor and delivery with the early placement of an epidural for analgesia and vigilant ICU care for the first 48 hours postpartum. Vaginal delivery should be the goal because maternal outcome may be better than with surgical delivery. This is especially true if the parturient has suffered a cardiac event in pregnancy. (19)

The Patient with Skeletal Deformities

Patients with achondroplastic dwarfism are more likely to require cesarean delivery (20).

Anesthetic concerns for these patients are multiple; craniofacial abnormalities, foramen magnum stenosis, and cervical spine abnormalities present scenarios for a potentially difficult airway. Respiratory complications are common, including chest deformities, sleep apnea, and upper-airway obstruction. These are complicated further by the decreased functional residual capacity accompanying pregnancy. These problems compound the respiratory compromise seen with high regional anesthetic levels or during emergence from general anesthesia. Spinal stenosis, lumbar hyperlordosis, and thoracolumbar kyphosis may be accompanied by neurologic impairment and may present technical challenges for regional anesthesia.

Preanesthetic assessment of these patients should include neck radiographs to assess cervical abnormalities and/or instability. Pulmonary function tests and an arterial blood gas test may be indicated. Based on the patient's condition, intrapartum use of an intraarterial catheter for blood pressure monitoring may be indicated.

The choice between general and regional anesthesia should be specific to the patient after airway assessment, respiratory assessment, and a neurologic examination are performed. The risk for difficult intubation may require awake intubation. General anesthesia may be indicated if the patient's respiratory status will not allow her to tolerate the supine position awake. Significant neurologic symptoms may preclude regional anesthesia.

Abnormal spinal anatomy in these patients increases the risk of technical problems, wet taps, and other minor complications with regional anesthesia. Single-dose spinal anesthesia may be associated with unpredictable spinal anesthetic levels; thus a catheter technique (epidural or continuous spinal), which allows for slow dosing, is preferred.

Osteogenesis imperfecta presents similar concerns for anesthetic care in labor. These patients also have spinal and airway abnormalities, which complicate anesthetic management. In addition, they are at risk for fractures as a result of fragile bones; they also may have bleeding abnormalities, which would preclude regional anesthesia. Prothrombin time, partial thromboplastin time, platelet count, and a bleeding time should be obtained prior to administering regional anesthesia.

Scoliosis and Spinal Surgery

Pregnancy is usually well tolerated in patients with scoliosis. Severe scoliosis is associated with cardiorespiratory compromise, which may worsen with the physiologic changes of pregnancy and require treatment in the peripartum period. Specific anesthetic concerns for patients with scoliosis are primarily technical. Placement of an epidural catheter in uncorrected scoliosis is technically more demanding. In corrected scoliosis the spine surgery may have obliterated the epidural space, resulting in patchy or nonexistent analgesia. Many patients have fused spines, leaving few interspaces uninvolved. X-rays and operative reports provide valuable information for the anesthesiologist in determining the most appropriate approach to the epidural space and should be obtained at the preanesthetic visit. If surgical delivery is necessary, again, the patient's cardiorespiratory status and her ability to tolerate the supine position are crucial to the choice of anesthesia.

Spinal Cord Injury

The majority of spinal cord injuries occur in the young, with a large number occurring in young females. Thus, pregnancy in patients with spinal cord injury is not uncommon. A woman's ability to carry and deliver a child largely is unaffected following spinal cord injury, although her disability may require interventions to ensure an uncomplicated labor and delivery. Abnormal presentation and failure to progress are more common in these patients and thus may increase the likelihood of cesarean delivery or assisted vaginal delivery. AH may occur in patients with lesions above T-10 (21). Antepartum consultation with an anesthesiologist for the early induction of epidural analgesia for labor is needed in these patients. If AH occurs before initiating analgesia, nitroprusside, hydralazine, or nitroglycerin should be used to control the blood pressure. AH despite epidural analgesia should be treated as indicated earlier and/or by "densening" the epidural blockade. Poorly controlled AH may necessitate an intraarterial catheter for blood pressure monitoring and aggressive antihypertensive therapy. There is no role for dilute solutions of epidural local anesthetics in these patients; solutions such as those listed in Table 13-7 are more appropriate. Spinal or epidural anesthesia should be administered in all patients with spinal cord injury for cesarean delivery,

Multiple Sclerosis

Multiple sclerosis is a demyelinating disease affecting the central nervous system, characterized by exacerbations and remissions over decades. It is twice as common in women than men. The rate of relapse during pregnancy is decreased, especially in the third trimester, and increases in the first 3 months postpartum. The changing neurologic picture in patients with multiple sclerosis must be appreciated when providing regional analgesic/anesthetic techniques. Spinal anesthesia has been implicated in exacerbations of multiple sclerosis, whereas exacerbations have not been reported with epidural anesthesia. Thus, spinal anesthesia should be avoided. If general anesthesia is elected for cesarean delivery, the exaggerated release of potassium with succinylcholine administration may occur. Also, prolonged response to nondepolarizing relaxants has been reported and is consistent with coexisting weakness (22,23).

SUMMARY

The anesthetic and analgesic choices for the disabled parturient are as diverse as those for women without comorbid disability. All patients should understand their analgesic options before parturition. This chapter serves as a review of analgesic/anesthetic options. A short list of specific disabilities is discussed. If a disabled parturient has concerns about her care, consultation with an anesthesiologist to develop an intrapartum analgesic plan is strongly recommended.

REFERENCES

1. American Society of Anesthesiologists. Statement of Pain Relief During Labor. Approved by the House of Delegates on October 13, 1999.
2. American Society of Anesthesiologists. Guidelines for Regional Anesthesia in Obstetrics. Approved by House of Delegates on October 12, 1988 and last amended October 18, 2000.
3. Wuitchik M, Bakar D, Lipshitz J. The clinical significance of pain and cognitive activity in latent labor. *Obstet Gynecol* 1989;73:35–42.
4. Palmer S, Lobo A, Tinnell C. Pain and duration of latent phase labor predicts the duration of active phase labor. *Anesthesiology* 1996;85:a858.
5. Halpern SH, Leighton BL, Ohlsson A, et al. Effect of epidural vs. parenteral opioid analgesic on the progress of labor. *JAMA* 1998;280:2105–2010.
6. Alexander, JM, Lucas MJ, Ramia SM, et al. The course of labor with and without epidural analgesia. *Am J Obstet Gynecol* 1998;179:516–520.
7. Bloom SL, McIntire DD, Kelly MA, et al. Lack of effect of walking on labor and delivery. *New Engl J Med* 1998;339:76–79.
8. Callis RE, Baxandall ML, Srikantharajah ID, et al. Combined spinal epidural (CSE) analgesia: technique, management, and outcome of 300 mothers. *Int J Obstet Anesth* 1994;3:75–81.
9. Honet JE, Arkoosh VA, Norris MC, et al. Comparison among intrathecal fentanyl, meperidine, and sufentanil for labor analgesia. *Anesth Analg* 1992;75:734–739.
10. Lydon-Rochelle M, Holt VL, Easterling TR, et al. Risk of uterine rupture during labor among women with a prior cesarean delivery. *New Engl J Med* 2001;345(1):3–8.
11. Hannah ME, Hannah WJ, Hewson SA, et al. Planned caesarean section versus planned vaginal birth for breech presentation at term: a randomised multicentre trial. *Lancet* 2000;356(9239):1375–1383.
12. Lumley J. Any room left for disagreement about assisting breech births at term? *Lancet* 2000;356(9230):1369–1370.
13. Hawkins JL, Gibbs CP, Orleans M, et al. Obstetric anesthesia work force survey, 1981 versus 1992. *Anesthesiology* 1997;87(1):135–143.
14. Reisner LS, Lin D. Anesthesia for cesarean section. In: Chestnut DH, ed. *Obstetric anesthesia: principles and practice,* 2nd ed. St. Louis: Mosby, Inc., 1999:465–492.
15. Lambert DH, Hurley RJ, Hertwig L, et al. Role of needle gauge and tip configuration in the production of lumbar puncture headache. *Reg Anesth* 1997;22:66–72.
16. Clark SL. Asthma in pregnancy. *Obstet Gynecol* 1993;1036–1041.
17. Chacko, KA. AHA medical/scientific statement 1994: Revisions to classifications of functional capacity and objective assessment of patients with diseases of the heart. *Circulation* 1995;92:2003–2005.
18. ASRA Consensus Statement 1998. Recommendations for Neuraxial Anesthesia and Anticoagulation. Developed from ASRA consensus conference, Chicago, IL, May 1998.
19. Hagay Z, Weissman A. Management of diabetic pregnancy complicated by coronary artery disease and neuropathy. *Obstet Gynecol Clin North Am* 1996(Mar);23(1):205–220.
20. Tyson JE, Barnes AC, McKusick VA, et al. Obstetric and gynecologic considerations of dwarfism. *Am J Obstet Gynecol* 1970;108:688
21. Obstetric management of patients with spinal cord injury. ACOG committee opinion. *Int J Gynecol Obstet* 1993;42:206.
22. Confareux, C, Hartchinson M, Houss MM, et al. Rate of pregnancy-related relapse in multiple sclerosis. *New Engl J Med* 1998;339:185–191.
23. Warren TM, Datta S, Ostheimer GW. Lumbar epidural anesthesia in a patient with multiple sclerosis. *Anesth Analg* 1982;61:1022–1023.

14

Baby Care Preparation: Pregnancy and Postpartum [1]

Judith G. Rogers, Christi V. Tuleja, Kris Vensand, and Through the Looking Glass

"Parenting is so difficult for anyone, so how does she do it?" "What a strong individual to be raising a child despite having a disability." Such statements from both professionals and laypersons convey a sense of worry as well as a sense of admiration when seeing a mother with physical disabilities. Her care for her baby may be perceived as beyond expectations and outside the norm.

However, for many women with disabilities having children is normal. In fact, it is often a lifelong dream just as it is for many nondisabled mothers. Nevertheless, many women who are disabled continue to encounter inadequate family and community support and/or inadequate access to useful resources and knowledgeable health care professionals. In fact, some women are pressured to terminate their pregnancies or relinquish their children by uninformed individuals unable to imagine how women with disabilities can care for their babies (1).

Despite social pressures and limited resources, numerous women with disabilities have cared for their infants successfully (2,3,4). Mothers with disabilities have been

and continue to be enormously resourceful about meeting their babies' needs. Regardless of how resourceful a mother may have been, most would have desired more support and resources during pregnancy, which is the time for planning and preparation. This chapter has been written to provide professionals with information about how to be a supportive resource for pregnant women with physical disabilities who are preparing to care for their new babies.

PREPARING THE PROFESSIONAL

A Supportive Approach: The "Can-Do Attitude"

Unlike most nondisabled women, women with disabilities usually do not receive a resounding "Congratulations!" when announcing their pregnancy to family, friends, and health care providers. Both directly and indirectly, many people convey disapproval and an unsupportive attitude. This is usually because, consciously or unconsciously, they have concerns about the woman's health or her ability to care for her baby. Some parents of women with disabilities may be concerned about the potential burden of caring for their grandchildren. They also may worry that their daughters will fail at baby care. Unfortunately, these reactions can undermine the confidence of the woman with a disability. Such women tend to avoid unsupportive individuals to maintain a sense of well-being during preg-

[1]This is a publication of the Research and Training Center on Families of Adults with Disabilities, and the National Resource Center for Parents With Disabilities, both funded by the National Institute on Disability and Rehabilitation Research of the U.S. Department of Education under grant numbers H133B30076-96 and H133A980001. The opinions contained in this publication are those of the grantee and do not necessarily reflect those of the U.S. Department of Education. Through the Looking Glass.

nancy and a positive and hopeful outlook on caring for their babies (1). Isolation can be one result of the lack of emotional support.

One important way a professional can support a woman with a disability is to recognize that she has the ability to be involved in the care of her baby. The importance of this "can-do attitude" is reflected in the findings of studies examining the impact of baby care adaptive equipment for parents with physical disabilities (5,6,7). At the end of the first study, parents were asked for general comments concerning the equipment intervention. A recurring theme was that parents found the occupational therapist's positive attitude refreshing because such responses to their parenting had been so rare. Additionally, this can-do attitude had an extremely powerful and positive impact on the parents' self confidence about their ability to care for their babies. A can-do attitude on the part of the professional when discussing the topic of baby care can be critical in forming a working relationship. Furthermore, if the woman feels supported she is more likely to share her baby care concerns, which makes mutual baby care planning more successful.

Visual History

To have a can-do attitude, professionals and laypersons may require a "visual history" of mothers with disabilities caring for their babies. A visual history is the accumulation of images of the various ways in which mothers with physical disabilities successfully perform baby care activities. These images often do not, but should, include the mothers using effective adaptive baby care equipment. Research has shown that parents with disabilities are more involved and more easily able to care for their babies with the use of appropriate adaptive baby care equipment (5,7,8).

The observer needs to be aware that an outsiders' perception of a mother's difficulty in providing care may be greater than the mother's self-perception. In two studies investigating the impact of baby care equipment on baby care activities for parents with disabili-

ties, occupational therapists tended to rate the level of parent difficulty or task demand while doing various activities as greater than the parents' self-ratings of the same task (5,7). One explanation for the differences between the perceptions of the parent and the person rating is the concept of "movement reference." Movement reference refers to internal kinesthetic memory created from years of using one's body in performing functional tasks. This gives us information such as, "My body moves this way when I diaper my child. Diapering usually feels easy." The observer appears to use her movement memory experiences as a reference point. Another reference point is visual history—that is, one's accumulated images of how it looks when other people do the same task. For example, when a person without a physical disability notices a person with a limp, they may interpret it in the following way: "I move in the usual way. Walking is easy. That person moves in a way that is different from my way. It appears awkward. Walking must feel different for them. It must be harder." Yet, the individual accustomed to walking with a limp internally feels her walking as normal for her and therefore not difficult.

However, if the observers perceive that they move similarly to the parent, the interpretation can be different: "I walk with a limp, it is not difficult for me, therefore it must not be difficult for them." In fact, this was noted in a study conducted in *Through the Looking Glass* (5) in which parents with physical disabilities were rated on various baby care activities. The occupational therapist with hemiplegic cerebral palsy perceived her movement style as similar to that of a parent she was rating. Her movement memory aligned with her observations (i.e., her one-handed diapering technique was similar to the way the mother completed diapering). With no *other* evidence of difficulty, the therapist rated the parent's level of difficulty as not very difficult. The rating seemed to be derived from the therapist's own movement memories. In contrast, the two nondisabled occupational therapists tended to rate the same diapering task as more challenging for the parent. Their reasoning process had much to do with the difference between what they observed and their personal movement references. This changed as both disabled and nondisabled therapists gained experience through direct intervention and indirect means (i.e., viewing videotapes). They relied less on their own movement references when assessing parent difficulty. Instead, the therapists relied more on behaviors, such as grimacing and/or wincing, which were interpreted as an indication of difficulty. This change may be evidence of the impact of visual history.

The professional who gains a visual history also will begin to internalize a can-do attitude. He or she should seek out disabled parents in the community to observe them doing baby care activities. In addition, professional resources (see "Resources" later in this chapter), such as videotapes of mothers with disabilities taking care of their babies, also can provide further opportunities for creating a visual history of parenting with a disability.

Assessing Baby Care and Parenting Abilities

A professional may be asked to assess the abilities of a mother with a disability to care for her baby. This is not a simple task, and a few important considerations need to be kept in mind. There are two aspects of parenting involved in such an assessment: the physical baby care and the psychologic or relationship potential.

The parent's ability to physically care for a baby can be assessed best when the parent has adaptive baby care equipment. Adaptive baby care equipment can decrease or eliminate environmental barriers so that the mother is able to care for her baby with more ease, less fatigue, and less chance of secondary injury (5,7,8). Lack of such equipment will give an inaccurate picture of the mother's ability to care for her baby.

Similarly, for a mother with a significant disability, the parent–child relationship can be properly assessed *only* if the mother has effective adaptive baby care equipment (3,9). Proper equipment allows the mother and the infant to get close enough to have the physical, visual, and verbal interactions that are necessary for the relationship to develop. Researchers investigating the impact of baby care equipment on parent–child interaction found that the baby care equipment decreased the physical demands of the baby care task on the parent. Further, this decrease in the physical demands of baby care was associated with an increase in positive parent–child interaction (5,7,8). Baby care equipment can increase physical proximity of the mother and child, and it can decrease the physical demands on the parent so that she is able to engage more freely with her child.

It is also important to remember when assessing a mother, with or without equipment and regardless of the degree of her disability, that she may elect not to be involved in some baby care activities. Her choice may be determined by her need to conserve energy for the more enjoyable tasks such as playing and feeding as well as a wish for her spouse or partner to do some of the baby care tasks.

If the professional is asked to assess a mother with a significant disability (such as quadriplegia), she or he needs to understand that the woman's involvement in her child's physical care can vary from being an orchestrator to being able to perform a number of tasks herself. In either case, the mother *can* establish and maintain a relationship with her child. In the latter case, the mother accomplishes this by interacting with her baby (e.g., playful eye contact, singing and talking to her baby) while someone else is physically performing tasks (3). By remaining present during the tasks the mother can orchestrate and control the baby care activities through directing the aide, and she also has an opportunity for eye contact and verbal interaction with her baby. In this way, the mother becomes a central focus for her baby during baby care activities, facilitating the parent–child relationship. (Having the mother orchestrate the activities is important so that the child learns to see the mother as the authority. This authority is crucial to her later being able to discipline her child.)

Discussing the Topic of Baby Care

The topic of baby care should be brought up early in a woman's pregnancy to provide an opportunity for her to share her concerns with respect to her role as a mother. Raising the topic of baby care can be challenging, however, because the pregnant woman may be feeling vulnerable if she has not experienced support from her general community and her family regarding her pregnancy.

A woman may have desired a child so much that thinking about potential barriers to her dream may be difficult to confront. The professional's supportive attitude, resources, and ability to build on the woman's ideas will help the woman begin to tackle obstacles one by one. As each baby care issue is handled or thought through, the pregnant woman's confidence will increase along with her problem-solving abilities. Usually, parents just need help initially to see that baby care problem-solving is no different from the every day problem-solving they already use when confronting environmental barriers.

The use of adaptive baby care equipment can make tasks possible or less demanding for most parents with disabilities. Bringing up the topic of baby care activities early in the pregnancy will allow the woman and her family enough time to have equipment adaptations made before the baby arrives. Finding the appropriate individual to make adaptations to baby care equipment may take time. In addition, it may take weeks and even months to complete the job. When equipment is made after the baby arrives, precious time has been lost in which the mother could have been more active in her infant's care or could have had more time for physical closeness and contact.

After the baby arrives, it is useful for the practitioner to be aware of psychosocial dynamics that may affect the woman's self-report of how things are going at follow-up visits. A mother initially may report that she is "having no problems," but on further conversation she may share that she is experiencing fatigue or muscle pain. Minimizing difficulties can be related to two phenomena: "supermom" and "disability accommodation."

The supermom pattern is familiar because it occurs with nondisabled as well as disabled mothers who push themselves to the utmost limits to appear capable of handling all situations or challenges both at home and at work. However, for the mother with a disability the need to be a supermom can be even more pronounced. A mother with a disability is less likely to receive social support or even may experience blatant prejudice with respect to parenting from the general community. This can add to her reluctance to report any difficulties she has with child care. This lack of support can pressure mothers with disabilities to try to appear completely capable of doing baby care activities without any assistance lest their parenting abilities be questioned.

Parents also may be reluctant to report true difficulties because of fear of being judged as inadequate and of having their children taken from them. Many parents with disabilities have heard frightening stories and seen media coverage of parents with disabilities who had children removed without an appropriate assessment (9). Therefore, in the clinical setting some parents initially may underreport their difficulties. These parents will need to be reminded that they really do not have to do *all* the baby care or to do it all perfectly to be good parents.

Another psychosocial influence that might lead to underreporting of baby care difficulties is the phenomenon of "disability accommodation." Disability accommodation develops in some people with a disability over time as they face numerous barriers in the environment. Despite resourcefulness at meeting the demands of the environment, some challenges usually remain. Individuals may learn to tolerate greater physical demands in many aspects of their lives. Therefore, their tolerance of frustration, pain, and difficulty may be higher during baby care and they may report only the most severe problems.

Some parents will be satisfied with their own baby care solutions. Consequently, it can be challenging to discuss with them a change that could make baby care easier, less fatiguing, or less painful. One way to approach this issue is to ask the parent to critique adaptive baby care equipment and/or an adaptive strategy. After using the equipment the parent may realize how difficult the task was without the equipment and may continue to use it. Each mother and situation is different. No one approach to inquiring about "how things are going" will be effective with all parents.

PRACTICAL BABY CARE PLANNING AND PREPARATION

Maintaining Physical Condition During Pregnancy

For many women, exercise to maintain physical conditioning may be essential to prevent loss of functioning or to ease a return to a pre-pregnancy level of functioning. Exercise also may increase range of motion and therefore facilitate a vaginal birth. In addition, it may maximize a mother's ability to care for her baby as well as prevent secondary injury during the baby care.

As important as exercise or physical therapy is, it may have negative connotations, reminding the woman of all the things she cannot do (1). This may be especially true for women who have a congenital disability and a history of physical therapy treatment. As a result, many women who have a disability do not exercise or seek treatment from a physical therapist. Explaining how an exercise program can later benefit her baby care skills may encourage her to start or maintain a physical regimen.

Performing exercises that maintain muscles needed to perform transitional baby care tasks (e.g., transferring, carrying/moving, positional changes) can be especially practical for facilitating the mother's skills. (The importance of transitional tasks is discussed later in the chapter.) Exercises focusing on the arms, trunk, and neck can strengthen transitional-task muscle groups.

Because of weight gain and the size of both the uterus and fetus, most women with disabilities will have their mobility and balance affected by pregnancy. Many women with disabilities are unable to walk or transfer themselves by the sixth month in the last trimester of pregnancy or in the beginning of the postpartum period. This change in mobility can put them at risk for falling. A fall in the beginning of the postpartum period can affect the mother's ability to participate in all aspects of baby care after the baby is born. Physical therapy intervention may help maintain safe walking and transferring functions. It may be necessary to discuss devices such as a motorized wheelchair, walker, or transfer board that can be used during pregnancy and postpartum.

Planning for Baby Care Equipment

Toward the end of pregnancy couples usually plan nurseries and receive baby care gifts. However, women who are disabled may need to guide family and friends toward considering their unique needs by purchasing "disabled-friendly" toys and equipment. Professionals can assist the mother and her family in deciding what baby care equipment might work. When deciding on baby care equipment the following should be considered: family roles, financial resources, home environment, and the mother's functional abilities.

The mother and her partner or other caregivers need to identify who will assume which baby care activities. Each family will have a unique way of sharing baby care that fits their lifestyle and their relationships. Some parents may work as a team to accomplish a particular task, whereas others will prefer to do them independently. Some mothers may rely on aides or extended family members to perform certain tasks.

In addition to role identification, the mother's or family's financial resources need to be considered when deciding to purchase or adapt a piece of equipment. Unless the family is able to utilize friends to do the service for free, the cost of an outside fabricator can be expensive when modifying or fabricating baby care equipment.

The mother and the professional also need to consider the physical layout of the home and any space restrictions before considering a piece of equipment. For example, this might make the difference between buying a standard crib and modifying it or making a larger one that has a diaper surface attached.

Most women who are disabled who have lived with their disabilities for a while know their bodies best and already may have a good deal of experience dealing with environmental barriers. Therefore, for the most part the professional can rely on the mother's feedback as to whether an equipment feature potentially will work for her. When the mother has a new injury or exacerbation, this process will be more one of trial and error. In general, a piece of equipment is assessed best in the home setting. Connecting the mother with professional resources in the community, particularly occupational therapists who are specialists in assessing functional daily skills and adapting equipment, can expedite this equipment development process. An alternative to finding an occupational therapist is to locate interested students at nearby occupational therapy or mechanical or rehabilitation engineering university departments.

Another valuable resource for a woman planning for baby care equipment is observing other parents with disabilities caring for their babies. This is similar to professionals, as this increases her visual history. Watching other parents doing baby care activities provides encouragement and stimulates problem-solving. The book *Adaptive Baby Care Equipment: Guidelines, Prototypes & Resources* and the videotape *Adaptive Babycare Equipment for Parents with Physical Disabilities* (see "Resources") can provide women with visual images of how parents accomplish various baby care activities using equipment. Locating other parents with disabilities in the community or obtaining videotapes of parents doing baby care activities can enhance the woman's self-confidence as well as provide practical solutions.

Importance of Transitional Tasks

Research indicates that problem-solving with respect to baby care activities should be-gin with "transitional tasks" (5,6,7). Transitional tasks (holding, transfers, carrying/ moving, and positional changes) are the essential movements within and between baby care activities (e.g., repositioning the baby for burping or transporting a child from the diapering surface to the highchair). Transitional tasks can be the most difficult aspect of care for parents and may impede the mother's ability to do most other baby care tasks from beginning to end. For example, one mother who has multiple sclerosis was able to do most of the baby care on the surface of her bed but found herself "a prisoner of her bedroom" because she was unable to hold and transport her baby in a safe and efficient way to other rooms. Equipment intervention gave her a means of securing her child on her lap and freed up her hands for functionally related tasks such as pushing her wheelchair, preparing bottles, and getting food for herself without leaving her child. After the parent and the professional have thought through equipment for transitional tasks, other potential baby care obstacles can be examined.

Commercial Baby Care Equipment

The mother and the health care professional first should investigate commercial baby care products as equipment solutions because they are less expensive and more available than specialized adapted equipment. Although not specifically designed for disabled users, some commercial products work well for mothers with disabilities or can be used in creative ways. For example, a bassinet Co-Sleeper on the market (see Right Start Catalogue in the "Resources" section) is open on one side and attaches to the parent's bed, thus eliminating the need to get out of bed to transfer the baby into the parent's bed. Reviewing baby care catalogues such as "One-Step-Ahead" or "Right Start" (see *Resources*) for the newest gadgets and changes in baby care products can be useful.

However, commercial products can prove to be, at best, frustrating to use or, at worst, an impediment to the mother's participation in the care of her baby. Much of what is commercially available is not designed for wheelchair users or people with reduced strength, reduced range of motion, standing balance issues, and/or lack of coordination. For example, the height of baby care surfaces such as cribs, highchairs, and diapering tables tends to be either too high or too low, making it difficult to transfer the baby from a wheelchair onto the equipment. Even able-bodied parents with normal range of motion and strength may have difficulty donning baby carriers and/or accessing cribs and highchairs while holding a baby. For this reason, new parents should be cautioned against buying standard baby care equipment and furniture without trying it out or considering how to overcome the equipment's limitations.

Modified or Newly Created Baby Care Equipment

Because most commercially available equipment does not meet all parents' baby care needs, the expectant mother likely will need to make alterations to generic equipment. For instance, a wheelchair user can change a baby's diaper on a standard table, desk, or card table with a foam pad and a child safety strap. A waist strap can be added to the portable nursing pillow made by Ecology Kid (for holding, feeding, and snuggling an infant on a mother's lap.)

Other solutions can be complex and require that the woman and trained professionals collaborate. For more technical adaptations or items made from scratch, one can use woodworkers, plastic manufacturers, seamstresses, welders, shoe-repair vendors, or sailmakers to modify existing products. Additionally, wheelchair repair companies employ individuals who have the skills and the interest in adapting wheelchair attachments. Finally, a rehabilitation or mechanical engineer can be another fabrication resource. The reader is referred to *Adaptive Baby Care: Equipment: Guidelines, Prototypes, and Resources* (Vensand et al. 2000), which has pictures and descriptions of more than 50 adaptive baby care prototypes that have been field-tested and effectively used.

Baby Care Techniques

Sometimes adaptive equipment alone may not be enough to reduce the physical demands of baby care. An adaptive technique in addition to equipment can be an important tool for making tasks easier or less demanding. Adaptive techniques are alternative ways of doing tasks and may include strategies for eliciting cooperation from the child. Appropriate baby care techniques can be practiced with a weighted doll during early pregnancy. Learning these techniques can provide the woman with additional strategies for physically managing her baby.

An occupational therapist can be a good resource for learning adaptive techniques for baby care. Many occupational therapists are familiar with one-handed techniques designed for adults who have had cerebral vascular accidents to use in daily living activities. These techniques can be applied to baby care tasks such as lifting and carrying the baby.

Transferring and transporting babies can be difficult tasks for women who have use of one arm, have limited upper-extremity strength and coordination, or are easily fatigued. Examples of techniques that can assist with transferring and transporting include the following:

Breaking down the task: To conserve energy and reduce task demand during transfers and transporting, mothers are encouraged to take time to rest and break the task down into smaller segments. Pausing between segments also may be beneficial.

Cueing: The parent is encouraged to cue the baby that a positional change or lift is about to occur. This can be done either verbally (e.g., saying the baby's name and counting "1, 2, 3") or by touching the baby to get his or her attention. This allows the baby to prepare for the lift or upcoming positional change. Some babies will become more still and compact (e.g., curl in a ball) to ease the lift for the parent (3).

One-armed lift: If the baby is lying supine with feet closest to the mother's chest, the mother leans forward and wraps her arm around the baby with support under the baby's head and neck. The mother then brings the baby to her chest and straightens up. This works best for a person with the use of one arm and without back problems.

Parents who cannot reposition or hold their babies up on their shoulders for burping can consider an alternative position and technique called *sit and lean*. For this technique, the parent holds the baby on her lap and faces the baby away from her body. Supporting the baby by placing one arm across the baby's chest, the parent then gently leans forward. This puts pressure on the baby's stomach and facilitates a burp.

Positioning the baby for diapering may be very challenging. The following techniques can assist with placing the diaper under the baby's bottom:

Cueing bottom up: As early as 1 month of age, some babies can begin to be taught to lift their bottoms up to assist the parent in placing the diaper under the baby's bottom. Initially, the parent cues the baby by moving the baby's bottom up and down and saying "up, up, bottom up." Young babies seem to enjoy having their bottoms moved up and down. Developmental changes—for example, the baby's discovery of his or her feet and increasing response to verbal cues—can decrease the need for the mother to actively assist in lifting.

Rolling to the side: Rolling the child to the side instead of lifting his or her legs to place the diaper can decrease the mother's need to lift the baby's legs.

Slide and lift: This technique is helpful for donning the diaper one-handed. With the baby's feet facing the parent, the parent places her palm up on an opened disposable diaper. While sliding the diaper under the baby, the parent lifts up the baby's bottom using the hand. The parent simultaneously cues the baby, "up, up, bottom up." This cueing begins to teach the baby to assist the parent during diapering.

PREPARING FOR A POSITIVE HOSPITAL STAY

A successful hospital experience can set the stage for the new mother to have more confidence in providing care for her baby. Supportive and knowledgeable staff can help relieve a mother's frustration at managing baby care tasks and help her cope by suggesting practical solutions. However, researchers investigating the impact of the health care delivery system on the care of the disabled pregnant woman found that there were few knowledgeable hospital staff who could give positive advice concerning baby care (10,11).

The occupational therapist and/or the mother may want to hold an in-service training prior to delivery for the hospital staff on techniques to assist the new mother in the care of her baby. Training can make the staff more aware of problems a mother who is disabled may face in the hospital setting. For example, a mother who does not have good grasp or strength may not be able to use the hospital's glass baby bottles. By being made aware of this problem, hospital staff can have alternative bottles available instead of questioning the mother's competency and the staff can feel more comfortable and confident in the mother's baby care ability. The in-service training should include a videotape of parents with disabilities doing baby care tasks as well as describing practical solutions (see "Resources," *Adaptive Babycare Equipment for Parents with Physical Disabilities*).

Practical issues not specific to baby care also need to be considered. These may include having durable medical equipment available during the hospital stay and asking the pregnant woman if she uses or needs a raised toilet seat or a shower chair so that the maternity ward can have them available for the new mother, thus making for a comfortable hospital stay.

Positioning for Holding and Nursing

Assistance may be needed at the time of delivery to facilitate closeness and physical contact between the mother and her newborn. After an arduous labor and delivery some mothers may shake uncontrollably, which can make holding the baby difficult. In addition, the reclining position of the delivery table can make it awkward for the mother to hold her baby on her chest. A new mother often has an intravenous line in her arm, which also can create challenges to holding and nursing the baby.

Having the father or the partner or the hospital staff assist the mother with holding her infant to her chest will allow the mother to focus on relating to her newborn rather than struggling to find a stable position for the infant.

After delivery some mothers may have problems holding and nursing their baby in the hospital bed because it lacks arm rests needed to help support or position the infant. For many people with disabilities arm rests provide the extra support needed for upper-extremity function. Therefore, providing a substitute for the arm rests such as sleeping pillows and/or nursing pillows may help the mother feel more confident because her baby is positioned more securely. Experimenting with a good position for holding and nursing is helpful for the hospital setting as well as for the home setting, especially if the mother is on bed rest.

For many mothers with a disability, the generally used "over the shoulder" burping position can be difficult or impossible because it requires muscle strength and coordination. The "sit and lean" technique discussed earlier in this chapter can be used to decrease the demands on the mother during burping.

For mothers who have had a cesarean section, the weight of the baby on the incision can cause pain. A new mother may feel so much pain and loss of mobility that she feels unable to hold her baby. Finding a comfortable position for the mother to hold and nurse her baby is especially important; one option is to have the mother lie on her side to nurse. The hospital stay is a good time for the mother to begin to understand her reaction to pain and its implication for baby care. Pain, whether it is from a cesarean section or from urination with an episiotomy, can trigger reactions such as increased spasticity or tremors, making baby care more challenging. One suggestion is to encourage the mother to schedule painful activities when the baby is sleeping so that she can recover from the pain before her baby needs her.

Breastfeeding Recommendations and Precautions

Women with a variety of disabilities can have special concerns related to nursing. Commonly reported breastfeeding discomforts for all nursing mothers are engorgement, infection, and the letdown reflex.

Dysreflexia can be triggered by physical discomfort in women with spinal cord injury with lesions at the level at T6 and above (12). *Mother To Be* (13) includes documentation of two women reporting dysreflexia during nursing: "For the first five minutes during the first month, my nipples were really sore and I could not hardly stand the pain, so when he first latched on it caused me to spasm really hard. My husband would have to stand there and hold my arms until I relaxed." Women who have a spinal cord injury at T6 and above should be aware of any dysreflexia symptoms and seek medical support.

Insufficient milk supply is another problem reported by women with upper-thoracic and cervical spinal cord injuries in *Mother To Be* (13). Some women may not have enough milk supply because of lack of sensation. For example, Sydney, who has a thoracic level 4/5 spinal cord injury, has sensation above the right nipple and below her left nipple. She was able to nurse from only her left breast. As she stated in her own words, "My milk dried up in my right breast and my right breast shrank back to normal two to three weeks after delivery."

There has been some controversy about whether breastfeeding can contribute to a multiple sclerosis exacerbation. A study done in 1998, however, "found breast feeding did not increase the risk of relapse or worsening of the disability in the postpartum period" (14).

In a study from the University of Manchester, researchers reported that women with rheumatoid arthritis might be susceptible to postpartum flareups, probably as a result of the increase of the hormone prolactin, which stimulates milk production. The researchers believe that "exposure to high levels of prolactin unaccompanied by correspondingly high levels of anti-inflammatory steroids could stimulate the development of RA in susceptible women" (15). Physicians may want to discuss this issue so women can be aware of this possibility when making choices about breastfeeding.

Nursing can be easier for women who have small breasts because it is easier for the baby to latch on and does not require as much use of one's hands. For women who have large breasts and limited hand use it is more difficult to provide breathing room for the baby's nose. Some women may find it easier to nurse if the bra cup is cut so the areola is exposed but the rest of the breast is held away from the baby's face.

Using an electric pump may be an issue for women with carpal tunnel syndrome. The vibration from the breast pump can cause wrist pain, making this procedure difficult.

POSTPARTUM FOLLOW-UP

The following are issues that many mothers with disabilities encounter as they care for their babies in the first few months of life. The professional can consider asking the mother about these topics directly or use the information presented here as background for discussions about how things are going for her at home.

Psychosocial Issues

Parents who have planned for practical, logistic issues before the baby comes home by having needed pieces of equipment and/or additional help may be better prepared for parental roles. However, some mothers with disabilities have expressed concerns about using adapted or modified equipment because it reminds them of the skills they do not have or are losing as a result of the progression of their disability. The adaptive equipment may be out of tune with their nursery fantasy if its appearance is unappealing.

Feeling incompetent is normal for most new mothers; however, for mothers with disabilities this feeling may be heightened. Mothers dealing with new or worsened disabilities, in particular, may worry that adaptive equipment or strategies will not provide "normal" experiences for their child or even might be detrimental to them. Many women can benefit from being introduced to other parents, perhaps in a support group with peers experiencing similar issues. Through the

Looking Glass, a nonprofit organization (see "Resources"), hosts a national parent-to-parent network that can connect mothers with disabilities who share similar experiences or face common barriers.

Another psychosocial issue that may emerge in the first 6 months relates to how family members accept equipment and support the new mother's independence and efforts to participate in the baby's care. Like professionals and parents with disabilities, families and friends of new mothers also may lack "visual histories." Therefore the families may have difficulty picturing how a baby care activity could be done in an adapted way. Furthermore, they may worry about the mother and/or baby's safety as well as the fatigue and stress mothers may experience. Sometimes a piece of equipment may threaten to usurp the grandparent's or other caregiver's self-perceived baby care role. Role divisions in the house are important to talk about because, although a piece of equipment may give parents with disabilities a new role, it also may take a role away from grandparents or other care providers.

When a piece of adaptive baby care equipment is introduced at or shortly after birth, a family system may not tolerate the quick change that it produces within the family. The possible simultaneous events of transitioning to motherhood and postpartum exacerbations can be more than families can handle. The baby care equipment temporally may be unused or refused until the family can adjust to changes more gradually (9).

Care Beyond Infancy—Staying One Step Ahead

Just as the mother settles into a routine at home with her infant and has become confident in using her adaptive infant care equipment, the child begins to grow and gain weight. This growth is accompanied by a series of relatively quick developmental changes such as rolling over, sitting up, climbing, and walking. These developmental changes may create new baby care equipment needs and/or new modifications to existing equipment. Continued involvement of an occupational therapist or another individual experienced in creating adaptive equipment and knowledge in adaptive techniques offers a crucial resource to the mother. An important task for the mother and the professional is to anticipate the child's growth and upcoming developmental changes. By anticipating the child's growth, equipment can be developed and ready in the home to assist the mother when needed.

It is important to note that as the specially designed equipment is being used, the families and/or professionals involved will need to monitor it for safety and continued appropriateness. Parts wear out and babies outgrow the equipment as they develop. These events may render the piece of equipment unsafe or impractical. Regular mechanical "tune-ups" (e.g., tightening bolts or replacing worn parts) are necessary to maintain adapted equipment's integrity.

One has to stay ahead of the baby's development and growth changes when providing equipment adaptations. Increasing mobility and weight can create challenges. However, in some respects, the physical care for the baby may become less demanding. For example, once the baby can climb from the floor onto the mother's lap, the need to lift is eliminated. Such cooperation may occur naturally or may be facilitated by intervention. In either case, development of the baby is fostered while physical demands on the parent are decreased.

Providing Developmentally Appropriate Experiences

For the child to develop properly he or she will need a variety of settings and experiences both within and outside the home. For some mothers, being able to provide these settings while maintaining access to their child can be a challenge. Mothers who are significantly disabled may decide to provide experiences to the child in one or two settings that are most accessible to them and safest for the child. For example, the mother might only allow the child access to a bedroom and the living room, which has been childproofed, while she is caring for the child. Another alternative is to build an elevated play center. The elevated play center is a large wooden playpen at a height accessible to a wheelchair rider (16). It can be used for baby care, for play, and to increase the baby's gross motor opportunities.

Floor time for the baby is important because it provides him or her an opportunity to develop motor and other skills. If the mother is unable to lift the baby up and down from the floor (with or without equipment) she will need to find others who can assist in providing this experience for the baby.

Companies are designing accessible parks and products that are increasing access into parks. Some portions of parks can still be inaccessible. The mother may need to bring another adult such as a friend or a mother's helper to assist with the physical lifting or monitoring of the child's safety in inaccessible areas. Using a walking harness also can provide the mother with security when in the community with her child (16). Adapting one's backyard may be a good alternative to playgrounds. Using a sand table that is accessible from a wheelchair instead of the low sandboxes found at playgrounds is one simple solution (17).

Home Support and Resources

Every new mother and family can benefit from extra help. It is therefore important to assess whether the family unit is overburdened. If the nondisabled partner already is doing extra work such as housework and a few baby care tasks, the family may want to find additional help. Although public policy usually precludes its use for direct baby care, many families may be eligible for outside support sponsored by the government such as in-home support services for help with housework and/or personal care assistance. If the family is not eligible for governmental support, setting up an alternative support system may be necessary. The family's religious affiliation may be a source for assistance to help with meals, household chores, and some baby care activities. A senior center is also another good resource for finding extra help because many seniors enjoy babies and also may need the extra income.

Although the extra support can be beneficial, it also can be a source of potential problems. A mother may be afraid to criticize the paid assistant for fear that the assistant will leave and she will be unable to find a replacement. For those families who have extra child care help, there is the possibility that the children will become more attached to the helper than to their parents. For this reason, it is important for the mother to maintain an active role in baby care so that the baby can see her as important and central to his or her well-being. For example, if someone else is diapering the child, the mother can be talking and playing with him or her during the task. The mother should direct the helper as to what clothes to put on, which food to eat, and what baby care task to do next. The use of adaptive baby care equipment can maximize the role of the parent and decrease the need for personal assistance.

Transportation for Mother and Baby

Some mothers who are disabled are unable to transfer their babies into safety car seats. Therefore, having knowledge of alternative forms of transportation can be important. Paratransit provides curb-to-curb service for individuals who use a wheelchair or other ambulatory assistive device. However, paratransit is not required to carry safety baby car seats or to transfer the baby into the safety car seat. This means that parents traveling with their babies must carry the baby car seat with them. Parents who use wheelchairs may find it impossible to carry a cumbersome car seat. Some parents have been successful at working with their local transit system to change the policies so that they will carry car seats and assist with transferring the baby into the car seats.

CONCLUSION

Both psychosocial and practical information are necessary to develop effective and supportive working relationships with disabled women during pregnancy. Adaptive

baby care equipment and support from a knowledgeable professional can provide women with disabilities a broader range of roles for involvement in baby care and help them achieve their dream of motherhood.

RESOURCES

The resources are current for 2003. Web sites and commercially available equipment keep changing. Check for new resources.

Organizations Serving Parents with Disabilities

Through the Looking Glass: The National Resource Center for Parents with Disabilities
2198 Sixth Street, Suite 100
Berkeley, CA 94710
(800) 644-2666
www.lookingglass.org

Charlotte Institute of Rehabilitation
1100 Blythe Boulevard
Charlotte, NC 28203
(704) 355-4300
www.carolinas.org/services/rehab/CIR/index.cfm

University of British Columbia, School of Nursing
Consultation Resource Services for Women with Disabilities
T201-2211 Wesbrook Mall
Vancouver, BC V6T 2B5 Canada
(604) 822-7444
www.school.nursing.ubc.ca/faculty/memberBio.asp?c=70.2993598832877

Woodrow Wilson Rehabilitation Center: Assistive Technology Services Division
Occupational Therapy Department
P.O. Box 1500
Fisherville, VA 22939
(800) 345-9972
www.wwrc.net/menuroot/AT-over-view.htm

Rehabilitation Institute of Chicago (RIC)
Health Resource Center for Women with Disabilities
345 East Superior Street, Suite 106

Chicago, IL 60611
(312) 238-1051
www.rehabchicago.org

Commercial Baby Care Equipment Catalogues

Perfectly Safe
7090 Whipple Avenue
North Canton, OH 44702
(800) 898-3696
www.perfectlysafe.com

One Step Ahead
P.O. Box 517
Lake Bluff, IL 60044
(800) 950-5120
www.onestepahead.com

The Right Start: Babies to Kids
5334 Sterling Center Drive
West Lake, CA 91361
(800) 548-8531
www.rightstart.com

Adapted Equipment (Mentioned in Chapter)

Co-Sleeper
Arm's Reach Concepts, Inc.
2081 North Oxnard Boulevard, P.M.B. #187
Oxnard, CA 93030
(800) 954-9353
www.armsreach.com

Bottle Holder "Baby Bundle"
Little Wonders
P.O. Box 728
Newfoundland, NJ 07435
(800) 639-2984
littlewonder@earthlink.net
www.littlewonders.com

Harness and Hand Strap
Gerber
45 Krupp Drive, Suite 30
Williston, VT 05495
(802) 862-4641, extension 22
info@kidsurplus.com
www.kidsurplus.com

The Kid Keeper
One Step Ahead Online Store
P.O. Box 517

Lake Bluff, IL 60044-0517
(800) 274-8440
questions@onestepahead.com
www.onestepahead.com

Kid Kozy Nursing Pillow
207 West Los Angeles Avenue, #190
Moorpark, CA 93021-1824
(866) 543-5699
sales@kidkozy.com
www.kidkozy.com

Phone Pal Phone Holder
Sammons Preston Rolyan (an AbilityOne Company)
4 Sammons Court
Bolingbrook, IL 60440-5071
(800) 323-5547
spr@abilityone.com
www.sammonspreston.com

Snugli Early Care Sling
Evenflo Company, Inc.
1801 Commerce Drive
Piqua, OH 45356
(800) 233-5921
parentlink@evenflo.com
www.snugli.com
Snugli Early Care Sling has been discontinued; used baby stores may carry.

Outdoor Recreation

Grounds for Play
1401 East Dallas Street
Mansfield, TX 76063
(800) 552-7529
www.grounsforplay.com

Mobi-Mat/RecPath
Recreation Dynamics, Inc.
10012 James Monroe Highway
Culpeper, VA 22701
(866) 221-6999
www.recreationdynamics.com/shots/single/2.php

The World Playground, Parks & Recreation Products and Services Web Directory-Accessible Equipment
List names of manufacturers that offer disability accessible playground equipment,

accessories, and components and products.
(800) 352-1137
www.playgrounddirectory.com/accessible.htm

Newsletters

Parenting with a Disability
Through the Looking Glass
2198 Sixth Street
Berkeley, CA 94710
(800) 644-2666
TLG@lookingglass.org
www.lookingglass.org/newsletter

Disability, Pregnancy & Parenthood International
National Centre for Disabled Parents
Unit F9, 89-93 Fonthill Road
London N4 3JH England
020 7263 3088
Fax: 020 7263 6399
info@dppi.org.uk
www.dppi.org.uk/journal/index.html

Resourceful Women
Health Resource Center for Women with Disabilities
345 East Superior Street, Suite 106
Chicago, IL 60611
(312) 238-1051
www.rehabchicago.org/community/hrcwd.php

Community Resources

Independent Living Centers (ILCs)
Directory from ILRU lists all ILCs in the country.
(713) 520-0232
www.ilru.org/silc/silcdir/index.html

Community Technology Centers' Network (CTCNet)
372 Broadway Street
Cambridge, MA 02139
(617) 354-0825
dschackman@ctcnet.org
www.ctcnet.org/mission.html

American Occupational Therapy Association (AOTA)
4720 Montgomery Lane

P.O. Box 31220
Bethesda, MD 20824
(301) 652-2682
www.aota.org

Rehabilitation Engineers of North America (RESNA)
1700 North Moore Street, Suite 1540
Arlington, VA 22209
(703) 524-6686
www.resna.org

Tetra Society of North America
Recruits skilled volunteer engineers and technicians to create assistive devises for people with disabilities.
770 Pacific Boulevard South
Box 27, Suite A304
Plaza of Nations
Vancouver, BC V6B 5E7 Canada
(877) 688-8762
info@tetrasociety.org
www.tetrasociety.org

Volunteers for Medical Engineering (VME)
2301 Argonne Drive
Baltimore, MD 21218
(404) 243-7495
vme@toad.net
www.toad.net/~vme

Videotapes/Publications: Parenting with a Physical Disability

Adaptive Baby Care Equipment: Guidelines, Prototypes & Resources
This publication provides guidelines for problem-solving baby care challenges; photographs and descriptions of over 50 pieces of baby care equipment prototypes; adaptive baby care techniques; adaptive baby care equipment safety checklist; commercial products; Commercial Product Safety Commission guidelines; and local and national resources.
Through the Looking Glass
2198 Sixth Street
Berkeley, CA 94710
(800) 644-2666
www.lookingglass.org/publications/pubdetails.php#ABCE

Adaptive Babycare Equipment for Parents with Physical Disabilities [10 min VHS]

Demonstrates how parents with physical disabilities have successfully used adaptive baby-care equipment and adaptive baby-care techniques.

Through the Looking Glass
2198 Sixth Street
Berkeley, CA 94710
(800) 644-2666
www.lookingglass.org/publications

Disability and Motherhood [25 min VHS]

Stories of three mothers with physical disabilities share their experiences of motherhood and disability and discuss public attitudes.

Films for the Humanities and Sciences
P.O. Box 2053
Princeton, NJ 08543-2053
(800) 257-5126
www.films.com/Films_Home/item.cfm?s=1& bin=5407

Positive Images [58 min VHS]

Women Make Movies
462 Broadway, Suite 500WS
New York, NY 10013
(212) 925-0606
www.wmm.com/catalog/pages/c130.htm

Childcare with Bilateral Transradial Amputations [15 min VHS]

Shows the level of independence that can be achieved by a motivated individual using prostheses. The person, a male in his twenties who sustained bilateral transradial amputations, demonstrates childcare with his initial set of cable-operated voluntary-opening split hooks and subsequently with his myoelectric prehensors.

Rehabilitation Institute of Chicago
LIFE Center
345 East Superior Street, First Floor
Chicago, IL 60611
(312) 238-5433
lifecenter.bitwrench.com/content/1965/?topic =3&subtopic=

REFERENCES

1. Rogers J, Matsumura M. *Mother to be: A guide to pregnancy and birth for women with disabilities.* New York: Demos Publications, 1991.
2. Garee B, ed. *Parenting tips for parents (who happen to have a disability) on raising children.* Bloomington, IL: Accent Special Publications; Cheever Publishing, Inc., 1989.
3. Kirshbaum M. Parents with physical disabilities and their babies. *Zero to Three* 1988;8(5):8–15.
4. Scheele C. Woman and SCI. Part 4: Motherhood–Three perspectives. *Paraplegia News* 1988;42(9):31–34.
5. Through the Looking Glass. *Developing adaptive equipment and adaptive techniques for physically disabled parents and their babies within the context of psychosocial services.* Berkeley: Through the Looking Glass, 1995.
6. Tuleja C, DeMoss A. Babycare assistive technology. *Technology and Disability* 1999;11:71–78.
7. Tuleja C, Rogers J, Vensand K, et al. *Continuation of adaptive parenting equipment development.* Berkeley: Through the Looking Glass, 1998.
8. DeMoss A, Kirshbaum M, Tuleja C, et al. *Adaptive parenting equipment: Evaluation, development, dissemination and marketing.* Berkeley: Through the Looking Glass, 2000.
9. Kirshbaum M. Babycare assistive technology for parents with physical disabilities: Relational, systems, and cultural perspectives. *American Family Therapy Academy Newsletter* 1997;67:20–26.
10. Lipson J, Rogers J. Pregnancy, birth and disability: Women's health care experiences. *Health Care for Women International* 1997;21(1):11–26.
11. Rogers J, Lipson J. *Final report: Pregnancy, birth and early postpartum among women with disabilities.* Berkeley: Through the Looking Glass, 1998.
12. Ozer M. *The management of persons with spinal cord injury.* New York: Demos Publications, 1998.
13. Rogers J, Matsumura M. *Mother to be: A guide to pregnancy and birth for women with disabilities,* 2nd ed. New York: Demos Vermande Publications, in press.
14. Confavreux C, Hutchinson M, Hours MM, et al. Rate of pregnancy-related relapse in multiple sclerosis. *New Engl J Med* 1998;339(5):285–291.
15. Barrett JH, Brennan P, Fiddler M, et al. Breast-feeding and postpartum relapse in women with rheumatoid and inflammatory arthritis. *Arthritis Rheum* 2000;43(5): 1010–1015.
16. Vensand K, Rogers J, Tuleja C, et al. *Adaptive baby care equipment: Guidelines, prototypes & resources.* Berkeley: Through the Looking Glass, 2000.
17. DeMoss A, Rogers J, Tuleja C, et al. *Adaptive parenting equipment: Idea book I.* Berkeley: Through the Looking Glass, 1995.
18. Charlifue SW, Gerhart KA, Menter RR, et al. Sexual issues of women with spinal cord injuries. *Paraplegia* 1992;30:192–199.
19. Jackson AB. Pregnancy and delivery. In: Krotoski D, Nosek M, Turk M, eds. *Women with physical disabilities.* Baltimore: Brookes, 1996:91–99.

15

Infertility Diagnosis and Treatment for the Disabled Woman

Natalie E. Roche and Gerson Weiss

There are between 4.5 million and 8 million infertile couples in the United States. This means infertility for one in 12 reproductive-aged couples and 15% of reproductive-aged women, according to the 1988 data from the National Center for Health Statistics and the National Survey in Family Growth.

There are approximately 28 million women who are disabled in the United States. There is currently no good estimate of the total number of women with disabilities who are infertile, but infertility rates are unlikely to be different from the general population. The standard definition of infertility is the inability to achieve pregnancy after 1 year of unprotected sexual contact. Fertility rates for women begin to decline after age 30, and this decline in fertility accelerates after age 38. Infertility diagnostic and treatment services for older women therefore are designed to address the issue of age-related infertility.

The desire for reproduction is a basic interest of most couples. The diagnosis of infertility can be a painful and difficult situation for all couples. The couples in which the female partner is disabled, however, face a unique set of concerns and barriers as they seek treatment for infertility. Those concerns and barriers include the distinct medical limitations imposed by an individual woman's medical condition. The woman who is disabled also may be subject to prejudice from family, friends, the medical community, and society at large as she attempts to achieve pregnancy. The woman who is disabled also may face economic barriers, including lack of health insurance, which may limit the options available for the diagnosis and treatment of infertility. It is imperative that those who give medical care to this patient population be sensitive to the additional stress placed on infertile couples when the female partner has a disability

CAUSES OF INFERTILITY

The causes of infertility in women who are disabled are similar to the general population. The most common causes of infertility in women are anatomic problems and hormonal problems. Infertility in women is caused to a lesser degree by impaired sexual function, unexplained infertility, cervical factors, and congenital anomalies of the reproductive tract. Male factor infertility is the responsible or contributing factor for infertility in 30% to 50% of infertile couples.

Male Factor Infertility

Male factor infertility frequently is overlooked and therefore is underdiagnosed and undertreated. The initial evaluation of the male partner is simple and straightforward. The evaluation should include a careful medical, surgical, family, and sexual history. In addition, a review of systems, list of current medications, and data regarding past fertility should be obtained. A complete physical examination with emphasis on evaluation of secondary sexual characteristics and the genitalia is mandatory.

The vast majority of infertility in males will be caused by the quality of the semen. Problems with the mechanics of placement of semen in the female can be a cause of male infertility but are generally a lesser factor.

The cornerstone of the laboratory evaluation of the male partner is semen analysis. Additional laboratory testing may be indicated including genital cultures, specialized semen evaluation, imaging studies, and genetic evaluation. The differential diagnosis of causes of male infertility include the following:

Infections: Mumps orchitis causes testicular atrophy; sexually transmitted diseases can cause scarring of the epididymis.

Structural: Cryptorchidism decreases sperm count; varicoceles obstruct the passage of sperm through the vas deferens.

Postsurgical: Prostatectomy and bladder-neck surgery can cause retrograde ejaculation.

Substance use: Alcohol, caffeine, marijuana, nicotine, cimetidine, and sulfasalazine can impair sperm production.

Genetic: Kallmann's syndrome (hypogonadotropic hypogonadism) can be a genetic factor.

Sexual behavior: Impotence is a factor; excessive intercourse and masturbation can decrease sperm counts.

The treatment of male factor infertility is directed toward the underlying cause. The success rates for treatment are diagnosis specific.

Female Factor Infertility

The most common causes of infertility in women are anatomic and hormonal. The anatomic causes of female factor infertility include tubal occlusion, endometriosis, structural abnormalities of the genital tract, and cervical factors. The hormonal causes of female factor infertility include ovarian dysfunction, hypothalamic dysfunction, and pituitary disease. Lesser causes of infertility in women include unexplained infertility and sexual dysfunction.

ANATOMIC CAUSES OF FEMALE INFERTILITY

The list of diseases associated with infertility in this category includes tubal occlusion, endometriosis, Asherman's syndrome, uterine septae/congenital anomalies of the reproductive tract, uterine and cervical polyps, and leiomyoma. All of these structural problems inhibit fertility by presenting a mechanical barrier to either fertilization or implantation.

Tubal occlusion is largely the late sequelae of pelvic infections and endometriosis. Pelvic inflammatory disease occurs in approximately 1.3 million American women each year. Infertility associated with pelvic inflammatory disease is estimated by Westrom to be 11.4% after a single episode, 23.1% after a second episode, and 54.3% after a third episode of infection. The diagnosis of pelvic inflammatory disease in women who are disabled can be complicated, according to Welner and Hammond. The reliability of classic signs and symptoms of pelvic infection can be limited in some women who are disabled. Women who are visually impaired may not be able to see genital lesions and discharge associated with sexually transmitted diseases. Other women who are disabled may have limited pelvic sensation. The usual findings of pelvic pain and cramping associated with pelvic infection may be absent, and spasticity and increased malaise may be the dominant symptoms. Delays in diagnosis of pelvic infection in some women who are disabled may predispose them to increased risk of tubal damage and infertility. Endometriosis commonly has been associated with pelvic pain and infertility. Tubal damage secondary to adhesions is a well-accepted mechanism for infertility in women who have endometriosis. The presence of peritoneal disease is less well accepted as an etiologic mechanism for infertility. The American Fertility Association classification of the severity of endometriosis correlates well with the likelihood of infertility. The more severe the diagnosis of endometriosis, the greater the chance of infertility. There is no evidence that women who are disabled are more likely to have endometriosis. They may be less likely to have a correct diagnosis and treatment of endometriosis because of fewer gynecologic encounters, atypical presentations, and lower index of suspicion by patients and practitioners.

Structural abnormalities are confined largely to polyps, leiomyoma, synechiae, and congenital anomalies of the female reproductive tract. The structural problems inhibit fertility by presenting a mechanical barrier to fertilization or implantation. There is no evidence at present that women who are disabled are at increased risk for problems in this category.

Hormonal derangements have the final common pathway of anovulation. The most common cause is ovarian dysfunction followed by hypothalamic dysfunction and pituitary disease. Some of the pathologic conditions seen in this category include polycystic ovarian disease, obesity, eating disorders, hyperprolactinemia, hypothalamic amenorrhea, premature ovarian failure, Cushing's disease, thyroid disease, and stress. Although data are limited, there is some information suggesting that women who are disabled may be at increased risk for hormonal derangement. Women with traumatic spinal cord and brain injuries have been reported to have oligomenorrhea and amenorrhea after their injuries. Elevated prolactins and galactorrhea have been noted for months after the acute insult in patients with brain injury. Women with autoimmune diseases including Sjögren's syndrome, scleroderma, lupus, rheumatoid arthritis, and multiple sclerosis have been documented to have menstrual irregularities, which are thought to be related to hypothalamic amenorrhea associated with chronic illness. Women who are disabled are also more likely than the general population to be exposed to medications that can interfere with ovulatory function.

The less common causes of infertility in women include anatomic derangements, cervical factors, drug use, sexual dysfunction, and unexplained infertility.

Drug use can interrupt normal ovulation. There is a long list of medications that have the potential to impair fertility. The woman

TABLE 15-1. *Drugs that can affect fertility*

Antipsychotics, anxiolytics, and hypnotics
Anticholinergics
Hormones
Antiandrogens
Antidepressants
Antihypertensives
Dopamine antagonists
H_2 antagonists
Psychotropic drugs

who is disabled may be at increased risk because she is more likely to be exposed to medications that have an impact on fertility. Prescription medications in this category that are used routinely by women who are disabled include antidepressants, steroids, and analgesic antiemetics (Table 15-1).

Sexual dysfunction can be a cause of infertility. The woman who is disabled may be at particular risk for this problem. The fatigue and pain associated with chronic illness may decrease the frequency of coital exposure in this population. The ability to have sexual intercourse three to four times per week is thought to optimize pregnancy rates, but may be difficult to achieve; some disabled women with spasticity and bladder and bowel control problems also may have diminished coital frequency. Women with paralysis may have impaired lubrication, and the use of lubricants, which impair sperm motility, may present a significant problem.

Cervical factors probably play an insignificant role in the problem of modern infertility treatment.

Unexplained infertility is a diagnosis of exclusion and is estimated to present in as many as one-third of infertile couples. There are no data to suggest that infertile women with disabilities are different than other women who have this diagnosis.

DIAGNOSTIC EVALUATION

The diagnostic workup for the woman who is infertile should be performed in an organized and cost-effective manner. The purpose of the evaluation is to identify correctly the cause(s) of infertility so that the most appropriate treatment plan can be formulated. Patients for diagnostic evaluation should be selected based on their inability to achieve conception after 1 year of unprotected intercourse. Patients who are appropriate for earlier evaluation are women age 35 years and older and those with infertility combined with other gynecologic abnormalities. Gynecologic abnormalities that warrant early infertility evaluation include the following:

1. Menstrual irregularities
2. Dyspareunia
3. History of pelvic inflammatory disease or ruptured appendix
4. Prior abdominal surgery
5. Endometriosis

The infertility evaluation should include careful history, physical examination, and laboratory tests. The data collected should include a medical, surgical, sexual, past fertility, and family history. A list of current medications and a review of systems should be included. Detailed preconception counseling is advisable, particularly when complex medical conditions are present. All patients should be offered screening for human immunodeficiency virus (HIV), rubella, and hepatitis B and should be offered folic acid supplementation.

Complete physical and pelvic examinations should be performed with emphasis on body hair distribution, body mass index, thyroid gland, secondary sexual characteristics, and the pelvic examination. The cornerstones of diagnostic testing for the infertile female are the determination of tubal patency, documentation of ovulation, and the endocrine evaluation.

Determination of tubal patency can be accomplished using hysterosalpingography, laparoscopy, hysteroscopy, or sonohysteroscopy. Each technique has its limitations. Hysterosalpingography is performed in the follicular phase of the menstrual cycle. Dye is injected into the uterus and will pass through patent fallopian tubes. This test can be used to diagnose pathology of the uterus and fallopian tube, including malformations and obstruc-

tion. When the test is positive for tubal occlusion, the use of a confirmatory test to establish the diagnosis is advisable.

Sonohysteroscopy can be used to diagnose uterine pathology by introduction of saline into the uterine cavity. This technique is very good for polyps, synechiae, and leiomyomas; it has limited value for evaluation of the fallopian tubes. *Hysteroscopy* can be used to diagnose uterine pathology. An advantage is that uterine pathology can be treated at the same time as diagnosis. It has limited value in the evaluation of the fallopian tubes.

Laparoscopy can be used to assess tubal patency when combined with chromotubation. It has the advantage that tubal pathology can be treated at the same time as diagnosis. It has limited value for initial evaluation of the infertile female. Intrauterine pathology cannot be evaluated. Laparoscopy for the evaluation of couples with unexplained infertility is not recommended because of the low yield for positive findings.

TABLE 15-2. *Autonomic dysreflexia*

Cause
Activation of the autonomic nervous system by painful stimuli from visceral organs. In patients with lesions above T6, signal from receptor travels up the spinal cord until it is blocked. Vasoconstriction causes blood pressure to rise, and parasympathetic discharge cannot travel down the spinal cord so blood pressure continues to rise.

Clinical Findings
1. Muscle spasms usually of the lower extremities
2. Headache
3. Labile hypertension
4. Sweating
5. Cardiac arrhythmias medicated by vagus nerve
6. Nasal congestion
7. Dilated pupils
8. Flushing

Severe Complications
1. Seizure
2. Intracranial hemorrhage
3. Coma
4. Death

Triggers
Uterine contractions, ovarian cyst rupture, urinary tract infection, distention of the urinary bladder, severe constipation, fecal impaction, ectopic pregnancy, decubitus ulcers, appendicitis, etc.

Treatment
Determine cause and remove painful stimulus, lower blood pressure (sublingual nifedipine).

The disabled woman can present a unique challenge when tubal patency is evaluated, especially with regard to positioning for the examinations. Patients with spinal cord injuries above T6 may develop autonomic dysreflexia during hysterosalpingography or sonohysteroscopy (Table 15-2). Careful monitoring and the ability to treat this potentially life-threatening complication are necessary. An alternative approach is to proceed to more invasive testing using hysteroscopy and laparoscopy with the patient under general anesthesia.

ASSESSMENT OF OVULATION

A thorough menstrual history is invaluable when it is time to assess ovulation. Simple diagnostic tests that can be used at home are part of the initial evaluation of ovulatory function. Basal body temperature (BBT) charting and ovulation prediction kits are easy to use. More invasive testing includes serum progesterone, serial transvaginal ultrasound, and endometrial biopsy.

Basal Body Temperature Charting

BBT is used to document the temperature rise, which is an indirect indicator of ovulation. The charting is limited because some ovulatory women do not demonstrate a temperature rise. Also, the timing of ovulation cannot be determined with accuracy, and BBT can be inconvenient to use for patients who travel or have inconsistent schedules. Women with visual impairments will require help to use BBT.

Ovulation prediction kits are used to identify the midcycle surge in luteinizing hormone (LH), which is an indirect measure of ovulation. More expensive than BBT, the accuracy of the kits varies. Kits can be difficult to use in patients with irregular cycles. Women with visual impairments will require help to use the ovulation prediction kits also.

Serum Progesterone

Serum progesterone can be used as indirect evidence of ovulation. When progesterone levels are more than 3.0 ng/mL, it is assumed that ovulation has taken place. The pulsatile nature of the progesterone release can make low, normal, and negative results difficult to interpret accurately. The test requires travel to a lab or the physician's office. The travel requirement is inconvenient for patients who are disabled, particularly those with limited mobility.

Transvaginal Ultrasound

Transvaginal ultrasound is used to evaluate the number, size, and architecture of developing follicles. This test is expensive and time consuming.

Endometrial Biopsy

Endometrial samples are taken 2 to 3 days before the expected period to evaluate the endometrium. The presence of secretory endometrium is evidence that ovulation has taken place. The test is expensive and inconvenient and may cause patient discomfort. The test rarely is used in the modern infertility evaluation. The only indication is for the evaluation of luteal phase defects. Women at risk for autonomic dysreflexia will require careful monitoring and the presence of staff who can manage this complication.

ENDOCRINE EVALUATION

Patients should have an evaluation of ovarian reserve. Common endocrine abnormalities that can affect fertility should be ruled out, including thyroid disease and prolactin disorders. Thyroid-stimulating hormone (TSH) and prolactin are sent as routine labs. Follicle-stimulating hormone (FSH) and estradiol are drawn on day 3 of the cycle. If FSH and estradiol are elevated, they indicate poor ovarian reserve, and poor response to treatment is anticipated. Clomiphene Citrate Challenge Test (CCCT) has proven to be efficacious in assessing ovarian reserve. Newer diagnostic tests include inhibin B, a member of the transforming growth factor β family. Inhibin B levels less than 45 pg/mL on day 3 of the cycle are associated with less favorable treatment outcomes. This is currently not clinically applicable as it is limited by expense and availability. (See Speroff, 1999.)

ASSESSMENT OF SEXUAL EXPOSURE

There is little role left for use of the postcoital test in the current evaluation of infertile couples. The use of techniques of intrauterine insemination has rendered this test passé. Certain women who are disabled may have significant enough physical limitations that the postcoital test may be useful to document the adequacy of intravaginal intromission.

The treatment of infertility is diagnosis specific. The diagnosis of infertility may be more difficult for some infertile women with disabilities, limiting treatment options. Initiation of folic acid supplementation and screening for HIV infection and rubella should be done prior to infertility treatment. Vaccination with rubella vaccine for women who are rubella susceptible is also recommended.

TREATMENT OF ANATOMIC CAUSES OF INFERTILITY

Treatment of Sexual Dysfunction

It is prudent for women who are disabled to attempt intercourse at the time of day when they have the least pain and fatigue. Use of pain relievers to diminish pain is indicated when timed intercourse is necessary. Slow, gentle movement of the lower extremities; careful positioning; stretching; and gentle massage during foreplay can help decrease spasticity in those at risk. The risk of autonomic dysreflexia triggered by sexual contact may be diminished by the same methods that decrease spasticity. The use of a routine to empty the bladder and bowel prior to intercourse and the use of Xylocaine gel on the perineum also may decrease autonomic dysreflexia in those at risk. Women who require the use of lubricants should use products that do not inhibit sperm motility (Table 15-3).

TABLE 15-3. *Lubricants*

Sperm motility diminished	Sperm motility unaffected
Petroleum jelly	Raw egg white
Saliva	Vegetable oil
	Replens douche

Treatment of Tubal Factors

The diagnosis of tubal occlusion may involve the use of laparoscopy, which allows the opportunity for treatment of tubal disease by the lysis of adhesions, fimbrioplasty, and removal of endometrial implants and endometriomas. Surgical intervention should minimize tissue manipulation and damage to pelvic organs.

Careful attention should be paid to the prevention of postoperative adhesions. The skilled surgeon makes intraoperative decisions that keep as the main priority the need to optimize fertility. All surgical treatment decisions must treat existing pathology while at the same time avoiding future impairment of fertility. In the current treatment of infertility, extensive surgical repair of damaged fallopian tubes is bypassed in favor of assisted reproductive technology.

Treatment of Structural Abnormalities of the Uterus

The diagnosis of structural problems of the uterus may be made by sonohysterography, hysterosalpingography, or hysteroscopy. The treatment of structural abnormalities is dictated by the type of abnormality present. The most common problems identified are endometrial polyps and uterine leiomyomas. Less common structural abnormalities include congenital anomalies such as the bicornuate uterus and uterine septae. The treatment of endometrial polyps with hysteroscopy and resection is minimally invasive and has been associated with improved pregnancy rates. The removal of uterine leiomyomas for infertility treatment requires the documentation of infertility or adverse pregnancy outcomes. The treatment options available include hysteroscopic resection of submucous leiomyomas, laparoscopic myomectomy, and myomectomy via laparotomy. The selection of method of treatment will depend on the location and size of the leiomyomas, operative skill of the surgeon, and patient preference. Myomectomy in infertile women with abnormal uterine cavities has been associated with improved pregnancy rates for selected patients. The most common congenital uterine anomaly is the uterine septae. As in the case of uterine leiomyomas, surgical intervention is not indicated unless there is documentation of adverse reproductive outcomes such as infertility or pregnancy loss. Abdominal metroplasty has been replaced by hysteroscopic resection. The use of laparoscopic guidance during operative hysteroscopy has been recommended to minimize traumatic injury to the posterior uterine wall. Use of laparoscopic guidance in the case of hysteroscopic surgery for the infertile patient is of particular importance. Avoidance of damage to the uterus and pelvic organs in this patient population is needed to prevent iatrogenic impairment of fertility.

TREATMENT OF HORMONAL DERANGEMENTS

Ovulation Induction

Prior to undertaking ovulation induction it is important to diagnose and treat pituitary, thyroid, and adrenal disorders. Patients should be screened with serum FSH, LH, TSH, prolactin, 17 hydroxyprogesterone, glucose, and insulin levels. The difficult problem of obesity also should be addressed, with recommendations for weight loss by exercise and dietary modifications. Weight loss improves the spontaneous pregnancy rates and improves responsiveness to ovulation induction. The importance of documenting adequate ovarian reserve cannot be overemphasized. This documentation is particularly vital for older infertile women (older than age 35 years) and for women who have a single ovary. Patients with a FSH level greater than 11 mIU/mL are unlikely to have a successful re-

sponse to ovulation induction and should be offered egg donation. Women older than 40 years of age have limited reproductive life. This population should be advised to avoid the delay associated with ovulation induction and also should proceed to egg donation. The process of ovulation induction is carried out in a stepwise fashion. The medication for initial treatment should be the simplest to administer, should be the least expensive, and should have the least side effects. Clomiphene citrate (Clomid) causes the hypothalamus to release gonadotropin-releasing hormone, which in turn stimulates the secretion of FSH and LH from the pituitary. FSH and LH promote the release of 17B estradiol in the ovary, which triggers ovulation. The results of clomiphene citrate treatment are the best in women who are young and have regular cycles. The results with clomiphene citrate are the worst for patients who have pituitary or ovarian failure or who have obesity with associated hyperandrogenism. Total pregnancy rates are improved when clomiphene citrate is combined with intrauterine insemination. The cost of clomiphene citrate is $10.00 per 50 mg.

The complications associated with the use of clomiphene citrate include ovarian cysts, bloating, weight gain, headache, visual disturbances, nausea, and multiple gestation (5% to 10%). Women who are disabled and at risk for autonomic dysreflexia may have significant complications with the use of clomiphene citrate. Intensive monitoring during clomiphene citrate cycles and the support of a physician with experience in the care of patients with autonomic dysreflexia is advisable. Multiple gestations may increase the risks of pregnancy for certain groups of women who are disabled. Women with severe musculoskeletal disorders, impaired mobility, and chronic illness affecting vital organ systems should avoid multiple gestations. Counseling prior to ovulation induction should address the issue of selective reduction for this high-risk population. Gonadotropins are used for ovulation induction but are more expensive, have higher complication rates, and are more complicated to administer. Gonadotropins usually are prescribed when ovulation induction with clomiphene citrate fails. Menotropins have been available for decades. They have the disadvantage of requiring large volume injections, which are uncomfortable. The newer, highly purified forms of FSH that are available on the market have the advantage of small injection volume and dosage consistency. The indications for the use of gonadotropins are similar to those for clomiphene citrate. Gonadotropins should not be used in women who have intracranial lesions including pituitary tumors, undiagnosed vaginal bleeding, ovarian cysts, or known hypersensitivity to gonadotropins. Women with ovarian failure will not respond to superovulation and should not be given gonadotropins. As in the case of clomiphene citrate, this patient population should be offered egg donation.

Treatment of Premature Ovarian Failure and Unexplained Infertility

The diagnosis of premature ovarian failure presents a difficult problem. The goal of most infertile couples is to achieve a pregnancy from their own genetic material. The review of premature ovarian failure by van Kasteren and Schoemaker evaluated 67 studies. They found a 5% to 10% pregnancy rate, which yielded 80% live births. They also found that all interventions used to treat this population of infertile women were equally ineffective.

Unexplained infertility is a diagnosis of exclusion. Couples who have this diagnosis have completed a standard infertility evaluation, and no cause of infertility has been identified. The treatment of unexplained infertility attempts to improve gamete number, quality, and interaction. Randolph has reported improved cycle fecundity with the use of gonadotropins and intrauterine insemination compared to clomiphene citrate and intrauterine insemination. In vitro fertilization has been recommended as the second line of therapy because of the invasive nature of the treatment and the cost. Watchful waiting has resulted in spontaneous pregnancies in couples with unexplained infertility, but most patients poorly accept this course of action.

RECURRENT PREGNANCY LOSS

Pregnancy loss is common in early pregnancy. A single episode of pregnancy loss in the first trimester does not increase the risk of poor outcome in future pregnancies. The loss of two consecutive pregnancies is defined as recurrent pregnancy loss and is associated with a 20% to 45% risk of pregnancy loss in the subsequent pregnancy. Recurrent pregnancy losses are caused by infections, uterine anomalies, genetic abnormalities, metabolic disorders, hormonal disorders, luteal phase defects, and immunologic factors.

The evaluation of couples with recurrent pregnancy losses requires a careful history, physical examination, and targeted special testing. The historical information gathered should focus on the pattern and timing of the pregnancy losses. Family history of pregnancy outcomes, screening for consanguinity in the couple, and evaluation of infections of the genital tract also must be obtained. A general medical history with emphasis on symptoms of autoimmune disease is mandatory. A general physical examination and pelvic examination are required, and the examiner should look carefully for signs of autoimmune disease, infectious diseases, and genital pathology.

The minimal diagnostic testing for this problem should include a screen for lupus anticoagulant and anticardiolipin antibodies, a screen for genital infections, and karyotyping for the couple. Endometrial biopsy and sonohysterography or hysterosalpingography should be strongly considered. The diagnosis and the presence of other factors that affect fertility, such as advanced maternal age, determine the treatment and term pregnancy rates.

SUMMARY

There currently are no available data to accurately calculate the problem of infertility in the population of women who are disabled. There is no evidence to suggest that women who are disabled are significantly different than women in the general population with regard to the frequency of infertility. There are also no data to suggest that the basic causes of infertility are different in women who are disabled compared to the general population. The standard evaluation of infertile couples should be the same for infertile women who are disabled. The providers of infertility care must be sensitive to the special needs of women with disabilities. Some women will require intensive preconception counseling. Other women will require assistance to complete some of the basic infertility diagnostic testing. Other women will be placed at risk by certain diagnostic testing and will require an alternative approach to minimize risk. All women will need additional time, thought, and counseling so that the diagnosis and treatment of infertility can be made in a way that is cost effective, safe, and acceptable to the patient.

SUGGESTED READING

American College of Obstetricians and Gynecologists. *2001 compendium of selected publications. Preconceptional care.* ACOG Technical Bulletin. Washington, DC: ACOG, 1995:205.

A Practice Committee Report. American Society for Reproductive Medicine. Optimal Evaluation of the Infertile Female. June 20, 2000.

Bajekal N, Li TC. Fibroids, infertility and pregnancy wastage. *Human Reprod Update* 2000;6:614–620.

Basson R. Sexual health of women with disabilities. *CMAJ* 1998;159(4):359-62.

Beckmann CR, Gittler M, Barzansky BM, et al. Gynecologic care of women with disabilities. *Obstet Gynecol* 1989;74:75–79.

Benshushan A, Shushan A, Paltiel O, et al. Ovulation induction with clomiphene citrate complicated by deep vein thrombosis. *Eur J Obstet Gynecol Reprod Biol* 1995;62: 261–262.

Bick RL. Recurrent miscarriage syndrome and infertility caused by blood coagulation protein or platelet defects. *Hematol Oncol Clin North Am* 2000;14(5):1117–1131.

Burns WN, Schenken RS. Pathophysiology of endometriosis-associated infertility. *Clin Obstet Gynecol* 1999; 42 (3):586–610.

Charlifue SW, Gerhart KA, Menter RR, et al. Sexual issues of women with spinal cord injuries. *Paraplegia* 1992;30: 192–199.

Daniluk J. Helping patients cope with infertility. *Clin Obstet Gynecol* 1997;40 (3):661–672.

Fody EP, Walker EM. Effects of drugs on the male and female reproductive systems. *Ann Clin Lab Sci* 1985;15(6): 451–458.

Furman LM. Institutionalized disabled adolescents: Gynecologic care. The pediatrician's role. *Clinical Pediatr* 1989;28(4):163–170.

Glass C, Soni B. ABC of sexual health sexual problems of disabled patients. *Br Med J* 1999;318:518–521.

Haywood JL, Goldenberg RL, Bronstein J, et al. Comparison of perceived and actual rates of survival and freedom from handicap in premature infants. *Am J Obstet Gynecol* 1994;171:432–439.

Hoeger KM, Guzick DS. An update on the classification of endometriosis. *Clin Obstet Gynecol* 1999;42(3):611–619.

Homer HA, Tin-Chiu L, Cooke I. The septate uterus: a review of management and Reproductive outcome. *Fertil Steril* 2000;73(1):1–14.

Jackson AB, Wadley V. A multicenter study of women's self-reported reproductive health after spinal cord injury. *Arch Phys Med Rehabil* 1999;80:1420 1428.

Kaplan D. Prenatal screening and its impact on persons with disabilities. *Clin Obstet Gynecol* 1993;36(3):605–612.

Korpelainen JT, Nieminen P, Myllyla VV. Sexual functioning among stroke patient's and their spouses. *Stroke* 1999;30(4):715–719.

Kump LM. Evaluating infertility: the basic workup. *Ob Gyn Manage* 2000:suppl 2–4.

Kutteh WH, Chao CH, Ritter JO, et al. Vaginal lubricants for the infertile couple: effect on sperm activity. *Int J Fertil Menopausal Stud* 1996;41(4):400–404.

Lalos A. Breaking bad news concerning fertility. *Human Reprod* 1999;14(3):581—585.

Lass A. The fertility potential of women with a single ovary. *Human Reprod Update* 1999;5(5):546–550.

Leibowitz D, Hoffman J. Fertility drug therapies: Past, present, and future. *J Obstet Gynecol Neonatal Nurs* 2000;29 (2):201–210.

Millsap D. Sex, lies, and health insurance: employer-provided health insurance coverage of abortion and infertility services and the ADA. *Am J Law Med* 1996;23(1): 51–84.

Norman RJ, Clark AM. Obesity and reproductive disorders: a review. *Reprod Fertil Dev* 1998;10(1):55–63.

Oei SG, Helmerhorst FM, Bloemenkamp KW, et al. Effectiveness of the postcoital test: randomised controlled trial. *Br Med J* 1998;317:502–505.

Penzias AS. Infertility Contemporary Office Based Evaluation and Treatment. *Obstet Gynecol Clin North Am* 2000; 27(3): 473–486.

Porter TF. Antiphospholipid Antibodies and Infertility. *Clin Obstet Gynecol* 2001;44(1):29–35.

Randolph RF. Unexplained infertility. *Clin Obstet Gynecol* 2000;43(4):897–901.

Reis JP. Advocate for disabled women. *Hosp Health Netw* 1993;67(14):46–47.

Slowey MJ. Polycystic ovary syndrome: new perspective on an old problem. *South Med J* 2001;94(2):190–196.

Speroff L, Glass RH, Kase NG. *Clinical gynecologic endocrinology and infertility,* 6th ed. New York: Lippincott Williams & Wilkins, 1999:1017–1019.

Spielvogel K, Shwayder J, Coddington CC. Surgical management of adhesions, endometriosis, and tubal pathology in the woman with infertility. *Clin Obstet Gynecol* 2000; 43(4):916–928.

Spitz A, Kim ED, Lipschultz LI. Contemporary approach to the male infertility evaluation. *Obstet Gynecol Clin North Am* 2000;27(3):487–516.

Stovall DW, Van Voorhis BJ. Immunologic tests and treatment in patients with unexplained infertility, IVF-ET, and recurrent pregnancy loss. *Clin Obstet Gynecol* 1999;42 (4):979–1000.

Surrey ES. Endoscopy in the evaluation of the woman experiencing infertility. *Clin Obstet Gynecol* 2000;43(4):889–896.

Szamatowicz M, Grochowski D. Fertility and infertility in aging women. *Gynecol Endocrinol* 1998;12(6):407–413.

Thornton KL. Advances in assisted reproductive technologies. *Curr Reprod Endocrinol* 2000;27(3):517–527.

van Kasteren YM, Schoemaker J. Premature Ovarian Failure: a systemic review of therapeutic Interventions to restore ovarian function and achieve pregnancy. *Human Reprod Update* 1999;5(5):483–492.

Van Voorhis BJ, Syrop CH. Cost-effective treatment for the couple with infertility. *Clin Obstet Gynecol* 2000;43(4):958–973.

Walbroehl GS. Sexual concerns of the patient with pulmonary disease. *Postgrad Med* 1992;91(5):455–460.

Wasser SK. Stress and reproductive failure: An evolutionary approach with applications to premature labor. *Am J Obstet Gynecol* 1999;180(1 Pt 3):S272–S274.

Weiss G. Fertility in the older woman. *Clin Consult Obstet Gynecol* 1996;8(1):56–59.

Weiss G. Ovulation induction strategies for the gynecologist. *Ob Gyn Manage* 2000;Suppl Nov:5–8.

Welner SL. A provider's guide for the care of women with physical disabilities & chronic medical conditions. North Carolina Office on Disability & Health, 1999.

Welner SL. Management of female infertility. In: Sipski ML, Alexander CL, eds. *Sexual function in people with disability and chronic illness.* Gaithersburg, MD: Aspen Publishers, 1997.

Welner SL. Infertility and management approaches for women with disabilities. *Sexuality and Disability* 1999;17(3):233–236.

Welner SL. Reproductive endocrinology and disability. The effect of disability on menstrual cyclicity and fertility. *Infertil Reprod Med Clin North Am* 1998;9(4):689–698.

Welner SL, Hammond C. Gynecologic and obstetric issues confronting women with disabilities. *Clinical gynecology.* Vol. 1, Chapter 102.

Weström L. Incidence, prevalence, and trends of acute pelvic inflammatory disease and its consequences in industrialized countries. *Am J Obstet Gynecol* 1980;138:880–892.

White MJ, Rintala DH, Hart KA, et al. Sexual activities, concerns and interests of women with spinal cord injury living in the community. *Am J Phys Med Rehabil* 1993;72:372–378.

Wingfield M, Healy DL, Nicholson A. Gynaecological care for the women with intellectual disability. *Med J Aust* 1994;160(9):536–538.

Witz CA. Current concepts in the pathogenesis of endometriosis. *Clin Obstet Gynecol* 1999;42(3):566–585.

Wolf LJ. Ovulation induction. *Clin Obstet Gynecol* 2000;43(4):902–915.

16

Osteoporosis: Unique Aspects of Pathophysiology, Evaluation, and Treatment

Rebecca D. Jackson, Laura E. Ryan, and W. Jerry Mysiw

Osteoporosis is one of the most pressing public health problems facing older people. It is defined as "a systemic skeletal disease characterized by low bone mass and microarchitectural deterioration of bone tissue, with a consequent increase in bone fragility and a susceptibility to fracture" (1). Although osteoporosis is a multifactorial disease, it is present in women a decade or two earlier than in men as a result of the impact of both a lower peak bone mass and accentuated menopause-related losses of bone. Thus, the greater risk for the development of osteoporosis in women has the potential to contribute to a progressively greater burden of illness and diminished quality of life as they age.

Bone mineral density (BMD) accounts for the majority of the variance in bone strength (2), but it is not the sole determinant of fracture risk and there is substantial overlap in BMD values between women who fracture and those who do not (3). In able-bodied women, other factors such as skeletal mineralization, bone geometry, and bone size can influence bone strength. It also has been recognized that environmental and other genetic factors play a role. However, superimposed on the environmental and genetic variation seen in able-bodied women, women with disabling conditions might have a range of other factors that could result in further accentuation of bone loss, changes in bone quality, or an increased risk for falls. Without recognition of the potential of a disabling condition to contribute further to the development of osteo-

porosis, the resultant increased risk for fractures could reduce the independence and subsequently the quality of life of the millions of women with disabling conditions.

PREVALENCE OF OSTEOPOROSIS

In able-bodied women, based on BMD measurements as a surrogate definition of osteoporosis, data from the National Health and Nutrition Examination and Surveys III estimates that 21% to 30% of postmenopausal white women in the United States have osteoporosis and an additional 54% have low bone density or osteopenia (4). In addition, 10% of postmenopausal African-American women and 16% of Mexican-American women have a hip BMD compatible with the definition of osteoporosis (5).

It has been estimated that osteoporosis is responsible for 1.5 million fractures annually. This includes approximately 300,000 hip fractures, 700,000 vertebral fractures, 250,000 wrist fractures, and more than 300,000 fractures at other skeletal sites (6). In the United States, a 50-year-old white woman has a 14% lifetime risk of suffering a hip fracture (7). When taking all fractures into account, more than 50% of postmenopausal white women will suffer at least one fracture as a result of osteoporosis during their lifetime. The rates for fracture in African-American women are approximately half as high (6).

The risk for fracture also increases with the presence of other risk factors. For example, as a woman ages, her 5-year risk for a hip fracture increases from 2.3% at the age of 50 years to a probability of 7.19% at age 75 (7). Other risk factors, including those that disproportionately affect women with disabilities, also might have an additive effect on fracture risk. The most substantial effect on fracture risk may be associated with the development of a mobility disability, and this is illustrated most dramatically in people with spinal cord injury (SCI). Although all patients with SCI have significantly increased rates of distal femur and proximal tibial fractures (8), the risk for fracture is greatest in the oldest individuals with SCI (from 14.5 to 45.7 fractures per 1,000 patient years for age intervals of 20 to 39 compared to 60 to 79 years) and in those people with the lowest BMD (9). Data on fracture prevalence in other disabled populations is incomplete or lacking, and there is a need for registry information to truly understand the magnitude of the impact of specific diseases or disability-associated risk factors for fracture.

PATHOPHYSIOLOGY OF OSTEOPOROSIS

The amount of skeletal bone mass at any time in adult life reflects the impact of the amount of bone attained during adolescence and the young adult years (peak bone mass) minus that which is lost through age, menopause, or secondary factors. Estrogen plays a decisive role in the initiation of bone growth and adolescent bone acquisition, but lifestyle factors including physical activity and nutrition are also important components to achieving peak bone mass. The maximum amount of attainable bone size is determined genetically. At the point peak bone mass has been achieved, men have a bone mass that is 10% to 15% greater than that of women. It is during this period of acquisition of peak bone mass that the skeleton has its first vulnerable window when inadequate dietary calcium, immobilization, or decreased exposure to reproductive hormones could diminish the peak

bone mass. This could manifest itself clinically years later as a lesser skeletal reserve to accommodate menopause- and age-related losses. Thus, disabilities that occur during the adolescent years can have an important adverse impact on acquisition of peak bone mass.

Bone mass remains relatively stable until about age 30 to 40 years, when bone loss slowly begins (10). Bone loss accelerates during menopause, the beginning of relative estrogen deficiency, with the greatest percentage of bone lost in the first 3 to 6 years, after which time it slows (2,11). After menopause, able-bodied healthy women can lose from 2% to 5% of bone mass per year. Bone loss continues through old age, and several studies suggest a second period of accentuated bone loss that occurs more than 20 to 25 years postmenopause.

This bone loss reflects an inefficient process of bone remodeling, a dynamic process of self-repair and renewal that occurs at discrete bone multicellular units (BMU) on the bone surface (12). The remodeling process has four basic steps: activation, resorption, reversal, and formation (13). Osteoclasts, cells that resorb bone in response to circulating cytokines to provide adequate extracellular calcium and phosphate levels, dig cavities in cancellous and cortical bone. The cell membrane that lays next to the bone forms a ruffled border that secretes acid onto the isolated bone surface to dissolve the bone mineral and enzymes to break down the organic matrix. This process also releases a chemical mediator(s) that recruits osteoblasts, the cells that regulate formation, to the bone surface through a coupled, coordinated process. During the slower process of bone formation, the osteoblast lays down collagen matrix (osteoid), which then is mineralized. For complete mineralization of the skeleton, an adequate supply of extracellular calcium and phosphate and sufficient $1,25 (OH)_2$ vitamin D must be present.

A single remodeling cycle takes 3 to 6 months to complete. At skeletal maturity, the amount of bone formed is equal to the amount resorbed and bone mass is stable. However, any disruption of the remodeling cycle (increased or decreased activation of bone modeling or enhanced resorption or diminished formation) can result in a net deficit in bone on completion of each cycle.

The process of bone remodeling is affected by both menopause and aging. As estrogen levels fall with menopause, there is an increase in release of interleukin-1 (IL-1) and tumor necrosis factor from peripheral blood mononuclear cells and IL-6 and both granulocyte and macrophage colony-stimulating factors from osteoblast and stromal cells (14). These cytokines and growth factors result in a stimulation of the BMU activation and an increase in resorption. There is concurrent uncoupling of bone remodeling, with formation falling behind resorption, further accentuating the net loss of bone mass (15).

As age advances, there are additional changes in bone remodeling that occur and further lead to bone loss. There is evidence that the depth and extent of the resorption cavity increases with age with decreases in the quantity of bone formed per remodeling cycle. This can lead to an ongoing loss of bone even when activation frequency is normal or diminished.

Changes in local or systemic cytokine expression can affect women with specific disabling conditions and put them at even greater risk for accentuating the menopause- and age-related losses. For example, women with rheumatoid arthritis have greater production of cytokines by the local inflammatory cells at the joint as well as peripheral blood mononuclear cells. This translates into accentuated severity of both periarticular and generalized osteoporosis.

Local changes in remodeling can have an impact on calcium balance that subsequently can affect the skeleton further. In early menopause, the net increase in bone resorption results in a transient increase in serum calcium levels, which subsequently suppresses parathyroid hormone (PTH) release.

The decrease in PTH secondarily results in a diminished 1-α hydroxylation of 25(OH) vitamin D with reduction in circulating 1,25(OH) vitamin D levels. These changes in calcitropic hormones then result in decreased enteral calcium absorption and enhanced renal calcium losses.

In contrast, with aging there is a decline in renal function with an inability to form adequate 1,25(OH) vitamin D. This results in diminished enteral calcium absorption and an appropriate compensatory increase in PTH. This secondary hyperparathyroidism increases bone resorption and contributes to the development of osteoporosis by increasing bone remodeling in a setting of low bone formation.

In women with disabilities resulting in mobility impairments, there is a large body of literature supporting an almost universal disruption in calcium homeostasis and changes in bone remodeling leading to the development of bone loss. The magnitude and duration of negative calcium balance seen in paralytic poliomyelitis is proportional to the degree and duration of the paralysis (16). The use of calcium radiotracers suggests that the negative calcium balance in patients with polio is primarily the result of a twofold to threefold increase in bone resorption with normal to twofold increase in bone formation rates (17). In contrast, following SCI there is an uncoupling of the rates of bone formation and resorption. Cancellous resorption surfaces increase by 78% by 16 weeks postinjury with a slow decline to normal by 40 weeks (18). Conversely, bone formation is depressed by 75% by the 10th week postinjury with return to low-normal levels by 40 weeks. Mineralization rates also are reduced to 25% of normal at 10 weeks; many still are depressed as many as 20 weeks postinjury. It has been postulated that these changes in remodeling reflect an increased longevity of the BMU with prolongation of the resorptive phase and a foreshortened formation phase leading to a net decrement of bone at each BMU.

Metabolic correlates of the changes in remodeling in women with disabilities, particularly those that affect mobility, accentuate some of the adverse changes in calcium balance seen with normal menopause and aging. Hypercalciuria is present in patients with virtually all causes of immobilization or mobility impairment. In SCI, this is present within 1 week after injury, peaks within 10 weeks at values between 350 to 400 mg/24 hours, and declines over the next 1 to 2 years (19,20). The maximal hypercalciuria observed in SCI is twofold to fourfold greater than that achieved in able-bodied subjects during bedrest (21), suggesting that neurologic injury either has some unique neurohumoral mechanism contributing to the bone loss or the loss of even normal muscle tone may have an additive adverse effect on bone metabolism. Associated with the hypercalciuria is concurrent suppression of PTH and 1, $25(OH)_2$ vitamin D (20,22) leading to diminished enteral calcium absorption and elevated calcitonin levels (23) in a compensatory attempt to diminish bone turnover.

In addition to the effect of these intrinsic changes in bone remodeling and calcium balance on the skeleton, optimal maintenance of bone mass in both able-bodied and disabled women requires avoidance of other factors that could affect remodeling adversely, such as inadequate mechanical strain through physical inactivity or deficiency in nutritional sources of calcium, phosphate, and vitamin D. Maintenance of bone mass requires meeting the skeletal requirements for all factors regulating skeletal mass, and a deficiency or adverse effect of any single factor cannot be compensated completely by attention to others. For women with disabling medical conditions, this becomes an important consideration when planning the appropriate prevention or treatment course.

RISK FACTORS FOR DEVELOPMENT OF OSTEOPOROSIS

Many factors have been described that adversely may affect the development of decreased bone mass and subsequent increase in fractures characteristic of osteoporosis. These have been best described for postmenopausal osteoporosis, but in women with disabilities these factors also may be important to consider. These risk factors can be subdivided into factors associated with low bone mass and those factors that independently increase the risk for osteoporotic fracture.

Risk Factors for Low Bone Mass

Low bone mass is an independent risk factor for fracture (24–29). Based on this fact, BMD is now used as a surrogate definition for osteoporosis. The factors contributing to low bone mass are many, and in any individual the cause of low bone mass is likely to be multifactorial (30–32). Traditional lists of risk factors that contribute to low bone mass often are divided into factors that are modifiable and nonmodifiable (Table 16-1) (33). The principal determinant of low bone mass is genetic; heritability accounts for 46% to 62% of the variance in BMD after adjustments for age, weight, height, and lifestyle (31,34). This genetic impact may be seen most dramatically during the acquisition of peak bone mass because bone formation rather than bone resorption appears to be strongly dependent on genetically determined factors. Although there have been intensive studies focusing on the elucidation of the genetic polymorphisms and candidate genes associated with osteoporosis, no one factor appears to explain a substantial portion of postmenopausal osteoporosis. It is more likely that this heterogeneous disease will have multiple different genetic factors that contribute to a similar phenotype. Although several of the genetic polymorphisms associated with osteoporosis also have been shown to be associated with a less positive outcome following neurotrauma (e.g., apolipoprotein E4 allelic variants), in general, the genetic factors contributing to osteoporosis in women with disabilities are unlikely to be substantially different than those identified in the general population of postmenopausal women.

Table 16-1. *Risk factors for low bone mass[a]*

Modifiable	Nonmodifiable
• Nutritional deficiency	• Gonadal steroid deficiency
Inadequate calcium intake[a]	Late menarche[a]
Inadequate vitamin D intake/synthesis[a]	Premature menopause[a]
Increased protein intake	Nulliparity[a]
Increased sodium intake	Secondary amenorrhea[a]
Increased caffeine intake	• Advancing age
High phosphate–containing carbonated beverages	• Low body weight[a]
• Lifestyle	• Genetic predisposition
Cigarette smoking	Female gender
Heavy alcohol use	White or Asian
Reduced physical activity[a]	Familial prevalence
	• Genetic polymorphisms

[a]Factor that can be potentially adversely affected by physical disabilities.

The second most important determinant of low bone mass is body weight; this accounts for 15% to 20% of the variance in BMD (31,32,35,36). Less than 3% of women weighing more than 70 kg will have osteoporosis. It is thought that some of the protective effects of high body weight are the result of the higher body fat in overweight and obese women, which can contribute to substantially higher estrogen levels and, thus, slower rates of bone loss. This same factor also may help to decrease the severity of osteoporosis in some women with disabilities where the attendant decrease in lean body mass with motor impairments may result in a higher percentage of fat mass. In contrast, however, rapid weight loss and malnourishment in women who suffer severe medical illnesses and in some cases of neurologic trauma may result in rapid concurrent bone loss that is never regained after recovery from the acute illness or other stressful event.

A reduction in estrogen levels such as occurs at menopause can result in increased rates of bone loss and lifelong exposure to estrogens in an independent factor relating to bone mass. Premature menopause results in bone loss occurring at a younger age, thus extending the period of life where a woman may have significant osteopenia or osteoporosis (37). Women with traumatic brain injuries may suffer panhypopituitarism that can result in early menopause (38). Secondary amenor-

rhea may occur in many women with disabilities as a result of medical complications, the underlying disease, or neurologic trauma. The severity of the impact of the secondary amenorrhea on the skeleton depends on the timing of the secondary amenorrhea (during peak acquisition of bone mass versus mid-adult years), the length of time that amenorrhea persists, and the trough of estrogen decline. Young-adult women with disabilities occurring early in their reproductive years have lower rates of pregnancy: this results in a lack of exposure to the high estrogen state of pregnancy and, thus, a lower bone mass. Parity and lactation (less than 1 year) have no effect on BMD (39).

Cigarette smoking (40,41) and alcohol intake (42) have adverse effects on bone mass; the mechanism of their impact has not yet been defined entirely. Women who smoke transition into menopause at a younger age, in part because of the more rapid metabolism of estrogens. Alcohol has direct adverse effects on the osteoblast and increases urinary calcium losses. Recent studies have suggested that heavy alcohol intake is deleterious to bone, whereas moderate alcohol intake is not.

Reduced physical activity can decrease bone mass dramatically, and the majority of women with disabilities that adversely affect motor function or endurance will have this risk factor for low bone mass. Mechanical strain modulates bone formation. This follows the principals of Wolff's law that states that the mass and distribution of mass (structure) will be modified in response to the perceived loads imposed on it (43,44). This is consistent with the patterns of bone loss seen following SCI, where the greatest decreases in bone mass are seen at skeletal sites where the decrease in the magnitude of mechanical strain is the greatest (e.g., the distal femur of proximal tibia), whereas skeletal sites such as the lumbar spine that still are loaded in the seated position are relatively maintained (45–49). Use of braces, casting, or other orthotic devices decreases the effect of active muscle contraction across specific regions of bone, and these devices have been associated with decrease in bone mass at those specific sites. If immobilization is brief (less than 10 weeks), recovery of BMD can occur (50). The devastating effect of prolonged immobilization has such a great effect on loss of bone mass that there appears to be little, if any, difference in BMD in patients with a neurologic injury based on gender.

Nutrition also plays a major role in the pathogenesis of osteoporosis. Low calcium intake in childhood and adolescence is associated with an increased risk of osteoporosis later in life, and may be associated with an increase in fracture risk as early as adolescence (51,52). Epidemiologic studies clearly have shown that lifelong calcium intake is correlated with BMD at all ages (53). Factors that adversely affect calcium balance also may increase the risk for low bone mass including excessive caffeine intake, high protein intake, or excessive sodium intake. There also has been great interest in exploring the more common acidogenic diet consumed by Americans and its adverse impact on enhancing bone resorption with resultant bone loss.

Risk Factors Directly Contributing to Risk for Fracture

Epidemiologic studies specifically addressing the older postmenopausal woman have identified a host of factors that, independent of bone mass, may enhance the risk for a fragility fracture; many of these factors may play a role in the increased risk for fracture in a woman with a disability. These can be broken into factors that affect the amount and quality of the skeleton directly, factors related to bone metabolism, factors that increase the frequency of falls, and the effect of the falls (Table 16-2) (26).

In addition to a decrease in bone mass, the quality of resultant bone may differ in some women with disabilities. In women with SCI, there is hypomethylation of the hydroxyproline, leading to reduced thermal stability and possibly leading to a greater risk for degradation (54). Bone geometry has a significant impact on fracture risk. In women who incur

Table 16-2. *Risk factors for osteoporotic fracture[a]*

Skeletal factors	Effect of falls
Bone mineral density and quality[a]	Strength and coordination[a]
Geometry of bone[a]	Height
Previous fracture[a]	Force and direction
Bone metabolism	Impact surface
Increased bone resorption rates[a]	**Other**
Low vitamin D stores[a]	Age
Frequency of falls	Maternal history of hip fracture
Strength and balance[a]	Low body mass index[a]
Reduced physical activity[a]	History of hyperthyroidism
Vision and neurologic function[a]	Resting pulse >80 bpm
Medications such as benzodiazepines[a]	Current cigarette smoking
Body mechanics[a]	Alcohol intake

[a]Risk factors for fracture (independent of bone mineral density) that could be affected by a disabling condition.

a mobility disability at a young age, lack of attainment of the normal bone size may affect fracture risk. For example, there may be geometric changes that occur at the hip (e.g., a shorter hip axis length) that might decrease the risk for hip fracture (55). At other sites, such as the spine, smaller vertebral endplates may result in higher vertebral pressures and, thus, an increased risk for spine fracture (56). Disabilities that occur after growth has ceased may affect the skeleton differently than a similar disability in children and adolescents. In adults who suffer a SCI, there are few significant adverse effects on geometric properties of the midshaft femur other than an increase in endosteal diameter (57). Similarly, in people with SCI who had never suffered a pathologic fracture of the lower limb, there were only minor changes in cross-sectional area of the tibia in comparison to able-bodied people, although those with SCI who suffered a fracture after their injury had a difference in all geometric properties studied (58). In contrast, analyses of apparent shear modulus and the flexural modulus of elasticity in the tibia from patients with SCI suggest that there are microstructural changes that occur after SCI that could alter mechanical properties and also lead to increased fracture risk (59).

Previous fracture is one of the greatest independent risk factors for fracture, and the common occurrence of a prior fracture in many women with disabilities may increase the subsequent risk for fracture. Postmenopausal women who sustain a vertebral fracture have a threefold to fivefold increased risk for a subsequent vertebral fracture within the preceding year (60,61). The presence of a vertebral fracture is associated with an increased risk of hip fractures (62), and the risk for any fracture is increased at least twofold among women who had a prior fragility fracture (61). If this relationship holds true for women with disabilities, the marked increase in prevalence of fractures in people with mobility disorders such as SCI might further increase the subsequent risk for additional fractures in women with disabilities.

Rates of bone resorption may independently predict risk for fracture, and in certain women with disabilities, the very rapid rates of bone resorption in women with underlying low bone mass may place them at the highest risk for fracture. Low vitamin D stores have been noted in women with multiple sclerosis (MS) and are associated with more rapid rates of bone loss than women with MS with normal vitamin D levels (63). Vitamin D deficiency is also frequently seen with other disabilities: 64% of men and women who had a cerebrovascular accident were vitamin D–deficient, and 76% had no sunlight exposure to enhance vitamin synthesis (64,65).

Because risk for fracture is a function of both the strength of bone and the severity of the force applied to bone, factors that increase the risk of falling or the amount of load sustained by the skeleton during the fall will affect the risk of fracture (66–68). Generalized weakness, poor balance, diminished depth perception or visual acuity, and certain medication use including the use of benzodiazepines and anticonvulsants are common in women with disabilities and may increase the probability of falls and reduce the likelihood of using effective protective reflexes. This increased likelihood of falling is confirmed by data showing an average of 1.4 falls per patient per year on a neurorehabilitation unit. Similarly, in women with rheumatoid arthritis (69) and MS (63), muscle weakness and atrophy resulted in a higher incidence of falls than in able-bodied age-matched controls. This is illustrated by the increased risk for fractures in patients with cerebrovascular accidents, where 79% of all hip fractures occur on the hemiparetic side (64).

In multivariate models of osteoporotic fracture, several other factors have been shown to contribute to fracture risk and should be considered (68). A family history of a fragility fracture has been associated with an increased risk for fracture possibly because of genetic factors contributing to skeletal geometry, bone mass, or bone quality. Several different variants of the Type I collagen gene have been

Table 16-3. *Secondary causes of osteoporosis*

Endocrinopathies	Other
Hyperparathyroidism	Radiation
Thyrotoxicosis	Immobilization
Cushing's syndrome	Systemic mastocytosis
Type I diabetes	Renal tubular acidosis
Hyperprolactinemia	Hypoxemia
Hypogonadism other than menopause	Medications
Anorexia nervosa	Thyroid hormone supplement
Panhypopituitarism	Glucocorticoids
Acromegaly	Anticoagulants
Adrenal insufficiency	Chronic lithium
Rheumatologic diseases	GnRH (gonadotropin-releasing hormone) agonists and
Rheumatoid arthritis	antagonists
Osteogenesis imperfecta	Anticonvulsants
Marfan's syndrome	Extended tetracycline use
Ehlers-Danlos syndrome	Cyclosporine A
Systemic lupus erythematosus	Loop diuretics
Gastroenterology	
Malabsorption syndrome	
Malnutrition	
Chronic liver disease	
Hematologic	
Thalassemia	
Multiple myeloma	
Leukemia/lymphoma	

identified in kindreds with multiple osteo-porotic fractures, suggesting that some families with increased risk for fracture may have qualitative, in addition to quantitative, defects in bone.

Although 80% to 85% of osteoporosis in women is the result of menopause- or age-related factors, there are a host of other medical conditions that may contribute to bone loss, qualitative abnormalities in bone, or increased risk for fracture and should be considered (Table 16-3). These are particularly important to consider in women with disabilities because many of these diseases may result in impairments in mobility, balance, or subsequent handicap. Most of these secondary causes of osteoporosis result in increased rates of bone resorption and subsequent bone loss. Diseases such as osteogenesis imperfecta and Ehlers-Danlos and Marfan's syndromes represent disorders of collagen that contribute to poor bone microarchitecture, whereas diseases such as the steroid excess in endogenous or exogenous Cushing's syndrome is associated with diminished rates of bone formation.

CLINICAL MANIFESTATIONS OF OSTEOPOROSIS

The surrogate use of BMD to define osteoporosis has important clinical utility because significant bone mass loss is likely to occur in women with disabilities prior to the first clinical manifestation. The hallmark of osteoporosis is the fracture. The classical fractures of postmenopausal osteoporosis occur first at the vertebrate (anterior wedge, end plate, or crush fracture) and the distal radius with later fractures noted at long bones and the hip. This pattern of fracture reflects the early estrogen-deficiency–associated cancellous bone loss in postmenopausal osteoporosis.

In women with disabilities, the location of greatest bone loss and, thus, the highest risk for fracture may be more because of loss of motor function and, thus, loss of mechanical strain. For example, in people who have incurred spinal cord injuries, there is an incremental risk for fracture with time postinjury that is localized primarily to the lower limbs (the distal femur and proximal tibia). In contrast, in people who have suffered a cerebrovascular accident with subsequent hemiparesis, although there is no significant increase in the cumulative risk for fracture compared to able-bodied controls, the majority of fractures occurred on the impaired side—in those limbs directly affected by a change in balance and coordination and resultant osteopenia due to a loss of normal mechanical strain (70).

Complications of fractures also contribute to the morbidity of osteoporosis and are specific to the site of fracture. With vertebral fractures, there can be the progressive development of kyphosis, decreased height, and back pain. As kyphosis becomes more severe, it may lead to the development of restrictive lung disease, early satiety, and constipation, further aggravating medical conditions that may be present in women with certain disabling conditions. Morbidity associated with hip fractures includes a further loss of mobility with change in gait pattern and a diminution in independence with activities of daily living (ADL). In people who are nonambulatory (such as in those with motor-complete SCI), fractures of the long bones may be associated with decreased rates of healing and the potential for autonomic hyperreflexia and pressure ulceration.

Osteoporotic fractures also are associated with a decrease in length of life, and there is no reason to suspect that the statistics that hold true for postmenopausal women without disability would not be similar if not worse for women with disabilities. There is a 2% decline in total life expectancy following spine fracture (71,72). Up to 12% to 20% of men and women who have a hip fracture die within 1 year of the fracture primarily because of the medical and nutritional state of the individual who fractures (73). Thus, the manifestations of osteoporosis in women with disabilities can be substantial, and only through early, aggressive intervention to recognize this disorder and prevent further bone loss can the morbidity and mortality associated with this disease be reduced.

CLINICAL EVALUATION OF THE WOMAN WITH A DISABILITY TO ASSESS FOR OSTEOPOROSIS

A medical history and physical and gynecologic examination should be performed on each woman with a disability as part of her evaluation for the prevention and treatment of osteoporosis. Because the current skeletal status reflects all factors that influence acquisition of peak bone mass (e.g., the timing of the disabling condition) or might accelerate rates of bone loss, the medical history must cover the entire lifetime. There should be detailed questions regarding lifestyle risk factors for osteoporosis including the presence of any restricted or unusual eating habits, lifelong intake of milk and dairy products, habitual physical activity including periods of immobilization and their timing, and the use of cigarettes and alcohol. A gynecologic history should focus on the course and timing of puberty, menstrual disruptions during adult life, pregnancy, and prolonged lactation (more than a 1 year). There should be careful determination of risk factors that might also independently affect the risk for fracture, including a history of previous fragility-related fractures in childhood or the adult years. Detailed medication history and questions to exclude secondary causes of osteoporosis also might point to issues that should be addressed specifically in the generation of an appropriate prevention and/or treatment plan. Questions regarding back pain or height loss may suggest the presence of a vertebral compression fracture, although most complaints of back pain are not related to osteoporosis and as many as one-third of all vertebral fractures are asymptomatic and only discovered after a change in height of more than 2.5 cm has been noted. Details of the impact of the disabling condition on ADL including a focus on weightbearing, postural stability; visual acuity; and risk for falls also might help to guide physical therapy and environmental recommendations.

The physical examination should focus on exclusion of secondary causes of osteoporosis and determination of the degree of neurologic impairment affecting strength, balance, and coordination. Assessment of generalized muscle strength, range of motion, postural stability, and gait may indicate a patient at increased risk for falls. Because vertebral fractures are always associated with a loss of height, measurement of height using a wall-mounted stadiometer should be performed annually. In women who cannot stand, assessment of seated height (coccyx to crown) or supine height can be performed. Thoracic vertebral fractures can lead to worsening dorsal kyphosis, whereas lumbar compression fractures may result in flattening of the normal lumbar lordotic curve. The presence of significant scoliosis might signal an individual who might benefit from aggressive prevention strategies. With more severe osteoporotic deformity, the abdomen may become more protuberant and eventually the ribs may rest on the iliac crest. Tenderness over a vertebrate might suggest a recent compression fracture, whereas generalized bone tenderness, particularly over the tibia and sternum, might suggest concurrent osteomalacia.

Although a careful history and physical examination should be part of every woman's routine preventive health care, unfortunately, a major contributor to poor bone health in women with disabilities is the lack of access to standard health care and preventive medicine. For example, up to 50% of women with MS do not get regular routine medical follow-up (74), and the statistics are even more humbling for women with cerebral palsy (75). Add to this that most women with osteoporosis have no signs or symptoms of osteoporosis until the first fracture occurs, and it becomes all the more imperative that paradigms for early diagnosis of this further disabling complication of many disabilities in women be developed and used routinely.

DIAGNOSTIC TESTING

Although low bone mass and fracture can conceptualize osteoporosis, the exact criteria for the diagnosis of osteoporosis by noninvasive measurements of bone mass remains problematic. Measurements of BMD account for 60% to 80% of the variance of the strength of bone (2), and low BMD is more effective at predicting fractures in postmenopausal women than blood pressure is at predicting the risk for stroke (76). However, there is substantial overlap of bone mass between patients with or without fragility fractures, and it is therefore necessary to take multiple factors into consideration rather than just using an arbitrary cutpoint for BMD to determine those women who might benefit from treatment (6). Use of specific risk factors independent of BMD that increase risk for fractures, consideration of aspects of the clinical examination that suggest a greater risk for falls, and use of certain biochemical testing including the potential for the utility of markers of bone turnover may help to identify those women at the highest risk for fractures.

Radiologic Assessment

BMD does predict fracture risk (26,29, 77–79), and estimates of relative risk for fracture typically are based on the number of standard deviations (SD) that the bone density falls below the mean for a normal young adult population. In able-bodied postmenopausal women, there is an exponential increase in fracture incidence starting one SD below the reference population (80). In general, for every one SD decrease in BMD, there is an approximate 1.8-fold to 2.2-fold increase in the relative risk for fracture at any skeletal site. However, this relationship may differ based on other factors; this is seen, for example, in steroid-induced bone loss where there is nearly a fourfold increase in fractures for each SD decrease in BMD. In SCI, each 1 standard deviation decrease in femoral neck BMD increased the risk of lower limb fractures 2.2-fold to 2.8-fold (81).

Using the well-defined relationship between the risk for fracture and bone mass, the World Health Organization developed three diagnostic categories based on the variance of the BMD from a normative population of young adults (the T score): normal (BMD that is no more than 1 SD below the young normal reference population), osteopenia (BMD between 1 and 2.5 SD below the reference population), and osteoporosis (more than 2.5 SD below the reference population) (82,83). However, it is important to realize that these criteria have significant limitations. They only have been validated against databases containing primarily healthy postmenopausal white women. They therefore may not have the same degree of accuracy in reflecting fracture risk for premenopausal women, women with secondary causes of bone loss such as steroid or other medication use, or women with disabilities.

To help categorize women as normal, osteopenic, or osteoporotic, measurement of BMD by any one of a number of absorptiometric techniques that vary in precision, accessibility, and discrimination can be made (Table 16-4). All these absorptiometric techniques are based on the principle that attenu-

ation of a radiation source (usually x-ray) will be related to the thickness and the composition of the tissue in the radiation path (83). All these techniques then derive three sets of clinically useful numbers: the BMD, the T score, and the Z score (a comparison of the individual patient's bone density to an age-, gender-, race-, and body weight-matched cohort) (Fig. 16-1).

To assess bone loss at central skeletal sites such as the spine and hip, which are locations of the most prevalent and clinically important fractures in postmenopausal osteoporosis, dual-energy x-ray absorptiometry (DEXA) has become the most widely used technique for assessment of osteoporosis (84). DEXA uses two beams of distinct energy to correct for differential soft-tissue attenuation, which allows for corrections for individual variability in soft tissue around the hip and spine. DEXA allows for measurement of bone mass in the axial skeleton, peripheral skeleton, and total skeleton. The results are expressed as bone mineral content or areal BMD (gm/cm^2). This areal measure-

Table 16-4. *Diagnostic tests for osteoporosis*

Radiologic tests	Purpose	Additional comments
Radiologic test		
Dual-energy x-ray absorptiometry	BMD of spine, femur, total body	Low radiation
Quantitative computed tomography	Spine	Pure trabecular bone
Quantitative ultrasound	Calcaneous	No radiation
Biochemical tests		
Calcium, phosphorus, magnesium	Adequate mineral for mineralization	Should be normal in involutional osteoporosis
Complete blood count	Exclude malignancy	Also can detect thalassemia
Serum alkaline phosphatase	Exclude osteomalacia	Also can be elevated with liver disease and some malignancies
TSH	Exclude subclinical hyperthyroidism	TSH <0.100 has adverse effect on skeleton
25 (OH) vitamin D	Exclude vitamin D deficiency	25(OH) vitamin D <30 ng/mL is insufficient
PTH	Exclude primary or secondary hyperparathyroidism	Must be interpreted in light of serum calcium
24-hour urine calcium	Exclude hypercalciuria	Helps to complete assessment of calcium homeostasis
Renal function	Assess safety for use of bisphosphonates	Also excludes renal osteodystrophy
Hepatic function	Assess safety of medication use	Also excludes chronic liver disease as secondary cause

BMD, bone mineral density; PTH, parathyroid stimulating hormone; TSH, parathyroid hormone.

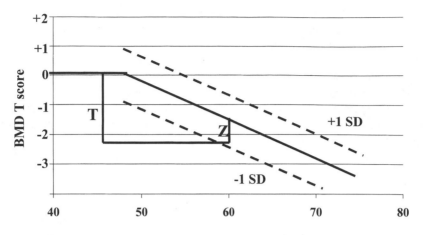

Fig. 16-1. Bone mass index—the relationship between T and Z scores.

ment can result in false lowering of the apparent BMD in individuals with very small bone volumes such as in women with mobility disabilities occurring prior to puberty. Overall, DEXA has excellent measurement precision and a low accuracy error that allows for serial follow-up for monitoring therapeutic efficacy or ongoing loss of bone. It has been used effectively to look at bone mass changes in a number of disabling conditions including SCI (85), MS (64,65), and stroke (86,87).

Quantitative computed tomography is the only diagnostic method that can determine true volumetric density and may play a role in assessing bone mass in women with very small (or conversely, very large) bone volume. It also can isolate trabecular and cortical bone content, and its greater sensitivity for detecting trabecular bone loss has made it a valuable research tool. Its improved ability to isolate pure trabecular bone mass has been shown to increase its sensitivity for detecting low spine BMD in SCI relative to DEXA (88). It has an *in vivo* precision error of 2% to 4% and an accuracy error of 5% to 15%, error rates that are much higher than those reported for DEXA. Although it is potentially widely available because it can be performed on a standard CT scanner, its higher radiation exposure and cost have limited its clinical use.

Recently, quantitative ultrasound (QUS) has been developed as a measure of bone quality. Because osteoporosis is a disease characterized by both reduction in bone mass and changes in microarchitecture, measurements of ultrasound transmission velocity that are affected by trabecular separation, connectivity, and elasticity could discriminate structural changes in osteoporosis. QUS does not use radiation, and recent studies support its potential efficacy in measuring acute bone loss in the early stages following a neurologic injury where traditional axial DEXA assessment may be limited by practical constraints (89).

All these techniques described readily differentiate between premenopausal and postmenopausal bone mass and can reflect age- and menopause-related bone loss (83). Likewise, all these techniques have been shown to differentiate between bone loss associated with disabling conditions, especially those associated with diminished mobility or weightbearing. Because osteoporosis is a systemic disease, measurements of bone density at one anatomic site are generally predictive of fracture risk at another. In addition, for menopause- and age-related osteoporosis, BMD at any skeletal site shows at least modest correlation with other skeletal sites (range from 0.5 to 0.8 at spine, regions of hip and forearm in women older than age 65) (90). Because rates of bone loss differ at different skeletal sites in women with many disabling conditions, the correlation between skeletal sites is likely to be even less robust.

The primary question that faces the clinician is what technique and, more importantly, what site should be measured to ensure the most accurate classification of fracture risk for a women with a disabling condition? Early in menopause (or with estrogen deficiency) there is accentuation of trabecular bone loss based on the greater rates of bone remodeling at these sites; measurements of bone mass at the spine will detect a greater number of women with menopause-induced bone loss than measurements at the hip. Later in life, the proportion of patients with osteoporosis detected by measurements at the hip or forearm is greater than the proportion identified at the postero–anterior spine. This reflects the greater likelihood of degenerative changes in the spine or vascular calcifications that can falsely elevate bone mass at the spine site.

Abundant data show that measurement of BMD at any skeletal site has some utility at predicting fractures at any other site. The hip BMD, however, is the best predictor of hip fracture and appears to predict all other types of fractures as equally well as measurements at any other site (26). Thus, for post-menopausal women, assessment of bone mass at the hip would be adequate for assessment of fracture risk with the addition of the spine BMD in younger early postmenopausal women (including those women with disabilities who suffer premature ovarian failure or secondary amenorrhea) to assess early trabecular bone loss.

For women in which immobilization associated with a disability might contribute to bone loss, bone loss is not universally lost below the site of the neuronal injury and the magnitude of loss is determined, at least in part, by the decrease in the extent of weight-bearing and/or mechanical strain postinjury. Therefore bone mass testing at skeletal sites that directly are affected by the disabling condition (e.g., hemiplegic side in patients with a cerebrovascular accident, distal femur or proximal tibia in SCI, or affected limb in reflex sympathetic dystrophy) might give information regarding the additive effect of the disability and other systemic factors on the bone mass, whereas analysis of bone mass at neurologically unaffected sites would give information regarding the underlying disability-independent effect of systemic factors on bone mass and skeletal health.

BMD should be assessed in women with disabilities to make an assessment of osteoporosis and, thus, fracture risk when the information obtained from the testing will affect therapeutic decision making. It can be used to diagnose osteoporosis when an atraumatic fracture is noted on radiographs (91). It can be useful in monitoring the course of metabolic diseases or medications that adversely affect the skeleton. Its role in monitoring therapeutic response is controversial, although there are data to suggest that therapies that result in stabilization or gains in BMD have the lowest incidence of fractures (92) and, thus, greatest efficacy. There are also data on the use of antiresorptive treatments to suggest that a reduction in BMD after 1 year often was followed by rapid gains in BMD in the second year, reflecting a regression to the mean rather than changes in treatment efficacy (7).

Biochemical Assessment

Biochemical testing (93) for renal and hepatic function, a complete blood count, serum calcium, phosphorus, and total alkaline phosphatase should be measured on all women with disabilities prior to initiating treatment (Table 16-4). In uncomplicated menopause or age-related osteoporosis, all these lab studies will be normal. In individuals in which the hip or wrist BMD is significantly lower than the spine BMD and in which immobilization can be excluded as the etiology of this disproportionately low BMD, measurements of PTH and 25(OH) vitamin D would be appropriate. In older women, because the presence of subclinical hyperthyroidism is common and may contribute to osteoporosis, a serum thyroid-stimulating hormone level should be obtained. If accelerated bone loss relative to age-matched controls is seen (Z score less than -1.5–2.0), additional testing as suggested by the history and physical examination should be performed to exclude secondary causes of osteoporosis.

It might be predicted that markers of bone resorption (e.g., N-telopeptide, C-telopeptide, pyridinoline, or deoxypyridinoline) and bone formation (osteocalcin, bone-specific alkaline phosphatase) would be helpful for assessing osteoporosis and guiding therapy choices, but to date, their role in management of clinical osteoporosis is limited. They correlate only weakly with magnitude of BMD response to treatment (94,95). The evidence report from the Agency on Healthcare Research and Quality stated that no single biochemical marker or group of markers identified individuals with osteoporosis or reliably identified people who would not respond to treatment (96). In women with disabilities, the biochemical markers theoretically could play a role in identifying premenopausal women with disabilities who have low bone mass who might be candidates for treatment if active bone remodeling is present because there are no data to suggest that treating patients with low bone mass where bone remodeling is balanced (or bone mass is stable) results in any benefit.

PRIMARY AND SECONDARY PREVENTION OF OSTEOPOROSIS

The goal of primary prevention of osteoporosis is to maximize attainment of the genetically determined peak bone mass and to minimize rates of bone loss with menopause and aging. Prevention strategies should include avoiding cigarettes, moderating alcohol consumption, minimizing the use of medications that contribute to a negative calcium balance or bone loss, and getting regular physical activity and adequate calcium and vitamin D intake.

Adequate calcium and vitamin D is necessary throughout the lifespan. Dietary sources of both of the nutrients are considered optimal, but it is widely accepted that very few American women achieve adequate stores by diet alone. Prior to menopause, women should take in 800 to 1,200 mg of calcium per day, increasing to 1,200 to 1,500 mg for postmenopausal women (7). The recommended vitamin D intake is 400 to 600 IU/d. Regardless of menstrual status, patients taking glucocorticoids should supplement their diet with the postmenopausal doses of calcium and vitamin D (97). If modifications in diet cannot be made to meet these recommended allowances successfully, calcium supplements may be used.

Calcium supplementation in childhood tends to result in small increases in BMD (98–100). When calcium supplements are used within the first 5 years of menopause, there is no substantial benefit in reducing rates of bone loss (101). In elderly men and women, a review of four randomized clinical trials (RCT) has demonstrated a decreased total fracture risk with calcium supplementation (102). In contrast, the administration of vitamin D_3 alone is not associated with a reduction in the incidence of hip and other nonvertebral fractures (103), although vitamin D_3 given together with calcium in a group of frail elderly people resulted in a reduction in the incidence of hip fractures (104).

Exercise stimulates osteoblastic bone formation, and weightbearing exercise contributes to the development and maintenance of bone mass. A systematic review of the efficacy of exercise for the prevention and treatment of osteoporosis among a diverse population of both premenopausal and postmenopausal women demonstrated trends suggesting that exercise increases or maintains bone density (105), whereas a meta-analysis limiting exercise trials to postmenopausal women failed to show any benefit (106). In contrast, exercise has been shown to decrease the risk of falls by improving neuromuscular function (107).

There are a number of medications available for the treatment of osteoporosis. The most efficacious agents prevent bone loss at both trabecular and cortical bone sites and reduce the risk of both vertebral and nonvertebral fractures. These agents can be divided conveniently into categories that maximize calcium balance, antiresorptive compounds, and anabolic agents (Table 16-5).

Calcitriol, or 1,25(OH) vitamin D, is not yet a recommended treatment for osteoporosis, although it is an important treatment option for certain types of osteomalacia. Its effect on reducing bone turnover and, thus, bone loss is through suppression of PTH. In at least one study, it has been shown to be effective at reducing vertebral deformity (108), but the higher risk for hypecalciuria and hypercalcemia limits its generalized use.

Hormone therapy, such as estrogen or estrogen/progestin (E+P), works by inhibiting osteoclast activity, thereby reducing bone turnover. In a study of estrogen alone, conjugated equine estrogen at doses of 0.625 mg/day resulted in gains in BMD at the spine and proximal femur of 5% and 2.5% over 3 years, respectively (109). In July 2002 the principal results of the Women's Health Initiative (WHI) double-blind, randomized, placebo-controlled E+P trial was terminated early after an average of 5.2 years of follow-up (110). This trial showed clear benefits with E+P use for osteoporosis with a reduction in hip and all clinical fractures by one-third and a 37% reduction in the rates of colorectal cancer. However, there were also substantial risks. E+P use was associated with a 29% increase in rates of coronary heart disease (CHD), a 41% increase in the rates of stroke, twofold greater risk of venous thromboembolic (VTE) disease, and a 26% increase in breast cancer. The CHD and VTE diverged from placebo almost immediately, and unlike data from the Heart and Estrogen/Progestin Replacement Study, in WHI there was no evidence that these risks disappeared with continued use. This resulted in an absolute risk per 10,000 person-years attributable to E+P of seven more CHD events, eight more strokes, eight more VTE, and eight more invasive breast cancers in contrast to absolute risk reductions of hip fractures and colorectal cancers of five and six fewer events, respectively. The absolute excess of risks versus benefits was 19 per 10,000 person-years of exposure. To date, subgroup analyses controlling for prior history of CHD or stroke, age, body mass index, or smoking status failed to define a higher (or lower) risk subgroup. Women reporting prior hormone use had higher rates of breast cancer than did women who never used postmenopausal hormones. Based on these results, although E+P is effective as a treatment for osteoporosis, one should consider use of alternative pharmacologic strategies with less serious risk profiles first. These results do not extend to estrogen alone; that arm of the WHI continues because the overall balance of risks and benefits is not yet clear. Those data should be available in the latter part of 2005.

Table 16-5. *Medications for the prevention and treatment of osteoporosis*[a]

Enhance calcium balance	Antiresorptive agents	Anabolic agents
Calcium	Estrogen plus progestin[b]	Exercise
Vitamin D	Estrogen alone	*Fluoride*
Calcitriol	Raloxifene	*Growth hormone*
Thiazide diuretics	Calcitonin	Parathyroid hormone[b]
	Etidronate	
	Alendronate[b]	
	Risedronate[b]	
	Zolendronate	
	Pamidronate	

[a]Medications in *italics* are considered experimental for the prevention and/or treatment of osteoporosis.
[b]These medications have been shown in randomized, controlled clinical trials to prevent bone mass loss or increase bone mass at both the spine and hip and to reduce the risk of both vertebral and nonvertebral fractures.

In an attempt to achieve some of the benefits of estrogen with lower risk for adverse events, the **selective estrogen receptor modulators (SERMs)** have been developed. Thus far, only raloxifene (RLX) has been approved for prevention and treatment of osteoporosis. At some target tissues such as the bone, RLX functions as an estrogen agonist, reducing bone turnover, increasing bone mass, and maintaining bony architecture. Like estrogen, it lowers LDL cholesterol, but there are little data available to assess its effect on CHD rates. At target tissues such as the breast and uterus, it is a potent estrogen antagonist, and use of RLX in women with a uterus does not require a progestin. In a prospective RCT of 7,705 women with osteoporosis, BMD at both the spine and hip modestly increased and the incidence of vertebral fractures decreased by approximately 50% (111,112). In women who had had an incident vertebral fracture prior to entry into the study (the highest risk for future fracture), RLX also decreased their risk for subsequent fracture by 30%. There are little data to support efficacy at reducing risk for nonvertebral fractures. There are data to suggest that RLX might reduce the incidence of breast cancer, notably estrogen-receptor positive cancers (113), and a large trial comparing the efficacy of RLX to tamoxifen in reducing breast cancer rates in women at high risk is under way. The side effects of RLX include an increased risk for VTE similar to that seen with estrogen and an increase in vasomotor symptoms and leg cramps.

All classes of **bisphosphonates** have been shown to both increase BMD and reduce the rate of fracture. They are potent inhibitors of osteoclasts; they reduce the rate at which new BMUs are formed, reduce the depth of the resorption cavity, and produce a positive bone balance at individual BMUs (114). This class of drugs is approved for the prevention and treatment of postmenopausal osteoporosis. Alendronate (115), risedronate (116), and cyclic etidronate (117) have been shown to increase BMD at both the spine and hip in a dose-dependent fashion. They also consis-

tently have resulted in a reduction in vertebral fracture incidence by 30% to 50%, with efficacy that starts as early as 6 to 12 months after initiating treatment. Benefits in fracture reduction have been noted in women with osteoporosis with or without a prevalent fracture and in patients taking glucocorticoids. Both alendronate and risedronate also decrease the rates of nonvertebral fractures (118,119).

Adverse effects of bisphosphonates mainly involve esophagitis; serious side effects can include esophageal erosions, ulceration, or inflammatory exudates (120). These adverse events are rare and typically occurred in patients who had not taken the pill with water, had taken it and then laid down, or who had previous esophageal pathology such as achalasia or delayed emptying. The intravenous bisphosphonates, pamidronate and zolendonate, have been shown in small studies to be effective at preventing bone loss and may be an option in patients who cannot tolerate oral bisphosphonates or who are unable to swallow effectively, such as those who have suffered strokes.

Calcitonin works by inhibiting osteoclast-mediated bone resorption. An RCT of postmenopausal women with osteoporosis showed that 200 IU calcitonin nasal spray daily resulted in modest increases in spine BMD (1% to 1.5%) and a 33% reduction in new vertebral fractures (121). However, its efficacy is limited; up to half the people taking calcitonin may not maintain BMD at the hip, and no study has found a significant reduction in nonvertebral fractures. Analgesic effects of calcitonin have been found to decrease osteoporotic bone pain in fracture subjects treated with calcitonin (122). Calcitonin may play a role in treatment of osteoporosis in women who cannot tolerate more potent and more effective treatment options.

Parathyroid hormone (1-34) is the first anabolic agent (bone formation stimulator) approved for the treatment of osteoporosis (123). It has been shown to increase the trabecular bone density in areas such as the vertebrae while causing no change or a modest reduction in BMD at skeletal sites primarily composed of cortical bone (124,125). An RCT of daily injectable PTH in women with postmenopausal osteoporosis showed reduction in vertebral and nonvertebral fractures by 60% after 20 months of treatment. Current recommendations limit use to 18 to 24 months to avoid risk for cortical bone loss with long-term treatment. Because the positive effects on BMD are lost after discontinuation, studies have focused on examining the use of PTH coupled with an antiresorptive agent with the hypothesis that the additional agent would potentiate the effect of the PTH after the PTH is stopped. When PTH is added to estrogen (124) or when PTH administration is followed by alendronate (126), the gains in BMD are greater than with the use of the antiresorptive agent alone and the resultant gain was maintained.

Other combination therapies have been suggested including the use of a bisphosphonate such as alendronate or risedronate together with either an estrogen or SERM. With each of these combination therapies, the resultant BMD gain is slightly higher than with either medication alone, but there are no data regarding the impact of combination therapy on either vertebral or nonvertebral fractures available. Therefore, based on the increased cost and potential for increased side effects associated with utilization of two concurrent medications, there are little data to support the need for combination therapy for osteoporosis in the majority of women with disabilities.

SUMMARY

In conclusion, osteoporosis is a common health problem facing women as they age. The attendant bone loss after menopause and with aging puts women at risk for fractures that have a major adverse effect on both the quality and length of life. In women with disabilities, the underlying disabling condition, the potential use of medications that could contribute to bone loss and a negative calcium balance, and neuromuscular deficits that could place them at risk for falls or result in reduced physical activity all further accentuate the risk for osteoporosis and subsequent further accentuation of the handicap associated with their disability. Recognition of risk factors for development of osteoporosis and risk for fractures combined with judicious use of bone mass testing using DEXA can help to identify those women who are likely to benefit from treatment. Based on the advances in diagnosis and treatment strategies over the past two decades and the intense investigations that are currently under way, the future is bright for the continued advancement of the most effective way to prevent the unwanted consequences of osteoporosis in women with disabilities.

REFERENCES

1. NIH Consensus Development Conference. Diagnosis, prophylaxis and treatment of osteoporosis. *Am J Med* 1993;94:646–650.
2. Riggs BL, Melton LJ III. The prevention and treatment of osteoporosis. *New Engl J Med* 1992;327:620–627.
3. AMA-CME Advisory Board. *Managing osteoporosis. Part 1: Detection and clinical issues in testing.* Chicago: AMA, 1999.
4. Melton LJ III. How many women have osteoporosis now? *J Bone Miner Res* 1995;60-A:930–934.
5. Looker AC, Johnston CC Jr, Wahner HW, et al. Prevalence of low femoral bone density in older U.S. women from NHANES III. *J Bone Miner Res* 1995;10:796–802.
6. Osteoporosis prevention, diagnosis and therapy. NIH Consensus Statement Online 2000 March 27–29, 17: 1–36.
7. National Osteoporosis Foundation. Osteoporosis: cost-effectiveness analysis and review of the evidence for prevention, diagnosis and treatment. *Osteoporosis Int* 1998;8(suppl 4):1S–88S.
8. Chantraine A. Actual concept of osteoporosis in paraplegia. *Paraplegia* 1978;16:51–58.
9. Frisbie JH. Fractures after myelopathy: the risk quantified. *J Spinal Cord Med* 1997;20:66–69.
10. Arlot ME, Sornay-Rendu E, Garnero P, et al. Apparent pre- and post-menopausal bone loss evaluated by DXA at different skeletal sites in women: the OLEFY cohort. *J Bone Miner Res* 1997;12:683–690.
11. Kanis JA. Estrogens, the menopause and osteoporosis. *Bone* 1996;19:185S–190S.
12. Frost H. A new direction for osteoporosis: a review and proposal. *Bone* 1991;12:429–437.
13. Baran RE. Anatomy and ultrastructure of bone. In: Fauvus MJ, ed. *Primer on the metabolic bone diseases*

    and disorders of mineral metabolism. Philadelphia: Lippincott-Raven, 1996.

14. Pacifici R. Estrogen, cytokines and pathogenesis of postmenopausal osteoporosis. *J Bone Miner Res* 1996; 11:1043–1051.

15. WHO Study Group. *Assessment of fracture risk and its application to screening for postmenopausal osteoporosis: report of a WHO Study Group.* WHO Technical Report Series 843, Geneva, Switzerland: World Health Organization, 1994:1–129.

16. Whedon GD, Shorr E. Metabolic studies in paralytic acute anterior poliomyelitis II: Alterations in calcium and phosphorus metabolism. *J Clin Invest* 1957;36: 966–981.

17. Heany RP. Radiocalcium metabolism in disuse osteoporosis in man. *Am J Med* 1962;33:188–200.

18. Minaire P, Meunier P, Edouard C, et al. Quantitative histological data on disuse osteoporosis: comparison with biological data. *Calcif Tissue Res* 1974;17:57–73.

19. Naftachi NE, Viau AT, Sell GH, et al. Mineral metabolism in spinal cord injury. *Arch Phys Med Rehabil* 1980;61:139–142.

20. Bergmann P, Heilporn A, Schoutens A, et al. longitudinal study of calcium and bone metabolism in paraplegic patients. *Paraplegia* 1977;15:147–159.

21. Claus-Walker J, Campos RJ, Carter RE, et al. Calcium excretion in quadriplegia. *Arch Phys Med Rehabil* 1980;302:701–708.

22. Stewart AF, Adler M, Byers CM, et al. Calcium homeostasis in immobilization: an example of resorptive hypercalciuria. *New Engl J Med* 1982;306:1136–1140.

23. Chantraine A, Heynen G, Fanchimont P. Bone metabolism, parathyroid hormone and calcitonin in paraplegia. *Calcif Tissue Int* 1979;27:199–204.

24. Black DM, Cummings SR, Melton LJ III. Appendicular bone density and a women's lifetime risk of a hip fracture. *J Bone Miner Res* 1992b;7:639–646.

25. Cummings, Black DM, Nevitt MC, et al. Appendicular bone density and age predict hip fractures in women. The Study of Osteoporotic Fractures Research Group. *JAMA* 1990;263:665–668.

26. Cummings SR, Black DM, Nevitt MC, et al. Bone density at various sites for the prediction of hip fractures. Study of Osteoporotic Fractures Research Group. *Lancet* 1993;263:665–668.

27. Gardsell P, Johnell O, Nilsson BE, et al. Predicting various fragility fractures in women by forearm bone densitometry: a follow up study. *Calcif Tissue Int* 1993;52: 348–353.

28. Hui SL, Slemenda CW, Johnston CC Jr. Age and bone mass as predictors of fracture in a prospective study. *J Clin Invest* 1988;81:1804–1809.

29. Hui SL, Slemenda CW, Johnston CC Jr. Baseline measurements of bone mass predicts fracture in white women. *Ann Intern Med* 1989;111:355–361.

30. Stevenson JC, Lees B, Davenport M, et al. Determinants of bone density in normal women: Risk factors for future osteoporosis. *Br Med J* 1989;298:924–928.

31. Slemenda CW, Hui SL, Longcope C, et al. Predictors of bone mass in perimenopausal women: a prospective study of clinical data using photon absorptiometry. *Ann Intern Med* 1990;112:96–101.

32. Bauer DC, Browner WS, Cauley JA, et al. Factors associated with appendicular bone mass in older women. *Ann Intern Med* 1993;118:657–665.

33. National Osteoporosis Foundation. Physicians guide to prevention and treatment of osteoporosis. Belle Meade, NJ: Excerpta Medica, 1998.

34. Slemenda CW, Christian JC, William CJ, et al. Genetic determination of bone mass in adult women: a re-evaluation of the model and the potential importance of gene interaction on heritability estimates. *J Bone Miner Res* 1998;6:561–567.

35. Franceschi S, Scinella D, Bidoli E, et al. The influence of body size, smoking and diet on bone density in pre- and post-menopausal women. *Epidemiology* 1996;7: 411–414.

36. Orwoll ES, Bauer DC, Vogt TM, et al. Axial bone mass in older women. *Ann Intern Med* 1996;124:187–196.

37. Kritz-Silverstein D, Barrett-Connor E. Early menopause, number of reproductive years and bone mineral density in post-menopausal woman. *Am J Public Health* 1993;83:983–988.

38. Lieberman SA, Oberol Al, Gilkison CR, et al. Prevalence of neuroendocrine dysfunction in patients recovering from traumatic brain injury. *J Clin Endocrinol Metab* 2001;86:2752–2756.

39. Stevenson JC, Lees B, Davenport M, et al. Determinants of bone density in normal women: risk factors for future osteoporosis. *Br Med J* 1989;298:924–928.

40. Kiel DP, Zhang Y, Hannon MT, et al. The effect of smoking at different life stages on bone mineral density in elderly men and women. *Osteoporosis Int* 1996;6:240–248.

41. Egger P, Duggleby S, Hobbs R, et al. Cigarette smoking and bone mineral density in the elderly. *J Epidemiol Community Health* 1996;50:47–50.

42. Felson DT, Zhang Y, Hannan MT, et al. Alcohol intake and bone mineral density in elderly men and women: The Framingham Study. *Am J Epidemiol* 1995;142: 485–492.

43. Wolff J. *The law of bone remodeling.* [Marquet P, Furlong R (translators)] New York: Springer-Verlag, 1986.

44. Simkin A, Ayalon J. *Bone loading: The new way to prevent and combat the thinning bone of osteoporosis.* London: Prion, 1990.

45. Sabo D, Blaich S, Wenz W, et al. Osteoporosis in patients with paralysis after spinal cord injury. A cross sectional study in 46 male patients with dual-energy X-ray absorptiometry. *Arch Orthop Trauma Surg* 2001;11:75–78.

46. Biering-Sorenson F, Bohr H, Schaadt O. Bone mineral content of the lumbar spine and lower extremities years after spinal cord lesions. *Paraplegia* 1998;26: 293–301.

47. Bloomfield SA, Mysiw WJ, Jackson RD. Bone mass and endocrine adaptations to training in spinal cord injured individuals. *Bone* 1996;19:61–68.

48. Garland DE, Maric Z, Adkins RH, et al. BMD about the knee in spinal cord injured patients with pathologic fractures. *Contemp Orthop* 1993;26:375–379.

49. Garland DE, Adkins RH, Stewart CA, et al. Regional osteoporosis in women who have a complete spinal cord injury. *J Bone Joint Surg Am* 2001;83: 1195–1200.

50. Hangartner TN. Osteoporosis due to disuse. In: Matkovic V, ed. *Physical medicine and rehabilitation clinics of North America: osteoporosis.* Philadelphia: WB Saunders 1995:579–594.

51. Heany RP. Nutrition and risk for osteoporosis. In: Mar-

cus R, Feldman D, Kelsey J, eds. *Osteoporosis*. San Diego: Academic Press 1996:483–505.

52. Chan GM, Hess M, Hollis J, et al. Bone mineral status and childhood accidental fractures. *Am J Dis Child* 1984;138:569–570.

53. Matkovic V, Koshal K, Simonovic I, et al. Bone status and fracture risks in two regions of Yugoslavia. *Am J Clin Nutr* 1979;32:540–549.

54. Chantraine A, Nusgens B, Lapier CM. Bone remodeling during the development of osteoporosis in paraplegia. *Calcif Tissue Int* 1986;38:323–327.

55. Faulkner KG, Cummings SR, Black D, et al. Simple measurement of femoral geometry predicts hip fracture: The study of osteoporotic fractures. *J Bone Miner Res* 1993;8:1211–1217.

56. Heany RP. Pathogenesis of osteoporosis. In: Fauvus MJ, ed. *Primer on the metabolic bone disease and disorders of calcium metabolism.* Philadelphia: Lippincott-Raven 1996:252–258.

57. Kiralti BJ, Smith AE, Nauenberg T, et al. Bone mineral and geometric changes through the femur with immobilization due to spinal cord injury. *J Rehabil Res Develop* 2000;37:225–233.

58. DeBruin ED, Herzog R, Rozendal RH, et al. Estimation of geometric properties of cortical bone in spinal cord injury. *Arch Phys Med Rehabil* 2000;81:150–156.

59. Lee TQ, Shapiro TA, Bell DM. Biomechanical properties of human tibias in long-term spinal cord injury. *J Rehabil Res Develop* 1997;34:295–302

60. Lindsay R, Silverman SL, Cooper C, et al. Risk of new vertebral fracture in the year following a fracture. *JAMA* 2001;285:320–323.

61. Klotzbuecher CM, Ross PD, Landsman PB, et al. Patients with prior fractures have an increased risk of future fractures: A summary of the literature and statistical synthesis. *J Bone Miner Res* 2000;18:721–739.

62. Black DM, Arden NK, Palmero L, et al. Prevalent vertebral deformities predict hip fractures and new vertebral deformities but not wrist fractures. *J Bone Miner Res* 1999;14:821–828.

63. Cosman F, Nieves J, Komar L, et al. Fracture history and bone loss in patents with MS. *Neurology* 1998;51. 1161–1165.

64. Sato Y, Fujimatsu Y, Kukyama M, et al. Influence of immobilization on bone mass and bone metabolism in hemiplegic elderly patients with long-standing stroke. *J Neurol Sci* 1998;156;205–210.

65. Sato Y. Abnormal bone and calcium metabolism in patients after stroke. *Arch Phys Med Rehabil* 2000;81: 117–121.

66. Johnell O, Gullberg B, Kanis JA, et al. Risk factors for hip fracture in European women. The MEDOS study. *J Bone Miner Res* 1995;10:1802–1831.

67. Dargent-Molina P, Favier F, Granjean H. Fall-related factors and risk for hip fracture. The EPIDOS prospective study. *Lancet* 1996;348:145–149.

68. Cummings SR, Nevitt MC, Browner WS. Risk factors for hip fractures in white women. Study of Osteoporotic Fractures Research Group. *New Engl J Med* 1995;332:767–773.

69. Bjilsma J, Jacobs J. Hormonal preservation of bone in rheumatoid arthritis. *Rhem Dis Clin NA* 2000;26: 112–115.

70. Melton LJ III, Brown RD Jr, Achenbach SJ, et al. Long-term fracture risk following ischemic stroke: a population-based study. *Osteoporosis Int* 2001;12: 980–986.

71. Cauley JA. Risk of mortality following clinical fractures. *Osteoporosis Int* 2000;11:556–561.

72. Kado DM, Browner WS, Palermo L, et al. Vertebral fractures and mortality in older women. Study of Osteoporotic Fractures Research Group. *Arch Intern Med* 1999;159:1215–1220.

73. Barrett-Connor E. The economic and human costs of osteoporotic fracture. *Am J Med* 1995;98:3s–8s

74. Shabas D, Weinreb H. Preventative healthcare in women with multiple sclerosis. *J Women's Health* 2000;9:289–395.

75. Turk MA, Scandale J, Rosenbaum PF, et al. The health of women with cerebral palsy. *Phys Med Rehabil Clin N Am* 2001:12:153–168.

76. Kanis JA. Diagnosis of osteoporosis. *Osteoporosis Int* 1997;7:S108–S116.

77. Melton LJ III, Atkinson EJ, O'Fallon WM, et al. Long-term fracture prediction by bone mineral assessed at different skeletal sites. *J Bone Miner Res* 1993;8: 1227–1233.

78. Wasnich RD, Ross PD, Heilbrun LK, et al. Prediction of postmenopausal fracture risk with use of bone mineral measurements. *Am J Obstet Gynecol* 1985;153: 745–751.

79. Gardsell P, Johnell O, Nilsson BE. Predicting fractures in women by using forearm bone density. *Calcif Tissue Int* 1989;44:235–242.

80. Miller PD, Bonnick SL, Rosen CJ, et al. Clinical utility of bone mass measurements in adults: Consensus of an international panel. *Semin Arthritis Rheum* 1996; 25:577–587.

81. Lazo MG, Shirazi P, Sam M, et al. Osteoporosis and risk for fracture in men with spinal cord injury. *Spinal Cord* 2001;39:208–214.

82. Kanis JA, Melton LJ III, Christiansen C, et al. The diagnosis of osteoporosis. *J Bone Miner Res* 1994;8: 1137–1141.

83. Genant HK, Engellae K, Fuerst T, et al. Non-invasive assessment and structure: state-of-art. *J Bone Miner Res* 1996;11:707–730.

84. Mazess R, Chesnut CH III, McClung M, et al. Enhanced precision with dual energy x-ray absorptiometry. *Calcif Tissue Int* 1992;51:14–17.

85. Robert D, Lee W, Caneo RC, et al. Longitudinal study of bone turnover after acute spinal cord injury. *J Clin Endocrinol Metab* 1998;83:415–422.

86. Lui M, Tsuji T, Higuchi Y, et al. Osteoporosis in hemiplegic stroke patients as studied by dual energy X-ray absorptiometry. *Arch Phys Med Rehabil* 1999;80: 1219–1226.

87. Ramnemank A, Nyberg L, Lorentzon R, et al. Progressive hemiosteoporosis on the paretic side and increased bone mineral density in the non-paretic arm the first year after severe stroke. *Osteoporosis Int* 1999;9: 269–275.

88. Liu CC, Theodorou DJ, Theodorou SJ, et al. Quantitative computed tomography in the evaluation of spinal osteoporosis following spinal cord injury. *Osteoporosis Int* 2000;11:889–896.

89. Warden SJ, Bennell KL, Matthews B, et al. Quantitative ultrasound assessment of acute bone loss following acute spinal cord injury: a longitudinal pilot study. *Osteoporosis Int* 2002;13:586–592.

90. Steiger P, Cummings SR, Black DM, et al. Age-related decrements in bone mineral density in women over 65. *J Bone Miner Res* 1992;7:625–632.

91. Holick MF. Metabolic bone disease. In: Noble J, ed. *Textbook of primary care medicine,* 3rd edition. St Louis: Mosby 2001:387–397.

92. Hochberg MC, Ross PD, Black DM, et al. Larger increases in bone mineral density during alendronate therapy are associated with a lower risk of new vertebral fractures in women with postmenopausal osteoporosis. *Arthritis Rheum* 1999;42:46–54.

93. Christiansen C. What should be done at the time of menopause? *Am J Med* 1995;98:56s–59s

94. Marcus R, Holloway L, Wells B. Turnover markers only weakly predict bone response to estrogen: The Postmenopausal Estrogen/Progestin Interventions Trial (PEPI) *J Bone Miner Res* 1997;12:S103.

95. Bauer DC, Black DM, Ott SM, et al. Biochemical markers predict spine but not hip response to bisphosphonates: The Fracture Intervention Trial (FIT). *J Bone Miner Res* 1997;12:s150.

96. Agency for Healthcare Research and Quality. *Osteoporosis in postmenopausal women: Diagnosis and monitoring: Summary.* Evidence Report/Technology Assessment: Number 28. AHRQ Publication Number 01-E031, 2001. Rockville, MD: AHRQ, 2001.

97. American College of Rheumatology Task Force on Osteoporosis Guidelines. Recommendations for the prevention and treatment of glucocorticoid-induced osteoporosis. *Arthritis Rheum* 1996;39:1791–1801.

98. Johnston CC Jr, Miller JZ, Slemenda CW, et al. Calcium supplementation and increases in bone mineral density in children. *New Engl J Med* 1992;327:82–87.

99. Lloyd T, Andon MB, Rollins N, et al. Calcium supplementation and bone mineral density in adolescent girls. *JAMA* 1993;270:841–844.

100. Lloyd T, Rollins N, Andon MB, et al. Enhanced bone gain in early adolescence due to calcium supplementation does not persist in late adolescence. *J Bone Miner Res* 1996;11:S154.

101. Dawson-Hughes B, Dallal GE, Krall EA, et al. A controlled trial of the effects of calcium supplementation on bone density in postmenopausal women. *New Engl J Med* 1990;323:878–883.

102. Cumming RG, Nevitt MC. Calcium for the prevention of osteoporotic fractures in postmenopausal women. *J Bone Miner Res* 1997;12:1321–1329.

103. Gillespie WJ, Avenell A, Herry DA, et al. *Vitamin D and vitamin D analogues for preventing fractures associated with involutional and postmenopausal osteoporosis.* (Cochrane Review). The Cochrane Library Issue 2. Oxford: Update Software, 2001.

104. Chapuy MC, Arlot ME, Rollings N, et al. Vitamin D3 and calcium to prevent hip fractures in the elderly woman. *New Engl J Med* 1992;327;1637–1642.

105. Ernst E. Exercise for female osteoporosis. A systematic review of randomized clinical trials. *Sports Med* 1998;25:359–368.

106. Berard A, Bravo G, Gauthier P. Meta-analysis of the effectiveness of physical activity for the prevention of bone loss in postmenopausal women. *Osteoporosis Int* 1997;7;331–337.

107. Province MA, Hadley EC, Hornbrook MC, et al. The effects of exercise on falls in elderly patients. *JAMA* 1995;273:1341–1347.

108. Gallagher JC, Goldgar D. Treatment of postmenopausal osteoporosis with high doses of calcitriol. A randomized controlled study. *Ann Intern Med* 1990; 113:649–655.

109. The Writing Group for PEPI. Effect of hormone therapy on bone mineral density: Results from the Postmenopausal Estrogen/Progestin Interventions (PEPI) Trial. *JAMA* 1996;276:1389–1396.

110. Writing Group for the WHI Investigators. Risks and benefits of estrogen plus progestin in healthy postmenopausal women: principal results from the Women's Health Initiative randomized controlled clinical trial. *JAMA* 2002;228:321–333.

111. Delmas PD, Bjarnason NH, Mitlak BH, et al. Effects of raloxifene on bone mineral density, serum cholesterol concentrations and uterine endometrium in postmenopausal women. *N Engl J Med* 1997:337: 1641–1647.

112. Ettinger B, Black DM, Mitlak BH, et al. Reduction of vertebral fracture risk in postmenopausal women with osteoporosis treated with raloxifene: results from a 3-year randomized clinical trial. *JAMA* 1999:282:637–645.

113. Cummings SR, Eckert S, Krueger KA, et al. The effect of raloxifene on risk for breast cancer in postmenopausal women: Results from the MORE randomized trial. *JAMA* 1999;281:2189–2197.

114. Fleisch H. Bisphosphonates: Mechanisms of action. *Endocrin Rev* 1998;19:80–100.

115. Liberman UA, Weiss SR, Broll J, et al. Effect of oral alendronate on bone mineral density and incidence of fractures in postmenopausal osteoporosis. Alendronate Phase III Osteoporosis Treatment Study Group. *New Engl J Med* 1995:333:1437–1443.

116. Harris ST, Watts GB, Genant HK, et al. Effects of risedronate treatment on vertebral and non-vertebral fractures in women with postmenopausal osteoporosis. A randomized controlled trial. *JAMA* 1999;282: 1344–1352.

117. Harris ST, Watts NB, Jackson RD, et al. Four-year study of intermittent cyclic etidronate treatment of postmenopausal osteoporosis: three years blinded therapy followed by one year open therapy. *Am J Med* 1993;95:557–567.

118. Black DM, Cummings SR, Karpf DB, et al. Randomized trial of the effect of alendronate on risk of fracture in women with existing vertebral fractures. *Lancet* 1996;348:1535–1541.

119. McClung MR, Geusens P, Miller PD, et al. Effect of risedronate on the risk of hip fracture in elderly women. *New Engl J Med* 2001;344:333–340.

120. DeGroen PC, Lubbe DF, Hirsch LJ. Esophagitis associated with the use of alendronate. *New Engl J Med* 1996;334:1016—1021.

121. Chesnut CH 3rd, Silverman S, Andriano K, et al. A randomized trial of nasal spray salmon calcitonin in postmenopausal women with established osteoporosis: the prevent recurrence of osteoporotic fractures study. *Am J Med* 2000;109:267–276.

122. Pun KK, Chan LWL. Analgesic effect of intranasal calcitonin in the treatment of osteoporotic compression fractures. *Clinical Ther* 1989;11:205–209.

123. Dempster DW, Cosman F, Parisien M, et al. Anabolic actions of parathyroid hormone on bone. *Endocr Rev* 1993;14:690–709.

124. Lindsay R, Nieves J, Formica C, et al. Randomised

controlled study of effect of parathyroid hormone on vertebral bone mass and fracture incidence among post-menopausal women on estrogen with osteoporosis. *Lancet* 1997;350:550–555.

125. Neer RM, Arnaud CD, Zanchetta JR, et al. Effect of parathyroid hormone (1-34) on fractures and bone mineral density in postmenopausal women with osteoporosis. *New Engl J Med* 2001;344:1434–1441.

126. Rittmaster R, Bolognese M, Ettinger M, et al. Enhancement of bone mass in osteoporotic women with parathyroid hormone followed by alendronate. *J Clin Endocrinol Metab* 2000;85:2129–2134.

17

Exercise and Physical Activity Options

Mayra C. Santiago

INTRODUCTION

A growing body of scientific research data has accumulated over the past 20 to 30 years indicating that physical activity and exercise are important modifiable behaviors in the prevention of major systemic diseases and the promotion of optimal physical and mental health. The great majority of these data are based on the results of epidemiologic and intervention studies in varied population groups of people without disability. Nonetheless, people with physical disabilities remain as one of the nationally targeted groups at risk of major disease processes directly or indirectly related to persistent low physical activity levels. Recently, attention has been directed at describing habitual levels of physical activity of women, yet data on women with physical disabilities is extremely sparse. Although based on limited research, findings on typical physical activity patterns of women with physical disabilities underscore the importance of enhancing levels of physical activity and/or exercise in this population.

This chapter will attempt to summarize key findings on the role of physical activity and exercise in the promotion of health and prevention of disease in the general population and target these findings as critically important to women with physical disabilities. Current understandings of habitual patterns of physical activity and exercise in women with physical disabilities are described. General and specific physical activity and exercise principles for women with physical disabilities are discussed. Some of the important disability-specific concerns during exercise are highlighted. Lastly, potential exercise-induced improvements will

be reviewed based on data from studies of people with physical disabilities.

A caveat to this chapter is that much of the knowledge that exercise physiologists, as well as other exercise specialists, and I have gained about promoting physical activity and exercise in people with physical disabilities is based on individualized attempts at applying general exercise physiology concepts to a diverse, disability-specific context of what is safe yet optimal for any one person. Because of the myriad of implications of any one primary physical disability and its related secondary conditions, no one "cookbook recipe" is appropriate for any one type of exercise. Any rule, principle, or method described in this chapter may need to be modified to address more safely and effectively the specific needs and implications of any given woman with any given physical disability. Nonetheless, it is the goal of this chapter to provide clinicians and health professional and practitioners with the following: (a) convincing evidence that increasing habitual levels of physical activity and/or exercise is a critical factor in enhancing the health and quality of life of their clients and patients, and b) basic guidelines for designing programs of physical activity and exercise with particular attention to how the nature of the program may be influenced by the type of physical disability of the client or patient.

PHYSICAL ACTIVITY, EXERCISE, AND HEALTH

Historically, exercise has played an important role in the health promotion and disease prevention agenda of the medical and other health-related professions. Early writings of preventive medicine pioneers such as Hippocrates included exercise as one of the key contributors to human health (1). Through contemporary times, physical movement was considered beneficial only if it was vigorous enough to significantly raise a person's breathing and heart rate. The American College of Sports Medicine (ACSM) published in 1978 the first set of guidelines on how much exercise is required to develop and maintain cardiorespiratory fitness and body composition in healthy adults (2). These early exercise guidelines were as follows:

1. The exercise mode is "aerobic" in nature and as such, uses large groups of muscles and is performed continuously.
2. The intensity of the exercise is at 60% to 90% of maximum heart rate (age limited) or 50% to 85% of maximal oxygen uptake.
3. The frequency of the exercise is 3 to 5 times per week.
4. The duration of the exercise is 15 to 60 minutes.

Recent exercise recommendations published by the ACSM (3,4) included the addition of muscular fitness (strength, endurance, and flexibility) exercises and the following modifications to the aerobic exercise guidelines: (a) to include a minimum of 20 minutes of either continuous or discontinuous exercise (with 10 minutes as minimum continuous duration), and (b) at a minimum intensity of 55% maximum heart rate (age limited) or 40% maximum oxygen uptake.

Physical "activity" did not enter into the national public health agenda until the late 1980s and 1990s, during which time a series of documents was published indicating that physical movement not need to be "vigorous" for it to be beneficial in promoting health, wellness, and disease prevention. "Physical activity" is distinguished from exercise as being any voluntary movement of the body that causes there to be an increase in energy cost. "Exercise" is described to be any type of physical activity that is planned, structured,

and performed with the intent of improving one or more physical fitness attributes and involves repetitive movements. In turn, "physical fitness" generally is defined as a set of attributes that allow a person to perform physical activities without undue fatigue, and as "health-related fitness," they include cardiorespiratory fitness, muscular fitness (strength and endurance), flexibility, and body composition (5).

Starting with the publication of *Healthy People 2000* by the U.S. Department of Health and Human Services (6) and continued with subsequent publications from the American Heart Association (7) and the Centers for Disease Control and Prevention (CDC) together with the ACSM (8), a capstone document was published in 1996 entitled *Physical Activity and Health: A Report of the Surgeon General* (9). This document reviewed the scientific data from the past 50 years on the amount of physical activity required to promote health and reduce disease and recommended that physical activity: (a) be "moderate" in intensity; (b) "...be performed regularly"; and (c) include a minimum of 30 minutes per day on "most, if not all, days of the week." Furthermore, the 30 minutes of moderate physical activity can be accumulated at different periods throughout the day (8).

"Moderate" physical activity is defined using units of metabolic equivalency of resting states or MET levels, such that 1 MET is equivalent to the required amount of metabolic energy for 1 kilogram (kg) of body weight to be maintained at resting states for 1 hour. "Moderate" physical activity requires a minimum energy cost (i.e., intensity) of 3 METs and up to a maximum of 6 METs and is the recommended amount of physical activity for health-related benefits. "Vigorous" physical activity or "exercise" is classified as reaching or exceeding a 6 MET level of intensity and is the recommended amount of exercise for physical fitness improvement or maintenance.

Publications such as *Healthy People 2010* (10) together with some of the previously described national health documents emphasize the link between major chronic diseases/conditions and low levels of physical activity, including cardiovascular disease (CVD; heart disease, stroke, hypertension, and peripheral vascular disease), type 2 diabetes, certain cancers, osteoporosis, and obesity. In *Healthy People 2000* (6) and continued in *Healthy People 2010* (10) people with disabilities remain as one of the main targeted subgroups of the general population for health-promoting interventions. The priority status for people with disability in national health objectives results from the higher risk for many chronic diseases and overall health disparities compared to people without disabilities.

Mortality rates from any cause in people of varied ages are described to be inversely related to levels of physical activity. In fact, an expert panel organized by the CDC and the ACSM report that habitual patterns of moderate physical activity can reduce mortality rates in the United States by approximately 250,000 per year (8). Participating in modest levels of physical activity that have a weekly energy cost of at least 1,000 kilocalories reduces the risk of all-cause mortality by 20% to 30% for adult men and women (11). After adjusting for the influence of other risk factors for all-cause and CVD mortality, low levels of cardiorespiratory fitness from physical inactivity have emerged as one of the primary and independent disease risk factors. In fact, low cardiorespiratory fitness levels in women predict all-cause mortality at levels similar to those of cigarette smoking (12). Women who exercise strenuously have 20% lower rates of invasive breast cancer as compared to women who do not exercise (13). Type 2 diabetes is a secondary risk factor for CVD, and women who exercise vigorously at least once a week have a significantly lower risk of developing this metabolic condition (14). Despite the preponderance of such data for the general population, no data have been published on the potential long-term health benefits from consistent patterns of moderate physical activity and/or exercise in people with physical

disabilities, such as reduction in disease risk or severity and/or mortality risk or rates. Nonetheless, there is a strong consensus among exercise and public health researchers and experts that such health benefits are at minimum equivalent for people with and without disabilities.

Clearly, these documented health benefits from regular participation in moderate levels of physical activity have a large potential impact for women with physical disabilities. Historically, physical movement in the form of exercise for people with physical disabilities was focused largely on the use of therapeutic exercise for rehabilitative outcomes of improved performance of activities or independent activities of daily living (ADL and IADL, respectively). Although the importance of therapeutic exercises remains undeniable, there has emerged an understanding among health practitioners of the importance of promoting physical activity and exercise in people with physical disabilities for the purpose of leisure, enjoyment, and overall physical and mental health benefits. This phenomenon has been referred to as a "paradigm shift" in the understanding of the role of exercise among health professionals and one that "persons with disabilities have demanded … and research supports " (15).

PATTERNS OF PHYSICAL ACTIVITY AND EXERCISE IN WOMEN WITH PHYSICAL DISABILITIES

Women in general report lower levels of physical activity than men do. National data on physical activity patterns in the general population indicate that approximately 29% of the population report a physically inactive lifestyle, 38% report no leisure-time physical activity (LTPA), 44% report insufficient levels of physical activity, and only 27% report recommended levels of physical activity. In these four categories of health guidelines for physical activity, women report higher levels of physical inactivity, no LTPA, and insufficient physical activity, as well as lower levels

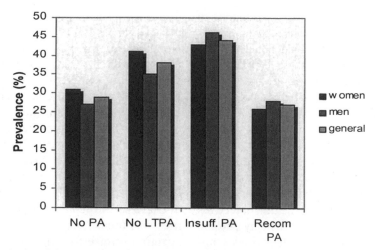

Fig. 17-1. Physical activity patterns of the general population. Based on national data from the Behavioral Risk Factor Surveillance System, 1990–1998, and the National Health Interview Survey, 1997–1998. (From Centers for Disease Control. Physical activity trends—United States, 1990–1998. *MMWR* 2001;50(9):166–169, with permission; Macera CA, Pratt M. Public health surveillance of physical activity. *Research Quarterly for Exercise and Sport* 2000;71(2 suppl):97–103, with permission; and Schoenborn CA, Barnes PM. Leisure-time physical activity among adults: United States, 1997–1998. *Advance Data from Vital and Health Statistics, Centers for Disease Control* 2002;325: 1–23, with permission.)

of recommended physical activity than men (see Fig. 17-1) (16–18).

Limited data are published on the physical activity patterns of people with disabilities. *Healthy People 2010* describes that people with disabilities report higher levels of physical inactivity (56% versus 36%) and lower levels of regular (27% versus 34%) and vigorous (10% versus 14%) physical activity than people without disabilities, respectively (see Fig. 17-2) (10).

Habitual patterns of physical activity in women with physical disabilities have been published to an even lesser extent. A 3-year research project funded by the National Institute of Child Health and Human Development and the National Center for Medical Rehabilitative Research allowed our research team at Temple University to collect data on the health needs, patterns, and behaviors of women with physical disabilities. In a survey of 165 women with physical disabilities, approximately 72% reported decreasing levels of physical activity in the past 10 years and al-

most 60% reported they "never to rarely" performed LTPA that was demanding enough to cause them to have an increase in their heart rate and breathing rate (19). Similarly, in a research project involving African-American women with mobility impairments, 92% of them reported that they did not participate in any type of LTPA (20). Yet, it is noteworthy that the majority of women in both of these research projects expressed a desire and interest to start a physical activity or exercise program.

Researchers in the area of physical activity assessments acknowledge that actual levels of physical activity may be underreported for women. This suspected underrepresentation might result from the use of survey instruments that query physical activity patterns with forms of movement that are not performed as typically by women as by men. For example, a woman may get most of her physical activity stimulus from non-exercise–related or non-sport–related activities such as household or dependent care activities. The

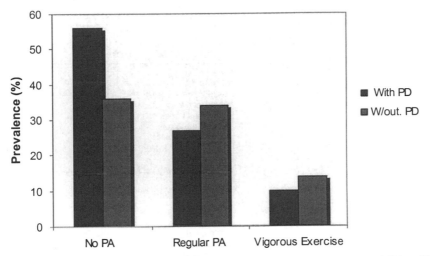

Fig. 17-2. Physical activity (PA) patterns in people with and without physical disabilities (PD). (From U.S. Department of Health and Human Services. *Healthy People 2010: Conference Edition, in Two Volumes.* Washington, DC: USDHHS, January 2000, with permission.)

previously described research project at Temple University used a modified physical activity assessment instrument that specifically addresses this consideration and found that levels of physical inactivity were pervasive throughout most life aspects of 126 women with physical disabilities (21). The majority of these women responded that they participated in no physically active household tasks or work-related tasks such as walking or standing. Additionally the majority also reported no LTPA and no exercise participation (Fig. 17-3).

PHYSICAL ACTIVITY AND EXERCISE PROGRAMS FOR WOMEN WITH PHYSICAL DISABILITIES

General Principles

Earlier in this chapter, moderate physical activity was distinguished from exercise as an activity that is performed at moderate levels of intensity (3 to less than 6 METs) and for the purpose of leisure, recreation, enjoyment, or daily tasks and chores. In contrast, exercise is an activity that is performed with the intent of improving one or more of the aspects of physi-

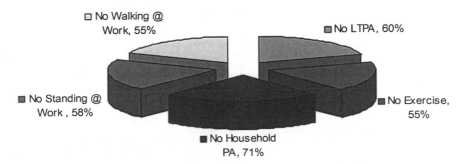

Fig. 17.3. Physical activity (PA) patterns in women with physical disabilities. (Based on data from Santiago MC, Cavanagh M, Thompson HC, Coyle CP. Physical activity patterns of adult women with physical disabilities. *Med Sci Sports Exerc*, 1998;30:S161, with permission.)

Table 17-1. *Estimate of energy cost of recreational/sports, physical activities, and exercises*

Activity	Intensity	Description of activity	# Kcals per kg of body weight per minute
Aerobics class		Low impact	0.083
		High impact	0.117
		Water aerobics/calisthenics, moderate effort	0.067
Badminton		Social singles or doubles games	0.075
Basketball		Wheelchair basketball	0.108
		Shooting baskets	0.075
		Nongame, general	0.100
Bicycling (outdoors)	<10 MPH (>6 min/mile)	Slow, leisure, for pleasure	0.067
	10–11.9 MPH (5–6 min/mile)	Slow, leisure with light effort	0.100
	12–13.9 MPH (4:18–5 min/mile)	Leisure with moderate effort	0.133
	14–15.9 MPH (3:48–4:18 min/mile)	Leisure, fast, vigorous effort	0.167
Bicycling (indoor stationary)	50 watts	Very light effort	0.050
	100 watts	Light effort	0.092
	150 watts	Moderate effort	0.117
	200 watts	Vigorous effort	0.175
Bowling		Recreational	0.050
Dancing		Ballroom, slow: waltz, foxtrot; samba, tango, cha-cha	0.050
		Ballroom, fast: folk, square, disco; line dancing, polka, country	0.075
		Ballet, modern, twist, jazz, tap, jitterbug	0.080
Canoeing, rowing		Light effort	0.050
		Moderate effort	0.117
Golfing		Using power cart	0.058
		Walking and pulling clubs	0.072
		Walking and carrying clubs	0.075
Hiking		Trails, cross-country	0.100
Horseback riding		Trotting	0.108
		Walking	0.042
Jogging	4.5 to <5 MPH (12–13 min/mile)	Combination of brisk walking and slow jogging	0.100
	5 MPH (12 min/mile)	Slow jogging pace	0.133
	5.2 MPH (11:30 min/mile)	Comfortable jogging pace	0.150
	6 MPH (10 min/mile)	Moderate jogging pace	0.167
	6.7 MPH (9 min/mile)	Fast jogging pace	0.183
Skating, roller		General, recreational	0.117
Skating, ice		General, recreational	0.092
Skiing, cross-country	2.5 MPH (24 min/mile)	Light effort	0.117
	4.0–4.9 MPH (12:15–15 min/mile)	Moderate effort	0.133
Snow shoeing		General, recreational	0.133
Softball/baseball		General, recreational	0.083
Swimming (laps)		Freestyle, light to moderate effort	0.117
		Freestyle, moderate to vigorous effort	0.167
Swimming (not laps)		Leisurely effort; in lake, river, or ocean	0.100
Table tennis (ping pong)		General, recreational	0.067
Tennis		Doubles game	0.100
		Singles game	0.133
Walking, outdoors (level ground)	<2 MPH (>30 min/mile)	Strolling	0.033
	2.0 MPH (30 min/mile)	Slow pace	0.042
	2.5 MPH (24 min/mile)	Comfortable pace	0.050
	3.0 MPH (20 min/mile)	Moderate pace	0.055
	3.5 MPH (17:08 min/mile)	Brisk pace	0.063
	4.0 MPH (15 min/mile)	Very brisk pace	0.083
	4.5 MPH (13:20 min/mile)	Very, very fast pace	0.105
	Up stairs	Moderate pace	0.083
Weight lifting		Free, nautilus, or universal type, moderate effort	0.050
Wheelchair propulsion		Pushing manual wheelchair for transportation	0.067
		Use of manual wheelchair propulsion as aerobic exercise training	0.133

(Estimates based on energy cost data published in Ainsworth BE, Haskell WL, Whitt ML, et al. Compendium of physical activities: an update of activity codes and MET intensities. *Med Sci Sports Exer* 2000;32:S498–S516, with permission.)

cal fitness (cardiorespiratory, muscular strength and endurance, flexibility) and at an intensity that meets or exceeds the 6 MET level. For benefits to be accrued from either type of physical movement, it must be performed in a consistent (habitual) manner. Simply put, only regular participation in moderate physical activity or exercise is going to produce desired benefits. These health or fitness benefits are produced because the human body adapts to any consistent physical movement stimulus in ways that allow it to respond to the same amount of movement with less physiologic effort and strain and thus less fatigue. When challenged by a new amount of movement that represents an "overload" demand to the working muscles and supporting cardiorespiratory system, the body systems once more adapt to this amount of effort to allow it to meet it with lesser physiologic strain and effort.

These overall benefits from regular participation in moderate physical activity or exercise are particularly important for people with physical disabilities because there is a high prevalence of fatigue as a secondary condition. Accelerated fatigue levels result directly from many disabling conditions and from persistent states of low physical movement asso-

ciated with the disability-induced impairments. In turn, such levels of fatigue may promote even less amounts of physical movement and thus increase physical deconditioning, which further aggravates fatigue rates. A recent survey of 165 women with physical disabilities, which used a combined score of frequency of endorsement and severity level, indicated that fatigue and physical deconditioning received the first and third highest ranking out of 32 self-reported secondary conditions (22). Only regular participation in moderate physical activity or exercise programs has the potential to break the "vicious cycle" caused and promoted by high levels of fatigue and physical deconditioning.

The potential amount of improvement that moderate physical activity or exercise programs can provide is proportional to the total amount of volume of movement that a person accumulates. Each activity effort contributes to this volume and typically is quantified by the amount of energy cost that it requires. Table 17-1 provides a sample listing of estimated energy costs for common types of physical activities and exercises that are performed for the purpose of recreation, leisure, sports, and/or fitness. Table 17-2 describes a

Table 17-2. *Estimate of energy cost of indoor and outdoor household physical activities*

Activity	Description of activity	# Kcals per kg of body weight per minute
Cleaning	Light effort: dusting, straightening up	0.042
	Heavy effort: windows, cleaning garage	0.050
	Sweeping floors/carpets	0.055
	Vacuuming, mopping	0.058
	Very heavy effort: scrubbing floors/bathroom	0.063
	Outdoor sweeping	0.067
Gardening	Trimming shrubs/trees with power cutter	0.058
	Trimming shrubs/trees with manual cutters	0.075
	Weeding, cultivating garden	0.075
	Digging, composting	0.083
Mowing lawn	Riding mower	0.042
	Walking with power mower	0.092
	Walking with hand mower	0.100
Raking lawn	Moderate effort	0.072
Snow shoveling	Riding snow blower	0.050
	By hand	0.100

(Estimates based on energy cost data published in Ainsworth BE, Haskell WL, Whitt ML, et al. Compendium of physical activities: an update of activity codes and MET intensities. *Med Sci Sports Exer* 2000;32:S498–S516, with permission.)

similar sample listing of common indoor and outdoor household physical activities. Using a person's body weight and the amount of time that they spend doing the specific activity allows for estimation of its required energy cost in calories or kilocalories (kcals). These energy cost estimates are used for documenting the accumulation of recommended amounts of physical activity/exercise to promote a person's overall health or physical fitness. More specifically, they also can be used to quantify the amount of potential movement-related energy deficits that can be established for people who are seeking to loose or maintain body weight by lowering their levels of body fat.

The use of these estimated energy cost values, however, needs to proceed with some cautionary comments. An important consideration is that almost all of these values were derived from research data gathered from people without physical disabilities. In fact, only three activities of the entire extensive listing in the actual publication (23), from which Tables 17-1 and 17-2 were developed, address the energy cost of using a wheelchair for locomotion (see listing for wheelchair basketball and wheelchair propulsion for transportation or aerobic exercise). Authors of the original publication pointedly identify the need that exists to evaluate the energy costs of physical movement in people with physical disabilities and the subsequent establishment of standards that will more accurately reflect this important health-affecting variable. These authors also acknowledge that any factor(s) that influence a person's gait efficiency will cause variations in energy costs. This cautionary note is particularly important for people with physical disabilities in which there are decreases in movement efficiency caused by the disabling condition, secondary conditions that may coexist, and/or use of assistive mobility equipment. Additionally, these authors warn that for people with high amounts of body mass (body weight), the listed energy costs of weightbearing activities may be an underestimation and non-weightbearing activities

may be an overestimation. Notwithstanding, this database is the most comprehensive and current data available regarding the measurement of the energy costs of human movement.

Tables 17-1 and 17-2 express estimated energy costs in kcals per kilogram of body weight per minute of the activity (kcals/kg/min). Any activity that is listed with an energy cost that is at least 0.050 kcals/kg/min meets national health promotion guidelines for moderate levels of physical activity (i.e., ≥ 3 METS). Any activity that is listed with an energy cost that meets or exceeds 0.100 kcals/kg/min represents intensities that promote improvements in physical fitness (i.e., ≥ 6 METS). Examples of how this database can be used are described as follows:

Example 1

Susan weighs 140 lbs and goes for a brisk walk for 35 minutes. You can calculate her estimated energy cost for the activity as follows (see Table 17-1):

1. Convert body weight from lbs to kg
   140 lbs divided by 2.2 = 63.64 kg
2. Look up activity in appropriate table:
   "brisk walking" = 0.063 kcals/kg/min
3. Calculate total kcals:
   Total kcals = 0.063 kcals/kg/min
   $\times$ 63.64 kg $\times$ 35 min
   $\cong$ 140 kcals (140.33 Kcals)

Example 2

Emily weighs 160 lbs and spends 1.5 hours doing general garden weeding. You can calculate her estimated energy cost for the activity as follows (see Table 17-2):

1. Convert body weight from lbs to kg:
   160 lbs divided by 2.2 = 72.73 kg
2. Look up activity in appropriate table:
   "weeding in garden" = 0.075 kcals/kg/min
3. Convert time in hours to minutes:
   1.5 hours $\times$ 60 min = 90 min
4. Calculate total kcals:
   Total kcals = 0.075 kcals/kg/min $\times$ 72.73 kg
   $\times$ 90 min $\cong$ 491 kcals (490.93 kcals)

Disability-Specific Considerations During Exercise

Each type of primary disability and its related secondary condition(s) will influence the concerns and safety factors that may need to be noted when a person exercises. Within any one type of physical disability, the level of disability severity and the potential for use of pharmacologic agents that may interact with an exercise response will modify further any listing of possible exercise concerns. Table 17-3 represents an attempt at providing a summary of some of the potential concerns that may exist for a listing of 11 types of physical disabilities common in women. The information in Table 17-3 was developed through a review of the exercise literature and with special contribution from two comprehensive exercise resource manuals published by the ACSM: *ACSM's Exercise Management for Persons with Chronic Diseases and Disabilities* (24) and *ACSM's Resources for Clinical Exercise Physiologist* (25). These resource manuals address exercise testing and training recommendations, potential contraindications, and pharmacologic considerations to exercise in detail by disability category. Regardless of the resource used to gain information about exercise considerations for women with physical disabilities, any described rule may need to be modified to address the individual needs of any one woman with a physical disability.

Cardiorespiratory (Aerobic) Exercise

An aerobic exercise stimulus is one in which the active muscles contract in a dynamic and repetitive manner and at low muscle tension intensities such that the contractions can be sustained for a "long" time (at least 3 to 5 minutes). Targeted goals are to sustain the movement for at least 10 to 15 minutes, with the opportunity to accumulate these amounts of exercise at different times throughout the day. The cardiorespiratory system responds to this type of movement with sustained increases in breathing and cardiac contraction rates to support oxygen and fuel delivery to exercising muscles and metabolite removal. Performing aerobic exercises at least two to three times per week is recommended. Typical types of aerobic activities are swimming, brisk walking, bicycling, and hiking (see Table 17-1 for other examples of activities that meet or exceed the energy cost of 0.100 kcals/kg/min or ≥ 6 METs).

The larger the amount of active muscle mass that participates in the aerobic exercise, the greater the systemic or "central" cardiorespiratory benefits, such as improved aerobic energy-producing capabilities in the active muscles, increased strength and endurance of respiratory muscles, and increased strength and vascularity of the heart. When there is a limited amount of muscle mass available to exercise aerobically, the benefits that are gained from regular participation are focused largely on local muscle tissue or "peripheral" improvements, including improved aerobic metabolic systems in muscle cells (i.e., enhanced mitochondrial structure and status) and increased vascular tissue density of the muscle bed. Systemic cardiorespiratory improvements are available to a lesser extent when small amounts of muscles are involved in the exercise effort. Although the amount of muscle mass that contributes to the exercise will vary with the type and severity of the disability, using as many muscle groups as possible in the aerobic exercise activity is an important consideration for maximizing overall cardiorespiratory fitness benefits.

Muscular Strength and Endurance Exercise

For improvement in muscle fitness (strength and endurance) muscle groups need to contract to produce tensions that exceed those typically required to carry out ADL and IADL. In contrast to aerobic exercises, muscle fitness exercises can be performed with small amounts of muscle, even

Table 17-3. *Potential concerns during exercise*

Disability	Overheating	Blood pressure	Heart rate	Respiratory limitations	Muscle spasticity and/or contractures	Muscle, joint, bone pain and/or damage	Muscle fatigue	Bladder and/or bowel problems	Impaired sensation	Balance, gait, and/or coordination problems
ALS					✓	✓	✓			✓
Arthritis (OA/RA)		✓	✓	✓ (RA)	✓	✓	✓	✓	✓ (RA)	✓
Fibromyalgia						✓	✓			
Cerebral palsy		✓	✓		✓	✓	✓			
Lupus		✓	✓	✓	✓	✓	✓	✓		
Multiple sclerosis	✓	✓	✓		✓	✓	✓	✓	✓	✓
Muscular dystrophy	✓	✓	✓	✓	✓	✓	✓			✓
Parkinson's disease		✓	✓	✓	✓	✓	✓	✓	✓	✓
Postpolio syndrome		✓	✓	✓		✓	✓		✓	✓
Spinal cord injury/spina bifida	✓	✓	✓	✓	✓	✓	✓	✓	✓	
Stroke/traumatic brain injury					✓	✓	✓		✓	✓

ALS, amyotrophic lateral sclerosis; OA, osteoarthritis; RA, rheumatoid arthritis.
(Table is a modification of data published in Coyle CP, Santiago M, Thompson H, et al. *Charting your course to health and wellness: a health promotion packet for women with physical-disabilities.* Philadelphia: Temple University, 1997, with permission.)

to the point of actually isolating specific muscle groups. In disabilities with muscle spasticity and/or contracture problems, it is recommended to start a program of muscle fitness by performing static muscle exercise in which there is not movement through the range of motion. As muscular strength and endurance improve, dynamic muscle exercises can be added to the program. Exercise recommendations center on performing 1 to 2 sets of 8 to 10 dynamic repetitions each, with at least a 3 to 5 minute rest period between sets, 2 to 3 times per week. The resistance or load used must overload the muscle to require tension production that modestly exceeds the tensions associated with the performance of ADL and IADL. Household items (such as a partially filled jug with a handle) can serve as the overload resistance as long as the object can be well gripped. Exercise bands also can be used for muscle fitness exercises and are helpful for women who have limited gripping ability. Rapping the exercise band around a hand, arm, or leg and attaching the other end to a fixed object creates an effective tension load for muscle fitness improvements.

Important considerations when performing muscle fitness exercises are to make the movements in a slow and controlled manner and to the full range of motion of the joint being exercised. This consideration is extremely important for women with disabilities at risk of spasticity, contractures, and/or joint pain (see Table 17-3). Additionally, movements never should be forced beyond the ranges established by the person's joint articulations and connective tissues. The two previously cited ACSM resource manuals (24,25) provide detailed disability-specific considerations for muscle fitness exercises.

Benefits that can be derived from participating in regular muscle fitness exercises are increases in muscular strength from improved neuromuscular recruitment abilities, increases in amounts of contractile muscle proteins, and increases in the strength and elasticity of connective tissues that contribute to muscle functioning. Together with improve-

ments in muscular strength also are increases in muscular endurance and thus reductions in muscle fatigue levels when performing demanding activities. Globally, these muscular strength and endurance benefits carry over to improving gait, coordination, and balance problems and significantly decreasing the risk of falls and movement-related injuries in general.

Flexibility Exercises

The purpose of performing flexibility exercises is to improve or maintain the ability to move through the full range of motion of a joint area. Benefits that are derived from regular flexibility exercises extend themselves to decreases in joint pain, muscular spasticity, and/or contractures and improvements in gait, balance, and coordination. As with muscle fitness exercises, stretching exercises need to be performed in a slow and controlled manner throughout the joint's full range of motion up to the point of joint articulation resistance; hold the stretch in that position for 10 to 20 seconds; then release the stretch in a slow, controlled manner back to resting position.

Overall Benefits from Exercise Programs

In each of the previous subsections, potential benefits were highlighted for each of the three types of exercises (cardiorespiratory, muscular fitness, and flexibility). Table 17-4 describes a summary of some of the common symptoms reported by women with physical disabilities and how these three types of exercise programs may affect the symptoms. Table 17-5 is a summary description of potential exercise benefits that have been published in the scientific literature for the 11 previously identified physical disabilities.

SUMMARY

Participation in regular programs of moderate physical activities and/or exercises will enhance the overall health, wellness, and

Table 17-4. *Potential benefits for symptoms by type of exercise*

Self-reported symptoms	Types of exercise		
	Flexibility exercises	Aerobic exercises	Muscular strengthening exercises
Excessive muscle weakness and/or fatigue	+	+	+
Decreased range of motion and/or pain in joints	+	+	++
Muscle spasticity and/or contractures[a]	+	++	++
Respiratory problems		+	
Circulatory problems (tingling, numbness in extremities)	+	+	
Overheat easily		+	
Balance, gait, and/or coordination problems	+	+	+

+This type of exercise can improve this particular symptom.

++This type of exercise may improve this particular symptom, yet should be done under clinical supervision.

[a]Muscle movements should be performed in slow, controlled manner; do static resistive exercises as initial muscle strengthening exercises before progressing to dynamic resistive exercises.

quality of life of women with physical disabilities. Although the capstone research has yet to be performed on how such improved patterns of habitual physical movement will improve the long-term mortality and morbidity risks of women with physical disabilities, the evidence is convincing that such benefits exist for women with physical disabilities as they do for women without physical disabilities. A critical piece of the puzzle on how to improve the participation of women with physical disabilities in such programs is the contribution from health providers and practitioners. Clinicians and health practitioners are vital players in the success of this important health behavioral modification by providing the encouragement, guidance, supervision, and support regarding increasing physical activity and exercise levels for women with physical disabilities.

Table 17-5. *Potential exercise effects by disability*

Disability	Potential exercise effects		
	Muscle strength and endurance effects	Aerobic/cardiorespiratory effects	Flexibility effects
ALS[a]	+	+	+
Arthritis (OA/RA)	++	++	++
Fibromyalgia	+[b]	+	+[b]
Cerebral palsy	+[b]	+[b]	+[b]
Lupus[c]		+[b]	
Multiple sclerosis	++	++	++
Muscular dystrophy[a]	+	+	+
Parkinson's disease[a]	+[b]	+[b]	+
Postpolio syndrome	++	++	++
Spinal cord injury	++[d]	++	++
Spina bifida[b]	+	+	+
Stroke/traumatic brain injury	+[d]	+	+

ALS, amyotrophic lateral sclerosis; OA, osteoarthritis; RA, rheumatoid arthritis.

+ Some level of documented improvements.

++ Significant level of documented improvements.

[a]Potential effects largely are aimed at minimizing loss of functioning or slowing down of the disease progress so as to maintain ability to perform activities of daily living and/or independent activities of daily living.

[b]Based on limited numbers of published studies on potential exercise training effects.

[c]Published literature on exercise training effects limited to aerobic effects.

[d]Muscle improvements limited to nonaffected muscles.

REFERENCES

1. Berryman J. The tradition of "six things non-natural": exercise and medicine from Hippocrates through antebellum America. In: Pandolf KB, ed. *Exerc Sport Sci Rev* 1989;17:515–559.

2. American College of Sports Medicine. The recommended quantity and quality of exercise for developing and maintaining fitness in healthy adults. *Med Sci Sports Exerc* 1978;10:vii–x.

3. American College of Sports Medicine. The recommended quantity and quality of exercise for developing and maintaining cardiorespiratory and muscular fitness in healthy adults. *Med Sci Sports Exerc* 1990;22:265–274.

4. American College of Sports Medicine. The recommended quantity and quality of exercise for developing and maintaining cardiorespiratory and muscular fitness in healthy adults. *Med Sci Sports Exerc* 1998;30:975–991.

5. Casperson CJ, Powell KE, Christensen GM. Physical activity, exercise, and physical fitness: definitions and distinctions for health-related research. *Public Health Rep* 1985;100:126–131.

6. U.S. Department of Health and Human Services. *Healthy People 2000: national health promotion and disease prevention objectives.* Washington, DC: U.S. Department of Health and Human Services, Public Health Services, 1991, DHHS Publication No. (PHS) 91-50212.

7. Fletcher GF, Blair SN, Blumenthal J, et al. Benefits and recommendations for physical activity programs for all Americans: a statement for health professionals by the Committee on Exercise and Cardiac Rehabilitation of the Council on Clinical Cardiology, American Heart Association. *Circulation* 1992;86:340–344.

8. Pate RR, Pratt M, Blair SN, et al. Physical activity and public health: A recommendations from the Centers for Disease Control and the American College of Sports Medicine. *JAMA* 1995;273:402–407.

9. U.S. Department of Health and Human Services. *Physical activity and health: a report of the Surgeon General.* Atlanta: U.S. Department of Health and Human Services, Centers for Disease Control and Prevention, National Center for Chronic Disease Prevention and Health Promotion, 1996.

10. U.S. Department of Health and Human Services. *Healthy People 2010: Conference Edition, in Two Volumes).* Washington, DC: USDHHS, January 2000.

11. Lee I-M, Skerrett PJ. Physical activity and all-cause mortality: what is the dose-response relation? *Med Sci Sports Exerc* 2001;33:S459–S471.

12. Blair SN, Kampert JB, Kohl HW, et al. Influences of cardiorespiratory fitness and other precursors on cardiovascular disease and all-cause mortality in men and women. *JAMA* 1996; 276:205-210.

13. Rockhill B, Willet WC, Hunter DJ, et al. A prospective study of recreational physical activity and breast cancer risk. *Arch Intern Med* 1999;159:2290–2296.

14. Manson JE, Rimm EB, Stampfer MJ, et al. Physical activity and incidence of non-insulin dependent diabetes mellitus in women. *Lancet* 1991;338:774–778.

15. Seaman J. Physical activity and fitness for persons with disabilitics. *Research Digest, President's Council on Physical Fitness and Sports* 1999;3(5):1–6.

16. Centers for Disease Control. Physical activity trends—United States, 1990–1998. *MMWR* 2001;50(9):166–169.

17. Macera CA, Pratt, M. Public health surveillance of physical activity. *Res Q Exerc Sport* 2000;71(2 suppl): 97–103.

18. Schoenborn CA, Barnes PM. Leisure-time physical activity among adults: United States, 1997–1998. *Adv Data* 2002;325:1–23.

19. Coyle C, Santiago M. *Promotion of health and wellness for women with physical disabilities: summary report.* Philadelphia: Temple University, 2000.

20. Rimmer JH, Rubin SS, Braddock D, et al. Physical activity patterns of African-American women with physical disabilities. *Med Sci Sport Exerc* 1999;31:613–618.

21. Santiago MC, Cavanagh M, Thompson HC, et al. Physical activity patterns of adult women with physical disabilities. *Med Sci Sport Exerc* 1998;30:S161.

22. Coyle CP, Santiago MC, Shank JW, et al. Secondary conditions and women with physical disabilities. *Arch Phys Med Rehabil* 2000;81:1380–1387.

23. Ainsworth BE, Haskell WL, Whitt ML, et al. Compendium of physical activities: an update of activity codes and MET intensities. *Med Sci Sport Exerc* 2000; 32:S498–S516.

24. Durstine JL., ed. *ACSM's exercise management for persons with chronic diseases and disabilities.* Champaign, IL: Human Kinetics Publishers, 1997.

25. Myers JN, Herbert WG, Humphrey R, eds. *ACSM's resources for clinical exercise physiology.* Philadelphia: Lippincott, Williams & Wilkins, 2002.

26. Coyle CP, Santiago M, Thompson H, et al. *Charting your course to health and wellness: a health promotion packet for women with physical disabilities.* Philadelphia: Temple University, 1997.

NIH funded project at Temple University for this article: *Promotion of Health and Wellness in Women with Physical Disabilities.* Grant # HD35059-01.

18

Nutritional Considerations

Jean Cassidy

"No amount of prevention will eliminate morbidity and overall deterioration if an individual's basic nutritional requirements are not satisfied."
Professional Nurse, 10/84

Nutrition is involved in the etiology, treatment, and prevention of at least six of the 10 leading causes of death in adults (1). Nutrition is a critical component of risk reduction and treatment and must be included in clinical and preventive services for women. During hospitalizations and/or initial rehabilitation treatment phases, education (if provided at all) is focused on lowering nutrition risk based on immediate concerns such as meeting nutritional requirements via nutrition support if there was a traumatic injury, stabilizing blood sugars, replenishing protein stores, and the like. Rarely is there adequate staff or time to discuss long-term nutritional issues. Therefore, there is a great need for health care professionals to be aware of the long-term nutritional issues and provide the necessary education.

MALNUTRITION

There are three types of malnutrition (2). One type is kwashiorkor or protein malnutrition. There are adequate calories from carbohydrates and fat but lower intake of protein. This person may appear well nourished. People who are obese often are not recognized as malnourished because of their size, but the diet actually may be quite poor. The second type is marasmus. This person eats protein, carbohydrate, and fat but in limited amounts; a person with marasmus appears thin. The

third type is a combination of these two, resulting from starvation.

WHAT CAN CAUSE MALNUTRITION?

Disability itself is a risk factor for malnutrition. Other risk factors that make optimal nutrition a challenging goal are depression, living alone, presence of multiple chronic conditions, poor or inadequate food choices, poor appetite from pain or pain medications, lack of finances or assistance, bad dentition, dysphagia or swallowing difficulty, and increased needs from illnesses or surgeries.

Well-known effects of malnutrition include a decreased muscle function, lower respiratory drive, lower cardiac function, loss of body tissue and muscle strength, decreased immune status, and decreased wound healing. It is important to screen clients for nutritional risk so these factors can be identified and appropriate referrals can be made. Many screening tools are available.

The Dietary Guidelines for Americans is a good foundation from which to start in the discussion of nutrition education. Special considerations for those with disabilities then can be emphasized. Inform your patients that the Dietary Guidelines for Americans 2000 (3) begin with the basics of the ABCs:

A = Aim for fitness. This means aim for a healthy weight and be physically active every day.
B = Build a healthy base. Follow the Food Guide Pyramid so that you get the vitamins, minerals, energy, and other healthful

substances from foods that your body needs each day.

C = Choose sensibly. Choose a diet that is low in saturated fat and cholesterol and moderate in total fat. Limit intake of sugars and salt.

BODY WEIGHT AND ADEQUATE NUTRIENT INTAKE

Most of your clients will be concerned about "calories" and weight management. Weight gain is often the result of a decreased calorie requirement as a result of a decreased activity level without the decreased calorie intake. Staying in a good weight range is important. However, other facets of good nutrition should not get lost in the goal of losing weight. Examples are preventing osteoporosis, maintaining good skin integrity, sustaining energy levels, avoiding constipation, and meeting the recommended dietary allowances (RDA) of vitamins and minerals. It is fine to cut back on calories, but also focus on choosing healthy calories.

It is important to differentiate between body weight versus body image. Help your clients do a self-assessment.

- Are they higher or lower than the ideal body weight range for the nondisabled population?
- Is their weight history of the past 6 to 12 months stable, or does it contain drastic fluctuations?
- What is their family history for being thin, heavy, pear shaped, etc.
- Is their weight interfering with transfers, ability to put shoes on, change leg bags, etc.?
- Are they needing a bigger wheelchair?

Always consider a psychologic consultation if someone appears to have a distorted body image or obsesses about gaining weight.

Patients may ask: "How many calories should I eat?" There is no quick answer. Many factors, including age, sex, height, weight, and activity level, are needed to give the best educated guess. If they really are interested in counting calories, they should count calories that they consume for 3 typical days. People tend to have better success with weight loss when they gradually cut their typical intake back by 200 to 500 calories instead of making a drastic decrease to a strict calorie level. This also can put up a red flag for those who are not getting nearly enough calories (e.g., 600 calories/day on a daily basis). A 3-day food record can be an invaluable tool to bring to a consultation with a registered dietitian (RD). The dietitian also can evaluate the intake of fat, protein, fluids, fiber, and vitamins and minerals.

WEIGHT GAIN

Occasionally you will see someone who needs to gain weight. Individuals will take this issue just as seriously as those who need to lose weight. It is imperative to take a detailed diet history to discover inadequate intake and/or poor habits. Meals should be at scheduled hours and should be planned. If oral intake meets estimated maintenance needs, an additional 500 calories per day is suggested to meet anabolic needs. Snacks between meals are usually more acceptable than larger meals. Some examples of ideas for an additional 500 calories are as follows:

1 cup low-fat milk, 2 slices bread, 2 oz. meat, 1 oz. cheese = 505 calories
Strawberry banana shake (see recipe at end of chapter) and 1 oz. walnuts = 505 calories
1 cup chili with beans, 1 corn muffin with 1 tsp. margarine = 525 calories
Munch mix (see recipe at end of chapter) ½ cup = 490 calories

Oral supplements also can be used if there is a lack of interest in food and in eating. There is no preparation involved, and they are easy to consume.

FIBER

Constipation is a common complaint of those with disabilities. There is an increased risk for constipation from immobility, certain medications, decreased gastrointestinal motility, lack of sensation, poor diet, or inadequate fluid consumption (4).

Eating more fiber and/or taking an over-the-counter fiber supplement often is advised. I have found that people need more information than this. It should be emphasized that any fiber supplement is a *supplement* and not a *replacement* for a high-fiber diet. High-fiber foods also provide many nutrients and are low in calories and fat. It is important for people to eat fiber *daily*. A high-fiber diet every few days actually can cause problems with alternating constipation and diarrhea. Consistency is critical. In the beginning, avoid overwhelming people by trying to distinguish whether foods are high in soluble or insoluble fibers. The emphasis should be on a variety of foods so they will be likely to get adequate amounts of both types.

For 2,000 calories, 20 to 35 grams of fiber is recommended. Again, the 3-day food record is a good assessment tool. If they only take in approximately 4 to 5 grams, it would be unwise to suddenly increase to 20 to 30 grams. Not everyone is an avid reader of nutrition information so be sure your clients know some good sources of fiber (Table 18-1). Label reading should be encouraged.

When fiber is increased in the diet, there also must be an increase in fluid intake because fiber pulls fluid from the body (6).

When the body gets too little water, it takes what it needs from internal sources such as the colon. The result is constipation.

FLUIDS

Water is considered to be one of the major nutrients bodies need. Water and other fluids play an important role in relation to skin, bladder management, bowel programs, and weight management. Water helps moisturize skin from the inside, preventing dryness. Adequate fluid intake is a key factor in avoiding urinary tract infections.

Alcohol and liquids with caffeine such as coffee, tea, and colas act as diuretics and cause the body to actually lose more water. These liquids and carbonated beverages also may irritate the bladder and should be limited.

Acidic urine is not the best environment for growing bacteria so it is desired. Drinking cranberry juice is a common practice to make the urine acidic. Although there is still some controversy about the benefit, if an individual claims it works for her, there is probably no harm.

A large amount of fluid dilutes urine, which helps prevent stones from forming. In the past, it may have been recommended that dairy products be avoided to help prevent kidney stones. Today it is recognized that dairy products, in moderation, can be a part of this high fluid intake.

Fluids often are overlooked as a source of calories. Regular soda, punch, and lemonade are loaded with sugar and can provide between 100 and 250 calories per serving. One to two servings of juice each day is fine, but a serving is only $\frac{1}{3}$ to $\frac{1}{2}$ a cup. If someone is drinking a quart of juice a day, this could be an extra 500 calories or more. Also, the body does not store the extra vitamin C; it is excreted in the urine. If an individual is prone to urinary tract infections, she should ask her doctor about a vitamin C supplement. If the cranberry juice or vitamin C is important to a client, diluting the juice with water will decrease the calories consumed. Cranberry tablets also are available.

Table 18-1. *Some high-fiber food choices*

Food choice	Fiber (g)
Cranberry sauce, ½ cup	2.9
1 dried fig	1.75
1 pear	4.6
5 dried prunes	4.0
Fresh raspberries, ½ cup	3.6
Oat bran, 1 tbsp	6.0
1 bean burrito	8.2
Peanut butter, 2 tbsp	2.4
Canned beans with franks, 1 cup	17.5
Canned peas, ½ cup	4.0
Oatmeal, 1 cup	4.1
Brown rice, 1 cup	3.3
Ham and swiss sandwich on rye	5.1

(Used with permission from ESHA Research, The Food Processor. http://www.esha.com.)

Water contains no calories, and it also offers other benefits. Water suppresses the appetite naturally and helps the body metabolize stored fat. It is easy to drink a lot of it. Today, in addition to tap water, there are flavored waters, mineral waters, and natural waters. Your patients should read the labels carefully because some have sugar added; they should buy the ones that state "no calories."

SKIN CARE AND NUTRITION

Risk factors for skin sores include immobility, poor transfers or positioning, inactivity, incontinence, aging, pressure sensation, body weight, and malnutrition (7). With obesity, there is a decreased maneuverability and prolonged contact with surfaces. There is also poor vascularization of adipose tissue. Inadequate protective padding and nutrient stores result from being underweight.

There are specific nutrients related to wound healing. One is protein. Low protein stores result in edema; this leads to less oxygen and nutrients being transported to the tissue cells and fewer waste products being removed. There is also decreased skin elasticity with low protein levels.

For women the RDA for protein is 48 grams/day. For a more individual assessment, the daily requirement for protein is 0.8 g/kg. This requirement is increased when certain medical conditions are present. Plus, there are direct protein losses through an open wound. As much as 1.5 g/kg may be needed to promote wound healing. When assisting your clients use Table 18-2 as a guide in determining whether they are consuming enough protein.

Do not underestimate the importance of complex carbohydrates and calories. If a high-protein diet is consumed yet calorie requirements are not met, the protein will be used for energy and not tissue repair.

Vitamin A increases collagen content and promotes overall immune response. Sources of vitamin A include dark-green vegetables, yellow-orange vegetables, apricots, cantaloupe, liver, fortified milk, and margarine.

Table 18-2. *Some high-protein food choices*

Food choice	Protein (g)
Milk, 1 cup	8
Meats, 3 oz (e.g., burger, pork chop, large chicken thigh)	21
Peanut butter, 2 tbsp	8
1 egg	7
Baked beans, ½ cup	6
Cottage cheese, ½ cup	12
Bread, 1 slice	3
Cheese, 1 oz	8
Oatmeal, ½ cup	5
Tuna fish, ¼ cup	12
Minestrone soup, 1 cup	6

Zinc is a necessary mineral for protein synthesis. It is difficult to measure tissue levels of zinc and imbalances of other nutrients can occur with high zinc absorption, so any supplementation should be done with a doctor's supervision. Food sources of zinc are meats, seafood, whole grains, and legumes.

Vitamin C is necessary for collagen production. It is widely available in fresh fruits, vegetables, and juices.

DYSPHAGIA

Dysphagia, defined as an inability to swallow or difficulty in doing so, is a result of many chronic medical conditions (8–10). This difficulty can lead to aspiration, or food going into the lungs. This then can result in aspiration pneumonia. A speech pathologist should be consulted if a client reports any of the following conditions:

1. Dry mouth—not able to moisten foods
2. A wet or hoarse voice after eating or drinking
3. Sensation of food sticking in throat, frequent clearing of throat
4. Coughing while eating or after eating
5. Pocketing of food
6. Poor tongue control
7. Needing excessive eating time

An RD should be consulted because people with dysphagia may not consume adequate amounts of food or liquids because it is difficult and this may not be reported. This can

Table 18-3. *Tips for dealing with dysphagia*

To make swallowing easier
Chew all food well.
Eat at a slower pace.
Take small bites.
Take a sip of liquid between bites—use liquids only after food has been cleared.
Eat when less fatigued.
Prepare easy-to-swallow foods.
Generally safe foods
Baked egg dishes
Meat or egg salad with mayonnaise
Soft or melted cheese
Pasta or rice casseroles
Meatloaf
Pudding
Hot cereal
Risky foods
Whole-grain breads
Plain rice
Ground meats without gravy
Dry cottage cheese
Peanut butter

lead to dehydration, constipation, or malnutrition. Weight should be monitored. Enteral feedings may be necessary for those who are not meeting calorie, protein, or fluid requirements by mouth.

Before seeing a speech therapist, the guidelines given in Table 18-3 may aid those who are suspected to have dysphagia.

TEXTURED DIETS

The swallowing process is complex, and foods eaten can have different effects depending on which phase of the swallow is problematic. Texture, cohesiveness, density, and viscosity of foods and liquids are considered. After a complete evaluation, a speech therapist will recommend a specific diet for those with dysphagia. Once the preferred texture is determined, the speech therapist, RD, and client should work as a team. This is an area that can be quite confusing.

Textured diets can have various names such as blenderized; pureed; dysphagia I, II, III diets; ground; mechanical soft; or soft. If a client has a handout or list from another facility, always review it or have a speech therapist review it because it can be different

from what your facility has and may need modifications.

Extra time should be spent obtaining food preferences and showing how they can be modified to fit into the diet prescription. It also would be time well spent to show the individual and/or caregivers how to blenderize or grind foods to the desired consistency.

For those with enough family or caregiver support, time, and energy there are some resources and cookbooks available to make appealing foods and meals. Use the RD as a resource too. He/she may have recipes and samples of food thickener. You also could call the dietary manager of a nursing home to see if they have any resources available to borrow.

For those with less time and energy, a strictly homemade blenderized diet may not be realistic. There are now some prepureed, frozen items available as well as prethickened liquids (juices, milk, and water). Again, doing a little research with your RD, local nursing home, or hospital may be worthwhile. Some companies may ship right to your home (see "Resources"). Because these items may be more costly and require freezer storage space, a balance between these convenience items and home-blended foods may be desirable. Please also see the section on oral supplements in this chapter.

GASTROESOPHAGEAL REFLEX DISEASE

Gastroesophageal reflex disease (GERD) also may cause aspiration (10). The reflex may cause stomach contents to go back into the esophagus. In severe cases, these contents could end up in the mouth, causing choking or pulmonary aspiration.

Individuals with GERD should be encouraged to do the following:

1. Avoid late-night snacks. Allow a few hours between eating and going to bed.
2. Decrease consumption of fatty foods, alcohol, and chocolate. These foods may lower the esophageal sphincter pressure.

3. Decrease consumption of coffee, foods containing large amounts of tomato, and orange juice because these can be irritating to the esophageal mucosa.

FATIGUE

Fatigue is a common complaint of the disabled population (4,11). Many factors can cause fatigue such as lack of sleep, pain, spasms, medications, caffeine consumption, anemia, or hypothyroidism. Just doing activities of daily living or other rehabilitation exercises can be fatiguing.

A well-balanced diet is important to help with energy levels. Five to six smaller meals or snacks may work better than three large meals. If possible, the patients should delegate some of the cooking or food preparation chores. If scheduling allows, most of the week's cooking can be done on one day; then, reheating is all that is required for the rest of the week. Another suggestion is to do large batches of items such as stew or spaghetti and freeze in small portions. Having "quick to go" foods on hand such as yogurt, raisins, bagels, trail mix, hard-boiled eggs, or cheese cubes should be encouraged. Frozen entrees are definitely convenient. They become part of a balanced meal if served with milk, fruit, and vegetable side dishes.

Meals should contain some carbohydrate, protein, and fat. A breakfast consisting of toast, juice, and fruit will not sustain someone as long as a breakfast consisting of buttered toast with 1 egg, juice, fruit, and skim milk.

ORAL SUPPLEMENTS

Oral supplements can be beneficial for many reasons. Extra nutrition for wound healing, a healthy snack if too tired to cook, or a high-calorie drink to curb weight loss are just a few reasons to consider them. See the RD because they often receive samples, coupons, and recipes for these products. Many are available at retail stores. Some of the major companies have home delivery programs as well (see "Resources").

ALTERNATIVE THERAPIES

The prevalence and expenditures of alternative medical therapy in the United States increased substantially in the 1990s. One article cites a 380% increase in the use of herbal remedies and a 130% increase in high-dose vitamin use from 1990 to 1997 (12). A low number of these uses are reported to the physicians, which means people are self-diagnosing and self-prescribing and harmful interactions may occur. Unfortunately, as a society we tend to believe in two misconceptions. One is that if something is in print or on the television, it must be true. The other misconception is that because a product is "all natural" it must be safe.

Those with physical disabilities use alternative therapies even more frequently than the general population. A survey of the general population reports 42.1% used one or more alternative therapies in 12 months. This included (among others) herbal medicine, lifestyle diets, megavitamin therapy, and commercial weight-loss programs. A survey of the disabled population showed that 57.1% used one or more alternative therapies in a 12-month period (13).

However, only between 37% and 62% of these unprescribed alternative therapies were discussed with the physician (13). With these unsupervised treatments (and even some supervised treatments) there is a risk of potentially dangerous herb–drug interactions, herb–herb interactions, or toxicities of certain vitamins or minerals. For example, it is becoming known that certain herbs should be avoided if someone is taking warfarin, heparin, nonsteroidal antiinflammatory drugs, aspirin, or other anticoagulants. This includes feverfew, gingko biloba, and ginseng, which are popular supplements. Also, chamomile and St. John's wort may inhibit iron absorption.

Health care professionals should become familiar with these practices and routinely ask patients or clients about them. Dialogue between the client and health care team is encouraged. We need to do what we can to help them become informed consumers. Another reason we should discuss the use of alternative therapies with our clients is the cost. We spent about $13.7 billion dollars for alternative therapies in 1990 (13). No doubt the current statistics are considerably higher. How much of this was spent on worthless treatments? There are people out there who will need to choose between prescription drugs, alternative treatments, or even possibly food because of limited finances. For further information on this topic, see references 12–14 and "Alternative Therapy Resources" (see below).

RESOURCES

Modified Convenience Foods

Med-Diet Inc.: 1-800-633-3438 or med-diet@med-diet.com
Home Net: 1-800-782-5569
AliMed Gourmet Puree: 1-800-337-2400 or *gourmetpuree.com*

Puree Cookbooks

Process Book for Pureed Meals. American Institutional Products, 2733 Lititz Pike, Lancaster, PA 17601
Creating Foods for Dysphagia and Pureed Texture Menus. Market Link, 2101 W. Rice, Chicago, IL 60622
Dysphagia Dining: A Handbook for People with Swallowing Disorders. Alta Bates-Herrick Hospital, Department of Nutrition and Food Services, 2001 Dwight Way, Berkeley, CA 97404
Puree Gourmet Cookbook. (See Home Net, earlier.)

Oral Supplements Home Delivery

Ensure Home Delivery: Ross Laboratories 1-800-986-8502 Monday–Friday 8 a.m. to 5 p.m. CST
Nutriline: Mead Johnson (Sustacal products) 1-800-247-7893 Monday–Friday 1 p.m. to 4 p.m. CST

Novartis Nutrition (Resource products): 1-800-828-9194 Monday–Friday 7 a.m. to 6:30 p.m. CST

Alternative Therapy Resources

National Council for Reliable Health Information: PO Box 1276, Loma Linda, CA 92354-1276.
The Honest Herbal (3rd ed., 1993) and *Herbs of Choice* (1994) by Varro Tyler, Ph.D., New York: Pharmaceutical Products Press, 1-800-342-9678
Environmental Nutrition Newsletter, http://www.environmentalnutrition.com
The American Dietetic Association Consumer Nutrition Hotline, 1-800-366-1655

HIGH-CALORIE, HIGH-PROTEIN RECIPES

Strawberry/Banana Yogurt Shake

½ cup strawberries
½ cup fortified milk (see below)
½ cup plain yogurt
1 tbsp. sugar
½ banana

Combine ingredients in blender and blend until smooth, about 30 seconds. Provides 325 calories and 14 grams protein.

Fortified Milk

1 cup nonfat dry milk powder
1 quart whole milk

Mix well and chill before using. One cup provides 220 calories and 15 grams protein. Use this in place of regular milk for drinking and cooking.

Munch Mix

½ cup toasted coconut
½ cup raisins
½ cup sunflower seeds
½ cup chocolate chips
1 cup peanuts

Mix well and store in an airtight container. Cashews, walnuts, pecans, and soy nuts, as well as various dried fruits, may be combined for this high-calorie, high-protein snack. One-half cup provides 490 calories and 13 grams protein.

Chocolate Milkshake

¼ cup chocolate syrup
1 ½ cups ice cream
½ cup nonfat dry milk powder
½ cup fortified milk

Combine ingredients in blender and blend until smooth. Makes approximately 2 cups. One cup of this recipe provides 415 calories and 15 grams protein.

Creamy Rice Pudding

2 cups cooked rice
2 tsp. margarine
2 cups fortified milk
½ tsp. cinnamon
¼ cup sugar

Combine all ingredients in saucepan. Cook over medium heat, stirring frequently until thickened to desired consistency, 10 to 15 minutes. Serve warm or cold. Makes 4 servings. One serving provides 260 calories and 9 grams protein.

REFERENCES

1. Endres JB. *Community nutrition: challenges and opportunities.* Upper Saddle River, NJ: Prentice-Hall, 1999.
2. Skipper A. *Dietitian's handbook of enteral and parenteral nutrition,* 2nd edition, Frederick, MD: Aspen Publications, 1998.
3. United States Department of Health and Human Services and the Department of Agriculture. "Nutrition and Your Health: Dietary Guidelines for Americans," May 2000. Available at http://www.health.gov/dietaryguidelines/#current.
4. Hickey JV. *The clinical practice of neurological and neurosurgical nursing.* 4th edition. Philadelphia: Lippincott, 1997.
5. ESHA Research – the Food Finder.
6. *Accent on Living.* Winter 1996:58–60.
7. Skipper A. *Dietitian's handbook of enteral and parenteral nutrition,* 2nd edition, Frederick, MD: Aspen Publications, 1998. SAME AS #2
8. Samuels MA. *Manual of neurologic therapeutics,* 6th ed. Philadelphia: Lippincott Williams, & Wilkins, 1999.
9. Hospital C. *Topics in spinal cord injury rehabilitation,* Vol. 2, Number 3. Frederick, MD: Aspen Publications, 1997.
10. American Dietetic Association. *Manual of clinical dietetics,* 6th edition. Chicago: American Dietetic Association, 2000.
11. Stolp-Smith KA, Carter J, Rohe DE, et al. Management of impairment, disability, and handicap due to multiple sclerosis. *Mayo Clin Proc* 1997;72:1184–1196.
12. Eisenberg DM, et al. Trends in alternative medicine use in the United States, 1990-1997. *JAMA* 1998:280 (18).
13. Krauss HH, Godfrey C, Kirk J, et al. Alternative health care: its use by individuals with physical disabilities. *Arch Phys Med Rehabil* 1998;79:1440–1448.
14. Miller LG. Herbal medicinals: selected clinical considerations focusing on known or potential drug-herb interactions. *Arch Intern Med* 1998;158:2200–2211.

19

New Perspectives on Hormonal Management of the Menopausal Woman with Disabilities or Chronic Disease States

Maureen Moomjy and Amalia C. Kelly

INTRODUCTION

Although it is a physiologic event, menopause can present with symptoms and disease risks of a pathologic nature for many women. Hypoestrogenism, although tolerated by some women, may result in symptoms or medical risks that qualify for treatment in others. There has been and continues to be an evolution of our understanding of the effects of estrogen deficiency, estrogen replacement, estrogen agonism, and estrogen antagonism. The most notable symptoms of estrogen deficiency are the hot flushes of vasomotor instability and the genitourinary dysfunction related to atrophy. Women with frequent hot flushes have disrupted sleep, with its associated fatigue, irritability, and impaired concentration. Women with genitourinary tract atrophy are more likely to suffer from dyspareunia, sexual dysfunction, chronic atrophic vaginitis, stress urinary incontinence, and frequent urinary tract infections. Additionally, a rapid decline of bone density occurs at the time of menopause given the absence of estrogen, which has been proved to inhibit bone resorption. Postmenopausal women are at increased risk of vertebral, hip, and wrist fractures if prolonged hypoestrogenism is untreated and if osteoporosis develops. Cardiovascular disease increases substantially after menopause such that it accounts for more than 45% of all deaths among women (1). The estrogen deficiency of menopause has been implicated in the development of unfavorable lipid profiles and impaired endothelial function and cardiovascular tone (2).

Quality of life may be affected positively by postmenopausal hormone replacement therapy (HRT) with its known effects of abatement of climacteric symptoms. Hormone replacement has been credited with stabilization of bone mineral density, resulting in a 50% or greater reduction of fracture risk, depending on duration of use (3). Prescription of HRT for relief of climacteric symptoms is limited by its association with an increased risk of breast cancer and an increased risk of clinically significant hypercoagulability. Any possible cardioprotective benefits of HRT have been refuted by randomized controlled trials (RCTs). The slow, steady evolution of information regarding the potential risks and benefits of postmenopausal HRT primarily derived from prospective cohort studies, such as The Nurses' Health Study, and numerous case-control studies have been challenged by prospective, randomized, controlled trials, primarily the Heart and Estrogen/progestin Replacement Study (HERS) and the Women's Health Initiative (WHI) study (4–10). Cardiac protection is not a benefit of HRT despite numerous earlier basic science and clinical cohort studies suggesting otherwise. In fact, there was a slight elevation of cardiovascular risk for women in the WHI trial taking a daily continuous estrogen and progestin regimen.

The risk-benefit analysis for women with disabilities must address whether the symptoms of the disease process itself might worsen when HRT is prescribed. Thus, alternative therapies may be necessary. Evaluation and consultation should be provided for all postmenopausal women, including those with chronic disabling conditions, regarding hormone replacement as well as other approaches to decrease morbidity and/or improve quality of life as they age. Women with chronic diseases or disabilities may have more risk factors for cardiovascular disease and osteoporosis because of their exclusion from participation in certain preventive behaviors such as weight-bearing activities and aerobic exercise. They also may have greater risk factors from thromboembolic events secondary to certain diseases and/or immobilization. This chapter will review the medical effects of HRT, outline similarities and differences between women with and without disabilities, discuss manifestations of menopausal effects that may be of special concern to the disabled population, and review contraindications for the use of hormone replacement therapies and alternative therapeutic options.

CARDIOVASCULAR DISEASE

Cardiovascular disease is the leading cause of mortality for women, claiming more than 500,000 lives annually, a twofold greater mortality than that attributed to all cancers (1). Any lifestyle change or medication that affects cardiovascular risk to any degree is of great importance because of the many people either at risk or currently suffering from cardiovascular disease. Although epidemiologic data from well-designed studies supported a 40% to 50% lower relative risk of cardiovascular disease for HRT users, the results of the WHI revealed no cardioprotective effect (4,10–12). In fact, the WHI estrogen and progesterone study found a hazard ratio of 1.3 for increased coronary heart disease for women randomly assigned to HRT. This marked contrast of findings has created great concern among women and their physicians.

There were many sound biologic studies revealing favorable estrogen effects on heart function and vascular tone, setting the stage for acceptance of epidemiologic studies showing reduction of cardiovascular disease. Animal studies have confirmed a distinct protective effect of estrogen on the development of atherosclerosis. Cynomolgus monkeys subjected to surgical menopause, fed high fat diets, and treated with estrogen replacement therapy (ERT) showed a significant reduction of coronary atherosclerosis compared to estrogen-deprived animals (13). However, regression of established atherosclerosis was not noted in relation to estrogen replacement. Measurements of high-density lipoprotein cholesterol (HDL-C), low-density lipoprotein cholesterol (LDL-C), and triglycerides for postmenopausal women participating in the Continuous Hormone As Replacement Therapy (CHART) study showed a positive impact of daily combined ethinyl estradiol and norethindrone acetate (14). Any reduction on cardiac events was not assessed by this 2-year study. The Postmenopausal Estrogen/Progestin Interventions (PEPI) trial found a range of positive effects on HDL-C for different hormone replacement regimens in comparison to the placebo group. Another prospective study analyzed lipid effects of transdermal estrogen therapy compared to oral estrogen therapy (both regimens involved cyclic medroxyprogesterone acetate). This group found a significant reduction of triglyceride levels only with transdermal estrogen treatment. The lower insulin levels associated with transdermal estrogen may be yielding the lower triglyceride levels (15). Longer-term comparative assessment of oral and transdermal ERT revealed a significant reduction of total cholesterol and LDL-C for both treatments, whereas no impact on HDL-C occurred for women receiving sequential estrogen and progestin therapy (16).

It has been demonstrated that estrogen binds to vascular endothelium and smooth muscle (17) and that it induces vasodilation for healthy and atherosclerotic vessels (18). Short-term intravenous infusions of ethinyl estradiol have been shown to decrease basal coronary vasomotor tone as measured by increased coronary flow and decreased coronary vascular resistance when compared with placebo for a group of healthy postmenopausal women (19). In an *in vitro* rabbit coronary artery ring experiment, estradiol-17β was shown to effect arterial relaxation. In this same model, increasing calcium concentrations increased arterial constriction as expected. This effect was blocked by estradiol in a dose-dependent manner (20). A significant improvement of cardiac function at rest and with exercise was noted for a group of healthy postmenopausal women taking ERT when compared to the same echocardiographic measures taken prior to initiation of treatment (21).

Despite the positive impact on many parameters of cardiovascular function when assessed in isolation, clinical cardiac endpoints are predicated on complex physiologic processes. Lack of cardioprotection and increased cardiovascular risk as determined by the WHI takes precedence over studies showing enhancement of any one aspect of cardiovascular function. The WHI included more than 27,000 healthy women, ages 50 to 79, divided into two main study groups according to whether the woman had an intact uterus. Those with an intact uterus were randomly assigned to either treatment with daily oral estrogen and progestin or placebo. Those without a uterus were randomly assigned either to treatment with daily oral estrogen or placebo. The daily estrogen plus progestin study, scheduled for completion in 2005, was halted in 2002 after 5.3 years. The advisory committee had determined that the cases of invasive breast cancer had exceeded a preestablished limit that indicated increased risk. The estrogen-only study group was permitted to continue. Relative risks for users of combined estrogen and progestin therapy were increased by 22% to 41% (10). Absolute risks are still small, with approximately eight new cases each of cardiovascular disease, thromboembolic events, stroke, and breast cancer for 10,000 women receiv-

ing combined hormone replacement for 1 year. Collectively, this can be interpreted as one adverse event for every 100 women receiving HRT over a 5-year period (22). Reduced osteoporosis and colon cancer rates were noted for the WHI participants, with a relative risk reduction of 24% to 34% for fractures and 37% for colon cancer. Absolute risk reduction is similarly small with six fewer cases of colorectal cancer and five fewer fractures for 10,000 women receiving treatment for 1 year (10). From a public health point of view, a medical intervention with serious small risks no longer can be considered preventive, and, as with most medications, the decision to take such medication requires assessment of potential risks and benefits for a given patient. It is noteworthy that the WHI excluded women with vasomotor symptoms and included women with an average age of 63 years. Older women without vasomotor symptoms are going to have less overall benefit from HRT and more overall risks as a result of age. Women with vasomotor symptoms may have lower circulating estrogen levels. They may or may not have the same risk profile in regard to exogenous HRT as the participants in the WHI. The WHI did not assess transdermal preparations or lower-than-standard-dose preparations.

The marked discrepancy between the epidemiologic studies and the RCTs highlight the significance of the "healthy user effect." Women who elect to use HRT have a healthier lifestyle; may be more likely to engage in exercise; and may visit the doctor more frequently, which may result in early identification and treatment of disease. Although prospective cohort studies have tried to control for this "healthy user effect," the true risk/benefit profile of various regimens of HRT only come from randomized controlled studies.

The potential secondary prevention of coronary events by HRT for women with established coronary disease has been refuted. Earlier studies suggested that women with known severe coronary artery stenosis who were current estrogen users had a better prognosis than nonusers (23). In contrast, daily combined continuous HRT, studied in a 4-year prospective RCT, the HERS Trial, did not show any significant benefit in reducing fatal or nonfatal cardiac events in women with established cardiovascular disease (8). It is interesting that a beneficial reduction of LDL-C and elevation of HDL-C was noted for the treatment group compared to the placebo group despite a lack of clinical benefit in this 4-year study. Additionally, a higher risk of nonfatal myocardial infarction (MI) or coronary disease death was noted in the first year for patients receiving treatment in comparison to placebo [relative hazard 1.52; confidence interval (CI) 1.01–2.29]. In subsequent years, the risk continued to decrease. The researchers noted that this time trend should be interpreted with caution given the level of significance. The HERS study suggested that the trend toward later benefit is consistent with other observational studies but that the finding of increased coronary events in the first year of treatment for women with established cardiovascular disease could be missed by observational studies. This group found a threefold increased risk of venous thromboembolic events and a slight increase of gall bladder disease for these patients with known coronary heart disease (24). Lack of a direct vascular effect for estrogen replacement has been reported for patients with established coronary artery disease who participated in the Estrogen Replacement and Atherosclerosis Trial. This was an RCT of 309 women with angiographically confirmed coronary artery disease at baseline. Women were randomized to unopposed estrogen replacement or daily combined estrogen and progestin replacement or placebo. This study revealed no difference between treatment and control groups of mean minimal coronary artery diameter as assessed by angiography after 3 years of treatment (7).

The American College of Obstetricians and Gynecologists recommends that estrogen and progestin therapy no longer should be recommended for the prevention of cardiovascular disease, and if previously prescribed for that purpose, it should be discontinued (25). Patients with chronic diseases or disabilities that limit mobility should be considered to have one risk factor for cardiac disease: a sedentary lifestyle. Women with chronic diseases that include vascular disease such as severe diabetes, lupus, and peripheral vascular disease may be at a similar low risk of increased cardiovascular disease with HRT as the women of the WHI or they may be at higher risk given their baseline disease. Although definitive data do not exist for women with vascular disease, it would be prudent to avoid HRT for this group if possible. Women with established cardiac disease and women with cardiovascular disease risk factors should consider other medical therapies in their pursuit of primary or secondary cardioprotection.

STROKE RISK

Estrogen plus progestin has been shown to increase the risk of ischemic stroke in older, healthy, postmenopausal women. The WHI revealed a 1.8% risk of all strokes for the women randomized to estrogen and progestin when compared to the 1.3% risk of stroke for women randomized to placebo (26). The WHI found a hazard ratio of 1.5, or a 31% increase in total stroke risk for estrogen and progestin users.

Epidemiologic cohort studies and case-control studies have shown no increase of the relative risk of stroke of any type among long-term users of estrogen-only replacement or combined hormone replacement (12,27–29, 29a). The Danish National Patient Registry was the largest case-control study, involving nearly 4,600 cases and controls. Only patients with nonfatal stroke were included as cases. Four subtypes of stroke were assessed including subarachnoid hemorrhage, intracerebral hemorrhage, thromboembolic infarction, and transient ischemic attack (TIA). HRT had no influence on the risk of hemorrhagic or thromboembolic strokes. There was, however, an increased risk of TIA among former users of HRT and among current users of unopposed ERT (28). The increased risk of TIA is consistent with the increased risk of ischemic stroke reported by the WHI. A recent extensive review of the literature of more than 40 reports of case-control and cohort studies revealed no increase of stroke risk for HRT users and a possibility of a moderately reduced risk of fatal stroke (30). This discrepancy with the WHI data most likely reflects differences attributable to the healthy user effect and possibly the older population of the WHI.

Duplex ultrasound assessment of the carotid arteries was used for women participating in the Cardiovascular Health Study to compare the possible vascular effects of estrogen-only replacement versus combined hormone replacement (30). This was a cross-sectional population-based study comparing internal carotid wall thickness and carotid stenosis between current HRT users and nonusers, for women older than 65 years of age. There was significantly less thickening of the carotid wall for current HRT users than nonusers. There was a lower odds ratio of carotid stenosis for current users of unopposed estrogen as well as users of combined estrogen and progestin replacement therapy when compared to nonusers of hormone replacement. Although the study controlled for lifestyle and risk factors, a healthy user effect still could exist.

Few studies have assessed the risk of recurrent stroke in stroke patients who are HRT users. An observational study of women in an aspirin trial who happened to use HRT revealed a reduced risk of stroke, retinal infarction, and death (31). Opposing results of increased risk, specifically a higher rate of ischemic stroke, was noted in another observational study of ERT use among stroke patients (33). For patients with a history of stroke, it is difficult to justify treatment with combined estrogen and progestin. The risk/benefit profile of estrogen-only therapy is pending on the completion of the estrogen-only arm of the WHI.

POTENTIAL FOR ALTERED COAGULATION

Oral estrogen is known to increase hepatic protein synthesis with a resultant increase of binding proteins, coagulation, and fibrinolysis factors. The overall clinical effect appears detrimental, although some benefit had been noted on studies of plasminogen-activator inhibitor type 1 (PAI-I) and homocysteine. PAI-1 is an antagonist of fibrinolysis and has been associated with increased risk of atherosclerosis and ischemic events. Oral conjugated estrogen, alone or in combination with progestin therapy, has been found to reduce PAI-1 levels by approximately 50% in postmenopausal women (34). In contrast to oral therapy, transdermal estrogen administration did not change PAI-1 levels. This is understandable because the liver is a major source of PAI-1. Homocysteine has been recognized as an independent risk factor for cardiovascular disease by precipitating endothelial damage and increasing atherothrombosis (35,36). Homocysteine appears to be influenced by sex hormones and has been demonstrated to be decreased during oral combined HRT and during transdermal estrogen-only replacement (37,38).

These findings of enhanced fibrinolysis are overshadowed by epidemiologic studies that link HRT to a twofold increased risk of pulmonary embolism (6) and a threefold higher risk of venous thromboembolism (39). The WHI documented a HR for pulmonary embolism of 2.13 (CI 1.39–3.25). According to the WHI, absolute excess risk for 10,000 women-years included eight more cases of pulmonary embolism attributable to combined estrogen and progestin treatment (10). This increased risk is consistent with most epidemiologic data. In a case-control study of women hospitalized for idiopathic venous thromboembolism, cases were twice as likely as controls to be current users of hormone replacement (40). These authors estimate the risk of venous thromboembolism to be one in 5,000 users per year (10). The WHI data suggest four cases of pulmonary embolism per 5,000 users per year. Dose-dependent increasing risk of thromboembolism was reported in a similar case-control study for women taking varying dosages of low dose estrogen (41). Given the extremely low incidence of spontaneous deep-vein thrombosis in postmenopausal women, the increased relative risk has evaded detection for many years. The absolute increase of morbidity is small, but the potential for a rare fatal outcome does exist.

For the women of the HERS study who were older and had established cardiovascular disease, the group receiving daily combined continuous hormone replacement had three times the rate of venous thromboembolic events as the placebo group (8). For individuals with a family history of arterial or venous thromboembolism, one could assess for hypercoagulability to identify specifically patients who should be excluded from ERT. Hypercoagulable states have been found in up to 10% of the patients with a history of unexplained venous thrombosis and in up to 40% of the patients with arterial thrombosis requiring surgical revascularization (42). Markers of hypercoagulability include low levels of protein C, protein S, and antithrombin III; genetic variants such as the factor V Leiden mutation, the prothrombin 20210A gene mutation, or the methylenetetrahydrofolate reductase (MTHFR) gene mutation; elevated homocysteine; or the presence of the lupus anticoagulant or antiphospholipid syndrome. This list may grow as numerous research advances in the arena of thrombophilias continue. Oral HRT has been associated with decreased levels of the natural anticoagulant antithrombin III in healthy women. Transdermal estradiol appears to have no impact on antithrombin III levels in healthy women (43). For women with a diagnosis of antithrombin III deficiency, HRT should be avoided.

In a case-control study of postmenopausal survivors of MI, the prothrombin 20210A gene variant was found to be a significant MI risk factor among postmenopausal women with hypertension. The risk was increased 11-fold if there had been use of HRT in this sub-group of women with hypertension and the prothrombin 20210A gene variant. No increased risk for MI was detected for women with the prothrombin 20210A gene variant in the absence of hypertension, nor for HRT users with factor V Leiden mutation, regardless of presence or absence of hypertension (44). As further studies are awaited, it is clinically justifiable to test for the prothrombin 20210A gene variant in women with hypertension contemplating initiation of HRT. Possible association of increased risk of pulmonary embolus with genetic-based thrombophilias was not assessed by this study.

It has been recommended by the American Heart Association Science Advisory Committee that HRT should be discontinued during episodes of hospitalization and/or complete immobilization and during an acute cardiovascular disease event. The decision to reinstitute HRT should be based on established noncoronary benefits and risks (45).

OTHER METABOLIC EFFECTS

Oral hormone replacement does not increase the risk of diabetes mellitus (46,47). A delayed insulin response to a glucose challenge, with an increased overall insulin response, has been noted for ERT, but whether this results in a clinically significant hyperinsulinemic effect remains to be determined (48,49). Because hyperinsulinemia is a marker of cardiac risk, any potential effect of hormone replacement on insulin resistance is of interest. An RCT that assessed glucose, insulin, lipoproteins, and sex-hormone–binding globulin levels for postmenopausal women with noninsulin-dependent diabetes mellitus in response to 3 months of treatment with daily 17β-estradiol and a single 10-day progestin withdrawal found a marked increase of sex-hormone–binding globulin and a reduction of free testosterone that was considered to be beneficial (50). Significant reductions of glycosylated hemoglobin, blood glucose, C-peptide, and LDL-C also were noted for these women with diabetes participating in this short-term RCT. In a similarly designed study of healthy postmenopausal women, glucose-tolerance testing and triglyceride levels were unchanged during HRT, whereas beneficial changes of lipoprotein profiles were documented (49). The transdermal route has been shown to reduce fasting plasma insulin levels and improve insulin sensitivity (51). Long-term risks and benefits of HRT for women with insulin-dependent or noninsulin dependent diabetes remain to be established. The physiologic studies published suggest that women with diabetes may experience relief of climacteric symptoms without compromise of glucose control.

MECHANISMS OF MAINTENANCE OF BONE DENSITY

Estrogen plays a vital role in the maintenance of bone density, helping to balance bone formation and bone resorption. Estrogen receptors have been localized to osteoblasts and osteoclasts (52). Estrogen positively affects calcium homeostasis with improved calcium absorption, reduced renal calcium loss, and possible inhibition of parathyroid hormone mediation of bone resorption (53). A postulated impact on bone marrow constituent cells also has been advanced (54). In the setting of hypoestrogenism, bone remineralization does not keep pace with bone resorption. Estrogen deficiency accelerates bone remodeling, which increases the chance of trabecular resorption and loss of the template for osteoblastic activity (55). Trabecular bone, found in the vertebrae and hip, is lost at a much faster rate (up to 5% to 8% per year) than cortical bone. If this accelerated bone loss is not halted, osteopenia and eventually osteoporosis develop. Hip, vertebral, and wrist fractures are a direct result of this estrogen-induced bone loss. In addition, lack of physical activity and insufficient calcium and vitamin D intake contribute to bone loss.

With estrogen replacement, bone formation and bone resorption are again in equilibrium with a slower rate of bone turnover and a significantly reduced rate of bone loss (56). In fact, in women with osteopenia or osteoporo-

sis, an increase in bone mineral density often is seen when HRT first is begun. Assessment of iliac crest biopsies for postmenopausal women with osteopenia or osteoporosis, before and after 2 years of HRT, revealed suppression of bone turnover and a reduction in the size of the resorption cavities (57). The Framingham study suggested that a long-term impact on bone density would require at least a 7-year period of treatment (58). Cessation of estrogen therapy is associated with a resumption of bone loss. A variety of oral and transdermal estrogens have been shown to be effective in reducing the rate of bone loss and fractures. In most studies, dosages equivalent to conjugated equine estrogen (CEE) 0.625 mg have been used. A number of investigators have sought to determine the lowest effective dose of estrogen that would be effective in maintaining bone density and lowering the rate of fractures. Serum estradiol levels maintained above 30 pg/mL were associated with maintenance or improvement of bone mineral density (59). Estrogen-replacement dosing of one-half or one-quarter the standard hormone replacement doses was associated with preservation of bone mineral density when used in combination with a daily calcium intake of 1,500 mg (60). In the RCT of ultra-low-dose HRT (the CHART study) a distinct increase of bone mineral density was noted with the addition of a daily dose of 1 mg of norethindrone acetate to ethinyl estradiol doses of 5 and 10 μg. Calcium supplementation in the absence of ERT is insufficient to reverse the rapid bone loss that is secondary to menopause, although calcium replacement reduces age-related bone loss (61). Smoking reduced bioavailable estrogen and would be expected to lessen the benefits of ERT. ERT has been shown to have a distinctive and additive impact on bone mineral density when used in combination with alendronate (62). After 2 years of treatment, patients in an RCT had significantly greater increases of bone mineral density at lumbar spine and femoral neck with combined therapy than with either alendronate or estrogen alone. Lack of impact on fracture risk reflected the short duration of this trial. Given the current risk profile of HRT according to the WHI, it seems prudent to start treatment for osteoporosis with bisphosphonates or raloxifene. Treatment of osteoporosis should not be the sole indication for the initiation of HRT unless the patient is not a candidate for bisphosphonates or raloxifene.

RELIEF OF CLIMACTERIC SYMPTOMS

A vast array of symptoms may result from the declining estrogen levels that accompany menopause. These include hot flushes and night sweats, disturbed sleep patterns, emotional lability, changes in cognitive function, vaginal dryness, dyspareunia, decreased libido, joint pains, and bladder dysfunction. Their severity can range from merely annoying to extremely debilitating. Often, control of these symptoms is the primary reason a woman chooses to begin HRT. Relief often is achieved with careful adjustment of the chosen drug regimen.

Hot Flushes

The hot flush is the most recognized symptom of menopause in this country. It is estimated to occur in 50% to 93% of menopausal women at some point during their transition (63,64). For many, flushes are a temporary condition lasting a few months to a few years. For others, they persist for decades. Subjectively, a flush is described as a sudden feeling of warmth, often arising from the chest and spreading to the face, associated with perspiration and sometimes followed by a chill. Physiologically it is characterized by an increase in skin temperature, peripheral vasodilatation, an increase in heart rate, and a marked decrease in skin resistance (65). Treatment with systemic estrogen (oral, transdermal, injectable, implants) is highly effective in relieving hot flushes. The efficacy is dose-dependent (66,67) and significantly better than placebo (66,68). There is, however, a profound placebo effect observed, making

placebo-controlled trials a necessity in studying any form of treatment for hot flushes. Other pharmacologic approaches to relieving hot flushes have been tried. Depot-medroxyprogesterone acetate was found to be significantly more helpful than placebo (69,70) and comparable to estrogen in effect. Although not as effective as estrogen, clonidine has been found to be significantly more effective than placebo in relieving hot flushes (71). More recently, the selective serotonin reuptake inhibitors (SSRIs) venlafaxine and paroxetine have been shown to reduce hot flushes by 50% to 70% (72,73).

Urogenital Atrophy

The changes that occur in the urogenital tract as a result of estrogen insufficiency have been well iterated. These include an increase in the pH, a decrease in moisture, a change in the vaginal flora, and a change in the vaginal maturation (74). Vaginal dryness and itching, dyspareunia, urinary urgency, and more frequent urinary tract infections result from these changes and often worsen, even after hot flushes have remitted.

Of particular interest to many women with disabilities is the potential benefit to the genitourinary system. Both systemic and topical (intravaginal) estrogen can relieve the symptoms of vaginal atrophy. Locally applied estrogen in very low doses has been shown to be effective. A silicone vaginal ring delivering 6.5 to 9.5 µg of estradiol daily restored the vaginal pH and maturation index and relieved symptoms in approximately 90% of women treated for 3 months (75). Vaginal tablets containing 25 µg of estradiol were found to be significantly more effective than placebo in relieving symptoms of dyspareunia and dryness. Of note, a marked placebo effect was observed (76). Intravaginal estrogen cream is significantly better than placebo in reducing the incidence of urinary tract infections (77). Urinary urgency and frequency often can be relieved with an extended course of estrogen replacement (78). A meta-analysis assessing the potential effect of estrogen therapy for women with a diagnosis of urinary incontinence found a significant positive effect of estrogen. An improvement of urethral closing pressures was detected by some of the studies reviewed (79). Women with multiple sclerosis, cerebrovascular accident, and post-polio syndrome may be uniquely susceptible to exacerbation of underlying bladder dysfunction. Thus, the superimposed deterioration during menopause can be especially troublesome.

There is minimal absorption of estrogen into the systemic circulation with vaginally delivered estrogen therapy (80). As such, transvaginal estrogen preparations should be used with great caution if a patient has a contraindication to systemic estrogen. Nonhormonal approaches to treating the symptoms of urogenital atrophy also have been used. Water-soluble vaginal lubricants and vaginal moisturizers can aid in making vaginal intercourse more comfortable. Regular sexual relations or vaginal dilatation also helps to maintain vaginal elasticity. Sexual desire and arousal have been found to be associated with plasma steroid levels and are enhanced in surgically menopausal women treated with androgen replacement (81).

POTENTIAL EMOTIONAL, NEUROLOGIC, COGNITIVE, AND NEUROMUSCULAR IMPACT OF HORMONE REPLACEMENT

Many other symptoms may be experienced during the menopausal period and the transition into menopause, although not all symptoms arise from estrogen deficiency. Depression is a problem reported by women in their menopausal years, but current evidence does not link major depression to lack of estrogen (82). Major depression is no more common in menopausal women (whether using HRT or not) compared to reproductive-aged women. Depressed mood is reported rather often, with a frequency of approximately 25% to 40%. Risk factors include a depressed mood before menopause and more severe and longer-lasting estrogen deficiency symptoms (83). Of special note, women with chronic illnesses

are at increased risk of depression and depressed mood (82,84).

Estrogen replacement has been found by some investigators to improve psychologic function (85). A meta-analysis concluded that women with climacteric symptoms had improvements of verbal memory, reasoning, motor speed, and vigilance with HRT (86). The prospective Rancho Bernardo study followed 800 women for 15 years to document estrogen use and assess any potential benefit of mood and of cognitive performance on eight standard instruments (87). Analysis of mood for these elderly members of the Rancho Bernardo study found no difference in depression for estrogen-treated women older than age 65 when compared with untreated women (88). Analysis of cognitive performance while controlling for age and education effects revealed no significant differences according to current use, past use, or never use. An insufficient number of women met criteria for the diagnosis of dementia to permit assessment of impact of estrogen replacement for this subgroup of women. The relative risk of developing Alzheimer's disease has been reported as significantly reduced for estrogen users in the prospective Leisure World Cohort Study (89). Risk reduction was greater for higher dose and/or longer duration of estrogen replacement. Animal studies reveal a plausible mechanism of action for estrogen on the acetylcholine system. In ovariectomized rats, estrogen was noted to increase acetylcholine synthetase (90). In another study of ovariectomized rats, learning and memory behavior was noted to be impaired in the estrogen-deficient state and normalized in the estrogen-replaced state (91). These researchers also reported a positive impact on acetylcholine synthesis as well as a decrease of acetylcholine uptake. The only two medications currently approved for treatment of Alzheimer's disease, tacrine and donepezil, exert their effects via central inhibition of acetylcholinesterase. In an RCT assessing efficacy of tacrine, it was found that women in the tacrine group who were incidentally receiving hormone replacement performed significantly better on cognitive tests than women taking tacrine who were not receiving hormone replacement (92). For women with established Alzheimer's disease, an RCT of 120 women showed no difference of cognitive function after 12 months of treatment. This study included a treatment with 0.625 mg/day of CEE versus 1.25 mg/day CEE versus placebo. This short course of two doses of estrogen did not appear to arrest progression of established Alzheimer's disease (93). The Women's Health Initiative Memory Study (WHIMS) reported no improvement of cognitive function for women randomized to daily combined conjugated equine estrogens and medroxyprogesterone acetate when compared to the placebo group (94). More concerning was an additional report from the WHIMS study documenting an increased risk of dementia with a hazard ratio of 2.05 for women receiving daily combined estrogen and progestin (95). There were 23 more case of dementia per 10,000 women years for the HRT group. The increased risk of dementia with HRT was noted in the first year of the study, suggesting that some participants had cognitive decline at the start of the study that may have been facilitated to progress with HRT. The authors suggest that the mechanism may be an increased risk of ischemic microinfarcts. The published WHIMS findings are specific for combined estrogen and progestin therapy. Reports on estrogen-only replacement therapy are pending at this time. Whether the same risk for increased dementia for younger women taking HRT exists remains to be determined.

To assess peripheral neuromuscular impact, an RCT compared estrogen replacement combined with calcium versus calcium alone for 116 middle-aged postmenopausal women, all of whom had suffered a recent fracture of the distal radius prior to entrance into the study (96). ERT of 4 years duration did not increase muscle performance, improve balance. or reduce falls for these middle-aged women with a history of wrist fracture.

Changes in muscle strength have been reported in studies looking at menstruating women. There was a suggestion that strength was maximal in the follicular phase when estrogen levels were highest and deteriorated with the progression of the cycle towards menses. Although some studies looking at muscle strength were unable to detect a difference in muscle strength in relation to HRT, one cross-sectional study of 273 subjects did note a reduction of muscle strength for men occurring at age 60 and for women occurring with menopause; a protective effect of HRT for postmenopausal women also was noted (97). Again, the healthy-user effect makes definitive conclusions difficult. The possible benefit of estrogen on muscle-wasting diseases, if any, requires further study.

RISK OF BREAST CANCER

Prior to the WHI report on risks and benefits of combined estrogen and progestin therapy, the effects of exogenous estrogen on breast cancer risk had been difficult to ascertain. More than 30 case-control and cohort studies have been published. Meta-analyses of the epidemiologic data suggest a small increase in breast cancer incidence related to estrogen replacement with extended use of 5 to 10 years (98,99). This increase in relative risk is most prominent when never users are compared to current users. A relative risk of approximately 1.3 is suggested by these meta-analyses, by the Nurse's Health Study, and by The Collaborative Group on Hormonal Factors in Breast Cancer (100,101). This translates into an increase from 11% to 15% in lifetime incidence of breast cancer and an approximate increase from 3% to 4% in lifetime breast cancer mortality. The WHI reported a hazard ratio for breast cancer of 1.26 for women randomized to treatment with daily combined estrogen and progestin in comparison to the placebo group. This translates into a 26% increase risk of breast cancer, or eight additional cases of invasive breast cancer for 10,000 women taking combined HRT for 1 year (10). Analysis of relevant risk factors for breast cancer revealed no change of the hazard ratio according to family history, race, parity, age of first birth, body mass index, or Gail-model risk score. There was an increased risk for women of the WHI who had reported previous treatment with HRT. The WHI group reported an interaction between breast cancer risk and total years of HRT use. For women without a history of previous HRT the hazard ratio for breast cancer was 1.06; for women with less than 5 years previous use, the HR was 2.13; and for women with more than 10 years prior use, the HR was 4.61. The Iowa Women's Health Study, a population-based 10-year survey study of more than 37,000 postmenopausal women found no increase in all types of breast cancer for short-term or long-term users. This study further assessed risk by type and histology of breast cancer. Breast cancer subtypes considered to have a favorable prognosis affected only 5% of the women who had breast cancer diagnosed during this study. However, in this subgroup of woman with favorable-prognosis breast cancer, there was a relative risk of 4.4 and 2.6 for less than 5 years of HRT use and more than 5 years of HRT use, respectively (102). Weighing the current evidence, the patient and physician must assess the potential benefits of estrogen as it relates to climacteric symptom relief and prevention of osteoporosis against its potential risks of breast cancer. Overall mortality for participants in the Nurses' Health Study revealed a lower relative risk of mortality (0.63) for current hormone users compared to never users (103). However, given the WHI data, it would appear that much of the reduced mortality is related to a healthy-user effect. There was no difference of breast cancer deaths for participants of the WHI. However, it is not possible to draw adequate conclusions given the relatively short duration of this study for the assessment of an endpoint such as breast cancer death. For patients electing treatment with HRT or ERT, shortened duration of use should be discussed and attempted.

IMPACT OF HORMONE REPLACEMENT THERAPY ON BREAST CANCER RISK: OPTIONS FOR WOMEN AFTER BREAST CANCER TREATMENT

The symptomatic woman with a previous diagnosis of breast cancer presents a particularly difficult therapeutic challenge. Estrogen may result in an increased risk to this patient, both in terms of recurrent and new disease. In general, whenever possible, alternative approaches for relief of climacteric symptoms and prevention of osteoporosis should be used. Climacteric symptoms yield less readily to alternative therapies. Hot flushes taper and disappear over time in most women, although the sleep and mood disturbances created in the interim may be intolerable. Atrophic vaginitis, unfortunately, tends to worsen with time, and local lubricants may be insufficient. Small doses of local estrogen, either as vaginal creams or as an estrogen-releasing silicon ring, may provide local relief with minimal systemic effects.

In trials assessing the efficacy of tamoxifen in the reduction of breast cancer recurrence, reduced rates of cardiac events were noted for tamoxifen users. Women prescribed tamoxifen should be made aware of the potential cardioprotection afforded by this medication (104–106). Despite these benefits, there may be an increase in endometrial pathology in tamoxifen users. Ultrasound surveillance has detected increased endometrial thickness for up to 28% of the tamoxifen users compared to 2% of the controls. However, endometrial pathology was noted for only 2% of those patients proceeding to biopsy: one case of carcinoma and one case of hyperplasia (107,108). Annual transvaginal ultrasound for tamoxifen users is a screening modality with high sensitivity but inadequate specificity. Criteria for proceeding to biopsy for a tamoxifen user will continue to evolve.

SPECIAL CONSIDERATIONS FOR WOMEN WITH DISABILITIES

Cardiac risk factors include obesity and a sedentary lifestyle. Women with disabilities are more likely than other women to be overweight and to have a sedentary lifestyle (109). Postmenopausal woman should be counseled that lifestyle modifications could be associated with a reduction of cardiovascular disease. Specific lifestyle modifications that are inversely associated with cardiovascular risk include smoking cessation, getting moderate exercise, consuming minimal amounts of alcohol, eating a heart-healthy diet, and having a body mass index of less than 25. Women who achieve low risk for three of these categories have a 44% risk reduction; women who achieve low risk in all five categories have an 80% risk reduction (110). The unfortunate reality is that only 3% of the women in the Nurses' Health Study achieved low risk in all five categories. Women with certain physical disabilities may need adaptations and supervision to avail them to moderate exercise or may not be able to achieve this lifestyle modification.

The decrease in skin collagen content observed in menopause is prevented consistently by estrogen replacement (111,112). Women with disabilities who use wheelchairs or other assistive devices are at risk for excessive pressure exerted on skin areas over prolonged periods. This excess pressure predisposes to irritation abrasion and possible skin breakdown. ERT may be beneficial in maintaining skin integrity for woman who use assistive devices or are otherwise at risk for skin breakdown.

Some chronic disorders result in impairment of respiratory function including poliomyelitis and muscular dystrophy. Because of reported bronchodilatory effects of estrogen in some studies, ERT may provide a unique benefit. Improved pulmonary function has been documented with an increase of forced expiratory volume in 1 second (FEV1) and a higher forced vital capacity (FVC) consistent with less pulmonary obstruction for HRT users compared to nonusers (113). This association of improved pulmonary function for HRT users persisted when assessed among subgroups of smokers, nonsmokers, and women without asthma. A study of 55 women with asthma using self-controls noted less exacerbations of severe asthma necessitating

glucocorticoid therapy during the 6 months of taking HRT (114). It is interest that there have been some data suggesting an increased risk of new diagnosis of asthma with long-term HRT use, especially with higher-than-standard doses of HRT (115).

The risk/benefit ratio of HRT for the patient with lupus continues to be debated. The few studies that exist regarding lupus flares during long-term HRT are divided as to whether flares are increased or unaffected (116–119). Others advocate that the influence of menopause with or without HRT on lupus is poorly understood and requires much more clinical data (120,121). Results of the SELENA trial (Safety of estrogens in lupus erythematosus-national assessment) should provide some much needed answers regarding the safety of HRT for women with lupus. The Nurses' Health Study reported an increased risk of 2.5 for the development of systemic lupus erythematosus for current users of HRT (122).

Rheumatoid arthritis has been associated with increased bone loss through a variety of mechanisms including direct effect of disease progression, long-term glucocorticoid steroid use, and decreased mobility and weightbearing (123). Improvement of markers revealing stabilization of bone density with HRT has been shown for patients with rheumatoid arthritis despite glucocorticoid use (123). An RCT assessing frequency of disease flare for patients with rheumatoid arthritis revealed that women who had adequate elevation of serum estradiol reflecting compliance with HRT were more likely to have improvement of some parameters of disease activity (124). Transdermal ERT, similarly studied in an RCT, showed reduction of disease symptoms, although laboratory evidence of a disease-modifying effect was not present (125).

Minimal publications exist for the potential impact of menopause with or without HRT on disease progression for women with multiple sclerosis. A pilot study that surveyed 19 postmenopausal women revealed that 82% reported worsening of symptoms with menopause and 75% of those who had tried

HRT reported an improvement of symptoms of multiple sclerosis (126).

For women with epilepsy, there are no retrospective or prospective published studies regarding effects of HRT. Information is largely anecdotal reporting beneficial effects, no effects, and adverse effects (127). Given the hepatic first-past effect, which may increase metabolism of anticonvulsants, utilization of transdermal estradiol would seem prudent. Initiation of HRT should be in consultation with the patient's neurologist. Quantitative assessment of the patient's baseline seizure activity or electroencephalogram activity could be considered with the intention to continue such specific evaluation during a pilot phase of HRT to facilitate HRT decisionmaking on a patient-by-patient basis.

IMPLEMENTATION OF HORMONE REPLACEMENT

Regimens for prescribing HRT vary widely and present an array of choices for the clinician and patient. Whether there is a difference of long-term benefits and risks according to regimen of hormone replacement remains to be established. However, symptom relief, side effects, and acceptability may vary significantly; therefore choice of preparation and regimen may affect compliance. Overall compliance has been estimated to be as low as 30% (128). It is worthwhile to be familiar with a variety of different preparations of HRT and alternative therapeutic approaches. Regardless of the dose of estrogen replacement, the presence of a uterus necessitates cyclic or daily progestin replacement to reduce the risk of endometrial cancer. In the CHART study, even ultra-low-dose replacement with unopposed ethinyl estradiol was associated with a significant increase in endometrial hyperplasia incidence (14). There are no data to suggest that progesterone confers any benefit to the woman who has undergone hysterectomy. The hysterectomized patient therefore should be treated with unopposed estrogen. All other women should be treated with a progestogen to prevent endometrial hyperplasia or carcinoma.

ESTROGEN

There is, at present, no evidence that different oral estrogen preparations, in equipotent doses, have any different biologic effects. The U.S. Food and Drug Administration (FDA)-approved oral estrogens include CEEs (Premarin), esterified estrogens (Estratab), micronized estradiol (Estrace), estrone estropipate (Ogen), and conjugated synthetic estrogens (Cenestin). Although some of these estrogens are biochemically manufactured from plant precursors, there is no evidence that this confers any particular benefit. Oral estrogen is absorbed through the hepatic portal system and therefore undergoes a high "first pass" through the liver. This results in a significantly increased renin substrate, binding globulins, and high-density lipoproteins, whereas transdermal estrogens do not have any of these effects (129). This hepatic effect may be considered to be beneficial in the patient with hypercholesterolemia and detrimental for the patient with cholelithiasis and for the patient with increased risk of thromboembolic phenomena. Active liver disease is an absolute contraindication for both oral and transdermal estrogen.

Nonoral estrogen can be prescribed as a transdermal delivery system containing estrogen only (Estraderm, Climara, Vivelle, Fempatch) or combined with norethindrone acetate (CombiPatch). Serum estradiol levels range between 50 and 80 pg/mL for the 0.1 mg transdermal patch; 40 to 75 pg/mL for the 0.05 mg transdermal patch; 20 to 50 pg/mL for 0.625 mg oral CEE; and 80 to 90 pg/mL for 1 mg of micronized oral estradiol. Serum estrone levels are approximately 50 pg/mL for the 0.05 and 0.1 mg transdermal patches and 60 to 180 pg/mL for 0.625mg oral CEE (129–131). Oral CEE, 0.625 mg, and 0.05 mg transdermal estrogen replacement provide comparable effects of improved vaginal epithelium, reduction of hot flushes, and reduction of urinary calcium and urinary calcium/creatinine ratios. Only oral CEE at a dose of 1.25 mg had a significant reduction of urinary hydroxyproline secretion, a marker of bone resorption. Neither the 0.05 mg nor 0.1 mg doses of transdermal estradiol reduced urinary hydroxyproline secretion (129). Skin patches are easy to use but may cause rashes or skin irritation in patients with sensitive skin. Patients with migraine headaches may find that the relatively constant release of hormone afforded by the transdermal delivery system causes decreases in hormonally sensitive migraines. Skin patches are also the preparation of choice for patients with cholelithiasis or familial hypertriglyceridemia.

Vaginal estrogens are absorbed systemically but have the advantage of offering relatively lower circulating levels for a given local vaginal effect (Premarin Vaginal, Vagifem, or Estring). They may be used appropriately in patients for whom vaginal dryness is a problem but for whom the least possible systemic dose is indicated. Vaginal CEE at a dose of 0.3 mg applied three times weekly has been shown to improve significantly vaginal cellular maturity, without any significant increase of serum estradiol levels (132). Although no changes were detected by sonographic assessment of the endometrium, there was one case of endometrial proliferation among the 20 women treated for 6 months. An RCT of 25 µg 17 β-estradiol vaginal tablets (Vagifem) compared with 1.25 mg CEE vaginal cream (Premarin Vaginal) demonstrated equivalent relief of symptoms of atrophic vaginitis. There was a higher mean serum estradiol level for women using the vaginal cream with more cases of endometrial proliferation or hyperplasia than for women using the vaginal tablets (133). The creams and tablets are given by vaginal applicator. The vaginal ring (Estring) is inserted at the back of the vagina and changed every 3 months. The vaginal ring delivery system has been documented to release 5 to 10 µg of estradiol every 24 hours (134). The systemic absorption is usually low with vaginal estrogens but may be increased significantly in patients with severe atrophic vagini-

tis or radiation injury to the vagina. In a comparative study of the vaginal ring with vaginal estrogen cream, a progestogen challenge test resulted in vaginal bleeding for 3% of the women with the vaginal ring delivery system and 20% with the vaginal cream treatment (135). Patient acceptability and compliance seem to be much greater with the vaginal estrogen ring than with vaginal creams (136). Estrogen-containing skin creams are available over the counter. However, there is as yet no consistent information available on absorption or bioavailability.

PROGESTOGEN

FDA-approved progestogens for HRT include medroxyprogesterone acetate (Provera, Cycrin), norethindrone (Aygestin), and micronized progesterone as an oral tablet (Prometrium) or suspended in a bioadhesive vaginal gel (Crinone). Oral micronized progesterone is quite well characterized with respect to endometrial protection and lipid effects. Skin creams containing progesterone, such as estrogen-containing creams, remain poorly characterized with respect to absorption and bioavailability. Progestogens may attenuate estrogen's beneficial effects on lipids. In some patients, they cause bloating and depression. In these patients, progesterone vaginal gel, or Prometrium tablets placed vaginally, may be used to maximize the local effect on the endometrium while minimizing systemic effects.

Regimen

In women with a uterus, estrogen and progesterone can be given cyclically or as a continuous combined regimen. Cyclic progesterone is given for 12 to 14 days every month in a dose equivalent to medroxyprogesterone acetate (5 or 10 mg) or micronized oral progesterone (200 mg) or progesterone bioadhesive vaginal gel (45 mg applied every other day). A withdrawal bleed may be seen at the end of the progestin phase. Alternatively, a progestin is taken daily throughout the month at a dose equivalent to medroxyprogesterone 2.5 mg or micronized oral progesterone 100 mg. Approximately 70% of women will be amenorrheic while taking continuous combined therapy, although it may take 12 to 24 months for the endometrium to become sufficiently atrophic to achieve this result. Ultra-low-dose continuous HRT yielded more than 80% amenorrhea at 3 months for participants in the CHART study. Continuous combined regimens may be particularly desirable in women with disabilities for whom vaginal bleeding may be more difficult to manage.

TESTOSTERONE

Small doses of testosterone may be added to the HRT regimen in women who complain of decreased libido or energy. Transdermal testosterone, 300 µg, has been shown in an RCT to improve sexual functioning and psychologic well-being for women who have undergone oophorectomy and hysterectomy (137). These benefits, however, were limited to women with impaired sexual function at baseline. The transdermal testosterone patch still is undergoing clinical testing and is not currently available for postmenopausal women. Testosterone also may be used as an addition to a "continuous combined" regimen to decrease spotting or bleeding. Androgen–estrogen replacement therapy has been associated with improved bone density in comparison to ERT for women with surgical menopause (138). Long-term effects of low-dose testosterone are at present unknown, so it should be used cautiously and with continuous assessment as to whether the desired benefits with respect to libido, energy, or amenorrhea have been achieved. Testosterone for hormone replacement is FDA approved as esterified estrogens combined with methyl testosterone (Estratest).

Patient Monitoring

Initiation of daily combined hormone therapy does result in irregular bleeding or spotting prior to amenorrhea. Such initial irregu-

lar bleeding needs to be managed clinically with patient education. Transvaginal ultrasound to check the endometrial thickness can assist the clinician regarding decisions of endometrial biopsy. Less studied replacement regimens, such as with micronized progesterone intravaginally or cyclic withdrawal every 2 to 3 months may be considered with increased surveillance of the endometrium. Transvaginal ultrasound assessment of the endometrial lining has become a widely respected screening test that assists the clinician. Because the majority of instances of postmenopausal bleeding are related to endometrial atrophy, unnecessary biopsies can be avoided with the additional information of endometrial thickness by ultrasound. The upper limit of thickness of the endometrium for a postmenopausal woman has been well debated in the literature. An RCT known as the Nordic trial assessed the predictive value of transvaginal ultrasound in the evaluation of the endometrium and established an endometrial thickness of less than or equal to 4 mm to provide the greatest sensitivity and specificity (139). Most other studies concur with a maximal endometrial thickness of 4 or 5 mm as being the upper limit of normal for a postmenopausal woman assessed early in the phase of a replacement cycle.

ALTERNATIVE MANAGEMENT OPTIONS FOR WOMEN IN WHOM ESTROGEN REPLACEMENT THERAPY IS POORLY TOLERATED OR IS CONTRAINDICATED

With some disabilities, estrogen may be poorly tolerated, may be contraindicated, or may require special monitoring. For women with disabilities and chronic diseases who cannot safely take ERT, health goals are better achieved using nonestrogen therapies such as bisphosphonates, lipid-lowering medications, and lifestyle changes. Another nonestrogenic alternative for menopausal patients in whom ERT is contraindicated or who prefer not to take ERT is raloxifene (Evista). As in other selective estrogen receptor modulators, such

as tamoxifen, raloxifene has both estrogen agonist and antagonist properties. Studies credit
raloxifene with a positive impact on bone
density that is comparable to HRT or to alendronate (140). In the Multiple Outcomes of
Raloxifene Trial (MORE), postmenopausal
women with osteoporosis were randomized to
treatment with raloxifene or placebo. The
women treated with raloxifene had a 76% decreased risk of invasive breast cancer during
the 3 years of treatment (141). There was no
increased risk of endometrial cancer consistent with the perceived estrogen antagonist
role of raloxifene on the uterus. In a short-
term RCT of raloxifene, a positive impact on
some biochemical markers of cardiovascular
risk was noted (142). In comparison to
placebo, raloxifene significantly lowered
LDL-C and increased HDL2-C and lowered
lipoprotein (a). Raloxifene did not significantly change HDL-C, PAI-1, or triglycerides.
The effects of raloxifene on markers of cardiovascular risk are similar to those reported
for tamoxifen, with an estrogen agonist effect
noted on LDL-C levels but not on HDL-C
levels. The risk for procoagulation is comparable to HRT; raloxifene is associated with a
threefold increased incidence of deep-vein
thrombosis (141). There is no improvement or
stabilization of cognitive function for raloxifene users in comparison to a placebo group
(143), and there is no abatement of vasomotor
symptoms. The SSRIs venlafaxine and paroxetine have been shown to reduce hot flushes
by 50% to 70% (72,73). Tibolone is a synthetic steroid that has estrogenic, progesto-
genic, and androgenic properties. It has been
shown to alleviate hot flushes and reverse
genitourinary atrophy and in animal studies
has been shown to have estrogen antagonist
effects on breast tissue and endometrium
(144). Long-term increase or decrease of
breast or uterine cancer risks as related to use
of tibolone remains unknown. Tibolone is currently available in the United Kingdom. It is
not available in the United States.

Additionally, treatments to prevent morbidity and to maximize health maintenance must
be developed with each woman involving a
multidisciplinary team approach of clinicians
with experience in disability who can advise
on physical activity regimens, lifestyle modification, dietary changes, and other modalities.

CONCLUSION

For all women, initiation of HRT for relief
of climacteric symptoms is a highly individualized decision that must weigh all the
risks and benefits and that should be focused toward short-term management of
menopausal symptoms with the lowest-dose
regimen possible. Women with disabilities
similarly should be given consideration for
treatment with estrogen or estrogen and
progestin therapy. Further data are needed
regarding the risk/benefit profile of estrogen only; the second arm of the WHI study
should provide more insights. Decisionmaking to initiate HRT as well as individualiza-
tion of formulation, dose, and route should
take into account the long-term health risks
apparent for a specific woman with her
unique medical history.

REFERENCES

1. American Heart Association. *1997 Heart and stroke
   facts: statistical update* . Dallas: American Heart Association, 1997.
2. Sullivan JM. Hormone replacement therapy and cardiovascular disease: the human model. *Br J Obstet Gynecol* 1996;103:59–67.
3. National Osteoporosis Foundation, Physician's guide
   to prevention and treatment of osteoporosis *Excerpta
   Medica* 1998;1–29.
4. Henderson BE, Paganini-Hill A, Ross RK. Estrogen
   replacement therapy and protection from acute myocardial infarction. *Am J Obstet Gynecol* 1988;169:
   312–317.
5. Stampfer MJ, Colditz, GA, Willet WC, et al. Postmenopausal estrogen therapy and cardiovascular disease: ten year follow-up from the nurses' health study.
   N Engl J Med 1991;325:756–762.
6. Grodstein KF, Stampfer MJ, Manson JE, et al. Postmenopausal estrogen and progestin use and the risk
   of cardiovascular disease. *N Engl J Med* 1996;335:
   453–461.

7. Herrington DM, Reboussin DM, Brosnihan KB, et al. Effects of estrogen replacement on the progression of coronary artery atherosclerosis. *N Engl J Med* 2000; 343:522–529.

8. Hulley S, Grady D, Bush T, et al. Randomized trial of estrogen plus progestin for secondary prevention of coronary heart disease in postmenopausal women. Heart and Estrogen/progestin Replacement Study (HERS) Research Group. *JAMA* 1998; 280:650-2.

9. Grady D, Herrington D, Bittner V, et al. Heart and estrogen/progestin replacement study follow-up (HERS II):1.Cardiovascular outcomes during 6.8 years of hormone therapy. *JAMA* 2002;288:49–57.

10. Writing Group for the Women's Health Initiative. Risks and benefits of estrogen and progestin in healthy postmenopausal women: principal results from the Women's Health Initiative randomized controlled trial. *JAMA* 2002;288:321–333.

11. Stampfer MJ, Colditz GA. Estrogen replacement therapy and coronary artery disease: a quantitative assessment of the epidemiologic evidence. *Prev Med* 1991;20:47–63.

12. Grodstein F, Stampfer JJ, Goldhaber SZ, et al. Prospective study of exogenous hormones and risk of pulmonary embolism in women. *Lancet* 1996;348: 983–987.

13. Clarkson TB. Estrogens, progestins, and coronary heart disease in cynomolgus monkeys. *Fertil Steril* 1994;62(Suppl 2):147s–151s.

14. Speroff L, Rowan J, Symons J, et al. The comparative effect on bone density, endometrium, and lipids of continuous hormones as replacement therapy (CHART Study). *JAMA* 1996;276:1397–1403.

15. Lobo RA, Ettinger B, Hutchinson KA, et al. Estrogen replacement, the evolving role of transdermal delivery. *J Reprod Med* 1996;41:781–796.

16. Whitcroft SI, Crook D, Marsh MS, et al. Long-term effects of oral and transdermal hormone replacement therapies on serum lipid and lipoprotein concentrations. *Obstet Gynecol* 1994;84:222–226.

17. Karas RH, Patterson BL, Mendelsohn ME. Human vascular smooth muscle cells contain functional estrogen receptors. *Circulation* 1994;89:1943–1950.

18. Collins P. Rosano GMC, Jiand C, et al. Cardiovascular protection by estrogen: a calcium antagonistic effect? *Lancet* 1993;341:1264–1265.

19. Reis SE, Gloth ST, Blumenthal RS, et al. Ethinyl estradiol acutely attenuates abnormal coronary vasomotor responses to acetylcholine in postmenopausal women.*Circulation* 1994;89:52–60.

20. Jiang C, Sarrel PM, Lindsay DC, et al. Endothelium-independent relaxation of rabbit coronary artery by 17β-oestradiol in vitro. *Br J Pharmacol* 1991;104: 1033–1037.

21. Pines A, Fisman EZ, Shapira I, et al. Exercise echocardiography in postmenopausal hormone users with mild systemic hypertension. *Am J Cardiol* 1996;78: 1385–1389.

22. Grady D. Postmenopausal hormones—therapy for symptoms only. *N Engl J Med* 2003;348:1835–1837.

23. Sullivan JM, El-Zeky F, Vander Zwaag R, et al. Effect on survival of estrogen replacement therapy after coronary artery bypass grafting. *Am J Cardiol* 1997;79:847–850.

24. Grady D, Wenger NK, Herrington D, et al. Postmenopausal therapy increases risk for venous thromboembolic disease. *Ann Intern Med* 2000;132: 689–696.

25. American College of Obstetricians and Gynecologists. Response to Women's Health Initiative Study Results, 2002. Available at *www.acog.com*. Accessed July 23, 2003.

26. Wassertheil-Smoller S, Hendrix SL, Limacher M, et al. Effect of estrogen plus progestin on stroke in postmenopausal women. The women's health initiative: a randomized trial. *JAMA* 2003;289:2673–2684.

27. Petitti DB, Sidney S, Quesenberry CP. Ischemic stroke and use of estrogen and estrogen/progestogen as hormone replacement therapy. *Stroke* 1998;29:23–28.

28. Pedersen AT, Lidegaard O, Kreiner S, et al. Hormone replacement therapy and risk of non-fatal stroke. *Lancet* 1997;350:1277–1283.

29. Fung MM, Barrett-Connor E, Bettencourt RR. Hormone replacement therapy and stroke risk in older women. *J Women's Health* 1999;3:359–364.

29a. Paganini-Hill A, Ross RK, Henderson BE. Postmenopausal oestrogen treatment and stroke: a prospective study. *BMJ* 1988;297:519–22.

30. Paganini-Hill A. Hormone replacement therapy and stroke: risk, protection or no effect? *Maturitas* 2001;38:243–261.

31. Jonas HA, Kronmal RA, Psaty BM, et al. Current estrogen-progestin and estrogen replacement therapy in elderly women: association with carotid atherosclerosis. *Ann Epidemiol* 1996;6:314–323.

32. American-Canadian Co-Operative Study Group. Persantine aspirin trial in cerebral ischemia—Part III: risk factors for stroke. *Stroke* 1986;17:12–18.

33. Hart RG, Pearce LA, McBride R, et al. Factors associated with ischemic stroke during aspirin therapy in atrial fibrillation. Analysis of 2012 participants in the SPAF I-III clinical trials. *Stroke* 1999;30: 1223–1229.

34. Koh KK, Mincemoyer RN, Bui MN, et al. Effects of hormone-replacement therapy on fibrinolysis in postmenopausal women. *N Engl J Med* 1997; 336: 683–690.

35. McCully KS. Vascular pathology of homocysteinemia: implications for the pathogenesis of arteriosclerosis. *Am J Pathol* 1969;111–128.

36. Welch GN, Loscalzo J. Homocysteine and atherothrombosis. *N Engl J Med* 1998;338:1042–1050.

37. Van der Mooren MJ, Wouters MGAJ, Blom HJ, et al. Hormone replacement therapy may reduce high serum homocysteine in postmenopausal women. *Eur J Clin Invest* 1994;24:733–736.

38. Mijatovic V, Netelenbos C, van der Mooren MJ, et al. Randomized, double-blind, placebo-controlled study of the effects of raloxifene and conjugated equine estrogen on plasma homocysteine levels in healthy postmenopausal women. *Fertil Steril* 1998;70: 1085–1089.

39. Varas-Lorenzo C, Garcia-Rodriquez LA, Cattaruzzi C, et al. Hormone replacement therapy and the risk of hospitalization for venous thromboembolism: a population-based study in southern Europe. *Am J Epidemiol* 1998;147:387–390.

40. Daly E, Vessey MP, Painter R, et al. Case-control

study of venous thromboembolism risk in users of hormone replacement therapy. *Lancet* 1996;348: 1027.

41. Jick H, Derby LE, Myers MW, et al. Risk of hospital admission for idiopathic venous thromboembolism among users of postmenopausal oestrogens. *Lancet* 1996;348:981–983.

42. Ray SA, Rowley MR, Loh AT, et al. Hypercoagulable states in patients with leg ischaemia. *Br J Surg* 1994;81:811–814.

43. Crook D. The metabolic consequences of treating postmenopausal women with non-oral hormone replacement therapy. *Br J Obstet Gynaecol* 1997;104: 4–13.

44. Psaty BM, Smith NL, Lemaaitre RN, et al. Hormone replacement therapy, prothrombotic mutations, and the risk of incident nonfatal myocardial infarction in postmenopausal women. *JAMA* 2001;285:906–913.

45. Mosca L, Collins P, Herrington DM, et al. Hormone Replacement Therapy and Cardiovascular Disease, *Circulation* 2001;104:499–503.

46. Satter N, Jaap AJ, MacCuish AC. Hormone replacement therapy and cardiovascular risk in postmenopausal women with NIDDM. *Diabetes Medicine* 1996;13:782–788.

47. Manson JE, Rimm EB, Colditz GA, et al. A prospective study of postmenopausal estrogen therapy and subsequent incidence of non-insulin-dependent diabetes mellitus. *Ann Epidemiol* 1992;2:665–673.

48. Godsland IF, Ganger K, Walton C, et al. Insulin resistance, secretion, and elimination in postmenopausal women receiving oral or transdermal hormone replacement therapy. *Metabolism* 1993;42: 846–53.

49. Crook D, Godsland IF, Hull J, et al. Hormone replacement therapy with dydrogesterone and 17 beta-estradiol: effects on serum lipoproteins and glucose tolerance during 24 month follow up. *Br J Obstet Gynaecol* 1997;104:298–304.

50. Andersson B, Mattsson LA, Hahn L, et al. Estrogen replacement therapy decreases hyperandrogenicity and improves glucose homeostasis and plasma lipids in postmenopausal women with noninsulin-dependent diabetes mellitus. *J Clin Endocrinol Metab* 1997;82: 638–643.

51. Lindheim SR, Duffy DM, Kojima T, et al. The route of administration influences the effect of estrogen on insulin sensitivity in postmenopausal women. *Fertil Steril* 1993;60:1176–1180.

52. Turner RT, Riggs BL, Spelsberg TC. Skeletal effects of estrogens. *Endocrin Rev* 1994;15:275–300.

53. Pilbeam CC, Klein-Nuelend J, Raisz LG. PTH stimulated resorption and prostaglandin production in cultured neonatal mouse calvariae. *Biochem Biophys Res Commun* 1989;163:1319–1324.

54. Lindsay R, Bush TL, Grady D, et al. Therapeutic controversy, estrogen replacement in menopause. *J Clin Endocrinol Metab* 1996;81:3829–3838.

55. Dempster DW, Lindsay R. Pathogenesis of osteoporosis. *Lancet* 1993;341:797–801.

56. Ettinger B. Prevention of osteoporosis: treatment of estradiol deficiency. *Obstet Gynecol* 1988;72: 12S–17S.

57. Vedi S, Compston JE. The effects of long-term hormone replacement therapy on bone remodeling in postmenopausal women. *Bone* 1996;19:535–539.

58. Felson DT, Zhang Y, Hannan MT, et al. The effect of postmenopausal estrogen therapy on bone density in elderly women. *N Engl J Med* 1993;329:1141–1146.

59. Genant HK, Lucas J, Weiss S, et al. Low-dose esterified estrogen therapy: effects on bone, plasma estradiol concentrations, endometrium, and lipid levels. *Arch Intern Med* 1997;157:2609–2615.

60. Quigley MET, Martin P, Burnier AM, et al. Estrogen therapy arrests bone loss in elderly women. *Am J Obstet Gynecol* 1987;156:1516–1523.

61. Ettinger B, Genant HK, Steiger P, et al. Low-dosage micronized 17β-estradiol prevents bone loss in postmenopausal women. *Am J Obstet Gynecol* 1992;166: 479–488.

62. Bone HG, et al. Alendronate and estrogen effects in postmenopausal women with low bone mineral density. *J Clin Endocrinol Metab* 2000;85:720–726.

63. McKinlay SM, Jeffreys M. The menopausal syndrome. *Br J Prev Soc Med* 1974;28:108–115.

64. Thompson B, Hart SA, Durno D. Menopausal age and symptomatology in a general practice. *J Biosoc Sci* 1973;5:71–82.

65. Sturdee DW, Wilson KA, Pipili E, et al. Physiological aspects of menopausal hot flush. *Br Med J* 1978;2: 79–80.

66. Jensen J, Christiansen C. Dose-response and withdrawal effects on climacteric symptoms after hormonal replacement therapy. A placebo controlled therapeutic trial. *Maturitas* 1982;5:125–133.

67. Callantine MR, Martin PL, Bolding OT, et al. Micronized 17B-estradiol for oral estrogen therapy in menopausal women. *Obstet Gynecol* 1975;46: 37–41.

68. Coope J, Thomson JM, Poller L. Effects of "natural oestrogen" replacement therapy on menopausal symptoms and blood clotting. *Br Med J* 1975;4: 139–143.

69. Bullock JL, Massey FM, Gambrell RD Jr. Use of medroxyprogesterone acetate to prevent menopausal symptoms. *Obstet Gynecol* 1975;46:165–168.

70. Lobo RA, McCormick W, Singer F, et al. Depo-medroxyprogesterone acetate compared with conjugated estrogens for the treatment of postmenopausal women. *Obstet Gynecol* 1984;63:1–5.

71. Edington RF, Chagnon J-P, Steinberg WM. Clonidine (Dixarit) for menopausal flushing. *CMA J* 1980;123: 23–25.

72. Loprinzi Cl, Pisansky TM, Fonseca R, et al. Pilot evaluation of venlafaxine hydrochloride for the therapy of hot flashes in cancer survivors. *J Clin Oncol* 1998;16:2377–2381.

73. Stearns V, Isaacs C, Powland J, et al. A pilot trial assessing the efficacy of paroxetine hydrochloride in controlling hot flashes in breast cancer survivors. *Ann Oncol* 2000;11:17–22.

74. Clayden JR, Bell JW, Pollard P. Menopausal flushing: double-blind trial of a non-hormonal medication. *Br Med J* 1974;1:409–412.

75. Hendriksson L, Stjernquist M, Boquist L, et al. A one-year multicenter study of efficacy and safety of a con-

tinuous, low-dose, estradiol-releasing vaginal ring (Estring) in postmenopausal women with symptoms and signs of urogenital aging. *Am J Obstet Gynecol* 1996; 174:85–92.

76. Eriksen PS, Rasmussen H. Low-dose 17B-estradiol vaginal tablets in the treatment of atrophic vaginitis: a double-blind placebo controlled study. *Eur J Obstet Gynecol* 1992;44:137–144.

77. Raz R, Stamm WE. A controlled trial of intravaginal estriol in postmenopausal women with recurrent urinary tract infections. *N Engl J Med* 1993;329: 753–756.

78. Smith P. Postmenopausal urinary symptoms and hormonal replacement therapy. *Br Med J* 1976;2:941.

79. Fantl JA, Cardozo L, McClish DK. Estrogen therapy in the management of urinary incontinence in postmenopausal women: a meta-analysis. First report of the Hormone and Urogenital Therapy Committee, *Obstet Gynecol* 1994;83:12–18.

80. Rigg LA, Hermann H, Yen SSC. Absorption of estrogens from vaginal creams. *N Engl J Med* 1976;298: 195–197.

81. Sherwin BB, Gelfand MM, Brender W. Androgen enhances sexual motivation in females: a prospective, crossover study of sex steroid administration in the surgical menopause. *Psychosom Med* 1985;47: 339–351.

82. Kaufert PA, Gilbert P, Tate R. The Manitoba Project: a re-examination of the link between menopause and depression. *Maturitas* 1992;14:143–155.

83. Avis NE, Brambilla D, McKinlay SM, et al. A longitudinal analysis of the association between menopause and depression: results from the Massachusetts Women's Health Study. *Ann Epidemiol* 1994;4:214–220.

84. Woods NF, Mitchell ES. Pathways to depressed mood in midlife women: observations from the Seattle Midlife Women's Health Study. *Res Nurs Health* 1997;20:119–129.

85. Ditkoff EC, Crary WG, Cristo M, et al. Estrogen improves psychological function in asymptomatic postmenopausal women. *Obstet Gynecol* 1991;78: 991–995.

86. La Blanc ES, Janowshk J, Chan BK, et al. Hormone replacement therapy and cognition: systematic review and meta-analysis. *JAMA* 2001;285:1489–1499.

87. Barrett-Connor E, Kritz-Silverstein D. Estrogen replacement therapy and cognitive function in older women. *JAMA* 1993;269:2637–2641.

88. Palinkas LA, Barrett-Connor E. Estrogen use and depressive symptoms in postmenopausal women. *Obstet Gynecol* 1992;80:30–36.

89. Paganini-Hill A, Henderson VW. Estrogen replacement and risk of Alzheimer's disease. *Arch Intern Med* 1996;156:2213–2217.

90. Luine VN. Estradiol increases choline acetyltransferase activity in specific basal forebrain nuclei and projection areas of female rats. *Exp Neurol* 1985;89: 484–490.

91. Simpkins JW, Green PS, Gridley KE, et al. Role of estrogen replacement therapy in memory enhancement and the prevention of neuronal loss associated with Alzheimer's' disease. *Am J Med* 1997;103(3A): 19–25S.

92. Schneider LS, Farlow M. Combined tacrine and estrogen replacement therapy in patients with Alzheimer's disease. *Ann N Y Acad Sci* 1997;826:317–322.

93. Mulnard RA, Cotman CW, Kawas C, et al. Estrogen replacement therapy for treatment of mild to moderate Alzheimer's disease. A randomized controlled trial. *JAMA* 2000;283:1007–1015.

94. Rapp SR, Espeland MA, Shumaker SA, et al. Effect of estrogen plus progestin on global cognitive function in postmenopausal women. The women's health initiative memory study: a randomized controlled trial. *JAMA* 2003;289:2663–2672.

95. Shumaker SA, Legault C, Rapp SR, et al. Estrogen plus progestin and the incidence of dementia and mild cognitive impairment in postmenopausal women. *JAMA* 2003;289:2651–2662.

96. Armstrong AL, Oborne J, Coupland CAC, et al. Effects of hormone replacement therapy on muscle performance and balance in post-menopausal women. *Clin Sci* 1996;91:685–90.

97. Phillips SK, Rook KM, Siddle NC, et al. Muscle weakness in women occurs at an earlier age than in men, but strength is preserved by hormone replacement therapy. *Clin Sci* 1993;84:95–98.

98. Colditz GA, Egan KM, Stampfer MJ. Hormone replacement therapy and risk of breast cancer. *Am J Obstet Gynecol* 1993;168:1473–1480.

99. Sillero-Arenas M, Delgado-Rodriguex M, Rodigues-Canteras R, et al. Menopausal hormone replacement therapy and breast cancer: a meta-analysis. *Obstet Gynecol* 1992;79:286–294.

100. Colditz GA, Stampfer MJ, Willett WC, et al. Prospective study of estrogen replacement therapy and risk of breast cancer in postmenopausal women. *JAMA* 1990;264:2648–2653.

101. Collaborative Group on Hormonal Factors in Breast Cancer. Breast cancer and hormone replacement therapy. *Lancet* 1997;350:1047–1059.

102. Gapstur SM, Morrow M, Sellers TA. Hormone replacement therapy and risk of breast cancer with a favorable histology. Results of the Iowa Women's Health Study. *JAMA* 1999;281:2091–2097.

103. Grodstein F, Stampfer MJ, Colditz GA, et al. Postmenopausal hormone therapy and mortality. *N Engl J Med* 1997;336:1769–1775.

104. McDonald CC, Alexander FE, Whyte BW, et al. Cardiac and vascular morbidity in women receiving adjuvant tamoxifen for breast cancer in a randomized trial. The Scottish Cancer Trials Breast Group. *BMJ* 1995; 311:977–980.

105. Rutqvist LE, Mattsson A. Cardiac and thromboembolic morbidity among postmenopausal women with early-stage breast cancer in a randomized trial of adjuvant tamoxifen, *J Natl Cancer Inst* 1993;85: 1398–1406.

106. Costantino JP, Kuller LH, Ives DG, et al. Coronary heart disease mortality and adjuvant tamoxifen therapy, *J Natl Cancer Inst* 1997;89:776–782.

107. Cecchini S, Ciatto S, Bonardi R, et al. Screening by ultrasonography for endometrial carcinoma in postmenopausal breast cancer patients under adjuvant tamoxifen. *Gyneco Oncol* 1996;60:409–411.

108. Powles TJ, Bourne T, Athanasiou S, et al. The effects

of norethisterone on endometrial abnormalities identified by transvaginal ultrasound screening of healthy post-menopausal women on tamoxifen or placebo. *Br J Cancer* 1998;78:272–275.

109. National Center for Health Statistics. *Healthy People 2000 review.* Hyattsville, MD: Public Health Service, 1997.

110. Stampfer MJ, Hu FB, Manson JE, et al. Primary prevention of coronary heart disease in women through diet and lifestyle. *N Engl J Med.* 2000;343:16–22.

111. Castelo-Branco C, Duran M, Gonzalez-Merlo J. Skin collagen changes related to age and hormone replacement therapy. *Maturitas* 1992;15:113–119.

112. Brincat M, Versi E, Moniz CF, et al. Skin collagen changes in postmenopausal women receiving different regimens of estrogen therapy. *Obstet Gynecol* 1987; 70:123–127.

113. Carlson CL, Cushman M, Enright PL, et al. Hormone replacement therapy is associated with higher FEV1 in elderly women. *Am J Respir Crit Care Med* 2001;163: 423–428.

114. Kos-Kudl B, Ostrowska Z, Marek B, et al. Hormone replacement therapy is postmenopausal asthmatic. *J Clin Phar Ther* 2000;25:461–466.

115. Ben Noun L. Drug-induced respiratory disorders: incidence, prevention and management. *Drug Safety* 2000;23:143–164.

116. Barrett-Connor E. Postmenopausal estrogen therapy and selected (less-often considered) disease outcomes. *Menopause* 1999;6:14–20.

117. Mok CC, Lau CS, Ho CT, et al. Safety of hormonal replacement therapy in postmenopausal patients with systemic lupus erythematosus. *Scand J Rheumatol* 1998;27:342–346.

118. Kreidstein S, Urowitz MB, Gladman DD, et al. Hormone replacement therapy in systemic lupus erythematosus. *J Rheumatol* 1997;11:2149–2152.

119. Arden NK, Lloyd ME, Spector TD, et al. Safety of hormone replacement therapy in systemic lupus erythematosus. *Lupus* 1994;3:11–13.

120. Le Thi Huong D, Weschler B, Piette JC. Effect of pregnancy, menopause and hormone substitution therapy on disseminated systemic lupus erythematosus. *Presse Medicale* 2000;29:55–60.

121. Lahita RG. The role of sex hormones in systemic lupus erythematosus. *Curr Opin Rheumatol* 1999:11: 352–356.

122. Sanchez-Guerrero J, Liang MH, Karlson EW, et al. Postmenopausal estrogen therapy and the risk for developing systemic lupus erythematosus. *Ann Int Med* 1995;123:961–962.

123. Hall GM, Spector TD, Delmas PD. Markers of bone metabolism in postmenopausal women with rheumatoid arthritis. Effects of corticosteroids and hormone replacement therapy. *Arthr Rheum* 1995;38: 902–906.

124. Hall GM, Daniels M, Huskisson EC, et al. A randomized controlled trial of the effect of hormone replacement therapy on disease activity in postmenopausal rheumatoid arthritis. *Ann Rheum Dis* 1994;53: 112–116.

125. MacDonald AG, Murphy EA, Capell HA, et al. Effects of hormone replacement therapy in rheumatoid arthritis: a double blind placebo-controlled study. *Ann Rheum Dis* 1994;53:54–57.

126. Smith R, Studd JW. A pilot study of the effect upon multiple sclerosis of menopause, hormone replacement therapy and the menstrual cycle. *J Royal Soc Med* 1992;85:612–613.

126a.Sherwin BB. Changes in sexual behavior as a function of plasma sex steroid levels in post-menopausal women. *Maturitas* 1985;7:225–33.

127. Lee MA. Epilepsy in menopause. *Neurology* 1999; 53:S41.

128. Witt DM, Lousberg TB. Controversies surrounding estrogen use in postmenopausal women. *Ann Pharmacother* 1997;31:745–755.

129. Chetkowski RJ, Meldrum DR, Steingold KA, et al. Biological effects of transdermal estradiol. *N Engl J Med* 1986;314:1615–1620.

130. Lobo RA, Brenner P, Mishell DR. Metabolic parameters and steroid levels in postmenopausal women receiving lower doses of natural estrogen replacement. *Obstet Gynecol* 1983;62:94–98.

131. Padwick ML, Endacott J, Whitehead MI. Efficacy, acceptability, and metabolic effects of transdermal estradiol in the management of postmenopausal women. *Am J Obstet Gynecol* 1985;152:1085.

132. Handa VL, Bachus KE, Johnston WW, et al. Vaginal administration of low-dose conjugated estrogens: systemic absorption and effects on the endometrium. *Obstet Gynecol* 1994;84:215–218.

133. Rioux J, Devin C, Gelfand MM, et al. 17β-estradiol vaginal tablet versus conjugated equine estrogen vaginal cream to relieve menopausal atrophic vaginitis. *Menopause* 2000;7:156–161.

134. Holmgren PA, Lindskog M, von Schoultz B. Vaginal rings for continuous low-dose release of oestradiol in the treatment of Urogenital atrophy. *Maturitas* 1989; 11:55–63.

135. Bachmann G, Notelovitz M, Nachtigall L, et al. A multicenter comparative study of the safety and efficacy of a low dose estradiol vaginal ring and conjugated estrogen cream for postmenopausal urogenital atrophy. *Prim Care Update Obstet Gyn* 1997;4: 109–115.

136. Bachmann G. Estradiol-releasing vaginal ring delivery system for urogenital atrophy: experience over the past decade. *J Repro Med* 1998;43:991–998.

137. Shifren JL, Braunstein GD, Simon JA, et al. Transdermal testosterone treatment in women with impaired sexual function after oophorectomy. *N Engl J Med* 2000;343:682–688.

138. Watts NB, Notelovitz M, Timmons MC, et al. Comparison of oral estrogens and estrogens plus androgen on bone mineral density, menopausal symptoms, and lipid-lipoprotein profiles in surgical menopause. *Obstet Gynecol* 1995;85:529–537.

139. Karlsson B, Granberg S, Wikland M, et al. Transvaginal ultrasonography of the endometrium in women with postmenopausal bleeding—a Nordic multicenter study. *Am J Obstet Gynecol* 1995;172: 1488–1494.

140. Santen R, Pinkerton JV. Alternatives to estrogen use in

post-menopausal women. *Menopausal Medicine* 1999; 7:1–7.

141. Cummings SR, Eckert S, Krueger KA, et al. The effect of Raloxifene on risk of breast cancer in post-menopausal women. *JAMA* 1999;281:2189–2197.

142. Walsh BW, Kuller LH, Wild RA, et al. Effects of ralox-ifene on serum lipids and coagulation factors in healthy postmenopausal women. *JAMA* 1998;279: 1445–1451.

143. Yaffee K, Krueger K, Sarkar S, et al. Cognitive func-tion in postmenopausal women treated with raloxifene. *N Engl J Med* 2001;344:1207–1213.

144. Rymer J. Menopause management: tibolone. *Meno-pausal Medicine* 2000;8:9–10.

20

Gynecologic Health Care for Developmentally Disabled Women

Elisabeth H. Quint

INTRODUCTION

Gynecologic health care for women with mental disabilities is often challenging for care providers. Normal gynecologic issues such as menstruation, sexuality, and contraception can become a cause of anxiety and concern for patients, caregivers, and parents. Puberty and the onset of the menstrual cycle mean significant adaptations from the patient, schools, parents, and other caregivers. Many clients live in smaller homes in the communities and attend regular schools and workplaces. This means that some behavior that is acceptable at home may need modification in these different settings. The primary care physicians can meet many of the patient's general medical needs (1). Some larger hospitals have established multidisciplinary clinics with an ethics committee that advises on the sensitive issues of contraception, abortion, and sterilization (2).

The main principle of all gynecologic care for women with disabilities should be that no gynecologic examination ever should be done by using force or inducement of fear. The patient's autonomy needs to be respected, and she should be allowed to participate in her own care as much as possible. Thorough evaluation of the patient's complaints with sensitivity toward abilities and disabilities, as well as adaptation of regularly used techniques, should enable the caregiver to perform a comprehensive gynecologic assessment of the patient with developmental disabilities and assess the need for preventive health care as well as any treatment or therapy.

REPRODUCTIVE HEALTH EVALUATION

Medical History

The extent to which a medical history can be elicited is dependent on two main factors. In the first place, it depends on the degree of handicap of the patient. Some patients can voice their own complaints or concerns, but often the parent or caregiver provides the history. Using basic language is very important if the patient is verbal. The second important component is the caregiver. If the client comes with a parent or a knowledgeable caregiver, then a full medical history will be available. Sometimes, however, the patient will come with a poorly informed attendant. It therefore is recommended to send a letter ahead of the visit to address the importance of information and an appropriate caregiver to accompany the patient. A request for menstrual and behavioral calendars (if indicated) may be included in this letter. If desired by the patient, trusted caregivers can accompany the patient to the visit to provide comfort during the examination.

Sexuality

Because sexuality in women with developmental disabilities is such an uncomfortable area for many people, it is important to discuss this at the visit with patients and caregivers. Patients with disabilities often are viewed as asexual (3), and therefore frequently have no access to appropriate services and counseling. The ability to reproduce is not necessarily affected by a mental or physical disability (4), so reproductive concerns need to be addressed. This includes assessing the patient's risk for abuse as well as her ability to have a consensual sexual relationship.

First, an assessment is done of the patient's knowledge of anatomy and sexual behavior with a discussion, pictures, slides, or anatomically correct dolls. Inquire about safety at school, work, and home, as well as possible behavioral problems, including public masturbation or hygiene issues. Second, a plan needs to be made to meet any unmet educational needs. The expression of sexual feelings, such as through masturbation, needs to be acknowledged and channeled into acceptable social norms.

For many teenagers who are disabled, dealing with the turmoil of adolescence can lead to enormous feelings of isolation. It is imperative that the teenager who is disabled has a chance to ask questions and learn about sexuality in a positive, constructive way at her own level. Sexual education can be done by the physician, a nurse, or a social worker with an interest in this area. Many schools offer a regular sexual education curriculum; however, the teens who are developmentally disabled often are excluded from that discussion. It is the duty of the health care team to assess the actual knowledge and understanding of the patients. Therefore, the evaluation should be started with simple questions to assess what the teenager knows and wants to know. It is also very important to address parental concerns. Often overwhelmed with day-to-day care of their handicapped child, the onset of puberty and menstrual cycles sends everyone out of balance. Requests often are made to stop cycles or to sterilize patients. These are tremendous concerns for the families and need to be addressed with the utmost consideration and concern.

For the woman who is mildly disabled, the emphasis is on education about periods, menstrual hygiene, sexual activity, and contracep-

tion. If the patient expresses a desire to become sexually active, then an assessment is made to address whether the patient can understand enough to consent to a sexual encounter as something that *she* desires. Most women who can perform their own toilet hygiene can be educated to manage their own menstrual hygiene. If the client wears diapers, the pad is inserted in the diaper to help with cleanliness and more frequent changes. Other areas of education deal with acceptable social behavior, including masturbation and the privacy of sexual activities. Time is spent on private and public body parts as well as learning to avoid situations that can lead to sexual abuse.

For the woman who is severely mentally disabled educational opportunities are more limited and include personal hygiene, avoidance of self-abuse, and acceptable social behavior.

Gynecologic Examination

The gynecologic examinations of women with developmental disabilities are complicated by several different factors. There may have been a history of abuse (5–7), or examinations may have been attempted with some force. This naturally will increase the anxiety of the patient. Often the verbal methods used during the pelvic examination to help relax a patient are not as successful in this population. Patients may have multiple physical handicaps, complicating the positioning and access to the vagina and abdomen; 45% to 55% of patients have neurologic abnormalities and 21% have some form of orthopedic problem (1).

Wearing a white coat is recommended, so the patient can clearly identify the caregiver. Allow a trusted caregiver or family member to be present, if the patient desires that. It may require several visits to a caregiver before the patient is comfortable and allows an examination. Some patients will benefit from practicing with gowns, instruments, and the examining table. Allow the patient some control over the examination by having her touch all the instruments and assist as much as possible. Sensitivity on the part of the caregiver is very important, and a hurried examination usually leads nowhere. When a pelvic examination is contemplated, it is important to realize whether it adds to the history and physical portion of the examination. If an examination is indicated, the approach needs to be individualized.

A gynecologic evaluation usually encompasses one or more of the following tests or examinations.

Breast Examination

The breast examination is usually well tolerated by the patient. Often they are used to their caregivers doing it on a monthly basis because this is often in the patients' care plan.

Pelvic Examination

The patient often will allow inspection of the external genitalia. Look for moles, hygiene, bruises, or tearing. If concerned about hygiene, bring that to the attention of the caregiver in a nonthreatening fashion. Sometimes patients will not allow help with hygiene or changing of clothes, and education may be needed. Before attempting an examination, assess the need for a pelvic examination and whether it adds to the history and general physical evaluation.

Because of physical handicaps, positioning the legs for a gynecologic evaluation may be difficult. Stirrups generally are not used. Options for positioning include the following:

1. Frog leg position with heels together in the midline and knees bend out to the side
2. V-position with both legs extended and slightly opened
3. Lying on the side with the legs bent but not separated
4. Elevating legs with knees slightly bent or not bent, without abduction of the hips. This position often works well because spreading of the legs may bring on a strong reaction from the patients.

In all these positions it is somewhat more difficult to perform an examination, but it certainly can be done (8). The sight of the speculum may cause concern for many patients, whereas others may want to feel it before use. Use a Huffman-Graves speculum (narrow, but long) as opposed to a pediatric speculum, which is narrow but too short for the adult woman. If it appears that a speculum examination is not possible, then use cotton-tipped swab Papanicolaou (Pap) test. One finger is placed in the vagina, and the cervix is located. Slide a moistened cotton-tipped swab or a soft-tipped plastic brush, if using liquid cytology, inside the vagina over the finger and place it inside the cervix. Although the results are generally suboptimal (9), this is often the only option. Bimanual examination, almost always with only one finger in the vagina, can be difficult because of lack of cooperation of the client and body position (such as with scoliosis). If the patient cannot relax, the abdominal rectus muscles stay very tight and palpation of the uterus and ovaries is limited. Deep, slow breathing can help relaxation of the abdominal wall; lowering the head of the patient onto the bed also helps. If the patient is unable to tolerate any vaginal examination, then a rectoabdominal examination can be performed, which can give some information regarding the pelvic organs. Obviously, this is a suboptimal examination. Many patients with mental disabilities have problems with their bowel elimination and therefore may have significant stool amounts in their rectum. A laxative or enema prior to an examination in a patient who has this particular problem can be very helpful. If the patient clearly states she cannot tolerate the examination, either by verbal or nonverbal language, her wishes should be respected. Some patients will have a very tight hymen, which may preclude an examination altogether.

Papanicolaou Smear (Pap Smear)

Because it is often impossible to verify past medical history, sexual activity, or sexual abuse, it is difficult to assess the risk factors for cervical cancer, although it seems that women with mental disabilities are probably not at unusually high risk for developing cervical cancer (9,10). Scientific data on Pap tests in women with mental disabilities is limited. One retrospective review of patients from a specialty clinic evaluated Pap tests and found the incidence of abnormal Pap tests to be 0.3% (9). Another study found three abnormal Pap tests out of 162 (1.8%) with one confirmed dysplasia in that group (10). There are no data on the newer liquid cytology techniques available for this population.

Several studies reveal that women with functional limitations (FLs) compared to women without FLs have fewer Pap tests and are somewhat less likely to undergo mammogram screening (11,12). These data do not specifically distinguish women with mental disabilities. The screening recommendations for Pap tests in the general population have changed to start at age 21 or within 3 years of the onset of sexual activity. After three normal annual test results in a low-risk woman, the frequency may be altered. (13)

The issue of sedation for Pap tests, as a preventive health care screening, is debatable. Some people have advocated this approach (14), but it never has been evaluated in a systematic fashion. Moreover, there are some concerns about the ethics of this approach (15). Review of data from a ketamine sedation program revealed that 14% of a study population of women with mental disabilities underwent sedation. Of these women, 25% still could not be examined with sedation. One of the main side effects from the sedation was nausea and vomiting, which potentially could lead to aspiration in this vulnerable population. There is no information on the emotional side effects of a pelvic examination in a sedated state. Therefore outpatient sedation only for preventive health care is debatable. If a patient needs a Pap test because of a previous abnormal result or a high-risk situation, the individual practitioner can consider sedation with oral agents in consultation with the patient's primary care provider.

Some large hospitals have programs set up with other services that may require anesthesia, such as dentistry. A combined dental procedure/gynecology examination, including a Pap test and bimanual examination, can be done under general anesthesia, if the anesthetic is indicated for the dental procedure.

Rectal Examination with Occult Blood Testing

Any woman older than age 50 years should have yearly rectal examinations and occult stool testing. Some women that will not allow a vaginal examination may allow a rectal examination. This also can be used for the rectoabdominal examination that can give information about the internal organs.

Pelvic Ultrasound

If an examination is impossible to be obtained, a pelvic ultrasound can be done to evaluate the uterus and adnexal structures. The optimal frequency for these examinations has not been established. It is not recommended as screening for the general population. Difficulty with ultrasonography includes patient cooperation and poor bladder filling. A discussion with the radiologist prior to these examinations with emphasis on the possible suboptimal nature of these examinations and that the goal is to rule out large abnormalities can be very helpful.

Mammograms

Mammograms for women who are disabled are recommended at the same age and frequency intervals as the general population. Clearly some patients have physical limitations as a result of body position and ability to tolerate the examinations. In discussion with the radiologist, the optimal imaging technique or place of service may be chosen.

MENSTRUAL ISSUES

Abnormal Uterine Bleeding

For the first 2 years after menarche, irregular anovulatory bleeding is very common (16), and reassurance is often all that is needed. If the bleeding is excessive or leads to hospitalization, a thorough workup is indicated. This includes a search for bleeding disorders, which are more common in those patients that have severe menorrhagia at menarche. Thyroid disease, both hyperthyroidism and hypothyroidism, can be associated with irregular bleeding and has a higher prevalence amongst patients with Down syndrome (17). Irregular bleeding is also common in women taking antiseizure medication or neuroleptics. Women with epilepsy have an increased incidence of reproductive endocrine disorders (18). The anticonvulsants (except valproic acid) increase the activity of cytochrome P-450 hepatic microsomal oxidative enzymes, resulting in a more rapid clearing of hormones. The neuroleptics and metoclopramide can cause hyperprolactinemia that leads to irregular bleeding or amenorrhea.

The initial approach focuses on the documentation of the problem, including menstrual calendars to document the regularity of the cycles and a thorough search for possible contributing factors, as outlined earlier. Blood work often includes hemoglobin, prolactin, thyroid-stimulating hormone (TSH), estradiol, and follicle-stimulating hormone (FSH), as indicated. Endometrial biopsy or dilatation and curettage, where anesthesia is required, should be considered for the same indications as in the general population, but caution about anesthetics is recommended.

It is important to have good documentation of the menstrual problem prior to initiating any treatment. This will help to assess the effectiveness of the treatment and to make sure it is not done solely for the convenience of the caregivers or for fear that the patient could become pregnant. If the cycles really interfere with daily life and cause problems to the extent where the patient cannot partake in her usual activities or cause her significant discomfort or anemia, then treatment needs to be considered. It is important to remember that once hormonal intervention is started, it often leads to lifelong treatment with unknown long-term effects.

Nonsteroidal antiinflammatory drugs (NSAIDs), when used in adequate doses, help with dysmenorrhea and lessen menstrual flow (19). If regularity or decrease in flow and cramping is desired, low-dose oral contraceptives are a good choice. If the patient has anovulatory cycles, another option is to use oral medroxyprogesterone, 10 mg/day for 10 days every month. If amenorrhea is the goal, depot medroxyprogesterone acetate, 150 to 250 mg every 9 to 12 weeks, has been used successfully. Side effects include weight gain, which can be up to 5 to 10 pounds per year, and osteoporosis (20,21). For women who may be dependent on other people for their transfers in and out of wheelchairs, significant weight increase may affect their life severely.

Other alternatives include endometrial ablation; however, this does not always cause amenorrhea and therefore may be less desired (22). Hysterectomy, although frequently requested, is only indicated for medical reasons. In some societies the vaginal hysterectomy for menstrual hygiene has been used, but this is not indicated in the United States (23). Abdominal surgery in women with mental disabilities has been associated with significant morbidity and should be done only after all medical options have been exhausted (24). The health care team, the patient, the parents, and sometimes the school or other caregivers need to work together to find the solution that is in the best interest of the patient.

Amenorrhea

Primary amenorrhea is usually genetically based or results from structural abnormalities. Secondary amenorrhea can result from anovulation, hyperprolactinemia, premature ovarian failure, or hypothalamic amenorrhea. In some patients who are severely disabled, weight fluctuations can lead to cessation of cycles. Neuroleptic use is another more common reason for amenorrhea associated with hyperprolactinemia. A thorough history; examination, including pelvic ultrasound in the case of primary amenorrhea; and some basic laboratory values, including TSH, prolactin, FSH, and estradiol, usually will lead to a diagnosis. The treatment depends on the findings. If the prolactin value is elevated, brain imaging is considered, except with mild elevations and use of prolactin-elevating medications. Many women who are disabled cannot tolerate the recommended computed tomography scan or magnetic resonance imaging, and a coned-down view of the sella is performed.

The premenopausal, young patient with low or absent estrogen, regardless of the etiology, should be considered for estrogen replacement therapy to prevent osteoporosis. The decision to start estrogen replacement therapy in every individual takes careful consideration. Often a discussion with caregivers and/or guardians is in order. An important consideration is the time that the woman has been hypoestrogenic. Reintroducing estrogen can lead to breast tenderness and vaginal bleeding, which can be traumatic to the patient. If estrogen is indicated, a very low dose of conjugated estrogens is given initially and is increased gradually to a full dose, combined with continuous progesterone to prevent any bleeding if possible. Calcium (1,000 to 1,200 mg/day) as well as vitamin D use should be encouraged. The patient with oligomenorrhea because of anovulation needs to be treated with cyclic progesterone or oral contraceptives.

CONTRACEPTION

Concerns around the topic of contraception often come from the parents when their daughter goes through puberty or from the caregivers if there is any concern about sexual activity. When this request is made, an assessment of the safety of the patient is in order. Why are the caregivers concerned? Often the request is made in a crisis situation: perhaps something has happened to the patient or to any of the patients in the group home. This may have made everyone acutely aware of the risk of abuse and hence the request. An open discussion with the patient, caregivers, and/or family is important. The caregivers' fears for pregnancy and abuse needs to be acknowledged, and the family, the patient, and the health care team need to work together to establish the best approach for the individual.

When the request for birth control comes from the patient herself, the care provider has to assess if this patient is able to have consensual sexual relations. This requires a complete evaluation of the patient's knowledge and understanding of the process of sexual activity. Often this cannot be obtained in one interview, and the help of a psychologist or social worker may be needed for private discussions with the patient. Discussions about sexually transmitted diseases and the use of condoms for safer sex are part of this process. Safety, efficacy, and ease of use are considered when choosing a contraceptive in any patient, and there are some special considerations in the patient who is developmentally delayed (4).

Oral contraceptives commonly are used in women with developmental disabilities because they reduce flow and cramping. A disadvantage is that they require daily intake, which may require supervision or daily reminders. Many patients with Down syndrome have significant flow abnormalities in the heart. This poses an increased risk in thrombus formation and should be considered when prescribing oral contraceptives. Immobility, resulting in increased deep-venous thrombosis risk, is another concern, especially in women in wheelchairs. Although there are no data available on this, caution should be used. Clients taking anticonvulsants, with the exception of valproic acid, may need a dose adjustment in the oral contraceptives because of the previously mentioned increased activity of the cytochrome P-450 enzymes. If persistent breakthrough bleeding occurs, an increase in estrogen content of the oral contraceptive is necessary (25). Progesterone-only oral contraceptives often are safe to use, although their contraceptive effect is slightly lower than the combined oral contraceptives and they can cause more irregular bleeding.

Intramuscular depot medroxyprogesterone acetate has been extensively used, both for contraception and for the cessation of menses (26). An initial month-long trial of oral progesterone is recommended before administering the intramuscular dose to assess for side effects or mood changes. After a 1-year period of intramuscular depot medroxyprogesterone acetate use, 50% of patients will be amenorrheic. Some patients may experience breakthrough bleeding. The side effects are discussed in the section on abnormal uterine bleeding. Calcium (1,000 to 1,200 mg/day) and vitamin D use should be encouraged.

The oral contraceptive patch has not been used in this population, but it may have the advantage of easy application. Detachment rates are around 4%, and that should be closely monitored by caregivers (27,28).

Barrier methods, such as the diaphragm and the cervical cap, require a high degree of personal initiative, intellectual understanding, and physical dexterity and therefore are not a good choice for most clients who are developmentally disabled. Condoms require a great degree of communication with partners, and patients may need help with that because the use of condoms for protection from sexually transmitted diseases is important.

The intrauterine device (IUD) traditionally has not been recommended in women with disabilities because of the inability for some patients to report symptoms as well as the need for an anesthetic at the time of insertion. The traditional copper-containing IUD, which increased bleeding and cramping, was not advocated in this group of women. However, with the advent of the levonorgestrel IUD, which decreases the menstrual flow significantly, this position may need to be reevaluated (29).

Patients and caregivers should be informed of the option of postcoital (emergency) contraception, which can be very useful in cases of contraceptive failure or rape (30).

Sterilization in women who are mentally disabled is a controversial topic. The American College of Obstetricians and Gynecologists presented a Committee Opinion on this issue in 1999 (31). The initial premise should be that nonvoluntary sterilization is ethically not acceptable because of the violation of privacy, bodily integrity, and reproductive rights. The parents, the guardians, and care providers of women with mental retardation may not agree with that sentiment (32). There are also widely varying federal, state, and local laws and regulations. If a very unusual situation arises, extensive consulting with an ethics committee (33), other physicians, social workers, clergy, or others is of the utmost importance (34). If a patient is mentally competent (35), then only after extensive consideration and counseling with the patient should a sterilization procedure be considered.

SEXUAL ABUSE

Sexual abuse in this vulnerable population is a big concern. Minimal data are available, and estimates range from 10% to 65% (6,7). A study comparing abuse in women with physical disabilities with a nonhandicapped group found that the overall incidence of abuse was similar in both groups (62% overall abuse, 30% sexual abuse) but that the handicapped women suffered more abuse by health care providers and attendants (36). Self-reported sexual abuse in adolescents with disabilities ranged from 19% to 24% (37). Overall, it is felt that women who are mildly or moderately developmentally disabled may be at the greatest risk (7). When performing a physical examination, care providers should be acutely aware of signs of abuse. Examine the patient for bruises, and ask for an explanation from the caregivers if any are found. Evaluation of external genitalia can be difficult because of the positioning limitations. It is difficult to use hymenal anatomy for positive evidence of sexual abuse, especially if the patient had pelvic examinations before. One study describes the difficulty in examining 35 severely handicapped women from an institution where one client was found to be pregnant (38). Any sexually transmitted disease is considered strongly suggestive of sexual abuse. If trichomonas is found on a Pap test, the patient needs to be reevaluated and the diagnosis needs to be made on a wet preparation; discharge possibly should be sent to the lab for diagnosis and preservation in case of further legal action. A full sexual abuse investigation should be started, although trichomonas possibly can be a contaminant from the bowel flora. The presence of human papillomavirus on a Pap test of a patient who is not known to be or have been sexually active should lead to a thorough evaluation.

CYCLIC BEHAVIOR CHANGES

Premenstrual syndrome (PMS) or menstrually related mood disorder occurs in up to 80% of women of reproductive age, causing 20% to 40% of women some difficulty regularly and 5% significant impact on work and lifestyle. PMS is a combination of behavioral and physical symptoms only occurring in the luteal phase of the menstrual cycle and disappearing after menses appear. If they occur at any other time, another source of these symptoms needs to be considered. In women with mental disabilities cyclic behavior changes is an often-heard complaint (39). There can be an exacerbation of previously present behavior or onset of new behavior. It may include aggression or self-mutilation. It can influence significantly the life of the patient, their caregivers, and the people they live with. Whether these behavior changes are indeed PMS is often difficult to discern. The behavior can be erratic and troublesome to interpret because a large number of these patients are nonverbal and also may have psychiatric disorders. Multiple medications often complicate the picture. The demonstration of true cyclicity of symptoms by means of daily charting and questionnaires to rule out underlying behavioral, mood, or psychiatric disorders is essential. For the patient in a group home this means a big commitment of time and observation from the caregivers. Daily symptom charts are used, focusing on the most trouble-

some behavior. If, after evaluation of several months of charts, the behavior appears clearly cyclic and only demonstrated in the second half of the cycle, treatment is initiated. The first line of treatment is an NSAID because some of the behavior may be related to dysmenorrhea (40). Other options include taking oral contraceptives, depot medroxyprogesterone acetate, or continuous oral progesterone. The success of these treatments in women with disabilities has not been studied in a prospective manner.

Fluoxetine, which is used as treatment for PMS in the general population (41), only sparingly has been used in women with mental disabilities. It has been prescribed for people with self-injurious behaviors to regulate their serotonin levels (42), and it may be an option for patients with persistent self-injurious behavior (43). This should be given in consultation with a psychiatrist and/or neurologist because of the potential for drug interactions (44).

REFERENCES

1. Minihan PM, Dean DH. Meeting the needs for health services of persons with mental retardation living in the community. *Am J Public Health* 1990;80:1043.
2. Elkins TE, Gafford LS, Wilks CS, et al. A model clinic approach to the reproductive health concerns of the mentally handicapped. *Obstet Gynecol* 1986;68:185.
3. Sulpizi LK. Issues in sexuality and gynecologic care of women with developmental disabilities. *J Obstet Gynecol Neonatal Nurs* 1996;25:609–614.
4. Haefner H, Elkins E. Contraceptive management for female adolescents with mental retardation and handicapping disabilities. *Curr Opin Obstet Gynecol* 1991;3:820.
5. Westcott H. The abuse of disabled children: a review of the literature. *Child Care Health Dev* 1991;17:243.
6. Blackburn M. Sexuality, disability and abuse: advise for life...not just for kids! *Child Care Health Dev* 1995;21:351.
7. Chamberlain A, Rauh J, Passer A, et al. Issues in fertility control for mentally retarded female adolescents: I. sexual activity, sexual abuse, and contraception. *Pediatrics* 1984;73:445.
8. Elkins TE, McNeeley SG, Rosen DA, et al. Clinical observation of a program to accomplish pelvic exams in difficult to manage patients with mental retardation. *Adolesc Pediatr Gynecol* 1988;1:195–198.
9. Quint EH, Elkins TE. The dilemma of cervical cytology in women with mental retardation. *Obstet Gynecol* 1997;89:123.
10. Jaffe JS, Timell AM, Eisenberg MS, et al. Low prevalence of abnormal cervical cytology in an institutional-

ized population with intellectual disability. *J Intellect Dis Res* 2002;46:569–574.

11. Use of cervical and breast cancer screening among women with and without functional Limitations— United States 1994–1995. *MMWR* 1998;47:853–856.

12. Nosek MA, Howland CA. Breast and cervical cancer screening among women with physical disabilities. *Arch Phys Med Rehabil* 1997;78(S):39–44.

13. Saslow D, Runowicz CD, Solomon D, et al. American Cancer Society guideline for the early detection of cervical neoplasia and cancer. *CA Cancer J Clin* 2002; 52(6):342–362.

14. Rosen DA, Rosen KR, Elkins TE, et al. Outpatient sedation: An essential addition to gynecologic care for persons with mental retardation. *Am J Obstet Gynecol* 1991;164:825.

15. Brown D, Rosen D, Elkins TE. Sedating women with mental retardation for routine gynecological examination: an ethical analysis. *J Clin Ethics* 1992;3:68.

16. Falcone T, Desjardins C, Bourque I, et al. Dysfunctional uterine bleeding in adolescents. *J Reprod Med* 1994; 39:761.

17. Prasher VP. Down syndrome and thyroid disorders: a review. *Down Syndr Res Pract* 1999;6(1):25–42.

18. Bauer J, Isojarvi JL, Herzog AG, et al. Reproductive dysfunction in women with epilepsy: recommendations for evaluation and treatment. *J Neurol Neurosurg Psych* 2002;73:121–125.

19. Chuong CJ, Brenner PF. Management of abnormal uterine bleeding . *Am J Obstet Gynecol* 1996;175:787–792.

20. Cromer BA, Blair JM, Mahan JD, et al. A prospective comparison of bone density in adolescent girls receiving depot medroxyprogesterone acetate (Depo-Provera), levonorgestrel (Norplant), or oral contraceptives. *J Pediatr* 1996;129:671.

21. Scholes D, LaCroix AZ, Ichikawa LE, et al. Injectable hormone contraception and bone density: results from a prospective study. *Epidemiology* 2002;13(5):581–587.

22. Wingfield M, McClure N, Marners PM, et al. Endometrial ablation: an option for the menstrual problems in the intellectually disabled. *Med J Aust* 1994;160:533.

23. Sheth S, Malpani A. Vaginal hysterectomy for the management of menstruation in mentally retarded women. *Int J Gynecol Obstet* 1991;35:319.

24. McNeeley SG, Elkins TE. Gynecologic surgery and surgical morbidity in mentally handicapped women. *Obstet Gynecol* 1989;74:155.

25. Back DJ, Orme MLE. Pharmacokinetic drug interactions with oral contraceptives. *Clin Pharmacokinet* 1990;18:472.

26. Kaunitz AM. Long-acting injectable contraception with depot medroxyprogesterone acetate. *Am J Gynecol* 1994;170:1543.

27. Gallo MF, Grimes DA, Schulz KF. Skin patch and vaginal ring versus combined oral contraceptives for contraception. *Cochrane Database of Systematic Reviews* CD003552. 2003;1.

28. Burkman RT. The transdermal contraceptive patch: a new approach to hormonal contraception. *Int J Fertil Womens Med* 2002;47(2):69–76.

29. French RS, Cowan FM, Mansour D, et al. Levonorgestrel-releasing (20 microgram/day) intrauterine systems (Mirena) compared with other methods of reversible contraceptives. *BJOG* 2000;107(10):1218–1225.

30. Grimes DA, Raymond EG. Emergency contraception. *Ann Intern Med* 2002;137(3):180–189.

31. American College of Obstetricians and Gynecologists. Sterilization of women, including those with mental disabilities. ACOG Committee Opinion 216. Washington, DC: ACOG, 1999.

32. Bambrick M, Roberts GF. The sterilization of people with mental handicap: the views of parents. *J Ment Def Res* 1991;35:353.

33. Elkins TE, Hoyle D, Darnton T, et al. The use of a societally based ethics/advisory committee to aid in decisions to sterilize mentally handicapped patients. *Adol Pediatr Gynecol* 1998;1:190.

34. Herr SS, Hopkins BL. Health care decision making for persons with disabilities. *JAMA* 1994;271:1017.

35. Morris CD, Niederbuhl JM, Mahr JM. Determining the capability of individuals with mental retardation to give informed consent. *Am J Ment Retard* 1993;98(2): 263–272.

36. Young MA, Nosek MA, Howland C, et al. Prevalence of abuse among women with physical disabilities. *Arch Phys Med Rehabil* 1997;78:S34.

37. Suris JC, Recsnick MD, Cassuto N, et al. Sexual behavior of adolescents with chronic disease and disability. *J Adol Health* 1996;19:124.

38. Elvik SL, Berkowitz CD, Nicholas E, et al. Sexual abuse in the developmentally disabled: dilemmas of diagnosis. *Child Abuse Neglect* 1990;14:497.

39. Kaminer Y, Feinstein C, Barrett RP, et al. Menstrually related mood disorder in developmentally disabled adolescents: review and current status. *Child Psych Human Dev* 1988;18:239.

40. Quint EH, Elkins TE, Sorg CA, et al. The treatment of cyclical behavioral changes in women with mental disabilities. *J Pediatr Adol Gynecol* 1999;12(3):139–142.

41. Steiner M, Romano SJ, Babcock S, et al. The efficacy of fluoxetine in improving physical symptoms associated with premenstrual dysphoric disorder. *BJOG* 2001;108 (5):462–468.

42. Gualtieri CT. The differential diagnosis of self-injurious behavior in mentally retarded people. *Psychopharm Bull* 1989;25:358.

43. Ricketts RW, Goza AB, Ellis CR, et al. Fluoxetine treatment of severe self-injury in young adults with mental retardation. *J Am Acad Child Adol Psych* 1993;32(4): 865–869.

44. Troisi A, Vicario E, Nuccetelli F, et al. Effects of fluoxetine on aggressive behavior of adult inpatients with mental retardation and epilepsy. *Pharmacopsychiatr* 1995;28:73.

21

Secondary Conditions: Physical Deconditioning, Fatigue, and Spasticity

Patricia C. Gregory, Ling-Ling Cheng, and Barbara J. de Lateur

INTRODUCTION

Disability is a prevalent problem in the United States. The Survey of Income and Program participation (SIPP), which uses a broad-based definition of disability, states that 20% of Americans (53.9 million) have a disability (1). Disability is defined as limitations in functional activities of daily living (ADL) or independent activities of daily living (IADL). Of those with disability, more than one half (53%), or 28.6 million, are women. Women also suffer more activity limitations compared to men (2). Across the spectrum, data based on the National Health Interview Survey (NHIS) indicate that activity limitation increases with age and that the prevalence among women increases disproportionately compared to men. Women also have a greater number of restricted activity days. They experience 18.2 days per year versus 13.6 per year for men. This may be partially explained by the fact that women have a greater burden of disability and disease comorbidity with advancing age (3,4). Diseases including heart disease, diabetes, hearing impairments, lung disease, and stroke have a greater prevalence in the most disabled population (3). That prevalence, however, also is associated with decline in instrumental and basic ADL (4). There is also a greater prevalence of pain in the disabled population (5); 30% of the severely disabled report pain. Risk factors for pain in the disabled population include advancing age and female gender. With women's increased life expectancy, there is a greater burden of older women with more physical disability. For minority women the picture is even bleaker. Native-American and African-American women have the highest rate of disability among women (2). Based on the SIPP, Native-American women have the highest rate of disability at 21.8%, followed closely by African-American women at 21.7%.

Disability, as defined earlier, is a prevalent and serious activity-limiting entity among women. Because of the impact of the disability, this population is at greater risk for a number of secondary conditions. Secondary conditions are defined as conditions experienced by an individual after a primary disability. There have been prior studies (2,6) that have focused on specific secondary conditions.

What further complicates the picture is that people often experience more than one secondary condition at a time. This makes it more difficult to treat and conquer the offending condition. One secondary condition may exacerbate another. Another secondary condition may be prevalent for a time, remit, and then relapse. The treatment for one secondary condition may exacerbate another secondary condition. All of these issues must be taken into consideration when attempting to treat specific secondary conditions. It is estimated that the impact of these secondary conditions is to limit their activities to fewer than 6 to 10 hours per week on the average (2). These conditions also are a significant predictor of overall health and independence (6). There are many secondary conditions, but this chapter focuses on three: physical deconditioning, fatigue, and spasticity.

PHYSICAL DECONDITIONING

Physical deconditioning is loss of physiologic reserves sufficient to cause activity limitation. Its prevalence is very high among the disabled population (2,6). Seekins and colleagues (6) found the prevalence in a rural population of disabled people to be 65%. This was higher than the prevalence of spasticity (59%) and close to the prevalence of pain (67% to 71%). Coyle and associates' (2) surveillance among disabled women described physical deconditioning to be among the most problematic secondary conditions. The impact of physical deconditioning can be described best in the arthritis population. Arthritis is hypothesized to exert its toll on task performance through what has been described clinically as the reluctant disuse cycle (Fig. 21-1) (7,8). In this cycle, subchondral bone erosions lead to pain. The hypothesized re-

sponse is to limit mobility to avoid the pain. This would lead to reduced range of motion, decreased exercise tolerance, and subsequent muscle atrophy and weakness. Secondary to disuse, the joint and surrounding muscles are at risk for further injury, which would lead to more pain and continuation of the cycle.

This pathway can be extrapolated to the disabled population (Fig. 21-2). Women with disabilities have reduced muscle mass (9), which leads to decreased strength (10) and worsening weakness. With aging they also will have a greater risk for sarcopenia (9,11). Sarcopenia is defined as a decline in muscle mass with an increase in intramuscular adipose tissue. It is more prevalent among women and is considered a normal part of aging. It involves loss of both type I and type II fibers. It is believed to contribute to morbidity by leading to decreased strength and aerobic and functional capacity and increasing frailty. It is believed to affect falls, rates of hospitalization, institutionalization, and mortality.

Among older women the disability experienced affects stair climbing, bathing, housework, and IADLs such as handling personal

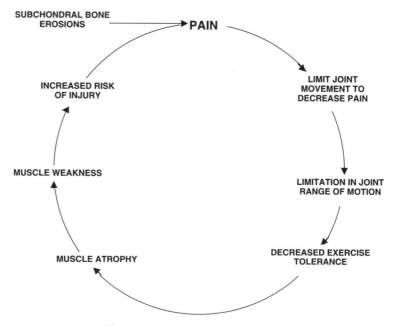

Fig. 21-1. Reluctant disuse cycle.

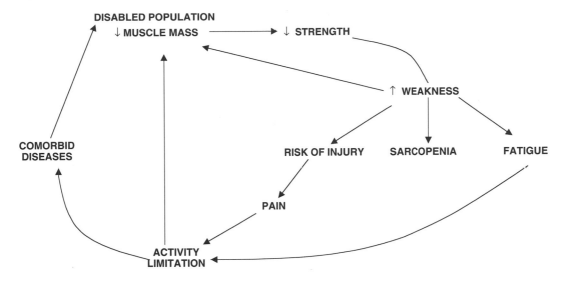

Fig. 21-2. Physical deconditioning cycle.

finances and using public transportation (12). All of this will lead to a greater risk of injury because of, for example, cumulative trauma disorders such as rotator cuff injury, lateral epicondylitis, and cubital and carpal tunnel syndrome (13). This then will lead to a greater prevalence of pain (5) and more activity limitation (1). This reduced activity limitation will lead to a risk of developing a greater number of comorbid diseases (1,3), all of which will lead to reduced muscle mass and repetition of the cycle.

People with disabilities have been shown to have reduced physical activity (PA) (2,6,14,15) and have been shown to be at risk for further physical deconditioning. These prior studies have shown that leisure-time physical activity (LTPA) is very low among people with disabilities. The NHIS (15) found that only 27% of people with disabilities engaged in regular moderate PA. Of this population, 30% reported no LTPA. The findings among African-American women are even more alarming. Only 10% of this population engaged in aerobic exercise three times per week, and only 8.2% reported any LTPA. This lack of PA has important implications. First, the benefits of regular physical exercise are

lost. This includes lowering blood lipids, arterial blood pressure, and blood clotting factors; increasing high-density lipoprotein levels; reducing insulin resistance; and preventing bone loss, venous thromboembolism, and weight gain. Secondly, regular physical exercise reduces the risk of other secondary conditions. Finally, regular physical exercise is tied to life satisfaction (16,17).

Women with disabilities have a lower rate of employment (1) and, therefore, do not reap the benefits of occupational PA (18). A prior study showed that even a moderate amount of PA on the order of 1.8 to 2.9 metabolic equivalents was protective against developing impaired mobility in a population cohort over 12 years.

Another implication of the reduced rate of employment is the barrier to health care access. Disabled women who are unemployed may not have insurance and therefore have limited access to medical care and follow-up. As previously mentioned, comorbid diseases have a role in declining functional status (3,4). Comorbid diseases not only exert their toll, as shown in Fig. 21-2; they also will cause more morbidity if they are not managed carefully.

The benefits of regular PA include preventing weight gain, reducing blood lipids, lowering blood pressure, helping prevent venous thromboembolic disease, reducing the complications of diabetes, reducing the effects of osteoporosis, and preventing the progression of sarcopenia (9). PA even at the low levels has been shown to slow the progression of disability (19).

FATIGUE

Fatigue is defined as any reduction in the maximal capacity to generate force or power output (20). There are many debates about how to measure fatigue. From an epidemiologic standpoint it can be defined as self-reported exhaustion (21) and is a risk factor for frailty. It is a particularly troublesome secondary condition among women with disability because it further compounds the reluctant disuse cycles and contributes to further functional decline. As mentioned before, women with disabilities have very low levels of PA (14,15). As a result they will have decreased strength and will be fatigued more easily with daily tasks. Figures 21-1 and 21-2 show that this is a cycle, which continues to spiral and inhibit function. The greater prevalence of chronic comorbid conditions among disabled women places them at greater risk for easy fatigability (22). They also have an increased metabolic cost to perform physical tasks because of the decreased muscle mass, inefficient locomotion, and abnormal posturing. They will have a decreased VO_2 max because of the limited PA and deconditioning. This also will result in greater fatigue at these low levels of activity. As previously mentioned, the high unemployment rate among these women does not allow them to reap the benefits of occupational PA. Women with disabilities as well as the disabled population attribute a large part of their difficulty to fatigue (2,6).

Treatment strategies to counteract the effects of fatigue should focus on measures to increase PA with an exercise program that includes strengthening and aerobic conditioning to improve the efficiency and power of muscle activity. Proper nutrition is important to supply the muscles with fuel to generate power.

SPASTICITY

Spasticity is a common secondary condition occurring after upper motor neuron injury in disorders such as multiple sclerosis, spinal cord injury, stroke, traumatic brain injury, and other progressive neurologic disorders. Disabilities resulting from such neurologic impairments account for the majority of disabling conditions, others impairments being arthritic conditions or pain syndromes (2). The impact of spasticity on function is variable and can be more debilitating in those with relative neurologic sparing, as in the case with incomplete tetraplegia compared with complete tetraplegia. Spasticity can lead to direct tissues changes (23) such as stiffness, contractures, atrophy, and fibrosis. Indirect consequences include loss of skin integrity; pain; and impaired sleep hygiene, gait, and function.

The pathophysiology of spasticity is not completely known. Decreased inhibitory inputs in response to usual stimulus and supersensitivity of remaining neuronal input have been described in the mechanism of spasticity (23). Lance defined spasticity as a motor disorder characterized by a velocity-dependent increase in tonic stretch reflexes (muscle tone) with exaggerated tendon jerks, resulting from hyperexcitability of the stretch reflex, as one component of the upper motor neuron

Table 21-1. *Positive and negative symptoms of spasticity*

Positive symptoms
Increased stretch reflexes
Released flexor reflexes (Babinski)
Exaggerated tendon jerks
Stretch reflex spread to extensor
Mass synergy patterns
Repetitive stretch reflex discharges (clonus)
Negative symptoms
Loss of finger dexterity
Weakness
Loss of selective control

Table 21-2. *The modified Ashworth scale*

0	No increase in tone
1	Slight increase in tone, catch, and release; minimal resistance at end range of motion
1+	Catch, followed by minimal resistance throughout the remainder (<50%) of the range
2	Marked increase in tone through most of the range of motion
3	Considerable increase in tone; passive movement difficult
4	Affected part is rigid in flexion or extension

syndrome (24). The upper neuron syndrome is comprised of negative and positive symptomatology (Table 21-1) (23). The positive or exaggerated symptoms are usually more amenable to treatment, whereas symptoms such as weakness and dexterity are much more difficult to alleviate and have a greater impact on function (23,25,26).

Spasticity is difficult to measure. No single measurement or tool can be used to describe an individual's spasticity completely (27,28). The Modified Ashworth Scale and the Penn Spasm Frequency Scale are common clinical scales. The Modified Ashworth Scale is an ordinal scale based on physical assessment of tone by an examiner (29). Although subjective, the Modified Ashworth Scale has been shown to be reliable and reproducible (30). The Penn Spasm Frequency Scale rates severity based on frequency of patient-reported spasms over a period of 1 hour (31) (Table 21-2) (29,30). More objective measures are needed. Current methods using biomechanical and electromyographic techniques are used primarily in research (26,32).

Options for treatment of spasticity are broad, ranging from prevention of noxious stimuli or use of physical modalities such as ice therapy to neurosurgical intervention (Table 21-3). A combination of interventions usually is needed to treat spasticity adequately. Decisions regarding which treat-

Table 21-3. *Treatment of spasticity*

Mechanical/physical
Pharmacologic
   Systemic
   Local (injections)
   Regional (intrathecal)
Surgical

ment option(s) to undertake depend on the severity of spasticity, its duration (whether and to what extent there are soft-tissue contractures), its distribution (whether it is global or localized), the site of central nervous system injury, other comorbidities, availability of support, and access to care (26,33). Because there is no cure for spasticity, goals of treatment should be discussed to guide type and intensity of treatment. Common goals are to improve function toward a specific task such as feeding or reducing leg adduction during gait, improve sleep, reduce pain, save time during ADL, and promote skin integrity by facilitating proper positioning.

Noxious stimuli such as that from acute cystitis, a new pressure sore, or bowel impact can lead to transient increase in spasticity or painful spasms. Mechanical and physical modalities commonly are used as an adjunct to systemic and local pharmacologic treatment. A daily or routine stretching program can facilitate self-care by reducing tone and has been shown to carry over (34,35). Ice or cryotherapy applied for 20 minutes can reduce spasticity temporarily (36). Splinting techniques can be used to prevent contractures, promote static stretch position, or reduce tone by decreasing afferent inputs that trigger synergistic movements (26,37). Weight bearing, tilt table standing, and electrical stimulation have been shown to reduce spasticity but with variable results (38–41).

Spasticity can be treated systemically with oral medications (Table 21-4), regionally with intrathecal baclofen (ITB), or locally using injection techniques. Gamma-aminobutyric acid (GABA) agonists are commonly the first line for spinal-mediated spasticity. Baclofen

Table 21-4. *Medications for spasticity*

Drug	Dosage range	Mechanism of range
Baclofen	10–150 mg	GABA agonist
Diazepam	2.5–60 mg	GABA agonist
Gabapentin	300–3,600 mg	Mimics GABA
Dantrolene	25–400 mg	Inhibits calcium release in skeletal muscle
Tizanidine	2–36 mg	Alpha-2 agonist

GABA, gamma-aminobutyric acid.

is the drug of choice for spinal-mediated spasticity; it has been shown to reduce flexor spasms and to improve range of motion and bladder control (42,43). The side-effect profile includes confusion and hallucinations. Withdraw seizure can occur if baclofen is withdrawn suddenly. Diazepam is efficacious in treating painful spasms (43) and can be used to prevent rebound increase in spasticity occurring in the morning after prolonged immobility. Dantrolene acts directly at the level of the sarcoplasmic reticulum and is effective in cerebrally mediated spasticity. Both dantrolene and tizanidine can cause hepatotoxicity. Gabapentin commonly is used for neuropathic pain and can reduce spasticity in slightly higher doses (44,45).

Chemoneurolysis (with motor point or nerve blocks) or chemodenervation (with botulinum toxin, or Botox) using injection therapy can be used to treat localized tone affecting a specific limb(s) and definable muscle(s). Antagonist muscles can be weakened to free agonist muscles to carry out a specific task such as feeding or improving gait. The techniques for injection have been described (46). Alcohol derivatives (such as phenol or ethyl alcohol) are used for both motor point and nerve blocks and when injected cause selective destruction of neural tissue. In a motor point block, phenol typically is injected at the greatest concentration of motor end plates of the involved muscle. Peripheral nerve blocks with injection of phenol or ethyl generally are preferred when problematic tone results from a group(s) of muscles innervated at a single nerve. Complications from injections include pain at the injection site and residual paresthesias (46).

Botulinum toxin reduces presynaptic release of acetylcholine from the motor axon (47). The use of botulinum toxin injections for treatment of spasticity is not yet approved by the U.S. Food and Drug Administration, but it is quite common and relatively safe (47,48). The technique is easier than that of nerve blocks. Electromyographic localization of motor end plates has been shown to produce better results (24,49,50). The effects of botulinum toxin dissipate over 3 to 5 months, unlike nerve and motor point blocks, which can last for several years. Cost can be prohibitive at $700 per vial, and repeated use can lead to formation of antibodies against botulinum toxin, which can lead to resistance. The use of botulinum toxin in pregnancy and during lactation is contraindicated (47).

ITB has been shown to reduce tone, improve function, allow intermittent catheterization, and improve sleep (30). ITB allows medication to be delivered directly to the subarachnoid space. The cerebrospinal fluid concentration achieved via the intrathecal route is four times that of the oral route (30,51). ITB therapy is considered in those with severe regional spasticity who have failed a combination of conservative measures or for those who are intolerant to effective doses of oral medications. ITB is contraindicated in pregnancy (24). Appropriate screening before pump and catheter placement commonly includes a discussion about access to follow-up medical and supportive care. Complications or limitations of ITB are related to hardware malfunction or malpositioning, maintenance care (refills and replacements), and expense of hardware and maintenance (52).

REFERENCES

1. Jans L, Stoddard S. Chartbook on women and disability in the United States. An InfoUse report. Washington, DC: U.S. Department of Education, National Institute on Disability and Rehabilitation Research, 1999.
2. Coyle CP, Santiago MC, Shank JW, et al. Secondary conditions and women with physical disabilities: a descriptive study. *Arch Phys Med Rehabil* 2000;81: 1380–1387.
3. Fried LP, Bandeen-Roche K, Kasper JD, et al. Association of comorbidity with disability in older women: the Women's Health and Aging Study. *J Clin Epidemiol* 1999;52(1):27–37.
4. Cho CY, Alessi CA, Cho M, et al. The association between chronic illness and functional change among participants in a comprehensive geriatric assessment program. *J Am Geriatr Soc* 1998;46(6):677–682.
5. Astin M, Lawton D, Hirst M. The prevalence of pain in a disabled population. *Soc Sci Med* 1996;42(11): 1457–1464.
6. Seekins T, Clay J, Ravesloot C. A descriptive study of secondary conditions reported by a population of adults with physical disabilities served by three independent living centers in a rural state. *J Rehabil* 1994;60:47–51.
7. Hicks JE. Exercise in patients with inflammatory arthritis and connective tissue disease. *Rheum Dis Clin N Am* 1990;16(4):845–870.
8. Dekker J, Boot B, van der Woude LHV, et al. Pain and disability in osteoarthritis: a review of biobehavioral mechanisms. *J Behav Med* 1992;15(2):189–214.
9. Heath GW, Fentem PH. Physical activity among persons with disabilities-a public health perspective. *Exercise Sport Sci Rev* 1997;25:195–234.
10. Langlois JA, Norton R, Campbell AJ, et al. Characteristics and behaviours associated with difficulty in performing activities of daily living among older New Zealand women. *Disabil Rehabil* 1999;21(8):365–371.
11. Evans WJ. What is sarcopenia? *J Gerontol Series A* 1995;50A(SI):5–8.
12. Laukkanen P, Sakari-Rantala R, Kauppinen M, et al. Morbidity and disability in 75- and 80-year-old men and women. A five-year follow-up. *Scand J Soc Med Suppl* 1997;53(3):79–106.
13. Cooper RA, Quatrano LA, Axelson PW, et al. Research on physical activity and health among people with disabilities: A consensus statement. *J Rehabil Res Dev* 1999;36(2):142–154.
14. Rimmer JH, Rubin SS, Braddock D, et al. Physical activity patterns of African-American women with physical disabilities. *Med Sci Sports Exerc* 1999;31(4): 613–618.
15. Heath GW, Fentem PH. Physical activity among persons with disabilities: a public health perspective. In: Holloszy JO, ed. *Exercise and sport sciences reviews*. Baltimore: Williams and Wilkins, 1997:195–234.
16. Tate DG, Riley BB, Perna R, et al. Quality of life issues among women with physical disabilities or breast cancer. *Arch Phys Med Rehabil* 1997;78(Suppl 5):S18–S25.
17. Kinney WB, Coyle CP. Predicting life satisfaction among adults with physical disabilities. *Arch Phys Med Rehabil* 1992;73:863–869.
18. Gregory PC, Gallo JJ, Armenian H. Occupational physical activity and the development of impaired mobility. The 12-year follow-up of the Baltimore Epidemiologic Catchment Area Sample. *Am J Phys Med Rehabil* 2001; 80:270–275.
19. Miller ME, Rejeski WJ, Reboussin BA, et al. Physical activity, functional limitations, and disability in older adults. *J Am Geriatr Soc* 2000;48(10):1264–1272.
20. Vollestad NK. Measurement of human muscle fatigue. *J Neurosci Methods* 1997;74(2):219–227.
21. Fried LP, Tangen CM, Walston J, et al. Frailty in older adults: evidence for a phenotype. *J Gerontol A Biol Sci Med Sci* 2001;56(3):M146–M156.
22. LaPlante M. *Disability risks of chronic illnesses and impairments*. Disability Statistics Report 2. San Francisco: University of California, Institute for Health and Aging, 1989.
23. Mayer, NH. Clinicophysiologic concepts of spasticity and motor dysfunction in adults with upper motorneuron lesion. *Muscle Nerve Suppl* 1997;6:S1–S13
24. Lance JW. Symposium synopsis. In: Feldman RG, Young RR, Koella WP, eds. *Spasticity: disordered motor control*. Chicago: Year Book Publishers, 1980: 485–494.
25. Young RR. The physiology of spasticity and its response to therapy. *Ann N Y Acad Sci* 1988;531:146–149.
26. Kirshblum S. Treatment alternatives for spinal cord related spasticity. *J Spinal Cord Med* 1999;22;3:199–217.
27. Pierson SH. Outcome measures in spasticity management. *Muscle Nerve Suppl* 1997;6:S36–S60.
28. Priebe MM, Sherwood AM, Thornby JI, et al. Clinical assessment of spasticity in spinal cord injury: A multidimensional problem. *Arch Phys Med Rehabil* 1996;77: 713–716.
29. Bohannon RW, Smith MB. Interrater reliability of a modified Ashworth Scale of Muscle spasticity. *Phys Ther* 1987;67:206–207.
30. Lee KC, Carson L, Kinnin E, et al. The Ashworth scale: A reliable and reproducible method of measuring spasticity. *J Neurol Rehab* 1989;3:205–209.
31. Penn RD, Savoy SM, Corcos D, et al. Intrathecal baclofen for severe spinal spasticity. *N Engl J Med* 1989;320:1517–1521.
32. Katz RT, Rovai GP, Brait C, et al. Objective quantification of spastic hypertonia: Correlation with clinical finding. *Arch Phys Med Rehabil* 1992;73:339–347.
33. Gormley ME, O'Brien CF, Yablon SA. A clinical overview of treatment decisions in the management of spasticity. *Muscle Nerve Suppl* 1997;6:S14–S20.
34. Burke D, Andrews C, Ashley P. Autogenic effects of static muscle stretch in spastic man. *Arch Neurol* 1971; 25:367–372
35. Guissard N, Duchateau J, Hainaut K. Muscle stretching and motor neuron excitability. *Eur J Appl Physiol* 1988;58:47–52.
36. Price R, Lehmann JF, Boswell-Bessette S, et al. Influence of cryotherapy on spasticity at the human ankle. *Arch Phys Med Rehabil* 1993;74:300–304.
37. Collins K, Oswald P, Burger G, et al. Customized adjustable orthoses: Their use in spasticity. *Arch Phys Med Rehabil* 1985;66:397–398.
38. Bohannon RW. Tilt table standing for reducing spasticity after spinal injury. *Arch Phys Med Rehabil* 1993;74: 1121–1122.
39. Kunkel CF, Scremin AM, Eisenberg B, et al. Effect of "standing" on spasticity, contracture, and osteoporosis in paralyzed males. *Arch Phys Med Rehabil* 1993;74: 73–78.

40. Franek A, Turczynski B, Opara J. Treatment of spinal spasticity by electrical stimulation. *J Biomed Eng* 1988; 10:266–270.

41. Bajd T, Gregoric M, Vodovnik L, et al. Electrical stimulation in treating spasticity resulting from spinal cord injury. *Arch Phys Med Rehabil* 1985;66:515–517.

42. Katz RT. Management of spasticity. *Am J Phys Med Rehabil* 1988;67:108–116.

43. Davidoff RA. Antispasticity drugs: Mechanisms of action. *Ann Neurol* 1985;17:107–116.

44. Mueller ME, Gruenthal M, Olson WL, et al. Gabapentin for relief of upper motor neuron symptoms in multiple sclerosis. *Arch Phys Med Rehabil* 1997;78:521–524.

45. Gruenthal M, Meuller M, Olson WL, et al. Gabapentin for the treatment of spasticity in patients with spinal cord injury. *Spinal Cord* 1997;35:686–689.

46. Gracies JM, Nance P, Elovic E, et al. Traditional Pharmacological Treatments for Spasticity Part I: local treatments. *Muscle Nerve Suppl* 1997;6:S61–S91

47. Brin MF. Botulinum toxin: chemistry, pharmacology, toxicology and immunology. *Muscle Nerve Suppl* 1997; 6:S146–S168

48. Jankovic J, Brin MF. Botulinum toxin: historical perspective and potential new indications. *Muscle Nerve Suppl* 1997;6:S129–S145.

49. Ajax T, Ross MA, Rodnitzky RL. The role of electromyography in guiding botulinum toxin injection for dystonia and spasticity. *J Neuro Rehabil* 1998;12:1–4.

50. O'Brien CF. Injection techniques for botulinum toxin using electrical stimulation. *Muscle Nerve Suppl* 1997; 6.S176–S180.

51. Abel NA, Smith RA. Intrathecal baclofen for treatment of intractable spinal spasticity. *Arch Phys Med Rehabil* 1994;75:54–58.

52. Gracies JM, Nance P, Elovic Elie, et al. Traditional pharmacological treatment of spasticity. Part II: General and regional treatments. *Muscle Nerve Suppl* 1997;6: S92–S120.

22

Disability and Depression

Rhoda Olkin

It is difficult to generalize about disability and depression because of the differences across the myriad types of disabilities. Even within broad categories of disability (e.g., physical or systemic, cognitive, sensory, developmental, and psychiatric) it is hard to draw firm conclusions about the incidence of depression. Depression would be expected to be differentially associated with disability factors such as degree of impairment, experiences of pain and fatigue, age at disability onset, relative degree of stigma, impact on quality of life, degree of uncertainty about future course of disability, and effects of disability on life expectancy. Furthermore, disability is a highly stigmatized condition and people with disabilities encounter discrimination, prejudice and oppression that together represent a significant long-term life strain (1). Such factors make it difficult to assess the association of depression and disability not confounded by other concomitant stressors.

Nonetheless, there are reasons to address the relationship of depression to disability. First, several studies suggest that people with disabilities have a markedly higher lifetime risk of disability than the general nondisabled population (1–3). Second, certain types of disabilities seem to carry higher risk of depression, even when compared with other chronic conditions and disabilities. Third, measurement of depression in people with disabilities is complicated by disability sequelae. For example, symptoms such as appetite change, insomnia, fatigue, attention to somatic complaints, constipation, and/or loss of libido can be attributed to some types of chronic conditions but also can be symptoms of depression (4). Fourth, studies consistently indicate that depression complicates recovery and rehabilitation, increases length of hospital stay, and reduces independence on activities of daily living (5,6). Thus depression should be considered a primary condition for treatment. Nonetheless, depression often is overlooked in rehabilitation admissions and treatment (7). Fifth, use of antidepressants [monoamine oxidase inhibitors, tricyclics, or selective serotonin reuptake inhibitors (SSRIs)] can be contraindicated for some specific disabilities or may exacerbate disability symptoms. For example, case reports on two women with cerebral palsy and depression indicate an increase in spasticity after treatment with SSRIs (8). Lastly, depression can affect not only the person with the disability but the family as well. For example, a study of wives of men who had experienced a stroke indicated a high rate of depression (about 70%) among the wives (9). A recent study found a similar effect between elders with visual impairments and their spouses, particularly with regard to depression (10). Thus the impact of depression is on both the person with the disability and his or her immediate environment, compounding the effects of the depression.

It is important to remember that "depression...is not an inevitable reaction to the onset of acquired physical disability" (11, p. 326). However, onset of disability, like other major stressors, does carry some risk of depression. It generally is estimated that about 30% (plus or minus 5%) of people with acquired disability will experience depression in the year after disability onset (7,12–15). The largest study to date that compared community samples of people with and without disabilities indicated rates of depression of 37% and 12%, respectively (3). Although rates of depression fell with age for both disabled and nondisabled people, the rates for disabled people were higher in each age group.

Specific disabilities may be associated with higher risk of depression. For example, estimates of depression after stroke range from 23% (15a) to 64% (9). Multiple sclerosis (MS) has higher rates of both depression and suicide than other disabilities (16–18). Two studies of depression among geriatric rehabilitation inpatients found that depression rates were unrelated to gender or ethnicity (7), and a study of depression after stroke found depression to be unrelated to gender, ethnicity, socioeconomic status, and marital status (15a). Because depression in the general population is higher for females than males and higher for some ethnic groups (e.g., Latino), we might expect these same factors to hold among people with disabilities, but this has not been well documented. It also is worthwhile noting the disparity of attention to depression and specific disabilities. For example, there are scores of references on depression associated with MS, but only four references in the past 6 years on depression associated with cerebral palsy.

Because of the difficulties just cited in making generalizations across disabilities, this chapter will review the literature related to depression and six specific disabilities: three physical disabilities [spinal cord injury (SCI), MS, and polio/post-polio syndrome (P/PPS)], two sensory impairments (vision and hearing), and one developmental disability (mental retardation). These disabilities were selected to illustrate differences in depression rates and manifestations across disabilities and a variety of issues that accompany diagnosis of depression among people with disabilities. The focus is mostly on more recent findings, from 1996 on, although in some cases more seminal work is included.

Several points should be kept in mind when reading these reviews. First, some disabilities involve pain, and pain *per se* is a risk factor for depression (19). Some of the increase in rates of depression among certain populations of people with disabilities may be the result of chronic pain rather than the disability. For example, in a study of 50 adults with cerebral palsy, pain was significantly positively associated with scores on the Center for Epidemiologic Studies–Depression Scale (20). Second, unemployment rates are high. The government generally cites a 76% unemployment rate. Other reports of rates of unemployment among specific disability groups include 39% unemployment among deaf people using state rehabilitation services (21), 80% among people with MS (22), 35% among people with mild disability, and 88% among those with more severe work limitations (4). Third, for each type of disability some specificity of depression criteria needs to be developed, such that assessment measures depression and not disability sequelae and that estimates of depression prevalence within the different disability types are established. Lastly, whether or not the disability is implicated in the development of depression, depression remains a treatable disorder (23,24).

THREE PHYSICAL DISABILITIES

Three physical disabilities were selected to illustrate important differences across the disabilities and the need for more disability-specific depression criteria. SCI, MS, and P/PPS share several features in common, notably significant fatigue and weakness, experience of pain, and uncertainty over future course of disability-related impairment as one ages. Two important differences among these three disabilities are the age of onset (typically late teens or early twenties for SCI, in the 30s or 40s for MS, and in childhood for P/PPS) and gender distribution (80% males for SCI, 55% to 80% females for MS, and no differences in P/PPS).

For each disability type we might ask two questions: (a) Does the disability *cause* depression? and (b) Is the disability *associated with* depression? The usual model for assessing these questions is as follows: The stressor (disability) is mediated by moderating variables (coping, social support) leading to an outcome (depression). This intrapersonal model has several problems. It focuses on disability itself as the stressor rather than stigma, prejudice, and discrimination. The model (a) is cross-sectional rather than across the life span, (b) often omits critical moderating and contextual variables, (c) is pathology oriented, and (d) confounds measurement of depression with disability sequelae and does not have for comparison norms for people with disabilities. These limitations should be kept in mind in evaluating rates of depression among people with physical disabilities.

Spinal Cord Injury

Perhaps because SCI involves such dramatic and profound physical and biologic changes, this disability, more than any other, has been saddled with the assumption of the stage model of response to disability. In the stage model, depression is seen as both normative and necessary for ultimate adaptation to SCI. However, "adaptation is unique to each person and does not follow predictable stages" (25, p. 72). It should be remembered that most people who sustain an SCI do not become clinically depressed in the first year after injury. Depression should not be viewed as inherent to SCI, although SCI may potentiate predisposition to depression. In a study of 11 pairs of monozygotic twins in which one of each pair had an SCI, there were no differences in scores on the Beck Depression Inventory or the depression scale of the Symptom Checklist–90, leading the authors to conclude that "SCI does not inevitably lead to increased depression" (26, p. 284). Indeed, one follow-up of a community sample from 1 to 5 years postinjury found only a 3% rate of depression at any one time and only 14% who rated their quality of life as poor (27). Nonetheless, there does seem to be some consensus that SCI carries increased risk of de-

pression (28). The empirical literature, however, is somewhat imprecise about prevalence in part because of the various ways in which the term depression is used. "Greater precision is recommended in distinguishing diagnosable depression from displays of negative affect, anxiety, distress, and dysphoria" (29, p. 816). The measurement of depression in people with SCI likewise needs greater refinement. A review of 64 empirical studies on depression and SCI from 1985 to 2000 (30) found the Beck Depression Inventory, which includes somatic items, to be the most commonly used measure, used in about one-third of the studies. A total of 16 different instruments were used, and virtually all of these measures included somatic symptoms, possibly artificially inflating the incidence of depression. Two studies have examined directly the issue of somatic items in assessment of depression using the Minnesota Multiphasic Personality Inventory-2 (MMPI-2) and found equivocal results (31,32). Thus at present there is no consensus on the best diagnostic criteria or tools to use to assess depression in people with SCI.

Almost all of the literature on psychologic responses to SCI pertains to adults with SCI, and there is a serious gap in the empirical literature, particularly prospective studies, related to children with SCI. Two retrospective studies of adults who sustained an SCI in childhood showed good acclimation and response to living with an SCI (33,34).

SCI often has sequelae that can increase the risk of depression. For example, sleep disorders after SCI are common (35,36) and are even more common than for people with traumatic brain injury (36). Pain is another complicating factor. Studies have found varying prevalence of pain: 23% of people with SCI 6 weeks after injury to 41% 1 year later (37); 25% of a community sample up to 5 years postinjury (27); and 79% of a community sample, of whom 39% describe the pain as severe (37a). In a study of 59 people with SCI, psychologic distress was moderately correlated with pain severity (38). Presence of pain has implications for psychosocial functioning – "neuropathic pain reduces quality of life, including mood and physical and social functioning" (39, p. S101). Although pain and depression were independent at admission for acute traumatic SCI patients, at discharge the two were significantly related (40). "Changes in pain affected depression more than changes in depression affected pain" (40, p. 329).

In addition to sleep difficulties and pain, bowel dysfunction is implicated in depression following SCI. There was a significant correlation between depression and time taken for a daily bowel management program, and bowel function was a source of distress for 54% of a group of 115 outpatients with SCI for a mean of 5 years (41). Thus SCI is associated with factors that in turn may be risk factors for depression.

Given the complications and methodologic issues cited earlier in this chapter, it is not surprising that there is great variation in findings related to prevalence rates for depression among people with SCI. A study of 85 people with SCI who were assessed from 6 to 24 weeks after injury found high levels of distress in 14% and concluded that this distress rate is comparable to that associated with other traumas (42). A similarly low rate, 16%, was found in 100 inpatients and outpatients followed for 1 year postinjury (43). In contrast, a survey of more than 1,000 outpatients with SCI at one rehabilitation hospital found that 48% had some clinically significant symptoms (not necessarily of depression) (44). Similarly, 60% of patients in rehabilitation, followed more than 3 years, had indications of depression on the Symptom Checklist–90, and 33% had persistent depressive scores in two assessment periods. In another study, rates of depression were higher among people with SCI (41%) than for people with post-polio syndrome (PPS) (22%) or no disability (15%) (45). Veterans with SCI appear to have depression (and substance abuse or dependence) at the same rate as veterans with other traumas not leading to SCI (46). Although two studies have found depression rates highest in the acute phase and leading up to hospital discharge (47,48), assessment of

depression should not be limited to those phases. Additionally, measurement of depression during the acute SCI treatment should be alert to false elevations as a result of somatic symptoms that stem from the injury.

In light of the wide variation in depression rates, much effort has gone into finding factors that might predict depression. The search for an SCI personality is fruitless, and of course "the way in which a person adjusts to a spinal cord injury reflects his or her long-standing, global perspective on life" (49, p. 26). Nonetheless, risk of depression after SCI may be associated with some variables. Although SCI among specific ethnic groups has not been surveyed extensively, those few studies that do exist clearly indicate higher risk for depression among ethnic minorities (44) and among certain ethnic groups [e.g., Latinos, compared with African-American and white people (50); American Indians (51,51a)].

As is true for nondisabled people, marriage is a buffer against stressors. Among 222 long-term SCI survivors in Britain, marriage was associated with less depression, greater life satisfaction and perceived quality of life, and better psychologic well-being (52). However, partners who provide some disability-related caregiving may incur some psychologic risk. A study of 124 spouses of long-term SCI survivors in Britain found that the nondisabled spouses fared worse psychologically than did the partner with SCI or spouses of nondisabled partners (53). In a study in Hong Kong, there were higher rates of depression in partners in marriages that preceded the SCI compared to postinjury marriages (54). Taken together, the literature suggests that assessment of psychologic status after SCI should extend to the marriage and the partner because partnership is a critical variable in psychologic outcome (55), as are relationships with peers with SCI (56).

Although it might seem intuitive that psychologic response to SCI would be affected by level of injury (quadriplegia versus paraplegia), mostly this has not proved to be the case. A study of 169 men with SCI found that exercise was associated with less frequency of depression and anxiety, but there were no psychologic measurement differences for those with paraplegia or quadriplegia, nor differences in modes of sports activities (57). A retrospective study of 86 adults with SCI onset prior to age 16 years found that depression was independent of level of injury (33). Also, a study of 65 people with SCI in rehabilitation in Portugal found no differences by level of injury. However, two studies of more specific variables did find differences. Sexual self-concept and prevalence of depression, but also overall adjustment to SCI, did differ in the expected direction for those with paraplegia versus quadriplegia (58). Conversely, suicide rates were twice as high for those with lesser degrees of disability as a result of SCI compared with people with quadriplegia (59).

Other factors that may be associated with depression post-SCI are lower levels of education (43), severe complications (43), lesser quality of social support (60), particular coping styles (61), and possibly younger age and male gender (62). Attribution style (63) and cognitive style have been examined (64–66). Although certain types of cognitions were associated with increased rates of depression among people with SCI, much as they are for those without disabilities, these types of cognitions were not more prevalent among people with SCI (66). Examining learned helplessness (which should correlate positively with depression) and self-efficacy (which should be negatively correlated with depression), both were found to have the expected relationship with depression for people with SCI and with MS, but it was the MS group that had significantly greater levels of depression and learned helplessness and lower levels of self efficacy than did those with SCI (65). Sustaining an SCI does not seem to directly alter one's cognitive style, but of course cognitive style will bear on response to SCI. At least one researcher (67) feels that "assessment of personality is an invaluable aid in predicting long-term outcomes after SCI and should remain a priority in diverse rehabilitation settings" (67, p. 118), but as yet no robust

set of variables has been found to be predictive in repeated studies. Furthermore, the investigation of correlates of depression after SCI should be broadened to include sociopolitical factors such as family, peers with disabilities, economics, discrimination, employment, housing, transportation, and other access issues. To continue the inquiry only into intrapsychic variables is to miss the profound alterations to one's social and political status post-SCI.

Issues of depression always carry implications for risk of suicide. Further, at least one study of more than 8,000 cases over 40 years found that 1.6% of cases of SCI were caused by a failed suicide attempt (68). For those 1.6% the gender ratio was equal, although a high proportion were single (49%) and unemployed (42%), and 33% had children. Depression (27%) and schizophrenia (33%) were the most likely psychiatric diagnoses.

A study of the incidence of suicidal *ideation* followed almost 500 patients with SCI for up to 2 years and found that 7.3% had suicidal ideation while in the hospital and 11.3% had suicidal ideation at some point after hospitalization (69). Earlier development of suicidal ideation was associated with more traditional risk factors such as previous psychiatric history and substance abuse, although depression also was associated with suicidal ideation for those who developed suicidal ideation either earlier and/or later. Two studies found high risk of suicidal *behavior* following SCI. An examination of all cases of SCI survivors in Denmark from 1953 to 1990 found that 10% of all deaths were from suicide, and 3% of all SCI cases living and deceased were from suicide attempts (59). This is a rate five times higher than expected in the Danish population and surprisingly was lower for men than for women. A second study examined suicide risk in three time periods (70). At time one, close to the time of injury, among 60 people with SCI, 12% had suicidal plans and one attempted suicide. The rate of suicidal plans was 11% at 3 months and 13% at 6 months. Thus it appears that suicide risk is not merely during the acute period of injury, and therefore should be assessed routinely along with other psychosocial factors, especially for those with depression, schizophrenia, and/or substance abuse.

As is true for other types of disabilities, there is no doubt that depression is associated with complications, such as secondary conditions, social isolation, and substance abuse (71); longer hospital stays (72); poorer overall health outcomes (72); and increased rehospitalization rates (13). Thus depression must not be thought of as a natural reaction to a major life stressor but rather as a serious primary condition that interacts synergistically and negatively with SCI, each complicating the response and treatment of the other.

Treatment of depression coinciding with SCI mostly mirrors treatment of depression with nondisabled people. However, there are a few caveats to keep in mind that are specific to this population. Although those with SCI might be viewed as clients who "will never get well" (73, p. 85), depression is a treatable disorder and no less so for people with SCI. As is true for other groups, the depression responds to cognitive behavior therapy (74) and possibly sports (57,75), but for people with SCI other forms of physical intervention also may prove effective (76,77). Some specific treatments necessitate caution. Treatment with Viagra for erectile dysfunction in 178 men with SCI in seven countries increased not only satisfaction with sex but also quality of life and decreased depression and anxiety (78; note that this study was funded by Pfizer, makers of Viagra). A case report of use of an SSRI for depression, however, warns about exacerbation of spasticity (79) [as was also the case for two people with cerebral palsy (8)]. Acupuncture for pain helped 46% of a sample of 22 people with SCI, but for 27% it increased pain that persisted for at least 3 months. A review of the use of electroconvulsive therapy (ECT) and a case example is available in the literature (80). As is true with all treatment for depression, screening for alcohol and substance abuse is critical but especially so for this population because alcohol and substance abuse affects physical health outcomes (81,82).

Multiple Sclerosis

The lifetime prevalence rate of depression among people with MS is approximately 50% (22,83,84), although a study in 2000 found a lower rate [23% lifetime prevalence for a small sample of 136 in Britain (85)]. Generally this 50% lifetime prevalence rate is higher than for other chronic illnesses (17, 86–88) or neurologic disorders (65,89,90). For example, Halbreich (88) noted that depressive episodes were more frequent in people with MS compared with the general population (with about a 15% lifetime prevalence of depression), people with other medical and neurologic illness, and people with disabilities not involving the central nervous system.

The point prevalence rate of depression found in studies of people with MS has varied widely, from 14% to 57% (22). This variation reflects several methodologic issues, including small numbers of participants sampled from differing populations and, as is true for SCI, lack of differentiation between depressive symptoms versus clinical disorders. Studies comparing point prevalence rates of depression for MS and other disorders yield mixed results. A study of 80 people with MS and 80 with SCI indicated that depression rates were higher and self-efficacy scores were lower for the MS group (65). However, depression rates were similar for 95 people with MS (19%) versus 97 people with rheumatoid arthritis (16.5%), and both were higher than the comparison group of 110 nondisabled people (4%) (91). Likewise, a comparison of 92 people with MS with 40 people with other motor neuron disorders found no differences in incidence or severity of depression (92).

The course and manifestations of MS are highly idiosyncratic, leading to a great deal of unpredictability and uncertainty in prognosis. Several authors have hypothesized that this uncertainty is one explanation for the increased depression rates (93–95). Despite the idiosyncratic nature of MS, there are some commonalities across cases and numerous

MS sequelae that are not infrequent. Most notable is the fatigue associated with MS (96). Point prevalence of fatigue was 52% to 58% in a sample of 55 people with relapsing-remitting MS (97), 85% in a sample of 68 consecutive outpatients with MS (98), and 46% of 50 people with MS (99). Fatigue is correlated with depression (98,100,101) and greater levels of impairment (99).

Cognitive decline or dysfunction is another common factor in MS, present in approximately 40% to 60% of people with MS (22). The pattern of symptoms varies greatly from person to person but often involves processing speed, attention, concentration, and verbal memory (22). MS can affect executive functioning (reasoning, sequencing, planning, and problem solving), and cognitive deficits early in the MS disease are associated with a greater number of cognitive deficits later in the disease process (22). Cognitive functioning can decline with disease exacerbations but also with treatment by corticosteroids used to ameliorate other MS symptoms. A study of cognitive changes over 2 years in 53 people with relapsing-remitting MS found that 28% worsened over the 2 years, although 9% improved and the rest remained stable (102). [See Mohr and Cox (22) for practical advice on neuropsychologic assessment of cognitive functioning in people with MS.]

Another feature sometimes associated with MS is pathologic laughing and crying (PLC), in which there are bouts of laughing, crying, or both in the absence of related stimuli or mood. This is estimated to occur with about 5% to 10% of people with MS and is associated with more physical and cognitive disability (22,103). PLC, coupled with the equanimity seen in about 5% to 10% of people with MS (consistent cheerfulness coupled with unawareness or unconcern with the disability), can complicate the diagnosis of mood states and easily can be misconstrued as patient denial or repression.

Other sequelae of MS include sexual dysfunction (91,104–106), bowel and bladder difficulties (22,91), and alterations to smell (105,107). It also must be remembered that MS is twice as common for women as for men, and women's other psychologic and health issues should not be overlooked. In one sample of 220 women with MS, most were not receiving appropriate preventive health care, and 9% reported sexual abuse and 28% reported psychologic abuse (108). These findings have obvious implications for the development and detection of depression.

Although the relationship between depression and disability is multifaceted and synergistic for most types of disabilities, the interface of depression and MS is especially complex. "Within the MS patient, depression can both result from and cause MS disease activity" (22, p. 491).

There are numerous studies examining the psychosocial and physiologic predictors of depression. Of particular note is that "rates of major depression in first-degree relatives of people with MS are the same for those with and without depression" (88, p. 40), and the high rate of lifetime depression in people with MS is not found in family members (84). Thus the depression is not simply an example of diathesis plus a stressor (MS). Instead, it appears that the depression is causally linked to properties of MS. In fact, a number of findings show that the depression concomitant to MS is caused by physiologic effects of the illness and that these effects may be somewhat distinct from the mechanisms that cause depression in people without MS. However, the nature of the particular physiologic changes that give rise to depression is not completely known. There are mixed findings on the relationship between depression in MS and immune factors (22,109,110). MS is associated with alterations in hypothalamic regulatory systems related to stress response and mood (111), but the extent to which this is associated with depressed mood in MS varies in different studies (112,113). Several studies suggest that MS is related directly to demyelination of white-matter pathways that project from subcortical to cortical structures (114,115) or corticocortical fibers projections such as the left arcuate fasciculus (116,117). Thus depression is associated with MS but also may be a direct symptom of MS (22). The depression then can affect compliance with treatment (118), which in turn can affect the disease process. Further, depression consistently is found to be the key predictor of the quality of life for people with MS, more so than the severity of impairment (83, 119–123a).

Type of coping (emotion focused or problem focused) generally is implicated in depression in response to a stressor, but the relationship of coping style and depression may be more complex for people with MS (93,124,125). MS is a disorder with an uncertain prognosis, usually degenerative, and is functionally impairing, with an 80% rate of unemployment (22). It may be that in light of these features of the disorder, styles of coping that serve the person well may not mirror those found for other types of stressors.

As with all depression, there is the risk of suicide, which seems to be higher among people with MS than the general population (16,18). Suicidal people with MS are "significantly more likely to live alone, have a family history of mental illness, report more social stress, and have lifetime diagnoses of major depression, anxiety disorder, comorbid depression-anxiety disorder" (16, p. 674). Nonetheless, one-third of those with MS who were suicidal had not received psychologic help (16). Treatment of depression, whether causally linked or merely associated with MS, should be a priority in management of MS. The depression associated with MS does seem to be amenable to improvement with cognitive-behavioral treatment (115,126); depression may not be self-limiting without treatment and, in fact, may worsen (23). [See Mohr and Goodkin (23) for a review of treatment of depression in MS.] Unfortunately, "depression in MS is more difficult to treat than previously thought. Only half the patients who received CBT showed clinically significant improvement, while more than 75% of patients receiving sertraline or group remained refractory to treatment" (22, p. 489). Thus, paradoxically, depression is associated strongly with MS and left untreated can

complicate the course of the disorder, is not self-limiting, and affects quality of life, but it also is recalcitrant to conventional treatment. It is not hard to see why Mohr and Cox (22) call for "more aggressive strategies for the treatment of depression in MS" (p. 489).

Polio/Post-Polio Syndrome

In addressing whether the rate of depression is higher among people with polio a key issue is the appropriate comparison group. Should the comparison be between people with polio with and without PPS, polio versus other physical disabilities, polio versus chronic pain, or polio versus no disability? [Post-polio syndrome typically occurs about 30 years after onset of polio and is characterized by increases in pain, fatigue, and new weakness. For further reading see Halstead (126a)]. The studies reviewed have varied in their comparison samples and thus have varying results. It should be noted that people with polio generally do experience both fatigue (127) and pain (128,129), both of which are associated with depression. Furthermore, because the onset of polio typically is in childhood, people with polio often have early histories of hospitalizations, surgeries, separation from parents, and medical trauma, which are risk factors for depression.

A few studies have examined rates of depression among people with polio with and without PPS. Because PPS was not identified until the mid-1980s, studies including people with PPS are all within the past 15 years. One of the earliest studies on polio and depression compared 93 people with polio (but not necessarily PPS) on a variety of psychologic symptoms including depression (130). Of the 93 people, 71 were a clinical sample and 22 were in a polio support group. Elevations in scores on the Symptom Checklist indicated depression in both samples, but exact rates were not given. Similarly, another early study compared 86 people with PPS and 20 controls without a disability (127). Results indicated that 27% of those with PPS had scores on the Beck Depression Inventory in the depressed range. However, it is curious that none of the control group had scores indicating depression because about a 1% to 3% point prevalence rate of depression in a community sample in the general population would be expected.

In contrast, at least two studies found little evidence of depression [Clark and colleagues (131) on 22 people with PPS and Schanke (131a) on 63 people with polio]. Further, a comparison of 121 people with polio and 60 age-matched controls found no differences in prevalence of depressive disorders between the two groups (132). Nonetheless, the prevalence of depression among those with polio was 28%. Notably, people with PPS had higher scores (greater severity of depression) than those with polio without PPS. Similarly, a comparison of people with polio with and without PPS likewise found higher levels of depression among those with PPS (133). One of the largest studies, on 121 people with PPS, used for comparison 177 people with SCI and 62 age-matched people with no disability (45). Results indicated clinically significant depression in 22% of those with PPS, 41% of those with SCI, and 15% of those without disabilities.

Addressing the question of predictors of depression, Tate and colleagues (128) found a 15.8% rate of depression among people with polio. There were several differences between those with and without depression, always in the expected direction: as for other populations, those people with polio who were depressed were more likely to live alone, be in worse health, report greater pain, be less satisfied with work and life, and cope less well.

It is important to note that a 5-year follow-up of 176 people with PPS found the participants to be less depressed, anxious, uncertain, and depressed than previously. Those with less psychologic distress made more accommodations to their PPS symptoms than did those with greater psychologic distress. This is an important finding for this particular disability because people with polio historically have been counseled to overcome the disability and push themselves. In contrast, responding to PPS is facilitated by realistic accommodation to the newer level of functional impairment.

If there is a physiologic or biochemical connection between polio and depression, there are two possible routes by which this occurs. The first is through changes to the reticular-activating system, which leads to alterations in the architecture of sleep. The second is through decreased serotonin, which is observed in people with chronic pain and in people with depression. For treatment purposes, however, it may not be useful to determine the cause of depression because depression in persons with polio generally responds well to treatment regardless of cause. Further, amelioration of depression tends to lessen the experience of pain (134).

TWO SENSORY IMPAIRMENTS

Although visual and hearing impairments are both referred to as sensory impairments, they share few features in common. However, they are each highly stigmatized and misunderstood conditions. It is hard for people with unimpaired hearing or sight to imagine coping with the loss of either sense. Yet those with sensory impairments from birth or an early age develop neural pathways and modes of functioning that incorporate the sensory deficit, not so much as compensatory measures but as alternate developmental patterns. In contrast, those who lose hearing or vision later in life have not developed these patterns and thus are disadvantaged by the sensory loss. Therefore it is important to make distinctions based on age of onset for both of these sensory impairments.

Visual Impairment and Blindness

A review of the recent literature (1996–2002) reveals approximately 20 studies related to visual impairments and depression. Most of these studies focus on late-onset visual impairment among the elderly (10, 135–141). In general these studies support the contention that visual loss later in life is a risk factor for depression. For example, out of 114 elderly adults with macular degeneration, 43% met criteria for depression (142). Another study of noninstitutionalized elderly people (mean age of 76 years) found that those with visual impairments were more likely than peers to have more than five depressive symptoms (139). In 70 elderly people attending a low-vision clinic, the rate of major depression was more than 39% (138,143). In a follow-up study of 31 elderly people with visual impairments (ages 71 to 84 years), 39% were depressed at baseline and 42% were depressed at follow-up 2 years later (144). Another study used a different measure of depression and found the rate of major depression to be 20% among people with visual impairment who were aged 75 years or older, compared to 15% of peers with no impairment (136). Importantly, in another study depression was a risk factor for falls in blind people aged 64 years or older (137). In a study of 40 elderly veterans (141), as in many of the studies cited earlier in this chapter, depression was associated with greater impairment in functioning. Further, depression in the spouse with the visual impairment predicted depression in the other spouse (10). Thus depression seems to be prevalent among older adults with visual impairments, and depression affects not just well-being but daily functioning. Taken together these studies suggest that depression should be assessed routinely along with visual status in medical and ophthalmology clinics.

The effects of diurnal and annual variations in light seem to affect people who are blind similarly to those with no visual impairment. For example, of 43 veterans aged 42 to 86 years, visual impairment did not have a significant effect on winter seasonality of depressive symptoms (144a). Similarly, visual acuity was not associated with poor sleep among 1,237 adult owners of guide dogs (144b). However, depression was associated with poor sleep—20% described their sleep quality as poor or very poor.

In one of the only studies on the relationship of ethnicity and visual acuity to depres-

sion, three groups of Hispanic adults with visual impairments (n = 2,432) were compared on rates of depression to people without visual impairments (144c). For Mexican Americans rates of depression were higher for those with at least moderate visual impairment. For Cuban Americans, the odds of a lifetime history of major depression were significantly higher for those with visual impairments. However, for Puerto Ricans, visual impairment was not associated with either current or previous depression. Thus studies need to be more specific not only about disability type and level of impairment but about ethnicity as well.

The studies cited earlier focus on people who lose visual acuity as adults. What about those who are congenitally blind? Three studies of adolescents with visual impairments yield mixed results. One study of 22 congenitally blind and 29 sighted adolescents (ages 12 to 18 years) used the Beck Depression Inventory to assess depression (145). Mean scores were more than 13 (moderate depression) for the blind adolescents and just higher than 7 (one point above the cutoff for no depression) for the sighted adolescents. However, two studies in Finland of adolescents with and without various impairments, including blindness (n = 54 and 115), found no differences in rates of depression (146,147). This was true despite more difficulties in friendships and greater feelings of loneliness among those with visual or other impairments. This suggests that those with early-onset blindness develop coping and resilience in the face of increased stressors and social isolation.

In sum, loss or impairment of vision later in life seems to be a significant risk factor for depression. The depression in turn affects level of functioning and risk of falls and injury. However, for early-onset visual impairment or blindness no conclusions can be made. Although there is some evidence of increased risk of depression, there also is evidence of increased coping and resilience in the face of social stigmatization and isolation.

Hearing Impairment and Deafness

Perhaps there is no group of people with impairments more diverse than those referred to variously as hearing impaired, hard of hearing, deaf, or deafened. Important distinctions include age at which hearing was lost, use of sign language, and attendance at schools for the deaf versus being mainstreamed in community schools and thus separated from deaf peers. A review of the recent literature (1996–2002) reveals that there has not been a cohesive body of research on depression and hearing impairment or loss, making it difficult to generalize or even to combine the findings of different studies. The 20 studies found tended to focus on people who are hard of hearing rather than deaf and generally support the contention that hearing loss as an adult, especially profound hearing loss, is a significant risk factor for depression (148–152). Hearing loss is a chronic stressor that places strains on family relationships and friendships, and the communication barriers reduce the person's access to the buffering effects of social support. Several studies indicate that for those who experience hearing loss, hearing aids (148,152) or cochlear implants (153,154) improve psychologic functioning and lessen depression.

Those who are prelingually deaf, for whom signing is their first (and perhaps only) language, and who identify with the deaf community are by convention referred to as *Deaf.* People who are Deaf generally do not consider themselves disabled but rather part of a Deaf community and culture. The risk of depression among this group has not been well established. One study of 50 Deaf and 50 hearing undergraduate students at four universities found higher rates of depression among the Deaf students on each of two different measures of depression (155). Another study using two different versions of a depression measure (written and signed versions of a language-simplified Beck Depression Inventory) with 48 Deaf adults found the two versions to be in concordance 54% of the time on category of depression severity (155a).

Leigh and Anthony (155b) also used the Beck Depression Inventory to assess depression among Deaf college students. They found good test–retest reliability for administrations 1 week apart and found that women showed more depression on both tests than men. These three studies focused on the reliability of measurement of depression among Deaf people and not the prevalence rate for depression among Deaf people. However, McGhee (155a) notes that approximately 16% of her sample of 48 Deaf adults had scores on either of the two versions of the Beck Depression Inventory (written or videotaped American Sign Language) that fell in the moderate to severe depression range [compared to 12% in the general population (156)]. A more recent study to examine incidence of depression among deaf people (both prelingually and postlingually deaf) found that rates were different between those with and without hearing loss but not as much as might be expected (150). Among the prelingually deaf, 27% of the men and 32% of the women showed indications of mental distress (not necessarily depression), compared to 22% and 27% of those without any hearing loss. For the postlingually deaf the rates were 28% for men and 43% for women.

At least two recent studies tried to demonstrate brain abnormalities (157) and electrocardiogram abnormalities (158) among Deaf people. These two references illustrate the seemingly widespread belief that inability to hear represents a biologic or neurologic deficit. However, the focus on deficits does not consider the alternate neurologic pathways that develop in the absence of usual pathways. It also should be noted that at least one study found indications of greater resilience and strengths among deaf people compared to hearing peers (149).

In summary, acquired hearing loss and adult-onset deafness carry a significant risk of depression. However, no conclusions can be drawn as yet about rates of depression among the prelingually deaf. Treatment for depression for those with hearing loss can be expected to be successful (158a). It is disturbing, however, that those who are deaf seem to receive differential diagnostic evaluations (159,159a) such that depression, a treatable disorder, is underdiagnosed and undertreated among people with hearing impairments.

A DEVELOPMENTAL DISORDER: MENTAL RETARDATION

The most common chromosomal cause of mental retardation is Down syndrome; thus it might make sense to review depression among this more specific population. However, this specificity is not possible because the literature fails to make distinctions based on etiology. Nonetheless, the distinction may be important: (a) Down syndrome carries specific risk of early-onset dementia of the Alzheimer's type (160–162); (b) people with Down syndrome usually have mild mental retardation and not severe to profound retardation; and (c) their risk of depression may not be the same as for those with mental retardation with different etiologies.

Varying terms are used to describe people with mental retardation, which can be confusing to readers. The term *developmental disabilities* includes a broad spectrum of disparate disorders, including autism, mental retardation, and cerebral palsy, and is insufficiently specific to use here. *Intellectual disabilities* is the more common term in Europe for mental retardation. *Learning disabilities* means intellectual disabilities in the United Kingdom and does not refer to the more specific learning disabilities unrelated to intelligence level as the term is used in the United States. In this review, the term mental retardation will be used to include mental retardation stemming from varying etiologies, including Down syndrome, and the more specific term Down syndrome will be used when applicable.

Of the approximately 130 articles on depression and mental retardation from 1996 to 2002, there is a remarkable lack of coherence to the literature. Topics emerge and are dropped, suggestions for future research are not heeded, and the call for more data goes

unanswered. Assertions are made and repeated but do not seem to be based on empirical data. A summary of the major issues follows.

Prevalence

"The high prevalence of psychiatric disorders in individuals with mental retardation is fairly well established" (162a). Indeed, an earlier study had found a 32% to 34% rate of psychiatric disturbance among 6,000 8-year-old German children with mental retardation and an 11% prevalence rate for depression in particular (163). Comparing older (ages 65 to 94 years) and younger (ages 20 to 64 years) individuals with mental retardation showed rates of psychiatric disorders, including depression, to be high in both age groups but significantly higher for the older group (62% versus 44%) (164). In a sample of 47 adults with mental retardation, 21% were found to have a depressive disorder (165). In a comparison of Down syndrome versus mental retardation with other etiologies, those with Down syndrome exhibited less psychiatric disturbance in childhood but were more prone to depression in adulthood (160). This increased rate of depression may reflect the skew toward milder mental retardation among people with Down syndrome because there is some evidence that people with milder mental retardation may exhibit more depression than those with more profound or severe mental retardation (166). It also is possible that the depression in Down syndrome is associated with the decline in cognitive functions and increased risk for dementia.

Among 70 institutionalized people with mental retardation who were referred for neuropsychiatric consultation, 20% of the referrals were for bipolar spectrum disorders and 9% were for depressive disorders (167). Of importance is the authors' observation of "a high occurrence of serious side effects of psychotropics or pharmacokinetic interactions" (167, p. 242). This observation is critical given the trend toward pharmacologic treatment of symptoms and disorders among people with mental retardation versus psychotherapy. Descriptions of clinical treatment with medication, electroconvulsive therapy, or light therapy (168–183) far outnumber the descriptions of therapy (184–191). Yet, as many references show, therapy seems to be an effective treatment for some people with mental retardation and definitely is indicated for the treatment of depression in this population. Pharmacotherapy should not be ruled out, however. In one study all 11 inpatients with severe mental retardation had remission of depressive symptoms within 5 weeks of medication treatment (192).

Symptoms and Diagnosis

Three questions arise throughout the literature on depression and mental retardation. These include: How can professionals recognize depression in people with mental retardation? Do symptoms of depression for people with mental retardation mirror those of people without mental retardation? What is the best way to assess and measure depression in people with mental retardation.

A critical issue is whether professionals accurately recognize depression in people with mental retardation. The concept of diagnostic overshadowing (193) refers to the probability of one prominent diagnosis (e.g., mental retardation) overshadowing a secondary diagnosis (e.g., depression) such that the latter is overlooked and symptoms are attributed to the former. Several studies have addressed whether diagnostic overshadowing occurs in practice. "The first and most important step in psychodiagnosis is to not view any symptoms or sign cluster as being based on the developmental disability itself" (194). Most studies indicate accuracy in recognition by professionals of depressive symptoms in people with mild, moderate, severe, or profound mental retardation (195–197), although at least one study indicated low overlap between self-report of symptoms by adults with mild to moderate mental retardation and ratings by others (198). Thus it would seem that diagnostic overshadowing has been minimized in the years since Reiss and associates (193)

first described the problem. However, the problem of overshadowing of depression still may exist. In one study staff directly involved in care of people with mental retardation were given vignettes of clients with mental retardation that varied by severity of mental retardation, gender, and presenting problem. Staff were significantly more likely to identify psychopathology and need for treatment in cases of aggressive disorder or psychosis than for depression. Also, despite similar rates of identification of diagnoses, cases with lesser degrees of mental retardation were more likely to be recommended for treatment and for verbal therapy rather than for medication (195).

A second critical question is whether the signs and symptoms of depression, and therefore the criteria for diagnosis of depression, are the same for people with mental retardation as for those without mental retardation, or whether there needs to be some "depressive equivalents" (199, p. 115). It would seem that for people with mild or even moderate mental retardation signs and symptoms of depression are along the lines of those cited in the DSM-IV (Diagnostic and Statistics Manual-IV). For example, a study of 12 people with mild mental retardation (ages 12 to 25 years) compared with children and adolescents without mental retardation found more similarities than differences for those with dysthymic disorder with and without mental retardation (200). The authors did note that the symptom profile of those with mental retardation fit somewhat more the profile of prepubertal children without mental retardation than adolescents without mental retardation. Regarding those with profound or severe mental retardation, it is harder to draw conclusions. One study found that, for 53 adults with severe or profound mental retardation divided into low mood and comparison groups, there were no differences between groups on self-injury, aggression, or disruption (symptoms considered as possible signs of depression) (201). Another study, on 22 people with severe to profound mental retardation and depression, found that scores on a depression symptom checklist were similar to core symptoms for diagnosis in DSM (199).

However, a study using DSM-III-R criteria for major depression with 89 people with severe or profound mental retardation (ages 18 to 51 years) living in a residential center examined utility of a DSM checklist (196). Total scores on the DSM checklist correlated with other observable behaviors not listed in DSM, but several behaviors were not in DSM but were in other measures (Aberrant Behavior Checklist and the Developmental Behavior Checklist).

The previously mentioned studies, taken as a group, would suggest that mental retardation does not radically alter the signs and symptoms of depression, but diagnostic accuracy could be increased with some attention to symptoms of depression more specific to people with mental retardation, especially severe or profound mental retardation. Although symptoms such as sleep disturbance, weight loss, crying, appetite changes, and social withdrawal can be seen in people with and without mental retardation, other symptoms such as screaming, aggression, loss of previous skills, and behavioral regression may be more specific to people with mental retardation.

A third question regards what measures or instruments are useful in evaluating presence of depression in people with mental retardation. The instruments examined included Swedish and French versions of the Reiss Screen for Maladaptive Behavior (202,203); the Aberrant Behavior Checklist (204); informant versus self report (205); Psychopathology Inventory for Mentally Retarded Adults (206); Diagnostic Assessment for the Severely Handicapped II (207); Kiddie Schedule for Affective Disorders and Schizophrenia (208); Rorschach Egocentricity Index (209); and Montgomery Asberg Depression Rating Scale (210). Each had utility in the context in which it was used, but three (Reiss, Kiddie SADS, and Aberrant Behavior Checklist) were the most frequently used.

Suicide

Only four articles in the past 6 years addressed the important area of suicide. The one empirical study compared the medical records of 11,277 people with Down syndrome versus 143,143 people with mental retardation with other etiologies (211). There were only four documented suicide attempts in the previous year for those with Down syndrome versus 1,142 (1%) attempts in the latter group. Consistent with this finding, but contrary to other studies (160,212), there was significantly less depression in people with Down syndrome versus those with mental retardation with other etiologies. Despite these data, an article on two cases of suicide attempts by people with Down syndrome asserts that "suicidal ideation and attempts are infrequent among patients with mental retardation" (212a). In fact, a study in the following year found a 20% rate of suicidal ideation, threats, or attempts among a clinical sample of children with developmental disabilities during one year period and asserts that suicidal ideation and attempts are underreported for this population (212b). The risks for suicide mirror those of the general population, including depression, posttraumatic stress disorder, and significant loss. Suicide attempts are less common among those with autism or severe or profound mental retardation than among those with mild mental retardation. Hanging is a more frequent method of suicide than for the general population, perhaps reflecting decreased access to firearms, driving automobiles, or self-administered medications.

CONCLUSIONS ABOUT DISABILITY AND DEPRESSION

Several conclusions about disability and depression can be drawn. The first is that different disabilities have received disparate amounts of research attention. This disparity reflects the vagaries of funding and ease of access to potential research participants more than the clinical needs of one group of people with disabilities over another. A second conclusion is that regardless of the cause of depression or the degree to which the depression is associated with the disability, depression remains a treatable disorder. Third, depression should not be considered auxiliary to disability; it should be thought of as a primary condition that can exacerbate and be exacerbated by the disability. Fourth, pain is a common and difficult component of disability and is associated with depression. More aggressive treatment and management of pain is necessary to alleviate depression in some people with disabilities. Fifth, medication effects and side effects interact with each disability type, and caution is urged in prescription and dosage of antidepressant medications for people with disabilities. Lastly, although many disabilities are not subject to much amelioration, depression remains a mostly treatable disorder and should be screened for routinely and treated.

REFERENCES

1. Turner RJ, Noh S. Physical disability and depression: A longitudinal analysis. *J Health Soc Beh* 1988;29: 23–37.
2. Neese RE, Finlayson FE. Management of depression in patients with coexisting medical illness. *Am Fam Phys* 1996;53:2125–2133.
3. Turner RJ, Beiser M. Major depression and depressive symptomatology among the physically disabled: Assessing the role of chronic stress. *The Journal of Nervous and Mental Disease* 1990:178(6):343–350.
4. Olkin R. *What psychotherapists should know about disability.* New York: Guilford Press, 1999.
5. Lai S, Duncan PW, Keighley J, et al. Depressive symptoms and independence in BADL and IADL. *J Rehabil Res Dev* 2002;39(5):589–596.
6. Silverstone PH. Changes in depression scores following life-threatening illness. *J Psychosom Res* 1990;34: 659–663.
7. Lichtenberg P. The DOUR project: A program of depression research in geriatric rehabilitation minority inpatients. *Rehabil Psychol* 1997;42:103–114.
8. Rone LA, Ferrando SJ. Serotonin reuptake inhibitor-related extrapyramidal side effects in two patients with cerebral palsy. *Psychosomatics* 1996;37(2):165–166.
9. Stein PN, Gordon WA. Hibbard M, et al. (1992). An examination of depression in the spouses of stroke patients. *Rehabil Psychol* 1992;37:121–130.
10. Goodman CR, Shippy RA. Is it contagious? Affect similarity among spouses. *Aging Ment Health* 2002; 6(3):266–274.
11. Elliott TR, Umlauf RL. Measurement of personality and psychopathology following acquired physical disability. In: Cushman LA, Scherer M, eds. *Psychological assessment in medical rehabilitation.* Hyattsville, MD: American Psychological Association, 1991.
12. Frank RG, Elliott TR, Corcoran JR, et al. Depression after SCI: Is it necessary? *Clin Psych Rev* 1987;7: 611–630.
13. Heinrich R, Tate D. Latent variable structure of the Brief Symptom Inventory in a sample of persons with spinal cord injuries. *Rehabil Psychol* 1996;41: 131–148.
14. Turner RJ, McLean PD. Physical disability and distress. *Rehabil Psychol* 1989;34:225–242.
15. Weissman MM, Myers JK. Affective disorders in a US urban community: The use of Research Diagnostic Criteria in an epidemiological survey. *Arch Gen Psychiat* 1978;35:1304–1311.
15a. Robinson RG. Diagnosis of depression in neurologic disease. In: Starkstein S, Robinson RG, eds. *Depression in neurologic disease.* Baltimore: Johns Hopkins University Press, 1993.
16. Feinstein A. An examination of suicidal intent in patients with multiple sclerosis. *Neurology* 2002;59(5):674–678.
17. Schubert D, Foliart RH. Increased depression in multiple sclerosis patients: A meta-analysis. *Psychosomatics* 1993;34(2):124–130.
18. Sadovnick A, Eisen RN, Ebers MD, et al. Cause of death in patients attending multiple sclerosis clinics. *Neurology* 1991;41:1193–1196.
19. Lagana L, Chen X, Koopman C, et al. Depressive symptomatology in relation to emotional control and chronic pain in persons who are HIV positive. *Rehabil Psychol* 2002;47(4):402–414.
20. Tyler EJ, Jensen MP, Engle JM, et al. The reliability and validity of pain interference measures in persons with cerebral palsy. *Arch Phys Med Rehabil* 2002;83 (2):236–239.
21. Larisgoitia DC. Factors that affect the employment status of adults who are deaf. *Diss Abs Int* 1997;58(3-A):0819.
22. Mohr D, Cox D. Multiple sclerosis: Empirical literature for the clinical health psychologist. *J Clin Psych* 2001;57(4):479–499.
23. Mohr D, Goodkin DE. Treatment of depression in multiple sclerosis: Review and meta-analysis. *Clin Psych* 1999;6(1):1–9.
24. Roberts SA, Kiselica MS, Fredrickson SA. Quality of life of persons with medical illnesses: Counseling's holistic contribution. *J Couns Dev* 2002;80:422–432.
25. Stiens SA, Kirshblum SC, Groah SL, et al. *Arch Phys Med Rehabil* 2002;83(3 Suppl 1):72–81, 90–98.
26. Tirch DD, Radnitz CL, Bauman WA. Depression and spinal cord injury: A monozygotic twin study. *J Spinal Cord Med* 1999;22(4):284–286.
27. Johnson RL, Gerhart KA, McCray J, et al. Secondary conditions following spinal cord injury in a population-based sample. *Spinal Cord* 1998;36(1):45–50.
28. Boekamp JR, Overholser JC, Schubert DS. Depression following a spinal cord injury. *Int J Psychiat Med* 1996;26(3):329–349.
29. Elliott TR, Frank RG. Depression following spinal cord injury. *Arch Phys Med Rehabil* 1996;77(8): 816–823.
30. Skinner AL, Armstrong KJ, Rich J. Depression and spinal cord injury: A review of diagnostic methods for depression, 1985–2000. *Rehabil Couns Bull* 2003;46 (3):174–175.
31. Barncord SW, Wanlass RL. A correction procedure for the Minnesota Multiphasic Personality Inventory-2 for persons with spinal cord injury. *Arch Phys Med Rehabil* 2000;81(9):1185–1190.
32. Rodevich M, Wanlass RL. The moderating effect of spinal cord injury on MMPI-2 profiles: A clinically

derived T score correction procedure. *Rehabil Psychol* 1995;40:181–190.

33. Gorman C, Kennedy P, Hamilton LR. Alterations in self-perceptions following childhood onset of spinal cord injury. *Spinal Cord* 1998;36(3):181–185.

34. Kannisto M, Sintonen H. Later health-related quality of life in adults who have sustained spinal cord injury in childhood. *Spinal Cord* 1997;35(11):747–751.

35. De Carvalho SA, Andrade MJ, Tavares, et al. Spinal cord injury and psychological response. *Gen Hosp Psychiat* 1998;20(6):353—359.

36. Fichtenberg NL, Zafonte RD, Putnam S, et al. Insomnia in a post-acute brain injury sample. *Brain Injury* 2002;16(3):197–206.

37. Kennedy P, Frankel H, Gardner B, et al. Factors associated with acute and chronic pain following traumatic spinal cord injuries. *Spinal Cord* 1997;35(12):814–817.

37a. Ravenscroft A, Ahmed YS, Burnside IG. Chronic pain after SCI. A patient survey. *Spinal Cord* 2000;38(10):611–614.

38. Bartok CE. The relationship between psychological distress and coping in a spinal cord injury population with severe chronic pain. *Diss Abs Int* 2002;62(12-B):5952.

39. Haythornthwaite JA, Benrud-Larson LM. Psychological aspects of neuropathic pain. *Clin J Pain* 2000;16(2 Suppl):S101–105.

40. Cairns DM, Adkins RH, Scott MD. Pain and depression in acute traumatic spinal cord injury: Origins of chronic problematic pain? *Arch Phys Med Rehabil* 1996;77(4):329–335.

41. Glickman S, Kamm MA. Bowel dysfunction in spinal cord injury patients. *Lancet* 1996;347(9016):1651–1653.

42. Kennedy P, Evans MJ. Evaluation of post traumatic distress in the first 6 months following SCI. *Spinal Cord* 2001;39(7):381–386.

43. Scivoletto G, Petrelli A, Di Lucente L, et al. Psychological investigation of spinal cord injury patients. *Spinal Cord* 1997;35(8):516–520.

44. Krause JS, Kemp B, Coker J. Depression after spinal cord injury: Relation to gender, ethnicity, aging, and socioeconomic indicators. *Arch Phys Med Rehabil* 2000;81(8):1099–1109.

45. Kemp BJ, Krause JS. Depression and life satisfaction among people ageing with post-polio and spinal cord injury. *Disabil Rehabil* 1999;21(5–6):241–249.

46. Radnitz CL, Broderick C, Perez-Strumolo L, et al. The prevalence of psychiatric disorders in veterans with spinal cord injury: A controlled comparison. *J Nerv Ment Dis* 1996;184(7):431–433.

47. Boekamp JR. Interpersonal and family factors in the course of depression following acute spinal cord injury: An investigation across hospital rehabilitation and 4 week post discharge follow-up. *Diss Abs Int* 1998;59(5-B):2412.

48. Kennedy P, Rogers BA. Anxiety and depression after spinal cord injury: a longitudinal analysis. *Arch Phys Med Rehabil* 2000;81(7):932–937.

49. Crewe NM. Life stories of people with long-term spinal cord injury. *Rehabil Couns Bull* 1997;41(1):26–42.

50. Kemp BJ, Krause JS, Adkins R. Depression among African Americans, Latinos, and Caucasians with spinal cord injury: An exploratory study. *Rehabil Psychol* 1999;44(3):235–247.

51. Krause JS, Coker JL, Charlifue S, et al. Depression and subjective well-being among 97 American Indians with spinal cord injury: A descriptive study. *Rehabil Psychol* 1999;44(4):354–372.

51a. Krause JS, Coker JL, Charlifue S, et al. Health outcomes among American Indians with spinal cord injury. *Arch Phys Med Rehabil* 2000;81(7):924–931.

52. Holicky R, Charlifue S. Ageing and spinal cord injury: The impact of spousal support. *Disabil Rehabil* 1999;21(5–6):250–257.

53. Weitzenkamp DA, Gerhart KA, Charlifue SW, et al. Spouses of spinal cord injury survivors: The added impact of caregiving. *Arch Phys Med Rehabil* 1997;78(8):822–827.

54. Chan RC, Lee PW, Lieh-Mak F. Coping with spinal cor injury: Personal and marital adjustment in the Hong Kong Chinese setting. *Spinal Cord* 2000;38(11):687–696.

55. McCormick MA. Family issues and outcomes of adjustment to spinal cord injury. *Diss Abs Int* 1996;56(8-B):4642.

56. King C, Kennedy P. (1999). Coping effectiveness training for people with spinal cord injury: Preliminary results of a controlled trial. *British J Clin Psych* 1999;38(1):5–14.

57. Muraki S, Tsunawake N, Hiramatsu S, et al. The effect of frequency and mode of sports activity on the psychological status in tetraplegics and paraplegics. *Spinal Cord* 2000;38(5):309–314.

58. Donelson EG. The relationship of sexual self-concept to the level of spinal cord injury and other factors. *Diss Abs Int* 1998;58(12-B):6805.

59. Hartkopp A, Bronnum-Hansen H, Seidenschnur AM, et al. Suicide in a spinal cord injured population: Its relation to functional status. *Arch Phys Med Rehabil* 1998;79(11):1356–1361.

60. Beedie A, Kennedy P. Quality of social support predicts hopelessness and depression post spinal cord injury. *J Clin Psych Medical Sett* 2002;9(3):227–234.

61. Kennedy P, Marsh N, Lowe R, et al. A longitudinal analysis of psychological impact and coping strategies following spinal cord injury. *Br J Health Psych* 2000;5(Part 2):157–172.

62. Laatsch L, Shahani BT. The relationship between age, gender and psychological distress in rehabilitation inpatients. *Disabil Rehabil* 1996;18(12):604–608.

63. Swanson F. Physical disability and learned helplessness and depression. *Diss Abs Int* 2001;62(3-B):1359.

64. Macleod L, Macleod G. Control cognitions and psychological disturbance in people with contrasting physically disabling conditions. *Disabil Rehabil* 1998;20(12):448–456.

65. Schnek ZM, Foley F, LaRocca N, G et al. Helplessness, self-efficacy, cognitive distortions, and depression in multiple sclerosis and spinal cord injury. *Ann Behav Med* 1997;19(3):287-294.

66. Tirsch DD. An empirical exploration of predictions arising from a cognitive-behavioral model of depression among persons with spinal cord injury. *Diss Abs Int* 2002;62(11-B):5396.

67. Krause JS. Personality and life adjustment after spinal cord injury: An exploratory study. *Rehabil Psychol* 1998;43(2):118–130.

68. Kennedy P, Rogers BA, Speer S, et al. Spinal cord injuries and attempted suicide: A retrospective review. *Spinal Cord* 1999;37(12):847–852.

69. Kishi Y, Robinson RG, Kosier JT. Suicidal ideation among patients during the rehabilitation period after life-threatening physical illness. *J Nerv Ment Dis* 2001;189(9):623–628.

70. Kishi Y, Robinson RG. Suicidal plans following spinal cord injury: A six-month study. *J Neuropsychiatry Clin Neurosci* 1996;8(4):442–445.

71. Groah SL, Stiens SA, Gittler MS, et al. Spinal cord injury medicine. 5. Preserving wellness and independence of the aging patient with spinal cord injury: A primary care approach for the rehabilitation medicine specialist. *Arch Phys Med Rehabil* 2002;83(3 Suppl 1):S82–89, S90–98.

72. Stoebner-May DG. Depression and health care utilization following long-term spinal cord injury. *Diss Abs Int* 2002;62(7-B):3390.

73. Allen-Wright S. Expanding health promotion to individuals with spinal cord injuries. *SCI Nursing* 1999;16 (3):85–88.

74. Craig AR, Hancock K, Chang E, et al. Immunizing against depression and anxiety after spinal cord injury. *Arch Phys Med Rehabil* 1998;79(4):375–377.

75. Foreman PE, Cull J, Kirkby RJ. Sports participation in individuals with spinal cord injury: Demographic and psychological correlates. *Int J Rehabil Res* 1997;20 (2):159–168.

76. Diego MA, Field T, Hernandez-Reif M, et al. Spinal cord patients benefit from massage therapy. *Int J Neurosci* 2002;112(2):133–142.

77. Guest RS, Klose KJ, Needham-Shropshire B, et al. Evaluation of a training program for persons with SCI paraplegia using the Parastep 1 ambulation system: Part 4. Effect on physical self-concept and depression. *Arch Phys Med Rehabil* 1997;78(8): 804–807.

78. Hulting C, Giuliano F, Quirk F, et al. Quality of life in patients with spinal cord injury receiving Viagra (sildenafil citrate) for the treatment of erectile dysfunction. *Spinal Cord* 2000;38(6):363–370.

79. Stolp-Smith KA, Wainberg MC. Antidepressant exacerbation of spasticity. *Arch Phys Med Rehabil* 1999;80 (3):339–342.

80. Hanretta AT, Malek-Ahmadi P. Successful ECT in a patient with hydrocephalus, shunt, hypopituitarism, and paraplegia. *J ECT* 2001;17(1):71–74.

81. Elliott TR, Kurylo M, Chen Y, et al. Alcohol abuse history and adjustment following spinal cord injury. *Rehabil Psychol* 2002;47(3):278–290.

82. Weingardt KR, Hsu J, Dunn ME. Brief screening for psychological and substance abuse disorders in veterans with long-term spinal cord injury. *Rehabil Psychol* 2001;46(3):271–278.

83. Courtney SW. Recognizing, understanding, and treating depression. *The Multiple Sclerosis Association of America's The Motivator.* Cherry Hill, NJ: MSAA, 2000:9–21.

84. Sadovnick A, Remick R, Allen J, et al. Depression and multiple sclerosis. *Neurology* 1996;46(3):628–632.

85. Patten SB, Metz LM, Reimer MA. Biopsychosocial correlates of lifetime major depression in a multiple sclerosis population. *Mult Scler* 2000;6(2):115–120.

86. Minden SL, Orav J, Reich P. Depression in multiple sclerosis. *Gen Hosp Psychiat* 1987;9:426–434.

87. Surridge D. An investigation into some psychiatric aspects of multiple sclerosis. *Br J Psychiat* 1969;115: 749–764.

88. Halbreich U, ed. *Multiple sclerosis: A neuropsychiatric disorder.* Washington, DC: American Psychiatric Press, 1993.

89. Rabins PV, Brooks BR, O'Donnell P, et al. Structural brain correlates of emotional disorder in multiple sclerosis. *Brain* 1986:109:585–597.

90. Whitlock FA, Sisking MM. Depression as a major symptom of multiple sclerosis. *J Neurol Neurosurg Psychiat* 1980;43:861–865.

91. Zorzon M, Zivadinov R, Monti-Bragadin L, et al. Sexual dysfunction in multiple sclerosis: A 2-year follow-up study. *J Neurol Sci* 2001;187(1–2):1–5.

92. Tedman BM, Young CA, Williams IR. Assessment of depression in patients with motor neuron disease and other neurologically disabling illness. *J Neurol Sci* 1997;152:S75–S79.

93. Kroencke DC, Denney DR, Lynch SG. Depression during exacerbations in multiple sclerosis: The importance of uncertainty. *Mult Scler* 2001;7(4):237–242.

94. Lynch SG, Kroencke DC, Denney DR. The relationship between disability and depression in multiple sclerosis: The role of uncertainty, coping, and hope. *Mult Scler* 2001;7(6):411–416.

95. Wineman NM, Schwetz KM, Goodkin DE, et al. Relationships among illness uncertainty, stress, coping, and emotional well-being at entry into a clinical drug trial. *Appl Nurs Res* 1996;9:53–60.

96. Krupp LB, Christodoulou C. Fatigue in multiple sclerosis. *Curr Neurol Neurosci Rep* 2001;1(3):294–298.

97. Bakshi R, Shaikh ZA, Miletich RS, et al. Fatigue in multiple sclerosis and its relationship to depression and neurologic disability. *Mult Scler* 2000;6(3): 181–185.

98. Ford H, Trigwell P, Johnson M. The nature of fatigue in multiple sclerosis. *J Psychosom Res* 1998;45(1 Spec No):33–38.

99. Vercoulen J, Hommes O, Swanink C, et al. The measurement of fatigue in patients with multiple sclerosis: A multidimensional comparison with patients with chronic fatigue syndrome and healthy subjects. *Arch Neurol* 1996;53(7):642–649.

100. Bakshi R, Czarnecki D, Shaikh ZA, et al. Brain MRI lesions and atrophy are related to depression in multiple sclerosis. *Neuroreport* 2000;11(6):1153–1158.

101. Kroencke DC, Lynch SG, Denney DR. Fatigue in multiple sclerosis: Relationship to depression, disability, and disease pattern. *Mult Scler* 2000;6(2):131–136.

102. Zivadinov R, Sepcic J, Nasuelli D, et al. A longitudinal study of brain atrophy and cognitive disturbances in the early phase of relapsing-remitting multiple sclerosis. *J Neurol Neurosurg Psychiat* 2001;70(6):773–780.

103. Feinstein A, Feinstein K, Gray T, et al. Prevalence and neurobehavioral correlates of pathological laughing and crying in multiple sclerosis. *Arch Neurol* 1997;54 (9):1116–1121.

104. Lottman PE, Jongen P, Rosier P, et al. Sexual dysfunction in men with multiple sclerosis - a comprehensive pilot-study into etiology. *Int J Impot Res* 1998;10(4): 233–237.

105. Zivadinov R, Zorzon M, Monti-Bragadin L, et al. Olfactory loss in multiple sclerosis. *J Neurol Sci* 1999; 168(2):127–130.

106. Zorzon M, Zivadinov R, Bosco A, et al. Sexual dysfunction in multiple sclerosis: A case-control study. I. Frequency and comparison of groups. *Mult Scler* 1999;5(6):418–427.

107. Zorzon M, Ukmar M, Bragadin L, et al. Olfactory dysfunction and extent of white matter abnormalities in multiple sclerosis: A clinical and MR study. *Mult Scler* 2000;6(6):386–390.

108. Shabas D, Weinreb H. Preventive healthcare in women with multiple sclerosis. *J Womens Health Gend Based Med* 2000;9(4):389–395.

109. Kahl K, Kruse N, Faller H, et al. Expression of tumor necrosis factor-alpha and interferon-gamma mRNA in blood cells correlates with depression scores during an acute attack in patients with multiple sclerosis. *Psychoneuroendocrinology* 2002;27(6):671–681.

110. Mikova, O, Yakimova, R, Bosmans E, et al. Increased serum tumor necrosis factor alpha concentrations in major depression and multiple sclerosis. *Eur Neuropsychopharmacol* 2001;11(3):203–208.

111. Michelson D, Gold PW. Pathophysiologic and somatic investigations of hypothalamic-pituitary-adrenal axis activation in patients with depression. *Ann N Y Acad Sci* 1998;840:717–722.

112. Fassbender K, Schmidt R, Mossner R, et al. Mood disorders and dysfunction of the hypothalamic-pituitary-adrenal axis in multiple sclerosis: Association with cerebral inflammation. *Arch Neurol* 1998;55(1):66–72.

113. Heesen C, Gold S, Raji A, et al. Cognitive impairment correlates with hypothalamo-pituitary-adrenal axis dysregulation in multiple sclerosis. *Psychoneuroendocrinology* 2002;27(4):505–517.

114. Berg D, Supprian T, Thomae J, et al. Lesion pattern in patients with multiple sclerosis and depression. *Mult Scler* 2000;6(3):156–162.

115. Mohr DC, Goodkin DE, Islar J, et al. Treatment of depression is associated with suppression of nonspecific and antigen-specific T(H)1 responses in multiple sclerosis. *Arch Neurol* 2001;58(7):1081–1086.

116. Pujol J, Bello J, Deus J, et al. Beck Depression Inventory factors related to demyelinating lesions of the left arcuate fasciculus region. *Psychiat Res* 2000;99(3):151–159.

117. Pujol J, Bello J, Deus J, et al. Lesions in the left arcuate fasciculus region and depressive symptoms in multiple sclerosis. *Neurology* 1997;49(4):1105–1110.

118. Mohr DC, Likosky W, Bertagnolli A, et al. Telephone-administered cognitive-behavioral therapy for the treatment of depressive symptoms in multiple sclerosis. *J Consult Clin Psychol* 2000;68(2):356–361.

119. Amato MP, Ponziani G, Rossi F, et al. Quality of life in multiple sclerosis: The impact of depression, fatigue and disability. *Mult Scler* 2001;7(5):340–344.

120. Fruehwald S, Loeffler S, Eher R, et al. Depression and quality of life in multiple sclerosis. *Acta Neurologica Scand* 2001;104(5):257–261.

121. Gulick EE. Correlates of quality of life among persons with multiple sclerosis. *Nurs Res* 1997;46(6):305–311.

122. Jonsson A, Dock J, Ravnborg M. Quality of life as a measure of rehabilitation outcome in patients with multiple sclerosis. *Acta Neurologica Scand* 1996;93(4):229–235.

123. Provinciali L, Ceravolo MG, Bartolini M, et al. A multidimensional assessment of multiple sclerosis: Relationships between disability domains. *Acta Neurological Scand* 1999;100(3):156—162.

123a.Wang JL, Reimer MA, Metz LM, et al. Major depression and quality of life in individuals with multiple sclerosis. *Int J Psychiat Med* 2000;30(4):309–317.

124. Aikens JE, Fischer JS, Namey M, et al. A replicated prospective investigation of life stress, coping, and depressive symptoms in multiple sclerosis. *J Behav Med* 1997;20(5):433–445.

125. Mohr DC, Goodkin DE, Gatto N, et al. Depression, coping and level of neurological impairment in multiple sclerosis. *Mult Scler* 1997;3(4):254–258.

126. Mohr DC, Boudewyn A, Goodkin D, et al. Comparative outcomes for individual cognitive-behavior therapy, supportive-expressive group psychotherapy, and sertraline for the treatment of depression in multiple sclerosis. *J Consult Clin Psychol* 2001;69(6):942–949.

126a.Halstead LS, ed. *Managing post-polio: A guide to living well with post-polio syndrome.* Arlington, VA: National Rehabilitation Hospital Press, 1998.

127. Berlly MH, Strauser WW, Hall KM. Fatigue in postpolio syndrome. *Arch Phys Med Rehabil* 1991;72:115–118.

128. Tate D, Forchheimer M, Kirsch N, et al. Prevalence and associated features of depression and psychological distress in polio survivors. *Arch Phys Med Rehabil* 1993;74:1056–1060.

129. Widar M, Ahlstrom G. Experiences and consequences of pain in persons with post-polio syndrome. *J Adv Nurs* 1998;28:606–613.

130. Conrady LJ, Wish JR, Agre JC, et al. Psychologic characteristics of polio survivors: A preliminary report. *Arch Phys Med Rehabil* 1989;70:458–463.

131. Clark K, Dinsmore S, Grafman J, et al. A personality profile of patients diagnosed with post-polio syndrome. *Neurology* 1994;44:1809–1811.

131a.Schanke AK. Psychological distress, social support and coping behaviour among polio survivors: a 5-year perspective on 63 polio patients. *Disabil Rehabil* 1997;19:108–116.

132. Kemp BJ, Adams BM, Campbell ML. Depression and life satisfaction in aging polio survivors versus age-matched controls: Relation to postpolio syndrome, family functioning, and attitude toward disability. *Arch Phys Med Rehabil* 1997;78:187–192.

133. Hazendonk KM, Crowe SF. A neuropsychological study of the postpolio syndrome: Support for depression without neuropsychological impairment. *Neuropsychiat Neuropsychol Behav Neurol* 2000;13(2):112–118.

134. Smith GR. The epidemiology and treatment of depression when it coexists with somatoform disorders, somatization, or pain. *Gen Hosp Psychiat* 1992;14:265–272.

135. Benn DT. The role of personality traits and coping strategies in late-life adaptation to vision loss. *Diss Abs Int* 1997;58(4-B):2151.

136. Lupsakko T, Jaentyjaervi J, Kautiainen H, et al. Combined hearing and visual impairment and depression in a population aged 75 years and older. *Int J Geriatr Psychiat* 2002;17(9):808–813.

137. Nakamura T, Kagawa K, Kakizawa T, et al. Risk factors for falls among blind elderly in a nursing home for the blind. *Arch Gerontol Geriatr* 1998;27(1):9–17.

138. Rovner BW, Shmuely DY. Screening for depression in low-vision elderly. *Int J Geriatr Psychiat* 1997;12(9): 955–959.

139. Rovner BW, Ganguli M. Depression and disability associated with impaired vision: The MoVIES project. *J Am Geriatr Soc* 1998;46(5):617–619.

139a. Galaria II, Casten RJ, Rovner BW. Development of a shorter version of the Geriatric Depression Scale for visually impaired older patients. *International Psychogeriatrics* 2000;12(4):435–443.

140. Shirley PSI, Leung YF, Mak WP. Depression in institutionalized older people with impaired vision. *Int J Geriatr Psychiat* 2000;15(12):1120–1124.

141. Upton LR, Bush BA, Taylor RE. Stress, coping, and adjustment of adventitiously blind male veterans with and without diabetes mellitus. *J Visual Impair Blind* 1998;92(9):656–665.

142. Casten RJ, Rovner BW, Edmonds SE. The impact of depression in older adults with age-related macular degeneration. *J Visual Impair Blind* 2002;96(6): 399–406.

143. Smuely DY, Rovner BW. Screening for depression in older persons with low vision: Somatic eye symptoms and the Geriatric Depression Scale. *Am J Geriatr Psychiat* 1997;5(3):216–220.

144. Rovner BW, Zisselman PM, Shmuely DY. Depression and disability in older people with impaired vision: A follow-up study. *J Am Geriatr Soc* 1996;44(2): 181–184.

144a. Oren DA, Zulman DM, Needham WE, et al. Visual impairment and patterns of winter seasonal depression: seeing the light? *J Visual Impair Blind* 2001;95(4): 226–229.

144b. Fouladi MK, Moseley MJ, Jones HS, et al. Sleep disturbances among persons who are visually impaired: survey of guide dog users. *J Visual Impair Blind* 1998; 92(7):522–530.

144c. Lee DJ, Gomez M, Orlando L, et al. Current depression, lifetime history of depression and visual acuity in Hispanic adults. *J Visual Impair Blind* 2000;94(2): 85–96.

145. Koenes SG, Karshmer JF. Depression: A comparison study between blind and sighted adolescents. *Iss Ment Health Nurs* 2000;21(3):269–279.

146. Huurre TM, Aro H. Psychosocial development among adolescents with visual impairment. *Eur Child Adol Psychiatr* 1998;7(2):73–78.

147. Huurre TM, Aro H. The psychosocial well-being of Finnish adolescents with visual impairments versus those with chronic conditions and those with no disabilities. *J Visual Impair Blind* 2000;94(10):625–637.

148. Cacciator F, Napoli C, Abete P, et al. Quality of life determinants and hearing function in an elderly population: Osservatorio Geriatrico Compano Study Group. *Gerontology* 1999;45(6):323–328.

149. Danermark B, Strom SL, Borg B. Some characteristics of mainstreamed hard of hearing students in Swedish Universities. *Am Ann Deaf* 1996;141(5):359–364.

150. DeGraaf R, Bijl RV. Determinants of mental distress in adults with a severe auditory impairment: Differences between prelingual and postlingual deafness. *Psychosomatic Med* 2002;64(1):61–70.

151. Kerr PC, Cowie RI. Acquired deafness: A multi-dimensional experience. *Br J Audiol* 1997;31(3):177–188.

152. Nehra A, Mann SBS, Sharma SC, et al. Psychosocial functions before and after the use of hearing aides in acquired hearing loss patients. *Indian J Clin Psych* 1997;24(1):75–81.

153. Knutson JF, Murray KT, Husarek S, et al. Psychological change over 54 months of cochlear implant use. *Ear Hear* 1998;19(3):191–201.

154. Proops DW, Donaldson I, Cooper HR, et al. (1999). Outcomes from adult implantation, the first 100 patients. *J Laryngol Otol* 1999;24(suppl):5–13.

155. Mulcahy RT. Cognitive self-appraisal of depression and self-concept: Measurement alternatives for evaluating affective states. *Diss Abs Int* 2002;62(10-B): 4796.

155a. McGhee H. An evaluation of modified written and American Sign Language versions of the Beck Depression Inventory with the prelingually deaf. *Diss Abs Int* 1996;56(11-B):6456.

155b. Leigh IW, Anthony TS. Reliability of the BDI-II with deaf persons. *Rehabil Psychol* 2001;46(2):195–202.

156. Beck AT, Rush AJ, Shaw BR, et al. *Cognitive therapy of depression: A treatment manual.* New York: Guilford Press, 1979.

157. Kral A, Hartmann R, Tillein J, et al. Delayed maturation and sensitive periods in the auditory cortex. *Audiol Neurootol* 2002;6(6):346–362.

158. Srivastava RD, Pramod J, Deep J, et al. Electrocardiographic changes following exercise in the congenitally deaf school children: Relationship with Jervell Lange Neilsen syndrome (the Long QT syndrome). *Indian J Physiol Pharmacol* 1998;42(4):515–520.

158a. Sherbourne K, White L, Fortnuni H. Intensive rehabilitation programmes for deafened men and women: an evaluation study. *Int J Audiol* 2002;41(3):195–201.

159. Pollard RQ. Public mental health service and diagnostic trends regarding individuals who are deaf or hard of hearing. *Rehabil Psychol* 1994;39:147–160.

159a. Tamaskar P, Malia T, Stern C, et al. Preventive attitudes and beliefs of deaf and hard-of-hearing individuals. *Arch Fam Med* 2000;9(6):518–525.

160. Hodapp RM. Down syndrome: Developmental, psychiatric, and management issues. *Child Adol Psychiatr Clin North Am* 1996;5(4):881–894.

161. Holland AJ. Down's syndrome. In Janicki MP, Dalton AJ, eds. *Dementia, aging, and intellectual disabilities: A handbook.* Philadelphia: Brunner/Mazel, 1999:183–197.

162. Thompson SB. Examining dementia in Down's syndrome (DS): Decline in social abilities in DS compared with other learning disabilities. *Clin Gerontol* 1999;20(3):23–44.

162a. Kahn S, Osinowo T, Pary RJ. Down syndrome and major depressive disorder: a review. *Ment Health Asp Develop Dis* 2002;5(2):46–52.

163. Linna SL, Moilanen I, Ebeling H, et al. Psychiatric symptoms in children with intellectual disability. *Eur Child Adol Psychiatr* 1999;8(Suppl 4):77–82.

164. Cooper SA. Psychiatry of elderly compared to younger adults with intellectual disabilities. *J Applied Res Intellect Disabil* 1997;10(4):303–311.

165. Davis JP, Judd FK, Herrman H. Depression in adults with intellectual disability. Part 2: A pilot study. *Aust N Z J Psychiatr* 1997;31(2):243–251.

166. Hardan A, Sahl R. Psychopathology in children and adolescents with developmental disorders. *Res Develop Disabil* 1997;18(5):369–382.

167. Verhoeven WMA, Tuinier S. Neuropsychiatric consul-

tation in mentally retarded patients: A clinical report. *Eur Psychiat* 1997;12(5):242–248.

168. Altabet S, Neumann JK, Watson-Johnston S. Light therapy as a treatment of sleep cycle problems and depression. *Ment Health Asp Develop Disabil* 2002;5(1): 1–6.

169. Aman MG, Collier-Crespin A, Lindsay RL. Pharmacotherapy of disorders in mental retardation. *Eur Child Adol Psychiatr* 2000;9(Suppl 5):98–107.

170. Carta MG, Hardoy MC, Dessi I, et al. Adjunctive gabapentin in patients with intellectual disability and bipolar spectrum disorders. *J Intellect Disabil Res* 2001;45(2):139–145.

171. Gensheimer PM, Meighen KG, McDougle CJ. ECT in an adolescent with Down Syndrome and treatment-refractory major depressive disorder. *J Develop Phys Disabil* 2002;14(3):291–295.

172. Hellings JA. Psychopharmacology of mood disorders in persons with mental retardation and autism. *Mental Retardation Develop Disabil Res Rev* 1999;5(4): 270–278.

173. Hemingway-Eltomey JM, Lerner AJ. Adverse effects of donepezil in treating Alzheimer's disease associated with Down's syndrome. *Am J Psychiat* 1999;156(9): 1470.

174. Matson JL, Bamburg JW, Mayville EA, et al. Tardive dyskinesia and developmental disabilities: An examination of demographics and topography in persons with dual diagnosis. *Br J Develop Disabil* 2000;46(91, Pt2):119–130.

175. Mikkelsen EJ, Albert LG, Emens M, et al. The efficacy of antidepressant medication for individuals with mental retardation. *Psychiat Ann* 1997;27(3):198–206.

176. Racusin R, Kovner-Kline K, King BH. Selective serotonin reuptake inhibitors in intellectual disability. *Mental Retardation Develop Disabil Res Rev* 1999;5 (4):264–269.

177. Ruedrich SL, Alamir S. (1999). Electroconvulsive therapy for persons with developmental disabilities: Review, case report and recommendations. *Ment Health Asp Develop Disabil* 2(3):1–9.

178. Schwartz-Mitchell JL. The effects of supported employment level on the psychosocial experiences of integrated workers with mental retardation. *Diss Abs Int* 2001;62(1-B):564.

178a. Stolker JJ, Heerdink ER, Leufkens H, et al. Determinants of multiple psychotropic drug use in patients with mild intellectual disabilities or borderline intellectual functioning and psychiatric or behavioral disorders. *Gen Hosp Psychiat* 2001;23(6):345–349.

179a. Tsiouris JA. Psychotropic medications. In: Janicki MP, Dalton AJ, eds. *Dementia, aging, and intellectual disabilities: A handbook.* Philadelphia: Brunner/Mazel, 1999:232–253.

180. Tsiouris JA. Drug treatment of depression associated with dementia or presented as "pseudodementia" in older adults with Down syndrome. *J Appl Res Intellect Disabil* 1999b;10(4):312–322.

181. Verhoeven WMA, Tuinier S. Cyclothymia or unstable mood disorder? A systematic treatment evaluation with valproic acid. *J Appl Res Intellect Disabil* 2001; 14(2):147–154.

182. Verhoeven WMA, Veendrik-Meekes M, Jacobs GAJ, et al. Citalopram in mentally retarded patients with de-

pression: A long-term clinical investigation. *Eur Psychiat* 2001;16(2):104–108.

183. Werry JS. Anxiolytics in MRDD. *Mental Retardation Develop Disabil Res Rev* 1999;5(4):299–304.

184. Ciechomski LD, Jackson KL, Tonge B, et al. Intellectual disability and anxiety in children: A group-based parent skills-training intervention. *Beh Change* 2001; 18(4):204–212.

185. Hand J. (1999). The care of individuals with mental retardation: Lessons from the New Zealand experience. *Int Rev Psychiatr* 1999;11(1):68–75.

186. Lunsky Y, Benson BA. Perceived social support and mental retardation: A social-cognitive approach. *Cogn Ther Res* 2001;25(1):77–90.

187. Meins W. Psychological treatment of mentally retarded adults with depressive disorders. *Nervenarzt* 1996;67 (3):216–218. (Only abstract is in English.)

188. Ruedrich SL, Hurley AD, Sovner R. Treatment of mood disorders in mentally retarded persons. In: Dosen A, Day K, eds. *Treating mental illness and behavior disorders in children and adults with mental retardation.* Washington, DC: American Psychiatric Publishing, 2001:201–226.

189. Schaya M, Galli-Carminati G. A pilot study on the evolution of a verbal group of eight patients in a day care hospital. *Revue Francophone de la Deficience Intellectuelle* 2000;1(2):137–147. (Only abstract is in English.)

190. Schulenberg SE. (2000). Depression in mental retardation: An additional direction for logotherapy. *Int Forum Logother* 2000;23(2):107–110.

191. Stoddart KP, Burke L, Temple V. Outcome evaluation of bereavement groups for adults with intellectual disabilities. *J Appl Res Intellect Disabil* 2002;15(1): 28–35.

192. Clark DJ, Gomez GA. Utility of modified DCR-10 criteria in the diagnosis of depression associated with intellectual disability. *J Intellect Disabil Res* 1999;43(5): 413–420.

193. Reiss S, Levitan G, Szyszko J. Emotional disturbance and mental retardation: Diagnostic overshadowing. *Am J Ment Defic* 1982;86:567–574.

194. Ruedrich SL, Hurley AD. Diagnostic uncertainty. *Ment Health Asp Develop Disabil* 2001;4(1):43–47.

195. Edelstein TM, Glenwick DS. Direct care workers' attributions of psychopathology in adults with mental retardation. *Mental Retardation* 2001;39(5):368–378.

196. Evans KM, Cotton MM, Einfeld SL, et al. Assessment of depression in adults with severe or profound intellectual disability. *J Intellect Develop Disabil* 1999;24 (2):147–160.

197. Munden AC, Perry DW. Symptoms of depression in people with learning disabilities. *J Learning Disabil* 2002;6(1):13–22.

198. Bramston P, Fogarty G. The assessment of emotional distress experienced by people with an intellectual disability: A study of different methodologies. *Res Develop Disabil* 2000;21(6):487–500.

199. Tsiouris JA. Diagnosis of depression in people with severe/profound intellectual disability. *J Intellect Disabil Res* 2001;45(2):115–120.

200. Masi G, Mucci M, Favilla L, et al. Dysthymic disorder in adolescents with intellectual disability. *J Intellect Disabil Res* 1999;43(2):80–87.

201. Ross E, Oliver C. The relationship between levels of mood, interest and pleasure and 'challenging behaviour' in adults with severe and profound intellectual disability. *J Intellect Disabil Res* 2002;46(3):191–197.

202. Gustafsson C, Sonnander K. Psychometric evaluation of a Swedish version of the Reiss Screen for Maladaptive Behavior. *J Intellect Disabil Res* 2002;46(3):218–229.

203. Lecavalier L, Tasse MJ. Translation and transcultural adaptation of the Reiss Screening Test for Maladaptive Behavior. *Revue Francophone de la Deficience Intellectuelle* 2001;12(1):31–44. (Only abstract is in English.)

204. Luiselli JK, Benner S, Stoddard T, et al. Evaluating the efficacy of partial hospitalization services for adults with mental retardation and psychiatric disorders: A pilot study using the Aberrant Behavior Checklist (ABC). *Ment Health Asp Develop Disabil* 2001;4(2):61–67.

205. Masi G, Brovedani P, Mucci M, et al. Assessment of anxiety and depression in adolescents with mental retardation. *Child Psychiat Hum Develop* 2002;32(3):227–237.

206. Balboni G, Battagliese G, Pedrabissi L. The Psychopathology Inventory for Mentally Retarded Adults: Factor structure and comparisons between subjects with or without dual diagnosis. *Res Develop Disabil* 2000;21(4):311–321.

207. Matson JL, Rush KS, Hamilton M, et al. Characteristics of depression as assessed by the Diagnostic Assessment for the Severely Handicapped - II (DASH-II). *Res Develop Disabil* 1999;20(4):305–313.

208. Masi G, Mucci M, Poli P, et al. Dysthymia in adolescents with mild mental retardation. *Psichiatria dell'Infancia e dell'Adolescenza* 1998;65(3):261–271. (Only abstract is in English.)

209. Colucci G, Pellicciotta A, Buono S, et al. The Rorschach Egocentricity Index in subjects with intellectual disability: A study on the incidence of different psychological pathologies. *J Intellect Disabil Res* 1998;42(5):354–359.

210. Masi G, Pfanner P, Marcheschi M. Depression in adolescents with mental retardation: A clinical study. *Br J Develop Disabil* 1998;44(87, Pt 2):112–118.

211. Pary RJ, Strauss D, White JF. A population survey of suicide attempts in persons with and without Down Syndrome. *Down Syndrome Q* 1997;2(1):12–13.

212. Collacott RA. People with Down syndrome and mental health needs. In: Bouras N, ed. *Psychiatric and behavioral disorders in developmental disabilities and mental retardation* New York: Cambridge University Press, 1999:200–211.

212a. Hurley AD. Two cases of suicide attempt by patients with Down's syndrome. *Psychiat Serv* 1998;49(12):1618–1619.

212b. Hardan A, Sahl R. Suicidal behavior in children and adolescents with developmental disorders. *Res Develop Dis* 1999;20(4):287–296.

23

Special Considerations for Using Psychiatric Medications

Jeffrey P. Staab and Dwight L. Evans

INTRODUCTION

Since 1990, more than 20 new psychiatric medications have been approved for use in the United States. Numerous other medications also have been investigated for psychiatric indications, including most new antiepileptic drugs (AEDs). For the most part, these agents are better tolerated than their predecessors. However, they are not free of adverse effects, and their common use by patients taking other medications increases the potential for unwanted drug–drug interactions. In this regard, women with physical disabilities are no different than other patients. They are more likely than ever before to receive medications for psychiatric illnesses. This is a welcome advance, but it exposes women with chronic physical ailments to the adverse effects of modern psychotropic agents, plus the potential for unfavorable interactions with their other medications. This chapter will review specific considerations in using common psychiatric medications and the potential interactions between psychotropic agents and several other classes of medications that are prescribed commonly to women with disabilities.

Older and newer psychiatric medications may cause difficulties for women with disabilities in three ways: (a) their adverse effects may exacerbate patients' medical symptoms, (b) their adverse effects may mimic or worsen the side effects of other drugs, and (c) their pharmacologic interactions with other medications may have untoward consequences. The first section of this chapter will focus on the adverse effects of psychiatric medications themselves. The second part reviews potential interactions between psychiatric medications and other drugs commonly used to treat physical disabilities.

ADVERSE EFFECTS OF PSYCHOTROPIC AGENTS

Antidepressants

Tricyclic Antidepressants

Tricyclic antidepressants (TCAs) are strong antagonists of cholinergic, histaminic, and α-adrenergic receptors. They also affect cardiac conduction in a manner similar to Type 1A antiarrhythmic agents (1). TCAs commonly cause constipation, urinary retention, drying of mucous membranes, sedation, and orthostatic hypotension. These side effects are greater at the doses needed to treat major depressive or anxiety disorders than at doses used for migraine prophylaxis or treatment of neuropathic pain (e.g., nortriptyline 75 to 125 mg/day versus 25 to 75 mg/day or amitriptyline 150 to 300 mg/day versus 25 to 100 mg/day, respectively). However, even at the lower doses, TCAs may add to the pharmacologic actions of skeletal muscle relaxants and antispasmodics (anticholinergic effects), sedatives and hypnotics (antihistaminic effects), antihypertensives (α-adrenergic effects), and antiarrhythmic agents. The anticholinergic effects may exacerbate cognitive deficits experienced by women with brain injuries, cerebrovascular accidents, or dementia. They also may worsen gastrointestinal hypomotility or neurogenic bladder dysfunction. The combined anticholinergic and antihistaminic effects may dry pulmonary secretions, making it more difficult for patients with respiratory illnesses to clear their airways. Patients may adapt somewhat to these side effects with time, but they also may persist for as long as the medications are being taken. These adverse effects do not preclude the use of TCAs when they are indicated and effective but call for closer monitoring of vulnerable patients.

Selective Serotonin Reuptake Inhibitors

Selective serotonin reuptake inhibitors (SSRIs) also cause adverse effects that may add to the physical problems experienced by women with disabilities. For most patients, SSRI side effects are transient problems lasting 3 to 7 days after the medications are started or the doses increased. Short-lived adverse effects include gastrointestinal upset (nausea, loose stools), sleep disturbance (insomnia or sedation), restlessness, and mild headache. Persistent sleep disturbances can be managed by adjusting the time of day that the medication is taken. Medications that cause insomnia can be taken early in the morning, whereas those that produce sedation should be taken in the evening. Low-dose trazodone (25 to 100 mg qhs) also may be helpful for persistent insomnia. If patients do not adapt to these side effects, a trial of a second SSRI is reasonable. However, our experience suggests that switching to a third or fourth SSRI is not likely to be successful for patients who have failed two of these medications.

The only long-term adverse effect common to all SSRIs is sexual dysfunction (2,3), which usually begins after 2 to 3 weeks of treatment. Women may experience decreased libido, reduced physical responsiveness to sexual stimulation, and anorgasmia. Mild sexual side effects may be transient or tolerable, but moderate to severe sexual dysfunction typically does not improve as long as patients

continue their medication. Fortunately, SSRI-related sexual dysfunction may be relieved by several pharmacologic antidotes (4) or by a switch to an antidepressant from another class. Sexual side effects often are not reported by patients but can be elicited by sensitive inquiry.

Most SSRIs appear to be neutral with regard to weight changes over the short term, but systematic assessments tracking patients' weight over several months or more generally are lacking. Loss of a few pounds is common during the initial weeks of therapy. After 1 year of treatment, most patients are within a few pounds of their premorbid weight. A small percentage of patients appears to be vulnerable to weight gain with SSRIs (5). The mechanism of this adverse effect is unknown, but the most troublesome pattern is an early and persistent increase in weight. Close attention to diet and exercise may mitigate this weight increase, but an aggressive diet and exercise program may not be practical for some women with disabilities. Therefore, women who gain more than a few pounds of unwanted weight in the first weeks of antidepressant therapy should be switched to another medication. In some cases, the weight gain may occur very gradually over several months.

Other Antidepressants

Among the other new antidepressants, venlafaxine and mirtazapine have side effects that are potentially noteworthy for women with disabilities. Venlafaxine may cause a clinically significant, dose-related increase in blood pressure in a small percentage of patients, especially those taking daily doses of 300 mg or more (6). This effect may be transient, with blood pressure gradually returning to baseline over several weeks of therapy (6). Mirtazapine seems to be more likely than other new antidepressants to cause weight gain. Some women will experience early and persistent weight gain, whereas others will see a gradual increase over several months (5,7).

Monoamine Oxidase Inhibitors

The monoamine oxidase inhibitors (MAOIs), phenelzine and tranylcypromine, are not used as much as they were in the past, but they remain potent medications for treatment-resistant anxiety and depressive disorders. Both may cause hypotension early in the course of therapy. Phenelzine tends to be sedating, whereas tranylcypromine may cause insomnia or restlessness. Both MAOIs have the potential for serious interactions with certain foods and medications (8). Hypertensive crises may occur when a patient being treated with an MAOI takes sympathomimetic medications or ingests food containing high levels of tyramine. Most processed foods today, including processed cheeses and meats, contain safe amounts of tyramine, but naturally aged foods and wines contain higher levels. Over-the-counter sympathomimetics, such as decongestants, appetite suppressants (including herbal preparations), and stimulants (e.g., caffeine products), may interact with MAOIs. Meperidine can have a potentially fatal interaction with the MAOIs. Serious adverse interactions have not been reported with other narcotics. Serotonergic medications, such as the SSRIs, venlafaxine, mirtazapine, and nefazodone, may cause the potentially lethal serotonin syndrome (delirium, increased muscle tone, autonomic instability) when combined with MAOIs. General anesthetics are difficult to administer to patients taking MAOIs, and pressor agents such as dopamine, dobutamine, and other sympathomimetics are incompatible with these drugs. MAOIs must be discontinued at least 2 weeks in advance of elective surgery for the body to rebuild its stores of monoamine oxidase. This makes the MAOIs difficult to use in women who may require multiple surgical procedures.

St. John's Wort

St. John's wort (hypericum perforatum) is a popular herbal supplement marketed for the treatment of depressed mood. Its precise mechanism of action is uncertain, but one of its chemical constituents may inhibit monoamine oxidase, whereas another appears to inhibit serotonin reuptake (9). The most common side effects of St. John's wort are nausea, somnolence, and restlessness. Adverse interactions, including the serotonin syndrome, have been reported with combinations of St. John's wort and SSRIs (9).

Antipsychotics

Typical Antipsychotics

The older generation of antipsychotics (often called typical antipsychotics or typical neuroleptics) may cause potentially troublesome extrapyramidal side effects (EPS) such as cogwheel rigidity of skeletal muscles, bradykinesia, masked facies, and tremor. The high-potency medications such as haloperidol and fluphenazine are more likely to cause serious EPS than low-potency drugs such as chlorpromazine and thioridazine. However, the lower potency medications possess stronger anticholinergic, antihistaminic, and α-adrenergic side effects, which were discussed earlier in the section on TCAs. Women suffering from spastic muscle conditions, contractures, and parkinsonism are likely to experience a worsening of these symptoms with typical neuroleptics, particularly the high-potency medications. Individuals with hypotension, cognitive deficits, gastrointestinal hypomotility, neurogenic bladder dysfunction, and viscous respiratory secretions may have more difficulty when prescribed lower potency typical antipsychotics. The antiemetic drugs, prochlorperazine and promethazine, are typical antipsychotics, despite the fact that they are used primarily to treat nausea. They may cause the same side effects as other typical antipsychotic agents.

All typical antipsychotics may cause akathisia, tardive dyskinesia (TD), neuroleptic malignant syndrome (NMS), hyperprolactinemia, and possibly ventricular dysrhythmias. Akathisia is a motor restlessness that manifests itself as uncontrollable fidgeting or pacing. For women confined to a bed or wheelchair, akathisia may present as vague discomfort in the larger skeletal muscles and a persistent desire to shift positions. Beta blockers and benzodiazepines can control this side effect, but the best intervention is a reduction in the antipsychotic medication, whenever possible, or a switch to a newer-generation antipsychotic medication. The risk for developing TD previously was thought to be proportional to an individual's total lifetime exposure to typical antipsychotics (i.e., high doses for long periods). Now it is recognized that a small percentage of patients (approximately 5%) may develop this chronic motor symptom within the first few months of treatment and that the incidence of TD may be 5% per year of typical antipsychotic exposure, up to a total prevalence of 20% to 25% in chronic users of these medications (10). The tongue fasciculation, lip smacking, chewing, facial grimacing, and spastic limb movements that characterize TD may be chronic (possibly permanent) once established. Therefore, clinicians should be alert to the development of involuntary movements in patients who regularly take typical antipsychotics, including the antiemetics. NMS is a rare but potentially lethal complication of antipsychotic use, marked by severe muscle rigidity, mental status changes, and autonomic instability. It usually requires stabilization in an intensive care setting (11). Hyperprolactinemia is caused by blockade of the dopamine D_2 receptor in the tuberoinfundibular region of the brain, which reduces the inhibitory effects of dopamine on lactotrophs in the pituitary. In women, antipsychotic-induced hyperprolactinemia may cause galactorrhea and irregular menstrual cycles, including amenorrhea. Lastly, several reports have linked typical neuroleptics, particularly thioridazine, to sudden cardiac death (12). Presumably, the causal mechanism is a prolongation of the QT interval (QTc more than 500 msec), with a resulting ventricular dysrhythmia. While further investigations are continuing, it may be prudent to use these agents cautiously in patients with known conduction abnormali-

ties and those taking other medications that affect cardiac conduction. When needed, doses of typical antipsychotics should be kept as low as possible, and intravenous administration should be kept to a minimum. In one retrospective, intensive care unit study (13), potentially lethal arrhythmias (e.g., Torsades de pointes) were found almost exclusively in patients who had been given more than 35 mg/day of intravenous haloperidol or equivalent doses of other typical antipsychotic medications.

Atypical Antipsychotics

The six newest antipsychotic drugs (called atypical antipsychotics or atypical neuroleptics) have side effect profiles that differ markedly from one another and from the typical agents. The most common side effects of risperidone are EPS, sedation, and hyperprolactinemia, although it is considerably less likely than the typical agents to cause these problems (14). Clozapine and olanzapine commonly cause weight gain (15,16). Recently, olanzapine has been linked to new-onset diabetes mellitus, exacerbations of preexisting diabetes, and impaired glucose tolerance in a series of case reports (17) and an investigation of a large general practice database in the United Kingdom (18). The prevalence and severity of these effects are not known. Therefore, firm conclusions cannot be drawn about the possible risks of prescribing olanzapine to women who have, or are at risk for, diabetes, coronary artery disease, or stroke. Clozapine has a 1% incidence of leukopenia, which requires weekly monitoring of blood counts for the first 6 months of therapy and then biweekly monitoring thereafter. Patients taking clozapine must be registered in a U.S. Food and Drug Administration (FDA)-mandated database to receive the medication. Additional clozapine side effects include tachycardia, fever, sialorrhea, and orthostatic hypotension (15). Despite these adverse effects, clozapine is the most potent of the atypical antipsychotic agents for treatment-resistant schizophrenia. Ziprasidone may be the most likely atypical antipsychotic agent to prolong the QTc interval. According to its package insert (19), it is contraindicated in patients with QTc intervals greater than 500 msec. There are insufficient data on interactions between ziprasidone and other cardiac medications, so it may be prudent to limit such coadministration until more information is available (20). Quetiapine appears to have the lowest overall side effect burden for women with disabilities, but it also has the widest therapeutic dose range and therefore requires the most clinical effort to titrate it optimally. Aripiprazole, the newest atypical antipsychotic, was approved by the FDA in December 2002. In premarketing trials, it caused extrapyramidal symptoms at about the same rate as risperidone (21). All six atypical antipsychotics have very low rates of TD, akathisia, and NMS.

Benzodiazepines

Benzodiazepines are highly effective anxiolytic and antispasmodic medications. Their most troubling side effects are cognitive impairment and physical sluggishness. They may increase the risk of falls in elderly patients and possibly in other patients with gait instabilities resulting from physical impairments. The addiction potential of benzodiazepines can be mitigated by careful patient selection and education as well as a conscientious plan to track the amount and frequency of prescriptions. Caution is warranted in patients who escalate their doses or need extra prescriptions for any reason. The biggest difficulty in using these medications for women with disabilities is their potential to exacerbate the cognitive and sedating effects of other central nervous system depressants such as narcotics and AEDs (e.g., phenobarbital). In addition, these medications must be tapered, not abruptly discontinued. For these reasons, antidepressants have supplanted benzodiazepines for long-term treatment of anxiety disorders (22). The TCAs, MAOIs, and particularly the SSRIs, venlafaxine, mirtazapine, and nefazodone, possess a wide spectrum of anxiolytic activity. They also treat the depressive symptoms that commonly coexist with anxiety in patients suffering from chronic physical illnesses.

MECHANISMS OF MEDICAL-PSYCHIATRIC DRUG–DRUG INTERACTIONS

Psychiatric medications interact with other drugs mostly through the cytochrome P-450 isoenzyme system in the liver. Psychiatric medications generally are not enzyme inducers, but some of them inhibit cytochrome P-450 isoenzymes to a pharmacologically important degree (23,24). Conversely, the serum concentrations of many psychiatric medications may be increased or decreased by drugs that inhibit or induce cytochrome P-450 isoenzymes.

Numerous *in vitro* studies have examined drug–drug interactions in isolated hepatic isoenzyme preparations in the laboratory. These investigations suggest many possible interactions, but only a few have been realized clinically because humans metabolize most drugs *in vivo* through multiple isoenzyme pathways. Therefore, drugs that inhibit a single isoenzyme may not cause as many *in vivo* interactions as *in vitro* studies suggest. Better sources of data about clinically important drug–drug interactions are pharmacokinetic and pharmacodynamic studies involving healthy human volunteers and targeted patient populations. Case reports illustrate potential interactions, but their significance depends on the number of cases that are reported compared to the prevalence of the medication combination in clinical practice. Case reports often are markers of isolated events in one or a few individuals, not widespread occurrences in the population as a whole. Unfortunately, case reports provide the only published data on interactions between many psychiatric medications and other drugs. The sections below emphasize prospective investigations wherever possible but otherwise synthesize information available from case reports.

POTENTIAL INTERACTIONS BETWEEN PSYCHIATRIC MEDICATIONS AND OTHER DRUG CLASSES

Immunosuppressive Agents

Cyclosporine

Cyclosporine is metabolized by CYP3A3/4 isoenzymes. Case reports have documented toxic levels of cyclosporine in patients prescribed fluoxetine (25), fluvoxamine, and nefazodone (26), all of which inhibit CYP3A4 isoenzymes to a moderate degree. In contrast, citalopram, which has minimal effects on cytochrome isoenzymes, did not interfere with cyclosporine metabolism (27). St. John's wort is a potent inducer of CYP3A4, capable of substantially reducing serum cyclosporine levels. This had produced unexpected rejection reactions in human organ transplantation (28). There are almost no data on the effects of cyclosporine on psychiatric medications. In one small study of nine patients undergoing kidney transplant, cyclosporine did not change the steady-state concentration of midazolam (29).

Tacrolimus

Tacrolimus, like cyclosporine, is metabolized primarily by the CYP3A group of hepatic isoenzymes. In one case report, the addition of nefazodone (a 3A4 inhibitor) caused tacrolimus toxicity, but paroxetine (a 2D6 inhibitor) did not (30). St. John's wort is likely to decrease tacrolimus levels significantly.

Corticosteroids

There are no significant adverse interactions between corticosteroids and psychiatric medications. In contrast, psychotropic agents may be used to manage the affective and psychotic side effects of corticosteroids, especially in patients who require recurrent treatment for severe exacerbations of pulmonary diseases, autoimmune illnesses, and other steroid-responsive conditions. The most common psychiatric effects of corticosteroids are alterations in mood, sleep, appetite, and energy level. Less often, psychotic symptoms in the form of an agitated, maniclike state may develop (31). Psychiatric side effects may occur at any dose of corticosteroids but are most common at doses greater than 40 mg/day of prednisone or its equivalent. They are most likely to develop during the first few days or weeks of treatment and are much less frequent with alternate day corticosteroid therapy (32). In two case reports, SSRIs were used to treat corticosteroid-induced mood and anxiety symptoms in patients who required ongoing corticosteroid treatment. In one case, sertraline relieved depression, agitation, and psychosis (33). In the other, fluvoxamine suppressed panic symptoms (34). We used the mood stabilizer divalproex to prevent recurrent mania in a patient who needed intermittent pulse steroid therapy despite a repeated history of steroid-induced manic psychosis.

Cytotoxic Agents

Cyclophosphamide

Cyclophosphamide is activated *in vivo* by the microsomal enzyme cyclophosphamide oxidase. In mice, chronic administration of the benzodiazepines chlordiazepoxide, diazepam, or oxazepam stimulated the activity of cyclophosphamide oxidase, producing a toxic accumulation of cyclophosphamide metabolites (35). Similar results occurred with the closely related compound ifosfamide (36). Although there are no clinical reports of cyclophosphamide–benzodiazepine interactions in humans, we encountered a case in which chronic benzodiazepine treatment may have been one of several factors contributing to a patient's unexpectedly high sensitivity to cyclophosphamide.

Antiepileptic Drugs

Spina and Perruca reviewed current information on the interactions between AEDs and psychiatric medications (37). The main interactions arise from the propensity of older AEDs, such as phenytoin, carbamazepine, and the barbiturates, to induce the metabolic activity of cytochrome P-450 isoenzymes. This reduces the serum levels of many psychotropic agents, including TCAs and typical and atypical antipsychotics. Another interaction is the result of the inhibition of cytochrome isoenzymes by some psychiatric medications, leading to an increase in serum levels of AEDs. Fluoxetine and fluvoxamine appear to be the most likely to cause this effect, probably because they inhibit multiple isoenzymes subtypes. Carbamazepine and phenytoin are the most susceptible to enzyme inhibition and the resulting clinical toxicity. There are no known interactions between AEDs and lithium.

Phenytoin

Phenytoin is a potent inducer of CYP3A4. The atypical antipsychotic, quetiapine, is largely metabolized by this isoenzyme. Quetiapine's clearance was increased fivefold in a group of psychotic patients also taking phenytoin, which necessitated higher than normal antipsychotic doses to maintain a therapeutic benefit (38). Interactions between phenytoin and the SSRIs mirror the inhibitory activity of each antidepressant on the cytochrome isoenzymes, especially CYP2C9, which appears to be the most important for phenytoin metabolism (39). Fluoxetine and fluvoxamine are more potent inhibitors of CYP2C9 than sertraline or paroxetine (40), whereas sertraline, paroxetine, escitalopram, and citalopram have minimal to no effect on this isoenzyme. There are case reports of increased phenytoin levels in patients prescribed fluoxetine or fluvoxamine (41). Furthermore, phenytoin levels dropped below the therapeutic range in a patient taking both phenytoin and fluoxetine after the fluoxetine was discontinued (42). A placebo-controlled study of 30 healthy males found no change in the pharmacokinetic or pharmacodynamic properties of phenytoin during a 24-day period of coadministration with sertraline at the maximum approved dose

of 200 mg/day (43). In a case report, two elderly women experienced a minor increase in phenytoin levels, without clinical toxicity, when prescribed sertraline (44). A single-blind, crossover trial found no effect from paroxetine on phenytoin levels or seizure control in patients with epilepsy (45).

Carbamazepine

Carbamazepine induces several cytochrome enzymes including CYP3A4 and 1A2. Several typical and atypical antipsychotics are metabolized by these isoenzymes. In a pharmacokinetic study of 11 healthy volunteers (46), olanzapine was cleared more rapidly after 2 weeks of treatment with carbamazepine than at baseline. The area under the curve (AUC) of the serum concentration of olanzapine over time was lower with carbamazepine cotreatment. Carbamazepine decreased the serum levels of clozapine (47) and risperidone (48) by more than 50%. The AUC and half-life of ziprasidone were modestly lower in nine healthy adults taking carbamazepine versus 10 taking placebo (49). Lower serum levels of haloperidol also have been reported with carbamazepine (50). Case reports suggest that carbamazepine may reduce serum levels and efficacy of the SSRIs. In two patients, serum citalopram levels increased after patients were switched from carbamazepine to oxcarbazepine (51). In another case, nonresponse to sertraline was blamed on coadministration of carbamazepine (52). Carbamazepine may have a small effect on clonazepam. In serum drug monitoring data from 183 patients (53) carbamazepine increased clonazepam clearance by 22%.

Several studies have demonstrated that certain psychotropic agents inhibit the metabolism of carbamazepine but not to a degree that has major clinical significance. Risperidone 1 mg/day was added to a stable, therapeutic dose of carbamazepine in eight patients with epilepsy and behavioral disturbances (54). The average carbamazepine levels increased from 6.67 to 7.95 mcg/ml (19.2%) after 2 weeks of cotherapy. Haloperidol appears to have a similar effect (50), and clonazepam reduced carbamazepine clearance by 20.5% (53). The SSRIs have even less effect on carbamazepine. Fluoxetine slightly increased the AUC of serum carbamazepine concentrations in six healthy males (55), but neither fluoxetine nor fluvoxamine changed the serum concentrations of carbamazepine in a series of 15 patients with epilepsy (56). Paroxetine had no effect on carbamazepine levels in a double-blind, placebo-controlled crossover trial in 20 patients with epilepsy (45). Sertraline did not change carbamazepine pharmacokinetics or cognitive side effects in 14 healthy male volunteers (57). There is one case report of nefazodone-induced carbamazepine toxicity (58). Nefazodone is a more potent inhibitor of CYP3A4 than any of the SSRIs.

Valproic Acid and Divalproex

The various forms of valproic acid have far fewer interactions with antipsychotics or antidepressants than phenytoin or carbamazepine. Coadministration of valproate to 10 patients taking risperidone did not alter the serum levels of risperidone or its primary metabolite (48). In one case, clozapine levels dropped after valproate was added (59), but two studies counter this report. The addition of valproate induced only minor changes in the serum levels of clozapine and its metabolites in six patients, and there were no significant differences in clozapine levels between 15 patients taking valproate and 22 taking placebo (60). Valproate caused a slight increase in peak lorazepam levels and AUC in 16 healthy subjects but no clinically significant changes in sedation (61). Paroxetine did not change the serum levels of valproate in a small number of patients with epilepsy (45), but fluoxetine reportedly decreased valproate levels in one case (62).

Antispasmodic Agents

Baclofen

There are no reports of interactions between the gamma-aminobutyric acid (GABA) type B receptor agonist, baclofen, and psychiatric medications in humans. In an animal model of GABA-B function, fluoxetine reversed the effects of baclofen (63). The exact nature of this interaction is unknown, and it is not known if fluoxetine might antagonise the clinical effects of baclofen in humans.

Anticholinergics

Anticholinergic drugs appear to have few pharmacokinetic interactions with other medications, but this is not an area that has received much investigation. In two studies, biperiden had no pharmacokinetic or pharmacodynamic interactions with the antipsychotics haloperidol (64) or perphenazine (65). Instead, the biggest problem with anticholinergic drugs is the fact that they often are used in combination with other medications that have significant anticholinergic side effects. A study done before the advent of SSRIs and atypical antipsychotics found that physicians were not selective in choosing medications with low anticholinergic potential (66). In two populations of patients particularly intolerant of anticholinergic effects, 60% of nursing home patients and 23% of elderly outpatients were taking at least one medication with anticholinergic side effects and 6% to 8% were taking three such medications. Strongly anticholinergic medications continue to have important therapeutic applications for women with disabilities. In addition to anticholinergic antispasmodics, TCAs are effective for chronic neuropathic pain and migraine headache and phenothiazines are excellent antiemetics. The anticholinergic burden of all medications that a patient is taking should be considered whenever anticholinergic agents are prescribed.

Benzodiazepines

Benzodiazepines are metabolized in the liver by two mechanisms. Lorazepam, oxazepam, and temazepam are conjugated with glucuronide. Other benzodiazepines are oxidized. Glucuronidation is much less affected by age and liver disease than oxidation. Therefore, fewer dose adjustments are needed in older patients or those with hepatic failure for the three benzodiazepines that are glucuronidated than for other medications in this class. However, valproate may inhibit glucuronidation. In eight healthy volunteers, valproate reduced the plasma clearance of lorazepam by 40% (67). Presumably, this also would affect the metabolism of oxazepam and temazepam, although there are no data on the combination of either of these medications with valproate. In contrast, lorazepam does not alter the metabolism of valproate (61). Tiagabine and triazolam did not interact in one pharmacokinetic, crossover study (68). There appears to be very little metabolic interaction between benzodiazepines and antidepressants. In crossover studies using healthy volunteers, there were no significant pharmacokinetic interactions between sertraline and diazepam (69), sertraline and clonazepam (70), nefazodone and lorazepam (71), or venlafaxine and diazepam (72). Fluoxetine inhibited the oxidation of alprazolam, but it did not affect the metabolism of clonazepam, which undergoes a nitrogenous reduction (73). Clozapine is not affected by benzodiazepines (47).

Analgesics

Opioids

There have been several studies of SSRI and opiate coadministration, which suggest that some of the SSRIs may modestly inhibit opiate metabolism. Sertraline increased methadone levels by an average of 26% in 31 depressed opiate addicts on methadone maintenance, but the effect was transient (74). Methadone levels gradually returned to baseline 6 to 12 weeks after sertraline was added. Paroxetine, a CYP2D6 inhibitor, increased methadone levels in eight patients who were homozygous for the CYP2D6 isoenzyme but not in two heterozygous patients who were less dependent on CYP2D6 activity (75). Case reports indicate that fluvoxamine may increase methadone blood levels (76–78), but fluoxetine did not affect morphine levels in a study of 15 healthy volunteers (79).

At least four case reports warn of the possibility that coadministration of SSRIs and tramadol may produce the serotonin syndrome. The R-isomer of tramadol inhibits serotonin reuptake, so the combination of an SSRI with this analgesic may increase substantially synaptic serotonin concentrations. The serotonin syndrome has been reported with tramadol plus fluoxetine (80), sertraline (81), and paroxetine (82,83).

The effects of opiate–SSRI combinations on pain control and antidepressant efficacy have been investigated. Acute administration of fluoxetine, 30 mg, increased the analgesic effect of morphine by 3% to 8%, while decreasing opiate side effects of sedation, nausea, and dysphoria in 15 healthy volunteers subjected to electrical tooth stimulation (79). However, in a double-blind, placebo-controlled investigation, fluoxetine, 10 mg administered for 7 days prior to surgery, shortened the duration of action of morphine for postoperative pain control (84). The efficacy of antidepressant treatment is unclear in patients receiving chronic opiates. In a study of opiate addicts on methadone maintenance, fluoxetine was no more effective than placebo for major depression (85). It is not clear if chronic opiate treatment similarly would impair the efficacy of antidepressants in other groups of patients such as those with chronic pain.

Nonsteroidal Antiinflammatory Drugs

The gastric side effects of nonsteroidal antiinflammatory drugs (NSAIDs) and aspirin are well known. de Abajo (86) and colleagues examined the association between upper gastrointestinal (UGI) bleeding or ulcer perforation and use of NSAIDs, aspirin, and SSRIs in the United Kingdom General Practice Research Database. They identified 1,899 patients with UGI bleeding or ulcer perforation and 10,000 matched control subjects to calculate the relative risks of gastrointestinal side effects among users of these medications. The odds ratio (OR) for developing UGI bleeding or ulcer perforation among users of SSRIs without NSAIDs or aspirin was 3.0, the same as for low-dose (81 mg/day) aspirin therapy—that is, patients taking either an SSRI or low-dose aspirin had three times the risk of UGI bleeding or ulcer perforation as patients taking neither of these medications. However, the risk was substantially higher in patients taking an SSRI with NSAIDs (OR = 15.6) or low-dose aspirin (OR = 7.1). These risks are not high enough to contraindicate the use of SSRIs with either NSAIDs or aspirin in women who may need these drugs. However, they suggest the need for increased vigilance regarding gastrointestinal symptoms when the combination is prescribed. The gastrointestinal risks from coadministration of NSAIDs or aspirin with other new antidepressants have not been studied.

NSAIDs may cause the kidneys to retain lithium. However, large differences exist in the potential for lithium toxicity among individual patients and the various NSAIDs (87). Some patients can take NSAIDs without much change in their lithium levels, whereas others will experience a profound effect. The first author (JPS) observed a patient who was on a stable, therapeutic lithium regimen develop lithium toxicity after a single 800-mg dose of ibuprofen. Patients who require chronic lithium therapy may take NSAIDs, but the lithium prescription may have to be adjusted whenever the NSAID dose is changed. Compliance with regular schedules of both medications is essential for their safe use together.

Anticoagulants

Warfarin

Warfarin is metabolized primarily by CYP2C9/10 and to a lesser extent by CYP1A2 and 3A4 (88). *In vitro* data suggest that fluvoxamine and fluoxetine may be more likely than other SSRIs to inhibit the metabolism of warfarin (89), and there are case reports of fluoxetine increasing warfarin anticoagulation (90,91). However, in a small prospective study, prothrombin times were not affected in six subjects who were admin-

istered fluoxetine 20 mg/day for 21 days while taking stable doses of warfarin (92). In another study, citalopram 40 mg/day did not alter the normal metabolism of a single dose of warfarin in 12 healthy subjects (87). The peak prothrombin time and the AUC of the prothrombin time were increased by less the 10%, a clinically insignificant change. Similarly, sertraline also caused only a clinically irrelevant increase of 7.9% over placebo in the AUC of the prothrombin time (93). Sertraline is highly bound to plasma proteins, but it caused only a small increase in unbound plasma warfarin compared to placebo. Citalopram, escitalopram, and venlafaxine have the lowest plasma protein binding among the newer antidepressants and do not significantly inhibit cytochrome isoenzymes (89). They would not be expected to change warfarin metabolism or prothrombin times.

Antiretrovirals

Protease Inhibitors

There are limited clinical data on potential interactions between antiretroviral agents and psychiatric medications. In one study, fluoxetine caused a clinically irrelevant increase of 19% in the AUC of ritonavir. No changes were recommended in ritonavir dosing during fluoxetine treatment (94). In contrast, venlafaxine reduced the peak serum concentration of indinavir by 36% and the AUC by 28% in nine healthy volunteers (95). The clinical significance of this change for patients with HIV/AIDS is unknown. St. John's wort, a potent CYP3A4 isoenzyme inducer, substantially increased the plasma clearance of indinavir. Trough indinavir levels decreased 81% and the AUC decreased 57% in eight healthy volunteers who were given St. John's wort (96). The magnitude of this change raises significant clinical concerns about reduced efficacy and the emergence of drug resistance in patients taking St. John's wort with indinavir.

Ritonavir induces CYP1A2 isoenzymes. In a study of 14 healthy volunteers, ritonavir doubled the plasma clearance rate of olanzapine, decreasing both peak concentrations and AUC by 50% (97). Increased vigilance for psychotic symptoms and olanzapine side effects may be needed whenever ritonavir doses are adjusted in patients taking olanzapine. *In vitro* studies suggest that indinavir inhibits CYP3A4, which may reduce the metabolism of trazodone, nefazodone, and alprazolam (99,100). Nelfinavir, ritonavir, and efavirenz decreased bupropion metabolism via inhibition of CYP2B6 in human microsomes (101). The clinical significance of these *in vitro* findings is not known.

Antibiotics

There are very few data on interactions between antibiotics and psychiatric medications. The macrolides, such as erythromycin, have received the most attention regarding potential interactions with other drugs, but there are only case reports about their interactions with antidepressants plus one small study with benzodiazepines. Delirium and possible serotonin syndrome were reported in cases where erythromycin was prescribed to patients taking serotonergic antidepressants (102,103). Erythromycin also increased serum levels and the AUC of diazepam and flunitrazepam but not to a clinically significant degree (104). Ciprofloxacin decreased the clearance of a single dose of diazepam and prolonged its half-life in 12 healthy volunteers but did not affect manual or cognitive measures of benzodiazepine effects (105). Ketoconazole strongly inhibits CYP3A4. *In vitro* studies suggest that it may reduce the metabolism of trazodone, nefazodone, and alprazolam (99–100). However, a crossover pharmacologic investigation in healthy volunteers found no significant interactions between ketoconazole and the atypical antipsychotic ziprasidone (106).

CONCLUSIONS

Psychiatric medications offer women with disabilities considerable relief from both psychiatric and physical symptoms. However, they may cause adverse outcomes in three ways: (a) their side effects may exacerbate patients' medical conditions, (b) they may increase the effects of other drugs, and (c) they may interact pharmacologically with other agents. Most drug–drug interactions are mediated by induction or inhibition of cytochrome P-450 isoenzymes in the liver. Phenytoin, carbamazepine, and the barbiturates are common enzyme inducers, whereas the macrolide antibiotics are common inhibitors. The doses of psychiatric medications may have to be adjusted when coadministered with these drugs. Conversely, the antidepressants fluoxetine, fluvoxamine, paroxetine, and nefazodone inhibit at least one cytochrome P-450 isoenzyme to a clinically significant degree, which may lead to an unwanted accumulation of other medications. There are a few noteworthy interactions that do not involve hepatic metabolism. These include the potential for an increased risk of UGI bleeding with SSRIs and NSAIDs or aspirin, the increased risk of lithium toxicity with NSAIDs, and the potentially fatal combination of meperidine and MAOIs. The coadministration of psychiatric and nonpsychiatric medications requires a thoughtful consideration of the benefits, risks, and available alternatives. In most instances, the benefits outweigh the risks. When this is not the case, effective alternatives are readily available. These facts should encourage the appropriate use of psychiatric medications for women with disabilities.

REFERENCES

1. Roose SP, Glassman AH. Antidepressant choice in patients with cardiac disease: lessons from the Cardiac Arrhythmia Suppression Trial (CAST) studies. *J Clin Psychiatry* 1994;55 Suppl A:83–87.
2. Montejo-Gonzalez AL, Llorca G, Izquierdo JA, et al. SSRI-induced sexual dysfunction: fluoxetine, paroxetine, sertraline, and fluvoxamine in a prospective, multicenter, and descriptive clinical study of 344 patients. *J Sex Marital Ther* 1997;23:176–194.
3. Clayton AH, Pradko JF, Croft HA, et al. Prevalence of sexual dysfunction among newer antidepressants. *J Clin Psychiatry* 2002;63:357–366.
4. Perlis RH, Fava M, Nierenberg AA, et al. Strategies for treatment of SSRI-associated sexual dysfunction: a survey of an academic psychopharmacology practice. *Harv Rev Psychiatry* 2002;10:109–114.

5. Fava M. Weight gain and antidepressants. *J Clin Psychiatry* 2000;61 Suppl 11:37–41.

6. Thase ME. Effects of venlafaxine on blood pressure: a meta-analysis of original data from 3744 depressed patients. *J Clin Psychiatry* 1998;59:502–508.

7. Thase ME, Nierenberg AA, Keller MB, et al. Efficacy of mirtazapine for prevention of depressive relapse: a placebo-controlled double-blind trial of recently remitted high-risk patients. *J Clin Psychiatry* 2001;62 (10):782–788.

8. Bernstein JG. *Handbook of drug therapy in psychiatry.* St. Louis: Mosby Yearbook, Inc., 1994.

9. Brenner R, Bjerkenstedt L, Edman GV. *Hypericum perforatum* extract (St. John's Wort) for depression. *Psychiatr Ann* 2002;32:21–28.

10. Kane JM, Woerner M, Lieberman J. Tardive dyskinesia: prevalence, incidence, and risk factors. *J Clin Psychopharmacol* 1988;8(4 Suppl):52S–56S.

11. Caroff SN, Mann SC. Neuroleptic malignant syndrome. *Med Clin North Am* 1993;77:185–202.

12. Hennessy S, Bilker WB, Knauss JS, et al. Cardiac arrest and ventricular arrhythmia in patients taking antipsychotic drugs: cohort study using administrative data. *BMJ* 2002;325(7372):1070.

13. Sharma ND, Rosman HS, Padhi ID, et al. Torsades de Pointes associated with intravenous haloperidol in critically ill patients. *Am J Cardiol* 1998;81(2):238–240.

14. Fleischhacker WW, Lemmens P, van Baelen B. A qualitative assessment of the neurological safety of antipsychotic drugs; an analysis of a risperidone database. *Pharmacopsychiatry* 2001;34:104–110.

15. Newer atypical antipsychotic medication in comparison to clozapine: a systematic review of randomized trials. *Schizophr Res* 2002;56:1–10.

16. Taylor DM, McAskill R. Atypical antipsychotics and weight gain—a systematic review. *Acta Psychiatr Scand* 2000;101:416–432.

17. Koller EA, Doraiswamy PM. Olanzapine-associated diabetes mellitus. *Pharmacotherapy* 2002; 22:841–852.

18. Newcomer JW, Haupt DW, Fucetola R, et al. Abnormalities in glucose regulation during antipsychotic treatment of schizophrenia. *Arch Gen Psychiatry* 2002;59:337–345.

19. Pfizer, Inc. Ziprasidone package insert. New York, 2002.

20. Haddad PM, Anderson IM. Antipsychotic-related QTc prolongation, torsade de pointes and sudden death. *Drugs* 2002;62:1649–1671.

21. McGavin JK, Goa KL. Aripiprazole. *CNS Drugs* 2002; 16:779–786.

22. Zohar J, Westenberg HG. Anxiety disorders: a review of tricyclic antidepressants and selective serotonin reuptake inhibitors. *Acta Psychiatr Scand* 2000;403:39–49.

23. Nemeroff CB, DeVane CL, Pollock BG. Newer antidepressants and the cytochrome P450 system. *Am J Psychiatry* 1996;153:311–320.

24. Owen JR, Nemeroff CB. New antidepressants and the cytochrome P450 system: focus on venlafaxine, nefazodone, and mirtazapine. *Depression Anxiety* 1998;7 (suppl 1):24–32.

25. Horton RC, Bonser RS. Interaction between cyclosporin and fluoxetine. *BMJ* 1995;311(7002):422.

26. Vella JP, Sayegh MH. Interactions between cyclosporine and newer antidepressant medications. *Am J Kidney Dis* 1998;31:320–323.

27. Liston HL, Markowitz JS, Hunt N, et al. Lack of citalopram effect on the pharmacokinetics of cyclosporine. *Psychosomatics* 2001;42:370–372.

28. Ernst E. St. John's Wort supplements endanger the success of organ transplantation. *Arch Surg* 2002;137: 316–319.

29. Li G, Treiber G, Meinshausen J, Wolf J, et al. Is cyclosporin A an inhibitor of drug metabolism? *Br J Clin Pharmacol* 1990;30:71–77.

30. Campo JV, Smith C, Perel JM. Tacrolimus toxic reaction associated with the use of nefazodone: paroxetine as an alternative agent. *Arch Gen Psychiatry* 1998;55: 1050–1052.

31. Brown ES, Suppes T. Mood symptoms during corticosteroid therapy: a review. *Harvard Rev Psychiatry* 1998;5:239–246.

32. Joffe RT, Denicoff KD, Rubinow DR, et al. Mood effects of alternate-day corticosteroid therapy in patients with systemic lupus erythematosus. Gen Hosp Psychiatry 1988;10(1):56–60.

33. Beshay H, Pumariega AJ. Sertraline treatment of mood disorder associated with prednisone: a case report. *J Child Adol Psychopharmacol* 1998;8:187–193.

34. Charbonneau Y, Ravindran AV. Successful treatment of steroid-induced panic disorder with fluvoxamine. *J Psychiatry Neurosci* 1997;22:346–347.

35. Sasaki K, Furusawa S, Takayanagi G. Effects of chlordiazepoxide, diazepam and oxazepam on the antitumor activity, the lethality and the blood level of active metabolites of cyclophosphamide and cyclophosphamide oxidase activity in mice. *J Pharmacobio-Dynamics* 1983;6:767–772.

36. Furusawa S, Fujimura T, Sasaki K, et al. Potentiation of ifosfamide toxicity by chlordiazepoxide, diazepam and oxazepam. *Chemical Pharmaceutical Bull* 1989; 37:3420–3422.

37. Spina E, Perucca E. Clinical significance of pharmacokinetic interactions between antiepileptic and psychotropic drugs. *Epilepsia* 2002;43 Suppl 2: 37–44.

38. Wong YW, Yeh C, Thyrum PT. The effects of concomitant phenytoin administration on the steady-state pharmacokinetics of quetiapine. *J Clin Psychopharmacol* 2001;21:89–93.

39. Nelson MH, Birnbaum AK, Remmel RP. Inhibition of phenytoin hydroxylation in human liver microsomes by several selective serotonin re-uptake inhibitors. *Epilepsy Research* 2001;44:71–82.

40. Ereshefsky L, Riesenman C, Lam YWF. Serotonin selective reuptake inhibitor drug interactions and the cytochrome P450 system. *J Clin Psychiatry* 1996;57 (suppl 8):17–25.

41. Mamiya K, Kojima K, Yukawa E, et al. Phenytoin intoxication induced by fluvoxamine. *Therapeutic Drug Monitoring* 2001;23:75–77.

42. Shad MU, Preskorn SH. Drug–drug interaction in reverse: possible loss of phenytoin efficacy as a result of fluoxetine discontinuation. *J Clin Psychopharmacol* 1999;19:471–472.

43. Rapeport WG, Muirhead DC, Williams SA, et al. Absence of effect of sertraline on the pharmacokinetics and pharmacodynamics of phenytoin. *J Clin Psychiatry* 1996;57 Suppl 1:24–28.

44. Haselberger MB, Freedman LS, Tolbert S. Elevated serum phenytoin concentrations associated with coad-

ministration of sertraline. *J Clin Psychopharmacol* 1997;17:107—109.

45. Andersen BB, Mikkelsen M, Vesterager A, et al. No influence of the antidepressant paroxetine on carbamazepine, valproate and phenytoin. *Epilepsy Research* 1991;10:201–204.

46. Lucas RA, Gilfillan DJ, Bergstrom RF. A pharmacokinetic interaction between carbamazepine and olanzapine: observations on possible mechanism. *Eur J Clin Pharmacol* 1998;54:639–643.

47. Jerling M, Lindstrom L, Bondesson U, et al. Fluvoxamine inhibition and carbamazepine induction of the metabolism of clozapine: evidence from a *Therapeutic Drug Monitoring* service. *Therapeutic Drug Monitoring* 1994;16:368–374.

48. Spina E, Avenoso A, Facciola G, et al. Plasma concentrations of risperidone and 9-hydroxyrisperidone: effect of comedication with carbamazepine or valproate. *Therapeutic Drug Monitoring* 2000;22:481–485.

49. Miceli JJ, Anziano RJ, Robarge L, et al. The effect of carbamazepine on the steady-state pharmacokinetics of ziprasidone in healthy volunteers. *Br J Clin Pharmacol* 2000;49 Suppl 1:65S–70S.

50. Iwahashi K, Miyatake R, Suwaki H, et al. The drug–drug interaction effects of haloperidol on plasma carbamazepine levels. *Clin Neuropharmacol* 1995;18: 233–236.

51. Leinonen E, Lepola U, Koponen H. Substituting carbamazepine with oxcarbazepine increases citalopram levels. A report on two cases. *Pharmacopsychiatry* 1996;29:156–158.

52. Khan A, Shad MU, Preskorn SH. Lack of sertraline efficacy probably due to an interaction with carbamazepine. *J Clin Psychiatry* 2000;61:526–527.

53. Yukawa E, Nonaka T, Yukawa M, et al. Pharmacoepidemiologic investigation of a clonazepam-carbamazepine interaction by mixed effect modeling using routine clinical pharmacokinetic data in Japanese patients. *J Clin Psychopharmacol* 2001;21:588–593.

54. Mula M, Monaco F. Carbamazepine-risperidone interactions in patients with epilepsy. *Clin Neuropharmacol* 2002;25:97–100.

55. Grimsley SR, Jann MW, Carter JG, et al. Increased carbamazepine plasma concentrations after fluoxetine coadministration. *Clin Pharmacol Ther* 1991;50: 10–15.

56. Spina E, Avenoso A, Pollicino AM, et al. Carbamazepine coadministration with fluoxetine or fluvoxamine. *Therapeutic Drug Monitoring* 1993;15: 247–250.

57. Rapeport WG, Williams SA, Muirhead DC, et al. Absence of a sertraline-mediated effect on the pharmacokinetics and pharmacodynamics of carbamazepine. *J Clin Psychiatry* 1996;57 Suppl 1:20–23.

58. Ashton AK, Wolin RE. Nefazodone-induced carbamazepine toxicity. *Am J Psychiatry* 1996;153:733.

59. Conca A, Beraus W, Konig P, et al. A case of pharmacokinetic interference in comedication of clozapine and valproic acid. *Pharmacopsychiatry* 2000;33: 234–235.

60. Facciola G, Avenoso A, Scordo MG, et al. Small effects of valproic acid on the plasma concentrations of clozapine and its major metabolites in patients with schizophrenic or affective disorders. *Therapeutic Drug Monitoring* 1999;21:341–345.

61. Samara EE, Granneman RG, Witt GF, et al. Effect of valproate on the pharmacokinetics and pharmacodynamics of lorazepam. *J Clin Pharmacol* 1997;37: 442–450.

62. Droulers A, Bodak N, Oudjhani M, et al. Decrease of valproic acid concentration in the blood when coprescribed with fluoxetine. *J Clin Psychopharmacol* 1997;17:139–140.

63. Kasture SB, Mandhane SN, Chopde CT. Baclofen-induced catatonia: modification by serotonergic agents. *Neuropharmacol* 1996;35:595–598.

64. Isawa S, Murasaki M, Miura S, et al. Pharmacokinetic and pharmacodynamic interactions among haloperidol, carteolol hydrochloride and biperiden hydrochloride. *Nihon Shinkei Seishin Yakurigaku Zasshi* 1999; 19:111–118.

65. Hansen LB, Elley J, Christensen TR, et al. Plasma levels of perphenazine and its major metabolites during simultaneous treatment with anticholinergic drugs. *Br J Clin Pharmacol* 1979;7:75–80.

66. Blazer DG 2nd, Federspiel CF, Ray WA, et al. The risk of anticholinergic toxicity in the elderly: a study of prescribing practices in two populations. *J Gerontology* 1983;38:31–35.

67. Anderson GD, Gidal BE, Kantor ED, et al. Lorazepam-valproate interaction: studies in normal subjects and isolated perfused rat liver. *Epilepsia* 1994;35:221–225.

68. Richens A, Marshall RW, Dirach J, et al. Absence of interaction between tiagabine, a new antiepileptic drug, and the benzodiazepine triazolam. *Drug Metab Drug Interact* 1998;14:159–177.

69. Gardner MJ, Baris BA, Wilner KD, et al. Effect of sertraline on the pharmacokinetics and protein binding of diazepam in healthy volunteers. *Clin Pharmacokinetics* 1997;32 Suppl 1:43–49.

70. Bonate PL, Kroboth PD, Smith RB, et al. Clonazepam and sertraline: absence of drug interaction in a multiple-dose study. *J Clin Psychopharmacol* 2000;20: 19–27.

71. Greene DS, Salazar DE, Dockens RC, et al. Coadministration of nefazodone and benzodiazepines: IV. A pharmacokinetic interaction study with lorazepam. *J Clin Psychopharmacol* 1995;15:409–416.

72. Troy SM, Lucki I, Peirgies AA, et al. Pharmacokinetic and pharmacodynamic evaluation of the potential drug interaction between venlafaxine and diazepam. *J Clin Pharmacol* 1995;35:410–419.

73. Greenblatt DJ, Preskorn SH, Cotreau MM, et al. Fluoxetine impairs clearance of alprazolam but not of clonazepam. *Clin Pharmacol Ther* 1992;52:479–486.

74. Hamilton SP, Nunes EV, Janal M, et al. The effect of sertraline on methadone plasma levels in methadone-maintenance patients. *Am J Addictions* 2000;9:63–69.

75. Begre S, von Bardeleben U, Ladewig D, et al. Paroxetine increases steady-state concentrations of (R)-methadone in CYP2D6 extensive but not poor metabolizers. *J Clin Psychopharmacol* 2002;22:211–215.

76. Alderman CP, Frith PA. Fluvoxamine-methadone interaction. *Aus NZ J Psychiatry* 1999;33:99–101.

77. DeMaria PA Jr, Serota RD. A therapeutic use of the methadone fluvoxamine drug interaction. *J Addictive Diseases* 1999;18:5–12.

78. Bertschy G, Baumann P, Eap CB, et al. Probable metabolic interaction between methadone and fluvoxamine

in addict patients. *Therapeutic Drug Monitoring* 1994;16:42–45.

79. Erjavec MK, Coda BA, Nguyen Q, et al. Morphine-fluoxetine interactions in healthy volunteers: analgesia and side effects. *J Clin Pharmacol* 2000;40:1286–1295.

80. Kesavan S, Sobala GM. Serotonin syndrome with fluoxetine plus tramadol. *J Royal Soc* Med 1999;92: 474–475.

81. Mason BJ, Blackburn KH. Possible serotonin syndrome associated with tramadol and sertraline coadministration. *Ann Pharmacother* 1997;31:175–177.

82. Egberts AC, ter Borgh J, Brodie-Meijer CC. Serotonin syndrome attributed to tramadol addition to paroxetine therapy. *Int Clin Psychopharmacol* 1997; 12:181–182.

83. Lantz MS, Buchalter EN, Giambanco V. Serotonin syndrome following the administration of tramadol with paroxetine. *Int J Geriatric Psychiatry* 1998;13: 343–345.

84. Gordon NC, Heller PH, Gear RW, et al. Interactions between fluoxetine and opiate analgesia for postoperative dental pain. *Pain* 1994;58:85–88.

85. Petrakis I, Carroll KM, Nich C, et al. Fluoxetine treatment of depressive disorders in methadone-maintained opioid addicts. *Drug Alcohol Dependence* 1998;50: 221–226.

86. de Abajo FJ, Rodriguez LA, Montero D. Association between selective serotonin reuptake inhibitors and upper gastrointestinal bleeding: population based case-control study. *BMJ* 1999;319(7217):1106–1109.

87. Finley PR, Warner MD, Peabody CA. Clinical relevance of drug interactions with lithium. *Clin Pharmacokinet* 1995;29(3):172–191.

88. Priskorn M, Sidhu JS, Larsen F, et al. Investigation of multiple dose citalopram on the pharmacokinetics and pharmacodynamics of racemic warfarin. *Br J Clin Pharmacol* 1997;44:199–202.

89. Duncan D, Sayal K, McConnell H, et al. Antidepressant interactions with warfarin. *Int Clin Psychopharmacol* 1998;13:87–94.

90. Woolfrey S, Gammack NS, Dewar MS, et al. Fluoxetine-warfarin interaction. *BMJ* 1993;307(6898):241.

91. Dent LA, Orrock MW. Warfarin-fluoxetine and diazepam-fluoxetine interaction. *Pharmacotherapy* 1997;17:170–172.

92. Ford MA, Anderson ML, Rindone JP, et al. Lack of effect of fluoxetine on the hypoprothrombinemic response of warfarin. *J Clin Psychopharmacol* 1997; 17:110 112.

93. Apseloff G, Wilner KD, Gerber N, et al. Effect of sertraline on protein binding of warfarin. *Clin Pharmacokinetics* 1997;32 Suppl 1:37–42.

94. Ouellet D, Hsu A, Qian J, et al. Effect of fluoxetine on pharmacokinetics of ritonavir. *Antimicrobial Agents Chemother* 1998;42:3107–112.

95. Levin GM, Nelson LA, DeVane CL, et al. A pharmacokinetic drug–drug interaction study of venlafaxine and indinavir. *Psychopharmacol Bull* 2001;35:62–71.

96. Piscitelli SC, Buratein AH, Chaitt D, et al. Indinavir concentrations and St. John's wort. *Lancet* 2000;35 (9203):547–548.

97. Penzak SR, Hon YY, Lawhorn WD, et al. Influence of ritonavir on olanzapine pharmacokinetics in healthy volunteers. *J Clin Psychopharmacol* 2002;22:336–370.

98. Zalma A, von Moltke LL, Granda BW, et al. In vitro metabolism of trazodone by CYP3A4: inhibition by ketoconazole and human immunodeficiency protease inhibitors. *Biol Psychiatry* 2000;47:655–661.

99. Rotzinger S, Baker GB. Human CYP3A4 and the metabolism of nefazodone and hydroxynefazodone by human liver microsomes and heterologously expressed enzymes. *Eur Neuropsychopharmacol* 2002;12:91–100.

100. von Moltke LL, Greenblatt DJ, Cotreau-Bibbo MM, et al. Inhibitors of alprazolam metabolism in vitro: effect of serotonin-reuptake-inhibitor antidepressants, ketoconazole, and quinidine. *Br J Clin Pharmacol* 1997; 43:315–318.

101. Hesse LM, von Moltke LL, Shader PI, et al. Ritonavir, efavirenz, and nelfinavir inhibit CYP2B6 activity in vitro: potential drug interactions with bupropion. *Drug Metabolism Disposition* 2001;29:100–102.

102. Lee DO, Lee CD. Serotonin syndrome in a child associated with erythromycin and sertraline. *Pharmacother* 1999;19:894–896.

103. Fisman S, Reniers D, Diaz P. Erythromycin interaction with risperidone or clomipramine in an adolescent. *J Child Adol Psychopharmacol* 1996;6:133–138.

104. Luurila H, Olkkola KT, Neuvonen PJ. Interaction between erythromycin and the benzodiazepines diazepam and flunitrazepam. *Pharmacol Toxicol* 1996; 78:117–122.

105. Kamali F, Thomas SH, Edwards C. The influence of steady-state ciprofloxacin on the pharmacokinetics and pharmacodynamics of a single dose of diazepam in healthy volunteers. *Eur J Clin Pharmacol* 1993; 44:365–367.

106. Micelli JJ, Smith M, Robarge L, et al. The effects of ketoconazole on ziprasidone pharmacokinetics–a placebo-controlled crossover study in healthy volunteers. *Br J Clin Pharmacol* 2000;49 Suppl 1:71S–76S.

24

Substance Abuse and Women with Disabilities

Jo Ann Ford, Margaret K. Glenn, Li Li, and Dennis C. Moore

Substance abuse has been a continuing problem in our society for many years. Increasing efforts have been made to understand why different populations become dependent on substances and to identify prevention and treatment models for different groups of people. For example, in recent years, there has been an emphasis on developing and evaluating treatment models specific to women. Although there has been some success in these efforts, people with disabilities, particularly women with disabilities, tend to be overlooked. This is despite a growing body of research indicating that people with disabilities use alcohol and illicit drugs as much as, if not more than, the general population (1–3).

Studies related to alcohol and other drug use have continued to show that women drink and use illicit drugs less than men do; however, there is still a concern related to the number of women who do use substances and to the consequences of their use. For example, women experience higher blood alcohol levels than men when equal amounts are consumed per pound of body weight, and they appear to develop health-related complications more rapidly than men with less alcohol intake (4). Women also are more likely than men to report psychoactive prescription drug use, and women who are polydrug abusers tend to be addicted to alcohol and prescribed drugs (5,6).

The 1999 National Household Survey on Drug Abuse (7) found that 36% of women ages 12 and older report a lifetime use of illicit drugs, with 9.6% reporting some drug use in the past year and 4.9% reporting some illicit drug use in the past 30 days. Just more than 41% of women reported current alcohol use; 13.1% reported binge drinking and 2.4% reported heavy alcohol use within the past month. Binge drinking was defined as consuming five or more drinks on one occasion at least 1 day during the past month, and heavy drinking was defined as consuming at least five drinks on one occasion at least 5 days in the past month.

The highest rates of illicit drug use were found in women between the ages of 18 and 25 (49% lifetime use, 25% use in the past year, and 13.1% use in the past month). The highest rates of alcohol use also were found in women who were between the ages of 18 and 25 (51.5%). Women in this same age group also reported binge drinking (28.1%) and heavy drinking (6.9%) more often than women in other age groups. Despite these high percentages of women reporting alcohol and illicit drug use, including binge drinking and heavy alcohol consumption, only 3.4% of women reported alcohol or illicit drug dependency, compared to 6% of men. Also, only 0.9% of women reported involvement in treatment during the past year, compared to 1.7% of men. These data support research findings that women, particularly women with disabilities, are still less likely to seek substance abuse treatment when problems arise (8–10).

In an epidemiologic study conducted by the Rehabilitation Research and Training Center on Drugs and Disability at Wright State University in Dayton, Ohio, a survey

Table 24-1. *Demographic characteristics of female participants (n = 1,671)[a]*

		Percentage	Number
Age	24 or younger	28.3	470
	25–34 years	22.3	371
	35–44 years	28.5	474
	45 or older	20.9	348
Race/ethnicity	Caucasian	72.0	1,162
	African American	18.1	292
	Native American	4.5	72
	Hispanic American	3.0	49
	Asian American	0.3	5
	Other/multicultural	2.1	33
Marital status	Never married	47.0	782
	Married	22.2	369
	Widowed/divorced/separated	29.4	490
	Other	1.4	24
Education	<12 years	13.0	216
	12 years	35.1	582
	>12 years	51.9	862
Income	Less than $5,000	23.8	372
	$5,000–$9,999	25.7	401
	$10,000–$19,999	21.7	339
	$20,000–$39,999	19.2	300
	$40,000 or more	9.5	148
Employment	Unemployed	40.8	675
	Work full time	11.6	192
	Work part time	16.6	275
	Student	18.8	310
	Supported/sheltered/temporary	7.3	120
	Other	4.9	81

[a]These data are from an epidemiologic study conducted between 1993 and 1999 by Substance Abuse Resources and Disability Issues (SARDI), Wright State University, Dayton, OH.

was used to determine the alcohol and drug use patterns of people qualifying for state vocational rehabilitation services. To qualify for these services, an individual must have a documented disability that significantly impairs her or his ability to obtain gainful employment without rehabilitation services. The study was conducted in a total of nine states between 1993 and 1999. There were a total of 3,173 respondents in this survey, 1,671 of whom were women. Table 24-1 describes the demographic characteristics of

Table 24-2. *Alcohol and illicit drug use, comparing women in the general population to women with disabilities*

	Women without disabilities (%)[a]	Women with disabilities (%)[b]
Lifetime use of illicit drugs	36	40.1
Use of illicit drugs in past year	9.6	14.5
Use of illicit drugs in past month	4.9	7.6
Current use of alcohol	41	31.4
Binge drinking in past month	13.1	9.6
Heavy drinking in past month	2.4	1.7
Combine alcohol and prescribed medications	—	26.7

[a]These data are from the 1999 National Household Survey on Drug Abuse, Substance Abuse and Mental Health Services Administration (SAMSHA).

[b]These data are from an epidemiologic study conducted between 1993 and 1999 by Substance Abuse Resources and Disability Issues (SARDI), Wright State University, Dayton, OH.

Table 24-3. *Percentage distribution of illicit drug use by women with disabilities (n = 1,648)[a]*

	Ever used	Used past year	Used past month
Marijuana	44.5	12.2	5.9
Cocaine	16.9	2.4	0.9
Crack	8.8	2.3	1.0
Inhalants	6.9	0.5	0.4
Hallucinogens	14.3	0.8	0.2
Stimulants	20.6	2.0	0.7
Sedatives/tranquilizers	18.1	3.5	1.6

[a]These data are from an epidemiologic study conducted between 1993 and 1999 by Substance Abuse Resources and Disability Issues (SARDI), Wright State University, Dayton, OH.

the women with disabilities who participated in this study.

Women with disabilities in this study reported higher rates of lifetime illicit drug use (40.1%), use of illicit drugs in the past year (14.5%), and use of illicit drugs in the past month (7.6%) when compared to women in the general population. Fewer women with disabilities reported current alcohol use (31.4%), binge drinking (9.6%), and heavy alcohol use (1.7%) when compared to women in the general population. It also should be noted that binge drinking in the Wright State University study was defined as "4 or 5 drinks" as opposed to "5 or more" defined by Substance Abuse and Mental Health Services Administration (SAMSHA) (7). This clearly indicated that women with disabilities are less likely to binge drink or drink heavily when compared to women in the general population (Table 24-2.) Women with disabilities also were asked if they had ever combined alcohol and prescribed medications with the intent of getting high or intoxicated, and 26.7% answered affirmatively. As shown in Table 24-3, marijuana is the most commonly used illicit drug for women with disabilities, followed by stimulants, and sedatives/tranquilizers.

Not surprisingly, women with chemical dependency as a primary disability were more likely to report illicit drug use in the past year than women with other disabilities. As shown in Table 24-4, women with mental illness were also more likely to have used illicit drugs, whereas women with developmental disabilities were the least likely to have used these substances in the past year. These findings support the literature in the field indicating that people with mental illness often have dual diagnoses and people with mental retardation are less likely to use alcohol or other drugs (11,12).

Table 24-4. *Percentage distribution of any illicit drug use (past 12 months) by disability (n = 1,489)[a]*

Primary disability	Illicit drug use in the past 12 months (%)	Total number
Mental illness	22.0	309
Physical disability	11.9	185
Sensory disability	11.0	145
Medical disability	13.3	421
Learning disability/mental retardation	4.6	216
Chemical dependency	34.5	50
Traumatic brain injury	16.7	66
Other	19.1	89
Total	14.5	1,489

[a]These data are from an epidemiologic study conducted between 1993 and 1999 by Substance Abuse Resources and Disability Issues (SARDI), Wright State University, Dayton, OH.

Women today still are faced with social stigma relating to their use of alcohol and other drugs. Continuing misconceptions about how alcohol effects women (e.g., making them more sexually aggressive or immoral) lead to negative stereotypes. This social stigma placed on women who abuse alcohol or other drugs is much greater than their male counterparts, resulting in feelings of guilt and shame as well as a poor self-image (13). Consistent with findings from a variety of studies, this negative stigma contributes to the large numbers of these women who are victims of aggression and violence and, in fact, may lead to the condoning of violence and other victimization of women who drink (14,15).

The reasons for using alcohol and other drugs and the risk factors associated with using drugs are different for men and women. Women report that they drink and use illicit drugs in a more medicinal way as an effort to relieve physical or psychologic pain (16–18). Women tend to seek treatment as a result of feelings of depression that are worsening. Women who do enter treatment identify high levels of depression, recurring guilt or shame related to substance use, and negative views of themselves. Women who abuse alcohol and other drugs report greater psychologic distress, more medical problems, and a greater level of addiction severity compared to men (19).

Studies related to substance use and abuse by people with disabilities emerged in the 1980s and 1990s. A growing number of studies have demonstrated that the presence of a physical, mental, or psychologic disability can elevate a person's risk for problems with the use of alcohol or other drugs (2,20). It has become more and more evident that people with disabilities have a higher rate of illicit drug use than the general population.

MENTAL ILLNESS

A dual diagnosis of mental illness and substance abuse is not uncommon in women seeking treatment for either an alcohol- or drug-related problem or for a significant mental disorder (21). In general, women show higher rates of dual diagnoses than men, and women reporting for treatment are more likely to be admitted to the hospital with affective disorders such as major depression (22). A study related to the prevalence of attention deficit/hyperactivity disorder (ADHD) among substance abusers found that overall, 19% of the women studied met the DSM IV (Diagnostic and Statistic Manual IV) criteria for the disorder; in addition, the women with ADHD reported a higher number of alcohol-related treatment episodes when compared to the women without ADHD (23). There also is evidence for higher rates of bulimia and other eating disorders among women seeking treatment for substance abuse (24) and in a national sample of women (25).

TRAUMATIC INJURIES

There have been many studies relating to alcohol abuse as a cause of trauma-related disabilities such as brain injury and spinal cord injury (SCI) (26–28). The patterns of drinking prior to traumatic injury also have been explored. Kreutzer and colleagues (29) looked at the preinjury and postinjury drinking patterns of 87 people with traumatic brain injuries and a noninjured control group. They found that a significantly higher proportion of consumers fell within the heavy drinker classification, although they drank less postinjury than the control group. A similar study found that a significant number of head trauma survivors with a history of substance abuse prior to the injury return to their previous patterns of alcohol and other drug use (30). Additionally, the average Michigan Alcoholism Screening Test (MAST) score for consumers with SCIs was 7, with 49% of the sample posting scores of 6 or higher, which can be indicative of alcohol dependence or abuse (31). Another study looked at college students with physical disabilities and found that those with congenital disabilities consumed much less alcohol than the general population, whereas those students with trauma-generated disabilities drank more than the estimates from the general population (32).

DEAFNESS AND HEARING IMPAIRMENTS

Studies related to the patterns of drinking and illicit drug use by people who are deaf or hearing impaired are difficult to conduct, and the results of the few available studies are varied. An early study (33) of individuals who are deaf reports drinking patterns that are similar to the general population, with the highest drinking rates reported by those individuals who had attended residential schools for the deaf. These results were substantiated in additional studies, which report that people with hearing impairments have substance abuse rates that are similar to the general population (34). An additional study of students in a residential school for the deaf found that the alcohol and illicit drug use patterns were similar to those of youth of the same age in the general population; however, legal problems related to drinking were much higher among the students who were deaf (35).

INTELLECTUAL DISABILITIES

Research related to individuals with intellectual disabilities consistently report that people with mental retardation are less likely to drink alcohol or use other drugs when compared to the general population (2,11,12,36). Additional information indicates that those individuals with intellectual disabilities who do drink and use illicit drugs were more likely to have an early onset of use and have experienced recurring episodes of intoxication by age 15 (11). There also is some evidence indicating that people with mental retardation who do drink experience recurring alcohol-related problems and consequences even with smaller amounts of alcohol (36,37).

HUMAN IMMUNODEFICIENCY VIRUS/ACQUIRED IMMUNE DEFICIENCY SYNDROME

Acquired immune deficiency syndrome (AIDS) is the fourth leading cause of death among women in their childbearing years (38). The rates of women infected with the human immunodeficiency virus (HIV) are growing at a faster rate than other populations. Many of these women are of minority background, poor, addicted to drugs, or sexually involved with drug users (38,39). Transmission of HIV is associated substantially with a number of substance abuse–related factors, including the use of contaminated or used needles to inject heroin and engagement of risky sex behaviors in exchange for powder or crack cocaine, among others. In addition, women may engage in these risky behaviors while they are under the influence of alcohol or other drugs or while they are under coercion (40). Once infected, continued alcohol and drug use will impact the progression of the disease as it weakens the immune system.

RISK FACTORS FOR SUBSTANCE ABUSE FOR WOMEN WITH DISABILITIES

Problems related to alcohol and other drugs are considered to be the number one public health problem in the United States. As such, it is essential that any efforts to treat this should consider the factors that make it possible for the disease to develop. One approach is to look at the contributing influences in lives of individuals that seem to occur statistically more often for those with substance abuse problems. These can be individual, family, and social/cultural characteristics.

People with disabilities could have a number of challenges in their lives that place them at risk for use and abuse of alcohol and other drugs that are similar to those faced by the general population. They include negative self-concept, family history of substance abuse, and peer pressure. One can view these circumstances as leading to an increase in physical, mental, and emotional vulnerability. This vulnerability could result in a setting where substances may be used to aid in coping.

There are many such issues associated with the presence of a disability in an individual's life. For example, compared to the general population, people with disabilities are more likely to experience medical problems; chronic pain; personal and social adjustment issues; unusual developmental experiences; excess free time; school and employment problems; higher incidence of poverty; and enabling by family members, school personnel, and health care providers. Additionally, the social stigma related to disability can make it easy to overlook substance abuse until the problems become more severe and significantly more difficult to treat (8).

Although both women with and without disabilities use alcohol and illicit drugs less than their male counterparts, they are more likely to experience problems such as depression, physical and sexual abuse and assault, unwanted pregnancies, sexually transmitted diseases, and marital difficulties. They often use alcohol and other drugs to cope with past abuse, and childhood sexual abuse has been linked with later problem drinking (41,42). Women also are at higher risk for developing physical health complications that can be attributed to substance abuse, such as cirrhosis of the liver and lung and breast cancer (43). Women are more likely to combine prescription drugs with alcohol (44,45).

Women with disabilities face many difficulties that contribute to or encourage alcohol and other drug use. These may be more severe than those encountered by women without disabilities. This problem may need to be examined in a number of ways. Women with disabilities confront challenges from at least two vantage points: that of being a woman and that of being disabled. They also may find themselves confronting factors that are related to their racial or cultural background,

their sexual orientation, or the environment in which they grew up. These begin to compound themselves into a picture of a group of individuals who are especially vulnerable to the problematic use of alcohol and other drugs.

Some of the more common substance abuse risk factors for women include peer pressure, low self-esteem, victimization, gender stereotypes, and family history of substance abuse (46,47). Some of the additional factors that place women with disabilities at risk–issues that require attention–are explained as follows.

Lack of Identification of Substance Abuse Problems

It is not unusual for family members, friends, and professionals to miss warning signs of substance abuse problems in women with disabilities. The behaviors that can be attributed to alcohol or other drug use could be attributed to the disability; therefore, substance abuse problems that develop may be less likely to be identified. The stigma associated with alcohol and drug abuse in women makes it more likely that women with disabilities will be overlooked as substance abusers even when symptoms are visible (48). In general, women are more likely to seek assistance for alcohol and other drug problems through informal routes such as suggestions of family and friends, and they are more likely to be referred to the mental health system (47), which may not consider substance abuse as a cause of the issues brought to their attention. By the time alcohol and other drug use problems are identified as the root of the challenges experienced by the woman with a disability, the substance abuse is likely to be very severe, making it less treatable.

Use of Prescribed Medications

Women with disabilities may take two or more prescribed medications, and many people with physical disabilities are likely to take up to five or more concurrent medications depending on age and the physical impairment (32,49). This increases their risk for the misuse or abuse of these medications, possibly using them for purposes other than those for which they were prescribed (45). In addition, the dangers in using alcohol and other drugs in conjunction with prescribed medications can be overlooked easily, particularly when medical professionals assume that women with disabilities do not drink alcohol or use illicit drugs. Some physicians also have the attitude that the disability is a condition that must be "fixed," and this attitude certainly is prevalent in today's society. With this "quick fix" attitude, women with disabilities may be offered additional prescription medications to alleviate their symptoms. These scenarios could create a variety of risks for substance use problems, including a compromised drug tolerance, addiction to prescription medications, and overmedication.

Some women with disabilities may be taking prescribed medications without understanding the potential side effects or the possible consequences of drinking or using other drugs in conjunction with these prescriptions. Additionally, some women with disabilities may not understand the specific nature of their disabilities or how their disabilities influence the way their bodies react to alcohol and other drugs. This lack of information coupled with the continued use of alcohol and other drugs can contribute to secondary disabilities or to reinjuries.

Self-medication for pain is a significant risk factor in disabilities of traumatic origin and for mental health conditions. Prescribed narcotic, antianxiety, and sedative medications are particularly dangerous, especially when used over a longer period. Women with disabilities who use these medications with other prescribed psychoactive medications and in combination with alcohol face significant health risks.

Marta, a young woman who experienced an SCI as a result of her alcohol and other drug use, described her misuse of medication: "When I left the hospital after my inpatient rehabilitation, I was still really depressed and was scared to death. The fears were more than I could talk about. Of course, I only knew one way to deal with fear—drinking and using drugs. I would call the doctor and put in my order: 'I need Quaaludes; I need Valium; I need codeine.' The doctor never questioned my requests. He would call in the prescriptions, and the pharmacy would deliver it to my house."

Atypical Social Experiences and Opportunities

Some women with disabilities are isolated from others outside their immediate families and service providers. They can be segregated into at-risk environments, often experiencing high levels of poverty, and lack access to services and social opportunities (50). Alcohol is still a common facilitator of social interactions, and some women with disabilities may have difficulty finding drug-free social alternatives. Some women with disabilities may find that peer groups that endorse drug use are the easiest to access because of these groups' acceptance of attributes that are different from the norms of society (51,52). The desire for social acceptance may reinforce alcohol and other drug use as a means of making the disability less noticeable.

Individuals with disabilities sometimes struggle with peer group and related social issues, especially in cases of congenital or early-onset disabilities. Women with these disabilities may be isolated from peers, with fewer opportunities to develop relationships. Frequent isolation, in some cases, can increase risk for substance abuse by depriving women of the opportunity to learn constructive peer interaction or to practice peer pressure resistance skills. Disabilities acquired later in life, including those affecting older women, also carry social consequences. The onset of a disability can necessitate a modification in social activities. It may include a greater likelihood for isolation, restricted mobility, or excess free time, all of which increase the risk for substance abuse.

> Leticia, a 43-year-old woman who experienced a traumatic brain injury at age 35, reported the following experiences after her injury: "My brother signed me out of the hospital after about 5 days. I had just come out of the coma. I don't remember very much of the next year other than I stayed in my house and was afraid a lot of the time. I wouldn't talk to any of my friends or go out if I thought that someone would see me. My brother would bring me groceries and check in on me. After about a year, I did start going back to the Alcoholics Anonymous meetings that I attended before my head injury. I wouldn't talk to anyone or tell anyone what I had gone through. My friends knew that I was different, and they avoided me too. I relapsed a number of times in this 2-year period."

Physical and Attitudinal Inaccessibility

Despite the passage of the Americans with Disabilities Act requiring equal access for people with disabilities, little progress has been made compared to the need. More buildings are becoming accessible, yet surveys indicate that significant numbers of treatment programs and service provider facilities such as shelters for battered women are not physically or otherwise accessible (53). In addition, many service providers have not had sufficient experience with people with disabilities to understand how to make their services fully accessible. The attitudes of professionals also can make the programs inaccessible to individuals with disabilities. For example, some people believe that all individuals who are deaf can read lips, refusing to see the need for interpreter services. Another scenario may be a treatment provider refusing admission to a woman who is using phenobarbital to control seizures because that particular medication has the potential to be abused.

Societal Attitudes Regarding Physical Perfection in Women

As is evident from advertisements and television, today's society continues to focus on physical perfection, particularly for women, creating the belief that women with disabilities are "imperfect" or "undesirable." In addition to experiencing discrimination, this contributes to poor self-image and feelings of shame about the disability. Women with disabilities often are encouraged, either overtly or subtly, to hide their disabilities, placing them in a situation where they may ignore obvious risk factors to fit in with their peers. To feel desirable or to find companionship, women with disabilities may use alcohol or other drugs as a means of initiating a physical or social relationship.

Entitlement

In part because of societal attitudes related to disability, family members, friends, and service providers sometimes make extraordinary accommodations for women with disabilities. Well-meaning individuals even may believe that a woman with a disability is more entitled to use alcohol or other drugs as a compensation for the disability. For example, many people without disabilities think or even say, "If I had a disability, I'd drink too." In addition, there is a pervasive belief that people with disabilities are sick and need medication to treat or cure their illness. Women with disabilities often are perceived by the uninitiated public as people who are entitled to additional compensation for what is viewed as a burden. This concept of "entitlement" also allows people with disabilities to avoid the consequences of substance abuse (54). It is a concept that exceeds the realm of "enabling," a common term in the substance abuse treatment field. Entitlement is believing that individuals with disabilities have more of a right to use alcohol or illicit drugs because of the disability. In contrast to the perception of others, people with disabilities do not tend to feel more entitled to use alcohol or other drugs because of the disability (32).

History of Victimization

The link between domestic violence, violence against women, and substance abuse is one of the strongest found in the research literature (14). The National Institute on Drug Abuse reports that up to 70% of women who abuse drugs have a history of physical and sexual abuse (45). Women with substance use disorders report childhood sexual abuse and other abuses more often than women who are not problem drinkers (45,55). There is a correlation between increased sexual assault and alcohol use that leads women to feel more responsible for what happened and men less so (56).

Women with abusive partners or who are sexually coerced are at higher risk for contracting sexually transmitted diseases including HIV infection (57,58). Women who are abused are also at increased risk for permanent disability including head trauma, physical disfigurement, and SCI (59).

Leticia described her experiences with two different partners, both of whom were abusive toward her. "I met a man when I was in residential treatment. I was single at the time, and I am one of those women who feel better and happier if I am in love. I fell in love with this man and moved in with him after treatment. On New Year's Eve, he went out with some friends. He came home high on crack and started attacking me. He hit me in the forehead with a baseball bat. That's all I remember of the incident, but I know that he threw me out of the second-story window. That's how I got my head injury. Several years later, I became involved with another man. He always would belittle me and make me feel badly about myself. At one point I went to donate blood at a local blood drive. A couple of weeks later, I got a phone call from the Red Cross telling me that I had tested positive for HIV. I told my boyfriend about the HIV, and he told me that he had it too."

Women with disabilities are more likely to be victimized than women without disabilities (53). This is often the result of segregation, poverty, and economic and social dependence on others (50). Women with various disabilities who experience abuse tend to have their experiences invalidated more often. For example, society tends to deny that women with disabilities are victims of violence by believing that the perpetrators act inappropriately as a result of being overtired or overworked because of the burden of caring for women with disabilities (50,60). In this way, violence toward women with disabilities is masked as socially acceptable behavior within families and institutions.

PREVENTION AND TREATMENT ISSUES

Addressing substance abuse issues is a difficult task in any population but especially for people with multiple stigmas associated with substance abuse such as women with disabilities. There are fewer social, programmatic, and recreational options for women with disabilities, especially when major changes in lifestyle are being attempted. For these reasons, assistance and additional resources are necessary to address substance abuse problems adequately.

There continues to be a significant lack of accessible and appropriate substance abuse prevention and treatment services for people with disabilities, particularly for women with disabilities. Women are less likely than men to be diagnosed with alcohol or other drug use problems and thus are less likely to be referred for any related treatment services. Additionally, women with physical challenges who are receiving disability services typically are not identified as having substance abuse issues even when they are displaying problematic behavior or other symptoms (8). In recent years there has been some interest in addressing substance abuse within social services and criminal justice systems, which have begun referring or even mandating that women participate in alcohol and drug addiction services. The women who are referred to treatment from this assistance appear to have higher rates of disability than do their male counterparts (61).

Prevention must occur at many levels beginning with community, consumer, and professional education and training. Some disability groups, such as people with traumatic injuries and people with mental illness, recently have been targeted for prevention efforts; however, all disability groups must be included in intervention outreach—not just those considered to be at the highest risk. In addition, prevention and treatment efforts still need to be focused on women with disabilities who frequently are disenfranchised.

A variety of prevention and treatment strategies are appropriate to consider, including child care, parenting education, financial counseling, suicide assessment, stress management services, vocational evaluation, and advocacy. These strategies may vary depending on the particular disability because, although some disability characteristics are similar, the specific substance abuse risks can be different. The following are some strategies that may assist women with disabilities:

Disability-Specific Support Groups

Support groups have been shown to be particularly effective for addressing a number of issues faced by women and by people with disabilities. Support groups can provide an opportunity to share feelings and experiences in an informal setting and can foster relationships outside of a treatment or therapeutic setting. Issues related specifically to disability management and lifestyle choices can be explored by people who share common experiences and similar functional impairments. Substance abuse issues also may be discussed within a disability-oriented context, allowing for the development of coping strategies that are practical and possibly more realistic.

Leticia states, "I get some of what I need in AA. I like the women's meeting that is here in town. I need more than this though. I see the same people in all the meetings because I live in such a small town. I want to talk about my disability, but I can't. People don't understand why I can't always remember stuff that I hear. I also can't talk about my HIV. I go through a lot of fear about my health, but being in a small town, I don't want everyone to know about my HIV. I wish that there was a place to get support for my disability and for my alcohol problems. I would even like to have a hotline or someplace to call where I could discuss things when I get depressed and it's related to my head injury or to the HIV."

Education About Medications

Consumers, pharmacists, physicians, and nurses can be valuable sources of information about how medications interact with alcohol and other drugs. All parties involved with women with disabilities need to have a thorough understanding of the implications for taking prescription medications including criteria for prescription misuse (62). The long-term effects of prescribed medication management also should be considered, and regular medication checks can be encouraged. These strategies can be beneficial in preventing overmedication, prescription medication misuse, and iatrogenic substance dependence.

Decisionmaking and Assertiveness Skills Training

Current mainstream prevention materials have some focus in this area, and many of these materials can be adapted or offered in different learning modalities for women with disabilities. Included in this component should be issues associated with accessing the community in the context of a disability. This training can include socialization skills and exploration of social activities that do not rely on alcohol or other drug use. Healthy activities to fill free time and to cope with a lack of social outlets also can be explored.

Substance Abuse Screenings for Behavior Problems and Traumas

When women with disabilities have experienced injury, a brief screening can be administered to determine whether substances were used at the time of the injury or if alcohol or other drugs were used on a regular basis. A screening also can be used for women with disabilities who are exhibiting behavior problems at school or in other social settings including work or rehabilitation. Legal problems, missed appointments, and absences from work or school are examples of behavior that may suggest the need for substance abuse screening.

> According to Marta, "At the age of 22, I decided to go for a motorcycle ride with a guy who apparently had been drinking all day. I had been drinking and was taking Quaaludes. We didn't get too far before we crashed. I was resuscitated and diagnosed with a broken neck and a broken back. The doctors told my family that I probably wouldn't live through the night. The only thing that I remember about that time was the horrible pain, and I was given large amounts of narcotic drugs. I had a hard time understanding that I now had a disability. I hadn't really seen a young person with a disability before, and I didn't understand why the hospital couldn't just fix me up and send me home. The doctor finally told me that I may never walk again, and I remember thinking that I need more drugs than they are giving me."

Training for Rehabilitation Professionals

The identification of substance abuse in people with disabilities is not occurring at the rate that current research suggests is needed, meaning that many women with disabilities are not being helped. Because of the complexity and uniqueness of problems associated with a dual diagnosis such as substance abuse and disability, consumers cannot be expected to always find their own adequate solutions. Rehabilitation professionals and primary care providers are in an excellent position to identify potential risks for substance abuse and to assist women with disabilities in addressing these risks. Learning about substance abuse and disability risks and recognizing the early signs and symptoms of drug and alcohol problems are valuable first steps to supporting and assisting women with disabilities in finding unique solutions to these problems.

Training for Substance Abuse Professionals

Training related to the implications and realities of the Americans with Disabilities Act is critical for substance abuse professionals. These clinicians also need to receive training in how to conduct activities to address alternative learning styles and in ways to adapt traditional treatment to accommodate women with disabilities. Substance abuse professionals also need to become aware of the risks for drug and alcohol abuse that may be prevalent in women with disabilities. This could improve communication when women with disabilities are identified as having substance abuse problems. Facts about disabilities and disability awareness training are also important areas for these professionals.

Training for Medical Professionals

Physicians do not routinely ask about alcohol and other drug use during office visits. Medical staff may be unaware of the risks for substance abuse associated with disability, and it is likely that many physicians inadvertently enable the continued use of alcohol and other drugs by women with disabilities. Providing training in identifying substance abuse risks and symptoms and implementing substance abuse screening should affect the medical outcomes for women with disabilities in a favorable way through earlier identification of substance abuse problems. When physicians make a referral for treatment and then provide follow-up care and support, women with disabilities may be more likely to either enter treatment or explore other alternatives to substance use.

Assessments

Assessments and interventions should consider a number of issues that may be prevalent for women with disabilities including issues related to mental health problems, suicidal tendencies, history of sexual and physical abuse, parenting concerns, and sexuality. Women who experience concerns related to past trauma may require therapeutic intervention immediately because these can lead to substance abuse. Issues related to early environmental stress, including sexual or other abuse, have been associated with lower self-preservation and higher suicidal ideation (63). Other mental health concerns to consider during an assessment relate to the feelings of shame and stigma associated with drinking for women, and women with disabilities have the added social stigma associated with disability. The assessment also should consider parenting skills and concerns because many women with disabilities have had poor role modeling or no role modeling for the parenting skills that they need, and they may feel overwhelmed or inadequate as parents (5). Both Marta and Leticia had suicidal ideations after becoming disabled. Leticia had tried to commit suicide one time at age 11 prior to the onset of any disability.

> Marta states, "I got so very depressed. I went to mental hospitals a number of times. I always felt like I didn't want to live, but I was too afraid to die."

Employment

Meaningful employment is very important to people with disabilities, particularly women. This population consistently faces difficulties with unemployment or underemployment. Women in general report to treatment with fewer marketable employment skills and lower income (19). Women who complete treatment programs report higher educational levels and more job experience than women who drop out of treatment prior to completion (64).

Alcohol and other drug use can be a way for some people to cope with boredom, excess free time, or feelings of inadequacy related to unemployment. By contrast, it has been shown that people with disabilities who have jobs are less likely to smoke marijuana (27). Additionally, women who were involved in educational or vocational programming in conjunction with treatment had longer periods of sobriety (65). For women with disabilities, treatment and prevention efforts should include opportunities for vocational rehabilitation, preemployment skills training, and job skills training. One promising program for people with traumatic brain injury and substance abuse provides a comprehensive assessment and intensive case management over at least a 1-year period (66). This program found that participants who received these services had better vocational rehabilitation outcomes and were more likely to abstain from the use of alcohol and other drugs.

Program Retention

The issues of program retention and utilization are ongoing concerns for substance abuse prevention and treatment programs. There is some research indicating that women are less likely to complete more intensive forms of programs; however, one recent study reported that women were more likely to be referred to intensive treatment settings because they report to treatment with a higher level of addiction severity (19). Another cause of program dropout may be illiteracy. Many traditional treatment programs rely on activities that involve reading and writing, and although they are designed to be therapeutic, they may cause additional stress and discouragement, leading to a sense of failure (64).

For some women with disabilities, an even greater sense of social isolation may occur during treatment. Feelings of isolation coupled with the family's lack of support for treatment often are associated with treatment dropout (64). Another obstacle is the fact that sometimes family members do not want the person with a disability to stop drinking or using other drugs or to gain in their independence. These family members may fear losing access to the benefits or to the income that the person with a disability has or losing access to prescribed medications or other drugs. If the person with a disability seeks treatment or other assistance, that person may choose to become more independent and leave an uncomfortable or risky environment.

Lack of adequate child care and feelings of responsibility related to family and home are also factors to consider in program retention for women with disabilities. In addition, some women actually may be fearful of seeking assistance for child care or related problems because alcohol and other drug abuse is looked on negatively by social service agencies. In this situation, women may feel a risk of loss of custody of their children and the threat of criminal prosecution for child endangerment (5).

Economic status, lack of insurance, or the disability condition itself sometimes may be factors for program dropout. A study conducted by Kropp, Manhal-Baugus, and Kelly (65) found that the majority of women who did complete treatment reported some means of income. Women who have been diagnosed with a severe mental illness tend to stay in treatment less time than those women without a mental illness (67).

Program Modifications

Prevention and treatment programs will need to make modifications to provide accessible and appropriate services for women with disabilities. For example, substance abuse treatment objectives may need to be adjusted for some women with physical challenges. Treatment programs often use cognitive therapies throughout all program activities. Communication problems, memory difficulties, and lower functioning levels all can complicate these approaches and lead to greater levels of stress for treatment participants. It is not uncommon for women with disabilities to present to treatment with low self-esteem, depression, and/or a low level of motivation to make changes. Some of the components of treat-

ment may need to include learning new ways to cope with disability, social situations, loss, anger, and sexuality. Skills training related to independent living also may be critical.

> Marta describes some of her experiences in residential treatment in the late 1980s: "I remember that I bathed on my own. I was not offered assistance with any of my personal care stuff, and I know I was not very clean during treatment. The patients all did exercises in the morning and, of course, there was no adaptation for me, so I just was not able to participate in that activity. I had to just sit and watch. Then, the staff wanted to teach us relaxation and it required us laying on the floor and deep breathing exercises, which could have been helpful for me. Again I was not offered any help to participate, so I didn't. That was depressing for me. I didn't ask for help. I wasn't in touch with my feelings and I was just trying to look as normal as I could and not set myself apart as different in any way. I wasn't in touch with what I really needed at the time, so I didn't ask for anything and I was not asked what I needed either. My disability was never talked about, and issues that I had relating to my disability were not addressed. I made it through treatment, but it was very hard. Some people with disabilities might have dropped out or never agreed to go in the first place."

CONCLUSION

In summary, substance abuse can be difficult to detect in women with disabilities, and the social stigma associated with both disability and with substance abuse only adds to the problem. Laurie's story in the following extract identifies a number of issues that women with disabilities may experience. It is not unusual for family, friends, and professionals to enable the use of alcohol and other drug use among women with disabilities, placing them at increased risk for health, social, and emotional consequences. There are a number of issues present in the lives of women at different developmental stages, in varying racial and cultural groups, and across economic barriers. Some of these are factors that place women with disabilities at risk for problems related to substance abuse. These factors are only indicators but can be extremely helpful in targeting services toward the women with disabilities who are most vulnerable. Not every woman who presents with these issues in her life will have a problem; however, an awareness and understanding of these issues will go a long way toward the early identification of substance abuse problems and toward finding solutions to the problems when they occur.

LAURIE'S PERSONAL STORY

Even though I'm disabled, my story is like most alcoholics. My mother is an alcoholic and I said I would never become like her. My mom was a single parent. She dealt with many stresses related to being a parent of two disabled kids. Regular child care services wouldn't accept my sister and I, so my mom had to pay for a private provider out of her minimum wage salary. These "providers" were usually 14-year-old girls from the neighborhood. My childhood was fairly unsupervised.

The same year my mother entered into recovery, I started drinking. I was 14. I began my drinking career at Muscular Dystrophy Summer Camp. The campers' parents were aware that we drank, but most considered it a rite of passage of adolescents. Parents seemed to find comfort in their children partaking in "normal" adolescent behavior.

I drank alcohol throughout high school. I had an older friend who bought it for me, and I would put it in small Perrier bottles and hide it around my room. Soon I discovered that I could purchase alcohol myself because I was rarely asked for my ID. I attribute this to the fact that I use a wheelchair; either cashiers assumed I was older or just felt sorry for me. In my senior year, I started using other drugs as well, cocaine, and marijuana, but I liked alcohol the best.

The summer after high school I came out as a lesbian. Although my disabled friends were accepting of my identity, they didn't really embrace it. I went to events and parties to meet other lesbians, but felt uncomfortable, mostly invisible. To feel more at ease in these settings, I would get drunk.

After high school, I moved to San Francisco to attend a state university. Most of my friends were other disabled folks who drank and got high a lot. The summer after my first year in college, my social network expanded greatly. I became involved in peace activism, which included doing civil disobedience and spending time in jail. Through this experience I made several friends, most of them other lesbians. We formed a tightly knit "affinity group" that did political work on various issues for 7 years. Today, two of these women are my best friends.

After my third year, I quit college. Blaming my poor academic performance on lack of transportation, I decided to earn some money and buy a van. I got a job at a disability public policy organization. When drinking interfered with my job, I was never put on notice or asked about it. Because the disability community is small, everyone was aware that I had a problem. Although no one at work ever confronted me, I was influenced by another disabled women, 20 years my senior, who is in recovery. Over lunch, she told me stories; embarrassing things she'd done while drinking and how recovery had really changed her life.

When I was 22, I began to spiral down pretty quickly. I endangered my life and others. One night while drunk, I was guiding two blind friends home. I proceeded to cross a very busy street. When they heard screeching brakes they stopped before cars would have hit us. Another night I was drunk and passed out. My roommate couldn't wake me up. She called an ambulance and they took me to the hospital with a blood alcohol level of .30%. Hospital staff monitored me, reviving me periodically with smelling salts. Once they were satisfied I was alert, they transported me back home. A month later, my doctor received the ambulance report and called my house but did not leave a message for me to phone her back, and she didn't take further action. I don't know what prevented her or the hospital staff from intervening when I was clearly in trouble.

A few months after that I got a call from a buddy from camp asking me to go to an AA [Alcoholics Anonymous] meeting with her. She didn't stop drinking, but I did. I was 24. I can't really put my finger on the pivotal factor. I think it was convergence of many factors, making the time just right. I had surrounded myself with people who didn't drink; some were in recovery, some were not. My two roommates didn't drink; the woman I was involved with was in recovery. I had just started working with an excellent therapist, a disabled women who forced me to be responsible for my behavior.

At AA meetings, I found a community of people who shared my stories. At first it was difficult for me to sit still and listen. I was caught up in judging them by their appearances. My political stance was always to view people who were not disabled, gay, working class, activists, or women as "other." The experience of recovery enabled me to see people beyond their shells. In listening to people share their fears, struggles, and triumphs, I was able to see the humanity in all people and begin to relate to others on that level.

My first year in recovery I made several changes in my life. I quit my job and started working for a private company that conducted disability-related research but was not run by people with disabilities. I ended a relationship that I recognized was harmful to me. I began seeing an acupuncturist who helped me look at how my diet affected my health and make changes. Today I eat a balanced diet and exercise three times a week. When I take care of my body, not only am I clear-headed and have more energy, but I feel able to take care of my life.

I was completely abstinent for the first 6 years of my recovery. A month shy of my 6-year anniversary, I had a "slip." I was under a lot of stress at work. One night I came home and my friend was gone for the night. I opened up a bottle of tequila and had a few shots. Within hours, I was devastated. Although it was late, I called a friend, completely freaked out. She calmed me down and convinced me to just go to bed. For a week, I was debilitated with self-loathing. I felt I had just thrown years of sobriety away and now I had to start all over. I was too humiliated to go to an AA meeting. Over time, I realized that recovery is a process and that I wasn't "starting over." No experience could erase all of the hard work I had dedicated to making healthy changes in my life.

For the first several years, I did not drink because I was afraid of alcohol. Drinking had caused my loved ones and me a lot of pain. Today, I do drink at times. A little over a year ago, on the spur of the moment, I split a glass of wine with a friend. I had always thought that if I drank again, I would immediately lose control and want to get drunk. But I didn't. I felt fine. I didn't feel a desire to get drunk. Since then, I have had a drink once in a while. When I decide to have a drink, I check in with myself to see how I'm feeling and what is going on with me. If I start to feel any of the old feelings or behaviors creeping up on me, I will know what to do and where I can seek help if I need it.

REFERENCES

1. Ford J, Moore D. *Substance abuse resources and disability issues: A training manual for professionals.* Dayton, OH: School of Medicine, Wright State University, 1992.
2. Greer BG. Substance abuse among people with disabilities: A problem of too much access. *J Rehab* 1986;Jan–Mar:34–37.
3. Moore D, Li L. Prevalence and risk factors of illicit drug use by people with disabilities. *Am J Addict* 1998; 2:93–102.
4. National Institute on Alcohol Abuse and Alcoholism. *Eighth special report to the U.S. Congress on alcohol and health.* Bethesda, MD: NIAAA, 1993.
5. Blume SB. Addictive disorders in women. In: Frances RJ, Miller SI, eds. *Clinical textbook of addictive disorders,* 2nd ed. New York: The Guilford Press, 1998: 413–429.
6. Niremburg TD, Gomberg ESL. Prevention of alcohol and drug problems among women. In: Gomberg ESL, Niremburg TD, eds. *Women and substance abuse.* Norwood, New Jersey: Ablex Publishing, 1993:339–359.
7. Substance Abuse and Mental Health Services Administration. *Summary of findings from the 1999 national household survey on drug abuse.* [DHHS Pub. No. (SMA) 00-3466]. Washington, DC: U.S. Government Printing Office, 2000.
8. Li L, Ford JA. Triple trouble: alcohol abuse by women with disabilities. *Applied Behavioral Science Review* 1996;4:99–109.
9. Ludeman E. Facing the barriers to treatment. *The Counselor* 1989;January/February:7–8.
10. Penniman LJ, Agnew J. Women, work and alcohol. *Occupational Medicine* 1989;4:263–273.
11. Westermeyer J, Phaobtong T, Nider J. Substance use and abuse among mentally retarded persons: A comparison of patients and a survey population. *Am J Drug Alcohol Abuse* 1988;14(1):109–123.
12. Edgerton RB. Alcohol and drug use by mentally retarded adults. *Am J Ment Deficiency* 1986;90(6): 602–609.
13. Weiner HD, Wallen MC, Zankowski GL. Culture and social class as intervening variables in relapse prevention with chemically dependent women. *J Psychoactive Drugs* 1990;22:239–248.
14. Substance Abuse and Mental Health Services Administration. SAMSHA studies alcohol-related violence and women. *SAMSHA News* 1995;3(4):12–13.
15. Blume SB. Alcohol and drug problems in women: Old attitude, new knowledge. In Milkman HB, Sederer LI, eds. *Treatment choices for alcoholism and substance abuse* Lexington, MA: Lexington Books, 1990: 183–200.
16. Clayton RR, Voss HL, Robbins C, et al. Gender differences in drug use: An epidemiological perspective. In Ray BA, Braude MC, eds. *Women and drugs: a new era for research.* Rockville, MD: National Institute on Drug Abuse, 1986:80–99.
17. Lex BW, Griffin ML, Mello NK, et al. Alcohol, marijuana, and mood states in young women. *Int J Addict* 1989;14:405–424.
18. Lex BW. Alcohol and other drug abuse among women. *Alcohol, Health & Research World* 1994;18:212–219.
19. Arfken CL, Klein C, diMenza S, et al. Gender differences in problem severity at assessment and treatment retention. *J Subst Abuse Treat* 2001;20(1):53–57.
20. Moore D, Li L. Substance use among applicants for vo-

cational rehabilitation services. *J Rehab* 1994;60:
48–53.

21. Pagliaro A, Pagliaro L. *Substance use among women. a reference and resource guide.* Philadelphia: Brunner/ Mazel, Edwards Brothers, 2000:182–190.

22. Westreich L, Guedj P, Glanter M, et al. Differences between men and women in dual-diagnosis treatment. *Am J Addict* 1997;6(4):311–317.

23. Schubiner H, Tzelepis A, Milberger S, et al. Prevalence of attention-deficit/hyperactivity disorder and conduct disorder among substance abusers. *J Clin Psych* 2000; 61(4):244–251.

24. Sinha R, O'Malley S. Alcohol and eating disorders: implications for alcohol treatment and health services research. *Alcoholism: clinical and experimental research.* 2000;24:1312–1319.

25. Dansky BS, Brewerton TD, Kilpatrick DG. Comorbidity of bulimia nervosa and alcohol use disorders: Results from the national women's study. *Int J Eating Disord* 2000;27(2):180–190.

26. Kolakowsky-Hayner S, Gourley E, Kreutzer J, et al. Pre-injury substance abuse among persons with brain injury and persons with spinal cord injury. *Brain Injury* 1999;13:571–581.

27. Heinemann A, Mamott B, Schnoll S. Substance use by persons with recent spinal cord injuries. *Rehab Psych* 1990;35:217–228.

28. Sparadeo FR, Gill D. Effects of prior alcohol use on head injury recovery. *J Head Trauma Rehab* 1989;4 (1):75–82.

29. Kreutzer JS, Doherty KR, Harris JA, et al. Alcohol use among persons with traumatic brain injury. *J Head Trauma Rehab* 1990;5(3):9–20.

30. Sparadeo FR, Strauss D, Barth JT. The incidence, impact, and treatment of substance abuse in head trauma rehabilitation. *J Head Trauma Rehab* 1990;5(3):1–8.

31. Heinemann A, Donohue R, Keen M, et al. Alcohol use by persons with recent spinal cord injuries. *Arch Phys Med Rehab* 1988;69:619–624.

32. Moore D, Siegal HA. Double trouble: Alcohol and other drug use among orthopedically impaired college students. *Alcohol, Health, and Research World* 1989;13(2): 118–123.

33. Isaacs M, Buckley G, Martin D. Patterns of drinking among the deaf. *Am J Drug Alcohol Abuse* 1979;6(4): 463–476.

34. Steitler KA. Substance abuse and the deaf adolescent. In: Anderson GB Watson D, eds. *The habilitation and rehabilitation of deaf adolescents.* Wagoner, AK: University of Arkansas, 1984.

35. Locke R, Johnson S. A descriptive study of drug use among the hearing impaired in a senior high school for the hearing impaired. In Schecter AJ, ed. *Drug dependence and alcoholism: social and behavioral issues.* New York: Plenum, 1981.

36. DiNitto DM, Krishef CH. Drinking patterns of mentally retarded persons. *Alcohol Health and Research World* 1984;8(2):40–42.

37. Westermeyer J, Kemp K, Nugent S. Substance disorder among persons with mild mental retardation: A comparative study. *Am J Addict* 1996;5(1):23–31.

38. Stevens SJ, Tortu S, Coyle SL. *Women, drug abuse and HIV infection.* Binghamton, NY: The Haworth Press, Inc., 1998.

39. Centers for Disease Control. *HIV/AIDS surveillance report.* Atlanta: U.S. Department of Health and Human Services, Public Health Services, Centers for Disease Control, 2001.

40. Center for Substance Abuse Treatment. *Substance abuse treatment for persons with HIV/AIDS. Treatment Improvement Protocol (TIP) Series 37* [DHHS Pub. No. (SMA) 00-3410]. Washington, DC: U.S. Government Printing Office, 2000.

41. Freeman RC, Collier K, Parillo KM. Early life sexual abuse as a risk factor for crack cocaine use in a sample of community-recruited women at high risk for illicit drug use. *Am J Drug Alcohol Abuse* 2002;28(1): 109–131.

42. Simpson TL, Miller WR. Concomitance between childhood sexual and physical abuse and substance use problems: A review. *Clin Psych Rev* 2002;22(1):27–77.

43. The National Center on Addiction and Substance Abuse. *Substance abuse and the American woman.* New York: Columbia University, 1996.

44. Lex BW. Women and illicit drugs: Marijuana, heroin, and cocaine. In Gomberg ESL, Nirenberg TD, eds. *Women and substance abuse.* Stamford, CT: Ablex Publishing Corp, 1993:162–190.

45. National Institute on Drug Abuse. *Women and drug abuse.* NIH Pub. No. 94-3732. Rockville, MD: NIDA, 1994.

46. Rousso H. *Girls and women with disabilities: An international overview and summary of research.* Oakland, CA: World Institute on Disability and New York: Rehabilitation International, 2000.

47. Blum LN, Nielson NH, Riggs JA. Alcoholism and alcohol abuse among women: Report of the council on scientific affairs. *J Womens Health* 1998;7(7):861–871.

48. Li L, Ford J. Illicit drug use by women with disabilities. *Am J Drug Alcohol Abuse* 1998;24(3):405–418.

49. Kirubakaran V, Kumar N, Powell B, et al. Survey of alcohol and drug misuse in spinal cord injured veterans. *J Stud Alcohol* 1986;47(3):223–227.

50. Waxman BF. Hatred: The unacknowledged dimension in violence against disabled people. *Sexual Disabil* 1991;9(3):185–199.

51. Jessor R, Jessor S. *Problem behavior and psychosocial development: A longitudinal study of youth.* New York: Academic Press, 1977.

52. Sweeney TT, Foote JE. Treatment of drug and alcohol abuse in spinal cord injury veterans. *Int J Addict* 1982; 17(5):897–904.

53. Beck-Massey D. Sanctioned war: Women, violence, and disabilities. *Sexual Disabil* 1999;17(3):269–276.

54. Li L, Moore D. Acceptance of disability and its correlates. *J Soc Psych* 1998;138(1):13–25.

55. Wilsnack S, Wilsnack RW. Epidemiology of women's drinking. *J Subst Abuse* 1993;3:133.

56. Abbey A, Ross LT, McDuffie D, et al. Alcohol and dating risk factors for sexual assault among college women. *Psych Women Q* 1996;20(1):147–169.

57. Kalichman SC, Williams EA, Cherry C, et al. Sexual coercion, domestic violence, and negotiating condom use among low-income African American women. *J Womens Health* 1998;7(3):371–378.

58. Monlina LD, Basinait-Smith C. Revisiting the intersection between domestic abuse and HIV risk. *Am J Public Health* 1998;88:1267–1268.

59. Miller BA, Wilsnack SC, Cunradi CB. Family violence and victimization: Treatment issues for women with al-

cohol problems. *Alcohol Clin Exp Res* 2000;24(8): 1287–1297.

60. Li L, Ford J, Moore D. An exploratory study of violence, substance abuse, disability, and gender. *Social Behavior and Personality* 2000;28(1):61–71.

61. LaPlante MP, Kennedy J, Kaye S, et al. Disability and Employment. *Disability Statistics Abstract,* Number 11. San Francisco, CA: Disability Statistics Center, 1997.

62. Kiley D, Brandt M. Issues and controversies in chemical dependence services for persons with physical disabilities. In: Heinemann AW, ed. *Substance abuse and physical disability.* New York: Haworth Press, 1993:259–269.

63. Hill EM, Boyd CJ, Kortge JF. Variation in suicidality among substance-abusing women. The role of childhood adversity. *J Subst Abuse Treat* 2000;19(4):339–345.

64. Kelly PJ, Blacksin B, Mason E. Factors affecting substance abuse treatment completion for women. *Issues Ment Health Nurs* 2001;22(3):287–304.

65. Kropp FB, Manhal-Baugus M, Kelly VA. The association of personal-related variables to length of sobriety: A pilot study of chemically dependent women. *J Addictions Offender Counseling* 1996;17(1):21–34.

66. Bogner JA, Corrigan JD, Spafford DE, et al. Integrating substance abuse treatment and vocational rehabilitation after traumatic brain injury. *J Head Trauma Rehab* 1997;12(5):57–71.

67. Brown VB, Melchior LA, Huba GJ. Level of burden among women diagnosed with severe mental illness and substance abuse. *J Psychoactive Drugs* 1999;31(1): 31–40.

25

Violence Against Women with Disabilities: The Role of Physicians in Filling the Treatment Gap

Margaret A. Nosek, Rosemary B. Hughes, Heather B. Taylor,
and Carol A. Howland

Primary care physicians and obstetricians–gynecologists have the power to make a significant difference in the lives of women with disabilities who are victims of some of the most obscure and brutal forms of violence, violence that is only possible because of the disability. Consider the following case study:

> Heather's husband John spit in her face, slapped her, tossed garbage on her bed, threw bags of dog feces at her, smeared food on her face, and locked her in a bedroom away from her children. Fighting back or escaping was not an option, not only because she was a C1-2 ventilator-dependent tetraplegic from a gunshot wound, but also because John's wealthy father was paying more than $250,000/year for her around-the-clock nurses. John's explosive anger upset Heather, making secretions build up in her tracheostomy. On numerous occasions, he refused to suction out the secretions, leaving her gasping for breath for hours until the next nurse arrived. Heather's weight dropped to 93 pounds, her blood pressure was soaring, and she had had pneumonia twice. A call from one of her nurses prompted investigations by the police, Child Protective Services, and Adult Protective Services, but Heather and her children were afraid to confirm that there was any problem. A year later, a clandestine call for help to her parents led to further investigations and the gathering of 1,000 pages of testimony from witnesses. Authorities recommended charges stemming from incidents that were corroborated by witnesses, including harassment, endangerment, aggravated assault, unlawful imprisonment, kidnapping, domestic violence, and vulnerable adult abuse. Sadly, to date, charges have not been filed. The city prosecutor claimed that Heather's credibility was in jeopardy because she previously had denied abuse. The County Attorney turned down the case for similar reasons. The governor and attorney general have not responded to her petition to prosecute this case and protect her safety, other than to refer her to victims' assistance organizations (1).

The facts of this case do not fit well with the textbook approach to domestic violence. The injuries were, on the surface, quite minor. Ventilator-dependent tetraplegia is such a rare condition that few people, especially those without medical training, understand the fragility that accompanies it or the potential lethality of delaying bronchial suctioning, smearing dog feces on the bed of someone who uses a Foley catheter, or forcing food in the mouth of someone with swallowing difficulties. Most women have to consider their financial dependence on the batterer before they can determine the best safety or escape plan. For Heather, escape was not a physical or a financial possibility. The only alternative to this terrorizing situation was to be placed in a nursing home, where abuse and incompetence would present in other ways. She was quite literally physically, emotionally, and financially trapped.

The criminal justice, human service, and medical systems failed Heather in many ways. Charges like harassment, endangerment, and vulnerable adult abuse do not even begin to represent the seriousness of John's actions. When someone refuses to perform a life-critical task such as bronchial suctioning with the intent to injure an individual who is physically unable to defend herself or perform the task unaided, it is quite a bit closer to attempted homicide than it is to endangerment. Human service workers also failed to recognize the lethality of this situation and did little to help Heather find other means of support. Perhaps the most insidious of these failures was how the medical systems obstructed the humane impulses of the nurses. Many who were eye-witnesses to these acts tried to report to the police and their own agency. If they were caught reporting, would John threaten to fire them or physically isolate them as he did Heather? The tyranny of his anger forced many of the nurses to quit; 40 different nurses had been in his employment in the course of 1 year. Those who went to the state nursing board for information and advice about what they should do were given little, if any, help, other than the suggestion to quit their job for their own protection. Heather had seen primary care and specialist physicians for her many health conditions during this time, yet nowhere in the records is there mention that any of them inquired about violence in her home.

Many physicians believe that it is not their responsibility to inquire about violence in their patients' lives or that there is no evidence to justify screening for abuse in clinical settings (2). There are many facts that support the error of this thinking. In this chapter, we will explain more about violence against women with disabilities, including its characteristics and prevalence, followed by our reasoning on why physicians have a special duty and opportunity to assist their patients who are victims of violence, especially those with disabilities, and our suggestions on what they can do to help.

DEFINITIONAL ISSUES: WHAT CONSTITUTES ABUSE

According to the American College of Obstetricians and Gynecologists (3) "abuse is forceful, controlling behavior that coerces a woman to do what the abuser wants without regard to her rights, body, or health. A woman is defined as abused if she has had intentional, usually repeated, physical or psychological harm done to her by a man with whom she is or has been in an intimate relationship." This definition is useful for the situation of most women, but it does not consider the life situation of many women with disabilities. A large segment of the population of women with functional limitations (52%) is not married. Women older than age 45 years with functional limitations are significantly more likely to live alone (4). Although intimate partner violence is the most prevalent type of violence experienced by women with disabilities, many are also victims of physical and sexual assault by personal care assistants and health care workers (5,6).

We have found the following definitions to be useful in our abuse research. *Emotional abuse* is being threatened, terrorized, severely rejected, isolated, ignored, or verbally attacked (7,8). *Physical abuse* is any form of violence against a woman's body, such as being hit, kicked, restrained, or deprived of food or water (9). *Sexual abuse* is being forced, threatened, or deceived into sexual activities ranging from looking or touching to intercourse or rape (9,10).

We identified certain types of abuse that are related specifically to disability (11,12). *Disability-related emotional abuse* often includes emotional abandonment and rejection or denial of disability. *Disability-related physical abuse* includes physical restraint or confinement; withholding needed orthotic equipment, medications, or transportation; or refusing to provide assistance with essential daily living needs, such as dressing or getting out of bed. *Disability-related sexual abuse* includes demanding or expecting sexual activity in return for help or taking advantage of physical weakness and an inaccessible environment to force sexual activity (11). Many of the incidents of abuse reported in this study occurred in *medical settings*. Certain acts are clearly abusive and punishable by law, such as rape by an orderly. Others, however, are not categorized so easily, such as excessively rough pelvic examinations, physical touch as part of psychotherapy, public stripping for examination, or restraints for patients who are agitated. It is sometimes difficult to draw the line between actions that are sanctioned as medically necessary and actions that in any other context would be considered abusive.

ISSUES OF PREVALENCE

Early studies reported that the rate of abuse among women with disabilities ranges from 31% to 83%, or double to quadruple the rate found among women in general (13,14). In our national study comparing women with physical disabilities to women without disabilities (5,6,12), rates of physical, sexual, and emotional abuse were equally high in both groups. The prevalence of having ever experienced physical or sexual abuse was 52% for women both with and without disabilities. Important differences between the groups, however, were that women with disabilities reported a larger number of perpetrators (with the most common being intimate partners, followed by family members) and the duration of the abuse was longer. They were also more likely to experience abuse by attendants, strangers, and health care providers. Compared to women without disabilities, women with disabilities were more likely to report more intense experiences of abuse, including the combination of multiple incidents, multiple perpetrators, and longer duration (15).

VULNERABILITY FOR ABUSE

Vulnerability for abuse is a product of the complex interaction of individual, intrapersonal, and societal/institutional factors (16). Certain characteristics of perpetrators and victims have been identified in retrospective studies of domestic violence. A review of research on risk factors for male-to-female domestic violence (17) identified younger age, less education, unemployment, pregnancy, childhood victimization, and mental illness as being associated with victimization. Some of these factors are known to be disproportionately characteristic of women with disabilities. Population statistics show their high rates of unemployment and poverty, lower education levels, and very high prevalence of depression (4). Abuse has been associated with depression and stress among women with disabilities in several of our recent studies (18–21).

In one study of women with physical disabilities, those who screened positive for abuse within the past year were younger, more educated, less mobile, and more socially isolated and had higher levels of depression (21). Longitudinal studies are needed to determine if variables such as social isolation and depression are risk factors for abuse or merely are correlated with it.

Other factors possibly contributing to increased vulnerability include the combined cultural devaluation of women and people with disabilities (22) often compounded by age-related devaluation (23), overprotection, and internalized societal expectations. Women with disabilities may have had fewer opportunities to learn sexual likes and dislikes and to set pleasing boundaries, perceiving celibacy or violent sexual encounters as their only choices, believing no loving person would be attracted to them (24). They often are perceived to be powerless and physically helpless (25).

Although women with severe disabilities face many barriers to the expression of their sexuality and, statistically, they are less likely to be married and more likely to live alone, many people mistakenly assume that all women with disabilities do not date, do not live with significant others, do not marry, do not have children, and do not desire such relationships, especially if they exhibit visible signs of disability such as disfigurement or use of a wheelchair. The assumption follows that an abnormal appearance makes such women undesirable to potential perpetrators of sexual assault. Findings from studies conducted at our center do not support these assumptions (12,25–26). Out of nearly 500 women with physically disabling conditions (e.g., spinal cord injury, cerebral palsy), 87% reported they had at least one serious romantic relationship or marriage, and more than half currently were involved in an intimate relationship. Level of sexual activity was found to be unrelated to the severity of the disability (27).

Vulnerability associated with the need for personal assistance and the problem of social isolation deserves special attention. The large majority of women who have significant functional limitations depend on family for personal assistance because assistance from outside the family is often expensive and not very reliable. In the event that the person providing the assistance is the perpetrator of abuse, the woman who is disabled may perceive that this is her only option and that abuse is the price she must pay for survival. As in the earlier case study, abusive actions by someone providing assistance may not be perceived as abusive by the uninformed observer. Several studies confirm a high prevalence of disability-related abuse perpetrated by personal assistants who were either intimate partners or hired attendants and provide evidence of its serious implications (13,20,28–31). The Centers for Disease Control and Prevention have identified social isolation as a key factor that must be addressed in delivering violence-prevention interventions to underserved communities (32). Each of the four types of isolation—geographic, economic, political, and social—is compounded by having a disability, thus elevating vulnerability for violence.

HEALTH CONSEQUENCES OF ABUSE

Women suffer adverse health consequences because of battering and other forms of abuse. As a result, domestic violence has been identified as a significant public health problem in the United States (33). The risk for abuse, effects of abuse on health, and barriers to seeking help for women who are disabled remain largely undocumented (31).

The literature on women in general indicates that domestic violence and other forms of abuse result in homicide (34), suicide (35), disability (36), emotional problems (37), medical complaints (38–40), drug and alcohol abuse

(35,38,41), and sexual dysfunction (37). Sexual abuse survivors may experience depression (42), chronic anxiety and tension (43), anxiety attacks and phobias, and sleep and appetite disturbance. Many survivors also have more medical complaints including pelvic pain (40), headaches, backaches, skin disorders, and genitourinary problems (38–39). It is important to note that many of these conditions are already more prevalent among women with disabilities, making it more likely for physicians to attribute causation to the disability and fail to pursue abuse as a possible cause. Survivors also experience exaggerated feelings of guilt and shame, negatively affecting their self-esteem and enhancing feelings of worthlessness (44). These feelings often result in poor body image, leading to obesity or eating disorders (39,45–46). Self-destructive behavior, self-mutilation, drug abuse, and alcoholism occur more frequently than among nonabused women (35,38,41). A history of abuse may have serious effects on a woman's relationship and sexuality issues, engendering lack of trust and feelings of passivity, powerlessness, and isolation. Left untreated, sexual abuse may lead to serious psychologic sequelae (37).

BEST PRACTICES IN ABUSE PREVENTION AND INTERVENTION

The development of more accessible resources and services for victims of abuse are key aspects of abuse intervention for women with disabilities (5,47). The National Domestic Violence Hotline keeps a database of battered women's programs throughout the country, with indications of their architectural accessibility and the availability of interpreter services. Guidelines are available for battered women's programs on implementing accessibility modifications according to the requirements of the Americans with Disabilities Act and increasing sensitivity and responsiveness among program staff to the needs of abused women with disabilities (48).

Although some battered women's programs have instituted excellent accessibility modifications, specialized programming, and outreach activities to meet the needs of abused woman with disabilities (47,49), the majority of programs are still essentially inaccessible and unaware of this problem. In a national survey of battered women's programs, we found that only a very small proportion of women with disabilities who are being abused, particularly those with physical or sensory disabilities, receive their services.

In summary, women with disabilities have a very high vulnerability for abuse and intimate partner violence, and this vulnerability increases in the presence of more severe mobility impairments, the need for personal assistance, social isolation, and depression. They are not only vulnerable to the same types of abuse all women face; they are vulnerable to a whole spectrum of abusive actions that are only possible because they have a disability. Most disabled women in abusive situations do not have the physical ability, independent mobility, financial resources, or social support to leave or even to seek help. The consequences of abuse on their physical and mental health may be extreme but most likely go unnoticed by health care professionals or are attributed to the disability itself rather than an abusive partner or personal assistant. The most inexcusable part of this scenario is that the systems established to help women who are being victimized—law enforcement, battered women's programs, and human services—are often inaccessible, unaware, and unresponsive to the needs of women with disabilities. Society at large and medical professionals in particular seem to still cling to the tragically false belief that no one would abuse a woman with a disability (50).

IMPORTANCE OF SCREENING FOR ABUSE IN CLINICAL SETTINGS

Whether patients in physicians' offices should be screened for abuse is an issue under debate in the literature. Ramsay and colleagues (2) reviewed 20 articles on screening for abuse in clinical settings and found that although a majority of women respondents felt it was acceptable, a majority of physicians and emergency department nurses were not in favor of it. Other than increased referral to outside agencies, the authors claim that little evidence exists for changes in important outcomes such as decreased exposure to violence. Despite their overall judgment of a poor-quality and inadequate body of literature, the authors leap to the conclusion that, although domestic violence is a common problem with major health consequences for women, implementation of screening programs in health care settings cannot be justified.

Reaction to this proclamation was quick and mostly negative. In the next issue of the *British Medical Journal* the editors reported receiving 28 letters responding to Ramsay and colleagues, with more than half agreeing that screening would require a culture shift to zero tolerance of domestic violence, as we have seen for child abuse (51,52). There was also general agreement that screening is a health professional's responsibility. Screening by a health professional "may be the first link in activating the chain of survival" (p. 1419) (51). One commentator took the stand that a physician's duty to report a crime should take precedence over the duty to maintain patient confidentiality (53). New regulations under the Health Information Portability and Accountability Act (54) undoubtedly will intensify this debate.

Medical organizations certainly have rallied in support of screening for domestic violence by health professionals. The American College of Obstetricians and Gynecologists and the International Federation of Gynecology and Obstetrics have issued statements encouraging their members to initiate screening in their practice and to take action to stop domestic violence (55). The *International Journal of Gynecology and Obstetrics* issued a supplement in September, 2002, dedicated to the problem of domestic violence, including proceedings of the International Conference on the Role of Health Professionals in Addressing Violence Against Women that was held on October 15, 2000, in Naples, Italy (55). Similar statements have been issued by the American Medical Association (56), the Institute of Medicine (57), American Association of Family Practitioners, Family Violence Prevention Fund, and Physicians for a Violence-free Society (58). Even the Joint Commission on Accreditation of Healthcare Organizations (59) requires written policies to improve identification and assessment of domestic violence victims, provider education, patient consent, and documentation of abuse. The standard of care for all medical, mental health, legal, and social work practitioners requires universal screening, basic safety planning, and appropriate referral to community resources (60).

Other reasons for screening patients for domestic violence, besides the ethical obligation to report a crime and liability for failure to report, are related to treatment outcomes. Lack of compliance with medical recommendations and unresponsiveness to treatment may not be the result of the woman's actions or attitudes. Special interviewing techniques are required to elicit relevant information from patients (61).

PRACTICAL GUIDELINES

It is understandable that physicians, like society in general, are uncomfortable talking about domestic violence. As in many other areas of behavioral inquiry, however, it is necessary, and guidelines have been developed with techniques for raising the subject and eliciting truthful responses. The first step in approaching this problem is to educate all medical personnel and staff in a clinical practice about the reality of domestic violence, including why

patients are reluctant to talk about it (Table 25-1) and why physicians are reluctant to ask about it (Table 25-2). The next steps have been outlined clearly by well-known prosecutor, advocate, educator, and survivor of domestic violence, Sarah Buel, who offers 10 recommendations for physicians related to their role in bringing about solutions to this problem (60). We have added comments to make these recommendations more relevant to abused women with disabilities.

1. Conduct universal screening. Considerable research has been done on the most effective means of identifying women who are victims of domestic violence. Studies have shown that women are more likely to disclose such stigmatizing experiences if screening is done by a nurse instead of asking patients to complete a brief written assessment (62). Computer-based health-risk assessment also has been shown to encourage more disclosure and documentation of abuse when patients receive computer-generated health advice and physicians receive patient risk summaries (63). Researchers at the Center for Research on Women with Disabilities (64) developed a tool for identifying women with disabilities who are in abusive situations, called the Abuse Assessment Screen–Disability (AAS–D) (Table 25-3). It is concise and relatively simple to administer in a clinical setting.

Table 25-1. *Why patients do not tell their doctors about abuse*

- She may fear retribution if the perpetrator learns the violence has been disclosed.
- She may be totally dependent on the perpetrator for personal care and have no other resources to tap.
- She may feel shame and humiliation that this is happening to her.
- She may think she deserved the abuse. She may think that, because of her disability, she cannot hope for better treatment.
- She may feel protective of her partner.
- She may have been told that no one else would have her or take care of her because of her disability.
- She may not fully comprehend her situation. She may not recognize that what she is experiencing is abuse, especially if she has been exposed to it most of her life.
- She may think her doctor is not knowledgeable or does not care about abuse.
- She may think her doctor is too busy to spend time talking about this problem.
- She may think her doctor cannot help her with this problem.

(From Nosek MA. *Guidelines for physicians on the abuse of women with disabilities.* Houston, TX: Center for Research on Women with Disabilities, 1996, with permission.)

Table 25-2. *Reasons physicians do not ask about abuse*

- They believe that abuse does not occur in the population of women with disabilities.
- The patient is tearful and uncooperative or she is intoxicated from intake of alcohol or other drugs, making it difficult to get the history.
- They think the woman provoked or deserved the abuse.
- They believe what happens in the home, in terms of domestic violence, is a private matter and, therefore, should not be discussed.
- They think she can just leave if she wants to.
- They know the assailant, and believe he or she is incapable of abuse.
- They do not know what to do if they uncover the abuse, or they believe it is the job of other professionals, such as social workers.
- They know what to do, but believe it will not help—"she just goes back to him anyway."

(From Nosek MA. *Guidelines for physicians on the abuse of women with disabilities.* Houston, TX: Center for Research on Women with Disabilities, 1996, with permission.)

Table 25-3. *Abuse assessment screen-disability (AAS-D)*

(Circle YES or NO)

1. *WITHIN THE LAST YEAR,* have you been hit, slapped, kicked, pushed, shoved, or otherwise physically hurt by someone?

   YES _____   NO _____

   If YES, who? (Circle all that apply)

   Intimate Partner   Care Provider   Health Professional   Family Member   Other

   Please describe _____

2. *WITHIN THE LAST YEAR,* has anyone forced you to have sexual activities?

   YES _____   NO _____

   If YES, who? (Circle all that apply)

   Intimate Partner   Care Provider   Health Professional   Family Member   Other

   Please describe _____

3. *WITHIN THE LAST YEAR,* has anyone prevented you from using a wheelchair, cane, respirator, or other assistive devices?

   YES _____   NO _____

   If YES, who? (Circle all that apply)

   Intimate Partner   Care Provider   Health Professional   Family Member   Other

   Please describe _____

4. *WITHIN THE LAST YEAR,* has anyone you depend on refused to help you with an important personal need, such as taking your medicine, getting to the bathroom, getting out of bed, bathing, getting dressed, or getting food or drink?

   YES _____   NO _____

   If YES, who? (Circle all that apply)

   Intimate Partner   Care Provider   Health Professional   Family Member   Other

   Please describe _____

(From McFarlane J, Hughes RB, Nosek MA, et al. Abuse Assessment Screen-Disability (AAS-D): Measuring frequency, type, and perpetrator of abuse toward women with physical disabilities. *J Womens Health Gend Based Med* 2001;10:861–866, with permission.)

2. Educate yourself and all staff about the dynamics of domestic violence. Ample information is easily available now through the literature cited, Websites of the medical organizations mentioned earlier, and local programs for battered women. These local programs often have staff that will come to a clinical site and conduct in-service training. Basic information on screening techniques, recognizing the signs and symptoms of abuse, follow-up interviewing, appropriate referrals, local resources, and measures to ensure the physical and emotional safety of your staff should be included in this training. It is essential to request and receive information specifically about women with disabilities as part of this type of training, given the many unique situations of dependence, physical limitations in self-defense, limited available helping resources, and the general lack of awareness or sensitivity to the vulnerability they face. Maintain contact with the Center for Research on Women with Disabilities through the abuse page on our Website (www.bcm.tmc.edu/crowd/) for materials and updates on current research and intervention programs. The American College of Physicians publication, *Violence Against Women,* contains a wealth of information on all of these topics, including violence against women with disabilities (50,65).

3. Develop a protocol for addressing domestic violence with patients who are victims and abusers. As required by the Joint Commission on Accreditation of Healthcare Organizations and as recommended by major medical organizations, every clinical setting should have a protocol for addressing domestic violence. At a minimum, this protocol should include a regular schedule of in-service training on the identification and management of cases where domestic violence is suspected, detailed screening and assessment procedures, staff assigned to conduct appropriate interviewing, information on local resources for reporting and referral, specific information about the accessibility and responsiveness of these resources for women with disabilities, and a plan for follow-up to discuss the abusive situation.

4. Document the victim's injuries, history of abuse, and identity of the batterer. In the case study that opened this chapter, justice was not served because of lack of documentation. What documentation did exist from the victim and her nurses was perceived as lacking credibility. Physicians are accustomed to preparing documentation for legal proceedings, and the credibility of their testimony is generally high. Therein lays the power of physicians to make a critical difference in the survival and well-being of abused women. With medical expertise combined with awareness of the dynamics of domestic violence, health professionals would be well equipped to disentangle the complexities of abuse in the context of disability. Specific information on recognizing the signs and symptoms of abuse in the medical history and medical examination can be found in Tables 25-4 and 25-5. In documenting evidence of suspected abuse, descriptions, photographs (with the woman's permission), and observations should be included. If abuse is suspected, statements to that effect should be written in the patient's record, whether or not discussion of this concern or any follow-up takes place.

One important detail in eliciting authentic abuse histories is to speak to the victim apart from the person who accompanies her. That person may very well be the perpetrator. Classic perpetrator behaviors in such settings include insistence on being with the patient at all times, speaking for the patient (a common behavior of many people toward women with disabilities, especially those with speech impairments), excessive expressions of concern, gestures of affection, and offers to help. For women with disabilities, these intimidating behaviors can

Table 25-4. *Clues from the medical history*

- A description of the incident that is not consistent with the kind of injury
- A time delay between injuries and presentation
- Blaming injuries on a disability-related cause, such as falling while transferring from a wheelchair to a tub
- An "accident"-prone history
- Suicide attempts or depression
- Repetitive psychosomatic complaints or recurring physical complaints with no physical signs of organic disease, including headaches, chest pains, heart palpitations, choking sensations, numbness and tingling, nervousness, dyspareunia, or pelvic pain
- Emotional complaints, including anxiety, panic attacks, sleep disorders, nervousness, depression, difficulty coping with parenting, or nonspecific complaints of marital problems
- Signs and symptoms of alcoholism or drug abuse
- Injury during pregnancy or "spontaneous" abortions, premature labor, low birthweight babies, and fetal injuries
- Other pregnancy-related problems, such as substance abuse, poor nutrition, depression, and late or sporadic access to prenatal care
- Signs and symptoms of posttraumatic stress syndrome: increased arousal, sleep difficulties, irritability, difficulty concentrating, and hypervigilance

(From Nosek MA. *Guidelines for physicians on the abuse of women with disabilities.* Houston, TX: Center for Research on Women with Disabilities, 1996, with permission.)

come not only from intimate partners but also from family members and personal care assistants. For disabled women with speech impairments, as often seen in cerebral palsy and other neurologic impairments, it is especially important to have someone take the time to communicate with them directly and privately.

5. Speak up with abuse victims and offenders. It takes a certain amount of courage to address suspected abuse with patients. Examination of one's own feelings and experiences is essential for approaching others on this topic with confidence. By entering into such discussions with patients, health care professionals bear witness to the violence and thereby have moral and legal obligations to take action while at the same time protecting their own physical and emotional well-being (66).

Buel (p. S52) (60) offers some useful language for talking with patients about suspected abuse. For victims, an effective way of beginning a discussion is, "I'm afraid for your safety," "It will only get worse," or "You don't deserve to be abused." If the victim has a disability, statements such as, "Yes, people with cerebral palsy often fall, but their bruises are not usually where yours are," or "Have you ever talked with family or

Table 25-5. *Clues from the physical examination*

- Examine the entire body, noting areas of tenderness, as well as areas with visible injuries.
- Injuries as a result of abuse may have a "central pattern"—that is, injuries to the face, neck, throat, chest, breast, abdomen, and genitals.
- Bear in mind that some injuries tend not to happen accidentally.
- Be suspicious of injuries suggestive of a defensive posture, such as bruises to the ulnar aspect of the forearm.
- Multiple injuries in various stages of healing suggest physical violence occuring repeatedly.
- Any injury during pregnancy should be explored to determine if it was sustained as a result of domestic violence.
- In patients who have difficulty communicating because of cognitive impairment, examine the genital area for signs of hematomas, bleeding, or the insertion of foreign bodies.

(From Nosek MA. *Guidelines for physicians on the abuse of women with disabilities.* Houston, TX: Center for Research on Women with Disabilities, 1996, with permission.)

friends who could help with your personal care needs if you felt unsafe?" will let them know that you are attuned to some of the issues they face. For batterers, you can say, "You can't keep doing this," "Most men are not violent with their partners and children," or "I wouldn't be doing you any favors to make excuses for the abuse; this is illegal and will likely land you in jail, possibly with a criminal record."

6. Provide safety planning and referrals. Assess the degree of danger the patient may be experiencing by asking if she is fearful at the moment, if the batterer is in a violent phase or under the influence of drugs or alcohol now, or if he has a weapon with him there at the clinic. For situations of extreme danger, contact the police and Adult Protective Services for the safety of the victim, your staff, the other patients in the clinic, and yourself.

The effectiveness of safety planning has been well documented in the literature (67). Research has begun on adapting traditional approaches to safety planning to the situation of women with disabilities (68). The basic components of safety planning are identifying family, friends, or church members the woman could stay with if her safety were threatened; developing a code system with a trusted person to signal for help; and keeping cash, keys, and other important documents at a safe location. We have added to these the disability elements of preparing plans for emergency accessible transportation; alternative means of communication; keeping extra medications, medical supplies, and (if possible) extra assistive devices at a safe location; and arranging for emergency backup personal care assistance. Planning is also appropriate on safety measures in medical settings, such as having trusted people accompany the patient and always keeping mobility devices within reach. Referral information should be on hand for the local police, Adult Protective Services, local battered women's programs, low-cost or free legal defense resources, and disability-related service providers such as the local center for independent living or home health care agencies.

7. Avoid victim blaming in all contacts with the victim and others. The remnants of traditional beliefs about domestic violence are, unfortunately, still very much with us. As recently as the 1970s, battering and rape were thought to result from agitation or seduction by women, and even children were blamed for provoking child abuse, giving rise to the oxymoronic concept of noninjurious abuse. Health care professionals must examine their own beliefs carefully and work to expunge any notion that victims are to blame for the violent actions of perpetrators. For the situation of women with disabilities, it is helpful to ask yourself whether, in any other context, such treatment would be acceptable. When people with disabilities who cannot tend to their personal needs are left without food or water, left to sit in feces, or confined to restricted areas of the home, that is not neglect; that is abuse.

8. Acknowledge that healing occurs at varying rates, and support the patient's method of coping. Solutions to abusive situations are much more difficult to identify for women with disabilities, particularly when financial dependence and the need for personal assistance serve to perpetuate the abuse. Alternatives, such as exploration of eligibility for government-funded benefit programs and natural supports in the woman's environment (family, friends, neighbors, church members), may take time to cultivate. Communication with local rehabilitation resources, disability rights organizations, or developmental disabilities support systems may open new avenues for changes to a nonviolent living arrangement.

Many women with disabilities survive intimidation, coercion, and violence by using denial. Although this is effective in the short term, it can lead to missed opportunities for intervention when intervention could be most effective. Pointing out the facts of a situation, the extent of injuries, the possible long-term effects of such injuries, and the impact on a woman's physical and emotional functioning can help her to understand her present and her future and encourage her to seek assistance.

9. Understand the liability implications for failure to intervene appropriately, including the duty to warn and reporting requirements. Many states have legislated mandatory reporting by health care professionals related to abuse of people with disabilities and older people who cannot speak for themselves. It is essential that physicians become familiar with these requirements just as they would for legislation related to the handling of controlled substances. Careful consideration must be given, however, to the woman's ability to speak and take action for herself, as well as the possibility of retaliation by the batterer. Women should be informed, involved, and consulted at every step of this process.

10. Understand the correlation between substance abuse and domestic violence. Research has shown a very strong correlation between substance abuse and domestic violence, mainly on the part of the perpetrator but also occasionally by the victim. Screening for substance abuse risk factors and behaviors should be conducted along with screening for domestic violence in the health evaluation of all patients. Abuse of prescription medicines, alcohol, or illegal substances is no more tolerable among people with disabilities than it is for anyone else. Disabled women who are victims of violence by substance abusing partners may have other avenues of relief in addiction rehabilitation service programs.

CONCLUSION

As a society, we have a long way to go before women with disabilities can live without fear of domestic violence. All women are vulnerable to violence in their home, but for women with disabilities, the financial disadvantages, the role entanglement of partner/personal care assistant, the stigmatization and devaluation of disability, and environmental barriers that limit access to battered women's resources make dealing with violence far more difficult. The range of "weapons" that can be used against women with disabilities is greater, the range of people who can disempower them is greater, and their natural defenses are fewer. With so many factors working against the feasibility of disclosing and resolving these problems, health care professionals have an even greater opportunity and duty to address violence against women with disabilities when it is suspected.

Solving the problem of violence against women with disabilities will require the involvement of segments of the community that traditionally have not been active in efforts to reduce domestic violence. It is essential that physicians prepare themselves and everyone involved in their practice to understand, identify, and respond appropriately to violence against the women they serve. By seeking training and becoming part of concerned networks of those working in the battered women's movement, the disability rights movement, disability service organizations, legal defense organizations, law enforcement, religious organizations, and health care, physicians can be effective agents of change. In this way we can expand the awareness and understanding of abuse in the context of disability and the critical importance of removing the barriers that face women with disabilities who are trying to eliminate violence from their lives.

REFERENCES

1. Silverman A. Paralyzed in paradise: Just when things couldn't get any worse for Heather Grossman–they did. *Phoenix New Times,* May 1, 2003. Available at www.phoenixnewtimes.com. Accessed July 23, 2003.
2. Ramsay J, Richardson J, Carter YH, et al. Should health

professionals screen women for domestic violence? Systematic review. *BMJ* 2002 Aug 10;325(7359):314.

3. Warshaw C, Ganley A, Saliber P. Improving the health-care response to domestic violence: A resource manual for health care providers. San Francisco: Family Violence Prevention Fund and Pennsylvania Coalition Against Domestic Violence, 1995.

4. National Center for Health Statistics. Healthy women with disabilities: Analysis of the 1994-1995 National Health Interview Survey: Series 10 Report [forward by F. Chevarley, J. Thierry, M. Nosek, C. Gill]. Atlanta: CDC/NCHS, in review.

5. Nosek MA, Howland CA, Young ME. Abuse of women with disabilities: Policy implications. *J Disabil Policy Studies* 1997;8:157–176.

6. Young ME, Nosek MA, Howland C, et al. Prevalence of abuse of women with physical disabilities. *Arch Phys Med Rehabil* 1997;78(12 Suppl 5):S34–S38.

7. Finkelhor D, Korbin J. Child abuse as an international issue. *Child Abuse Neglect* 1988;12:3–23.

8. Claussen AH, Crittenden PM. Physical and psychological maltreatment: Relations among types of maltreatment. *Child Abuse Neglect* 1991;15:5–18.

9. Soeken K, McFarlane J, Parker B, et al. The abuse assessment screen: A clinical instrument to measure frequency, severity and perpetrator of abuse against women. In: Campbell JC, ed. Empowering survivors of abuse. Thousand Oaks, CA: Sage, 1998:195—223.

10. Cole SS. Facing the challenges of sexual abuse in persons with disabilities. *Sex Disabil* 1984;7:71–88.

11. Nosek MA, Foley CC, Hughes RB, et al. Vulnerabilities for abuse among women with disabilities. *Sex Disabil* 2001;19:177–189.

12. Nosek MA, Howland CA, Rintala DH, et al. National study of women with physical disabilities: Final report. *Sex Disabil* 2001;19(1):5–39.

13. Sobsey D, Doe T. Patterns of sexual abuse and assault. *Sex Disabil* 1991;9:243–260.

14. Sobsey D. Violence and abuse in the lives of people with disabilities: The end of silent acceptance? Baltimore, MD: Paul H. Brookes Publishing Co., 1994.

15. Nosek MA, Walter LJ, Young ME, et al. Lifelong patterns of abuse experienced by women with physical disabilities, unpublished manuscript.

16. Hamby SL, Koss MP. Violence against women: Risk factors, consequences, and prevalence. In: Liebschutz JM, Frayne SM, Saxe GN. *Violence against women: A physicians guide to identification and management.* Philadelphia: American College of Physicians, 2003:3–38.

17. Schumacher JA, Feldbau-Kohn S, Smith-Slep A, et al. Risk factors for male-to-female partner physical abuse. *Aggr Viol Beh* 2001;6:281–352.

18. Hughes RB, Swedlund N, Petersen N, et al. Depression and women with spinal cord injury. *Topics Spinal Cord Injury Rehabil* 2001;7:16–24.

19. Hughes RB, Taylor HB, Robinson-Whelen S, et al. Perceived stress and women with physical disabilities. In: Nosek MA, Hughes RB, Taylor HB. Violence against women with physical disbilities: Final Report. Houston, TX: Center for Research on Women with Disabilities, 2002:60–71.

20. Hughes RB, Taylor HB, Shelton ML, et al. Dynamics of violence against women with disabilities: a qualitative study. In: Nosek MA, Hughes RB, Taylor HB. Violence against women with physical disbilities: Final Report.

Houston, TX: Center for Research on Women with Disabilities, 2002:14–29

21. Nosek MA, Taylor HB, Hughes RB, et al. Demographic, disability, and psychosocial characteristics of abused women with disabilities. In: Nosek MA, Hughes RB, Taylor HB. Violence against women with physical disabilities: Final Report. Houston, TX: Center for Research on Women with Disabilities, 2002:46–59

22. Belsky J. Child maltreatment: An ecological integration. *Am Psychol* 1980;35:320–335.

23. Kreigsman KH, Bregman S. Women with disabilities at midlife: [Special issue: Transition and disability over the life span]. *Rehab Counsel Bull* 1985;29:112–122.

24. Womendez C, Schneiderman K. Escaping from abuse: Unique issues for women with disabilities. *Sex Disabil* 1991;9:273–280.

25. Howland CA, Rintala DH. Dating behaviors of women with physical disabilities. *Sex Disabil* 2001;19(1):41–70.

26. Rintala DH, Howland CA, Nosek MA, et al. Dating issues for women with physical disabilities. *Sex Disabil* 1997;15(4):219–242.

27. Nosek MA, Rintala DH, Young ME, et al. Sexual functioning among women with physical disabilities. *Arch Phys Med Rehabil* 1996;77(2):107–115.

28. Curry M., Hassouneh-Phillips D, Johnston-Silverberg A. Abuse of women with disabilities: An ecological model and review. *Violence Against Women* 2001;7:60–79.

29. Powers LE, Curry MA, Oschwald M, et al. Barriers and strategies in addressing abuse: A survey of disabled women's experiences. *J Rehab* 2002;68(1):4–13.

30. Saxton M, Curry MA, Powers LE, et al. "Bring my scooter so I can leave you": A study of disabled women handling abuse by personal assistance providers. *Violence Against Women* 2001;7:393–417.

31. Hassouneh-Phillips D, Curry MA. Abuse of women with disabilities: State of the science. *Rehab Counsel Bull* 2002;45:96–104.

32. Centers for Disease Control and Prevention. Webcast: Sexual violence prevention: Building leadership and commitment to underserved communities. Available at: http://www.phppo.cdc.gov/PHTN/webcast/svprev/default.asp. Accessed April 3, 2003.

33. U.S. Department of Health and Human Services. Disability and secondary conditions. In: *Healthy People 2010.*Washington, DC: U.S. Department of Health and Human Services, 2000.

34. Kellerman A, Mercy J. Men, women, and murder: Gender-specific differences in rates of fatal violence and victimization. *J Trauma* 1992;33:1–5.

35. Finkelhor D, Araji S, Baron L, et al. Sourcebook on child sexual abuse. Newbury Park, CA: Sage, 1986.

36. Murphy PA. Taking an abuse history in the initial evaluation. *NARPPS* 1992;7:187–190.

37. Ratican KL. Sexual abuse survivors: Identifying symptoms and special treatment considerations. *J Counsel Dev* 1992;71:33–38.

38. Faria G, Belohlavek N. Treating female adult survivors of childhood incest. *Social Casework* 1984;65:465–471.

39. Courtois CA, Watts DC. Counseling adult women who experienced incest in childhood or adolescence. *Personnel Guidance J* 1982;60:275–279.

40. Cunningham J, Pearce T, Pearce P. Childhood sexual abuse and medical complaints in adult women. *J Interpers Viol* 1988;3:131–144.

41. Briere J, Zaidi LY. Sexual abuse histories and sequelae in female psychiatric emergency room patients. *Am J Psychiatry* 1989;146:1602–1606.

42. Browne A, Finkelhor D. Impact of child sexual abuse: A review of the research. *Psych Bull* 1986;99:66–77.

43. Briere J, Runtz M. Symptomatology associated with childhood sexual victimization in a nonclinical adult sample. *Child Abuse Neglect* 1988;12:51–59.

44. Bradshaw JS. Healing the shame that binds you (Cassette Recording No. 1-55874-043-0). Deerfield Beach, FL: Health Communications, 1989.

45. Gordy PL. Group work that supports adult victims of childhood incest. *Social Casework* 1983;64:300–307.

46. Kearney-Cooke A. Group treatment of sexual abuse among women with eating disorders. *Women Ther* 1988; 7:5–21.

47. Swedlund NP, Nosek MA. An exploratory study on the work of independent living centers to address abuse of women with disabilities. *J Rehab* 2000;66:57–64.

48. National Coalition Against Domestic Violence. *Open minds, open doors: Technical assistance manual assisting domestic violence service providers to become physically and attitudinally accessible to women with disabilities.* Denver, CO: National Coalition Against Domestic Violence, 1996.

49. Howland CA. *Serving women with disabilities: A directory of abuse intervention services.* Houston, TX: Center for Research on Women with Disabilities, Baylor College of Medicine, 1999.

50. Nosek MA, Howland CA. Women with disabilities. In: Liebschutz JM, Frayne SM, Saxe GN. *Violence against women: A physician's guide to identification and management.* Philadelphia: American College of Physicians, 2003:201–210.

51. Twisselmunn, B. Summary of responses [to Ramsay et al]. *BMJ* 2002 Dec 14;325(7377):1419.

52. Nurse J. Culture shift is needed. *BMJ* 2002 Dec 14;325 (7377):1417.

53. Davies P. Doctor's duty of confidentiality may not be in patient's or community's interest. *BMJ* 2002 Dec 14;325 (7377):1418.

54. Health Insurance Portability and Accountability Act of 1996 Public Law 104-191, Aug. 21, 1996. Available at http://aspe.hhs.gov/admnsimp/pl104191.htm. Accessed July 23, 2003.

55. Jones RF 3rd, Horan DL. The American College of Obstetricians and Gynecologists: responding to violence against women. *Int J Gynaecol Obstet* 2002 Sep;78 Suppl 1:S75–77.

56. American Medical Association. Diagnostic and Treatment Guidelines on Domestic Violence. Chicago: American Medical Association, 1992.

57. Cohn F, Salmon M, Stobo J, eds. *Confronting chronic neglect: the education and training of health professionals on family violence.* Washington, DC: Institute of Medicine, 2002.

58. Bauer ST, Shadigian EM. Screening for violence makes a difference and saves lives. *BMJ* 2002 Dec 14;325 (7377):1417.

59. Joint Commission on Accreditation of Healthcare Organizations (JCAHO). *Comprehensive accreditation manual for hospitals,* Update 3. Oakbrook Terrace, IL: JCAHO, 1997:PE-10-PE-34.

60. Buel SM. Treatment guidelines for healthcare providers' interventions with domestic violence victims: experience from the USA. *Int J Gynaecol Obstet* 2002 Sep;78 Suppl 1:S39–44.

61. Varjavand N, Cohen DG, Novack DH. (2002) An assessment of residents' abilities to detect and manage domestic violence. *J Gen Intern Med* 2002 Jun;17(6):465–468.

62. McFarlane J, Christoffel K, Bateman L, et al. Assessing for abuse: self-report versus nurse interview. *Public Health Nurs* 1991 Dec;8(4):245–250

63. Rhodes KV, Lauderdale DS, He T, et al."Between me and the computer": increased detection of intimate partner violence using a computer questionnaire. *Ann Emerg Med* 2002;40:476–484.

64. McFarlane J, Hughes RB, Nosek MA, et al. Abuse Assessment Screen-Disability (AAS-D): Measuring frequency, type, and perpetrator of abuse toward women with physical disabilities. *J Womens Health Gend Based Med* 2001;10:861–866.

65. Liebschutz JM, Frayne SM, Saxe GN. Violence against women: A physicians guide to identification and management. Philadelphia: American College of Physicians, 2003.

66. Saxe GN, Liebschutz JM, Edwardson E, et al. Bearing witness: the effect of caring for survivors of violence and health care providers. In: Liebschutz JM, Frayne SM, Saxe GN. *Violence against women: A physicians guide to identification and management.* Philadelphia: American College of Physicians, 2003:157–166.

67. McFarlane J, Malecha A, Gist J, et al. An intervention to increase safety behaviors of abused women: results of a randomized clinical trial. *Nurs Res* 2002 Nov–Dec;51 (6):347–354.

68. Taylor HB, Hughes RB., Mastel-Smith B, et al. Developing and determining the feasibility of a safety planning intervention for women with disabilities. In: Nosek MA, Hughes RB, Taylor HB. Violence against women with physical disbilities: Final Report. Houston, TX: Center for Research on Women with Disabilities, 2002:81–92

69. Nosek MA. *Guidelines for physicians on the abuse of women with disabilities.* Houston, TX: Center for Research on Women with Disabilities, 1996.

26

Sexuality Issues

Beverly Whipple and Sandra L. Welner

SEXUALITY ISSUES IN WOMEN WITH A DISABILITY OR CHRONIC ILLNESS

We are all sexual beings from the time we are born until the time we die. Women with disabilities and chronic illnesses are, of course, sexual beings; however, they may need to make some adjustments to continue to receive pleasure from sensual and sexual intimacy. Such individuals may have to redefine the meaning and purpose of sexuality in their lives and will have to appreciate their own value in a world that may invite them to feel less worthy because of their disability or chronic illness (1).

Women with chronic or disabling conditions retain the right to make decisions about their sexuality, whether these decisions steer the woman to be more or less active sexually, or perhaps to express her sexuality in different ways than she did prior to the onset of her disability or chronic illness (2). Physical limitations can threaten a woman's feelings of self-determination in all activities, including sexual expression. These women will need to find the delicate balance between independence, dependence, and interdependence (1). The realization that women can continue to be attractive sexual beings and that their disability or chronic illness does not eradicate this part of the human experience will help to enforce a more positive self-concept.

SEXUALITY AND SEXUAL EXPRESSION

Before specifics can be discussed concerning sexuality and women with a disability or chronic illness, it is important first to define sexuality. In the past, sexuality was viewed as having one purpose, and that purpose was reproduction (3). Today, sexuality is conceptualized as an important aspect of health and human behavior; it enhances the quality of life, fosters personal growth, and contributes to human fulfillment (4). Sexuality refers to the totality of a being; it does not just refer to the genitals and their function. This holistic view of sexuality encompasses human qualities and includes all of the components—biologic, psychologic, emotional, social, cultural, and spiritual—that make people who they are. People have the capacity to express their sexuality in any of these areas without necessarily involving the genitals (5).

Another area that must be considered in terms of sensuality and sexuality is a woman's self-concept and body image, which can influence how a woman with a disability or chronic illness may interact with others. The response of significant others to the woman also may influence her self-concept and body image. The ways in which the woman with a disability or chronic illness perceives her body will influence her sexual self-concept and her sexual behaviors (1). The relationship between body satisfaction and self-satisfaction is particularly strong among females because society places so much emphasis on attractiveness as an important indicator of female worth and value (6). Therefore, an alteration in a person's appearance or even the perception of a person's body may have far-reaching social consequences (5).

Another consideration in terms of sensuality and sexuality is what the health care professional and/or the woman or the couple view as their goal of sexual expression. There are two views of sexual expression (7). The goal-oriented view is analogous to climbing a flight of stairs. The first step is touching, the next step is kissing, followed by caressing, vagina–penis contact, intercourse, and then the top step of orgasm. The goal of one or both partners is orgasm. If the sexual experience does not lead to the achievement of that goal, then one or both partners do not feel satisfied with the experience (5). The second view is pleasure-oriented, which is analogous to a circle, with each expression on the perimeter of the circle considered an end in itself. Whether the experience involves kissing, oral sex, or holding, each experience is an end in itself and each is satisfying to the couple. There is no need to have this form of expression lead to anything else (5). Problems may occur if one person in a relationship is goal-oriented and the other person is pleasure-oriented and they are not aware of their focus or they do not communicate their views to each other. If the health care provider is "genital-orgasm goal-oriented" he or she may have difficulty suggesting alternative forms of sexual expression to a woman with a disability or chronic illness (1).

MODELS OF SEXUAL RESPONSE

A number of models of sexual response have been proposed since Masters and Johnson first published their arbitrarily chosen phases of excitement, plateau, orgasm, and resolution (8). Kaplan (9) added desire as a first phase. Reed's Erotic Stimulus Pathway model has been superimposed on the Kaplan model. Reed's model has four phases: seduction, sensations, surrender, and reflection (1).

Whipple and McGreer expanded Reed's model to explain how a woman's sexual response is circular and not linear, like male sexual response (1,30). In other words, the triphasic model of Kaplan, on which the common classifications of sexual dysfunctions are based, is based on the male linear model of desire, arousal (erection), and orgasm. The

sexual experience of many women does not necessarily follow this linear progression. Women often report a high level of sexual satisfaction despite the absence of orgasm or vaginal lubrication (30). A model must assign significance to nonbiologic components such as pleasure and satisfaction. In the expansion of Reeds Erotic Stimulus Pathway model (Fig. 26-1), how a woman feels immediately after a sexual experience will act as feedback for future sexual experiences with that person or with other people. If the immediate reflection is positive (i.e., warm, loving, and pleasurable), then the desire will be stimulated for another time. If the reflection is negative (i.e., the woman did not feel pleasure or satisfaction), then the feedback will act to lower desire for another time. Reflection appears to be the beginning of the next sexual experience and considers the components that are important to the woman.

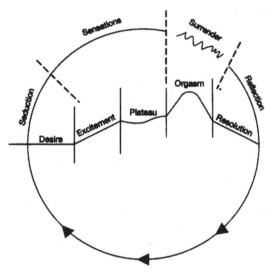

Fig. 26-1. Whipple and McGreer's expansion of Reed's Erotic Stimulus Pathway model. The reflection phase leads to the seduction phase of the next sexual experience, when the experience results in pleasure and satisfaction for the woman. (From Whipple B, Brash McGreer K. Management of female sexual dysfunction. In: Sipski ML, Alexander CJ, eds. *Sexual function in people with disability and chronic illness.* Gaithersburg, MD: Aspen Publishers, 1997:527, with permission.)

Currently the triphasic model of desire, arousal, and orgasm is used as a basis for defining sexual function and dysfunction in women with and without disability and chronic illness. This model does not reflect the sexual experiences of women and inaccurately will render pathologic what seems normal and natural for many women (30).

PATTERNS OF SEXUAL RESPONSE

In addition to models of sexual response, the health care provider has to be aware of the various patterns of female sexual response that have been described. Masters and Johnson reported that there is one reflex pathway in female sexual response. The clitoris is reported to be the major source of sensory input, the pudendal nerve is its sensory pathway, and the "orgasmic platform" undergoes myotonic buildup and discharge during orgasm (8). Perry and Whipple described a second pathway that included the Grafenberg spot (or G spot) as the major source of stimulation and the pelvic nerve and hypogastric plexus as its major pathway. The major myotonic responder consisted of the musculature of the uterus, bladder, and urethra; the contractile elements associated with the paraurethral glands; and the proximal portion of the pubococcygeus muscle (10). Perry and Whipple claimed that this double-reflex concept could account for the reported ability of some women to selectively experience "vulval," "uterine," or "blended" orgasm (11).

Women also have reported that they could achieve orgasm from fantasy alone, without touching their bodies. In a laboratory study designed to document this occurrence, orgasm from either self-induced imagery or genital self-stimulation was associated with significant increase in blood pressure, heart rate, pupil diameter, and pain thresholds over resting control conditions (12). On the basis of these findings, it is evident that physical genital stimulation is not necessary to produce a state that is reported to be an orgasm.

Knowledge of the various models of sexual response and the variety of ways women experience sexual pleasure is important for health care providers who are counseling women with disabilities or chronic illnesses about their sexual concerns (32). It is also important for the health care provider to be aware that there is no right or wrong way to experience sexual pleasure and that each person is unique and responds differently depending on many variables (1).

DISABILITIES AND CHRONIC ILLNESS

Many disabilities alter neurologic function that can affect areas of the brain and spinal cord, which in turn can result in some degree of sexual dissatisfaction. Such conditions include head injury, stroke, psychomotor epilepsy, spinal cord injury (SCI), and multiple sclerosis.

Vascular disorders affect the circulatory system and appear to be more disabling for males because erection depends on blood flow. However, these syndromes may be just as disabling for women in terms of sensation, lubrication, and orgasm. These diagnoses include disorders of blood vessels and the heart, such as thromboembolic disorders, cardiac disease, and sickle cell anemia, and may alter sensation, lubrication, and orgasm.

Endocrine imbalances disturb hormonal stability. Any problem that results in lowered levels of testosterone may affect sexual desire and response. Changes in sexual function also can be noted in diabetes and other endocrine disorders.

Debilitating conditions such as cancer, lung disease including asthma and chronic obstructive pulmonary disease, and degenerative disorders exemplified by some forms of arthritis that produce general ill health and affect sexual responsiveness through fatigue, malaise, and illness-focused environments (1,9,13).

Medications that women with disabilities and chronic illness take to manage common problems can cause sexual dissatisfactions and dysfunctions. Examples of such medications include tranquilizers, antidepressants, antihypertensive drugs, cholesterol-lowering drugs, antispasmodics, ulcer medications, and many more (33). Alcohol, heroin, and sedatives such as barbiturates also may cause sexual problems. And antihistamines may result in decreased vaginal lubrication (1).

Psychosocial factors, such as communication problems, sexual misinformation, unhealthy relationships, and childhood or historical traumas, also can influence sexual function (1,3,4).

Therefore, there are many areas to be considered when discussing sexuality with a woman with a disability or a chronic illness. Generalizations should not be made purely on the nature of the physical challenge or chronic condition. It is important to evaluate the totality of a woman's symptoms when working with sexual dissatisfactions in a woman with a disability or chronic illness.

PLISSIT MODEL

One way to determine what level of counseling is needed by a couple or a woman with a disability or chronic illness is to use the PLISSIT model developed by Annon (31). This model is used by health care providers to determine if they are able to provide the sexuality information and counseling needed or if they should refer to a certified sex therapist. The P-LI-SS-IT model is divided into levels, depending on the amount and type of intervention that is needed. The first level of the model is *Permission*; level two is *Limited Information*; level three is *Specific Suggestions*; and level four is *Intensive Therapy*. Theoretically, each succeeding level of the model requires increasing degrees of knowledge, training, and skill on the part of the health care provider. The model offers guidelines to help the health care provider distinguish between problems that she or he can handle and those that require greater knowledge, training, and skill.

According to Annon, the first level, *permission,* basically is letting clients and their significant other know that it is all right to continue doing what they have been doing. With many women or couples, this is all that

is needed. Annon defines *limited information* as providing clients with the specific factual information directly relevant to their particular sexual concerns. *Specific suggestions* is the level requiring the health care provider to make an in-depth analysis of the concern, to relate a breadth of knowledge to the behavioral and sexuality areas to the concern, and to use transmittal skills to make the specific suggestions relevant and acceptable to the woman and/or her partner. When *intensive therapy* is needed, referral usually is made to a sex therapist certified by the American Association of Sex Educators, Counselor and Therapists (AASECT) (31). (See contact information at end of this chapter.)

SEXUAL EXPERIENCES

A woman with a disability or a chronic illness may need to make specific adjustments to have or resume good sexual experiences (14). Family members and friends, as well as the health care provider, can encourage the woman to gain new strategies for positive interactions in all settings. Sexual adaptations may present new challenges to couples. It is crucial to foster creativity and open dialogue for experimentation. Such experimentation may include different positions; new ways of arousing or stimulating the partner; or use of sexual aides such as feathers, dildos, or the like (Fig. 26-2). Open communication between partners and a sense of humor can help minimize embarrassment from bowel and bladder accidents or involuntary movements from muscle spasms that may result in discomfort (16).

Incorporating sexual adaptations into sex play (what some still call foreplay) can be particularly useful. For example, as a partner positions spastic legs, stroking and massaging may improve spasticity while stirring sexual closeness between partners. Many women with chronic conditions experience fatigue, pain, or stiffness, which may be worse at certain times of the day (17). Acknowledging these timing issues and fostering closeness and caring during these less optimal periods

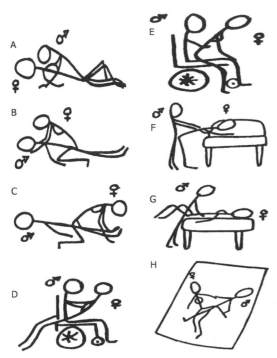

Fig. 26-2. Suggested coital positions for people with a disability or chronic illness. (From McCormick GP, Riffer DJ, Thompson MM. Coital positioning for stroke-surviving couples. *Rehabil Nurs* 1986;11(2):17–19, with permission of the Association of Rehabilitation Nurses, 4700 W. Lake Avenue, Glenview, IL 60025-1485.)

can maximize opportunities for sexual intimacy at times of peak energy and nadirs of pain. Taking analgesics or medication to control specific symptoms prior to sexual interactions may be helpful.

Thus, sexual pleasuring need not be restricted to the able-bodied but is an enjoyment that can be shared by all individuals. Societal stereotypes may work against spontaneity and sensual exploration; therefore, it is essential to support and validate women with disabilities or chronic illnesses in their quest for sexual fulfillment (18).

ADULT-ONSET DISABILITY OR CHRONIC ILLNESS

Physical challenges and longstanding medical conditions that have their onset in adulthood may challenge many of the woman's established behavioral patterns including psychologic, social, and sexual interactions. The ideal "sexy woman" is stereotypically slender, agile, and physically attractive, although many women in all cultures never match these stereotypes and still are able to find positive sexual identity within themselves. Women with physical disabilities or chronic illnesses may be more threatened and devalued by negative stereotypes. Not only do they not fit "into the mold," but they also may have muscle spasms, sit in wheelchairs, use adaptive mobility aides, and need assistance with activities of daily living. These disability-related changes may challenge a woman's sexual identity. A woman's previous sexual experiences can be a handicap or an asset to readjustment, depending on her mindset. A sense of humor can be the most valuable attribute in making flexible adjustments to physical limitations. There is a paucity of supportive literature targeted at issues of body image, self-esteem, and physical attractiveness in women with disabilities and chronic illnesses. However, these gaps are starting to be bridged by creative activist pioneers and researchers in advancing the cause of sexuality for women with physical disabilities and chronic illnesses (34).

Health care providers caring for a woman with acquired disabilities or chronic illnesses should recognize these issues and provide encouragement for adaptive intimacy strategies and support the natural quest of women to maintain sexual desirability (1,35). Facilitating pleasure between couples is an essential part of intimacy, and couples may benefit from counseling with knowledgeable professionals to support, enable, and validate their need to develop individual ways of giving and receiving sexual pleasure (19). Health care providers should refer individuals and couples to AASECT certified sex counselors or sex therapists for help with sexual and intimacy concerns that are beyond the scope of their expertise. (See contact information at the end of this chapter.)

SPECIAL CONCERNS

Unfortunately, this less-than-stable body image and shaky self-esteem may put women with disabilities or chronic illnesses at risk for sexual exploitation and abuse (20,21). They may welcome somebody, anybody, who would want to be with them in a sexual way, and they may adopt the "beggars can't be choosers" philosophy. Health care providers working with these women should address these issues preemptively, as close to the onset of disability or chronic illness as possible, to discuss this danger and provide avenues for supportive counseling.

Our culture tends to overvalue spontaneity and undervalue planning (1). In certain circumstances, planning can make the difference between an unpleasant, stressful encounter and a romantic interlude. Simple things such as transferring onto a steady, stable surface; providing a warm, romantic, and private environment; timing medications to minimize pain or spasticity; propping pillows and cushions in areas that require extra support; and positioning limbs in such a way as to facilitate masturbatory activities or a sexual encounter with a partner in the most relaxed, comfortable fashion possible can create the aura of "planned spontaneity" (1).

Sometimes disability may lead to behavioral changes in the affected woman, which although understandable because of her situation, may make her interactions with others more difficult. She may become more demanding and assume the role of a martyr, attempting to generate guilt feelings from her caregivers to prevent the unspoken fear of rejection and/or abandonment. This unfortunately may have the opposite effect, causing her caregivers to become overstressed and reluctant to interact with her because of this excessively demanding behavior. Although some of these issues can be worked out through family therapy, continuous demands on the caregiver are clearly not eliminated through counseling. The Well Spouse Foundation is a national resource whose focus is to balance the needs of the "patient" and the "caregiver" (1). (See contact information at the end of this chapter.) Each partner, and indeed every member of the family system, has special and universal needs for breaks in routines, adequate rest, and appreciation. All need to be empowered by the health care provider to assert their own needs while respecting the needs of other members of the unit.

AGING

The aging process results in a natural decline in agility and flexibility in all individuals, although in people with preexisting disabilities or chronic illnesses these changes may be accentuated (22). Menopause may bring alterations in sexual function such as decreased desire, delayed orgasm, and decreased vaginal lubrication. Women with disabilities and chronic illnesses may experience these changes as well as changes related to their condition and the medications they are taking. In addition to antihypertensives, lipid-lowering agents, diuretics, and antidepressants widely prescribed in the general population of menopausal women, other commonly prescribed medications such as immunosuppressive agents (e.g., corticosteroids), anticonvulsants (e.g., carbamazepine), anticholinergics-urinary tract agents (e.g., Ditropan), and antispasmodics (e.g., baclofen and diazepam) also should be considered as affecting sexual function (33).

Adaptations for maximizing flexibility and well-being are essential components of daily living for a woman with a disability or chronic illness. Exercise should be done to maintain range of motion, especially in hips and the lower back because these areas commonly are involved in sexual positioning. Exercise also should be done after corrective surgery for the same reasons. Changing sides in bed also can be helpful to emphasize utilization of functional and intact extremities, such as the unaffected side of a stroke patient (5,23) (Fig. 26-2). The health care provider must be aware that there are times when the woman's partner fears causing discomfort or injury to the women and this can be a deterrent to resuming sexual activities. If this fear is not verbalized, the woman may interpret her partner's reluctance as rejection rather than protection. Counseling for the couple and not just the woman is very important here (5).

SPINAL CORD INJURY

One area of disability and chronic illness, SCI, will be used as an example in terms of new research findings concerning sexuality and sexual expression. There is very little known about sexual response in women with SCI, and literature regarding women with SCI concerning orgasm is scant. However, promising new research is being conducted in these areas. Sipski and her colleagues (24) studied women with incomplete SCI and Whipple and her colleagues (26–29) studied women with complete SCI. Studies are reporting that women with SCI can respond to audiovisual stimulation similarly to able-bodied women in those functions that are controlled neurologically above the levels of their injuries, whereas genital vasocongestion may not occur because the neurologic pathway is interrupted. In contrast, reflex genital vasocongestion can occur in women with SCI despite a lack of subjective arousal (24). It has been reported that "although vaginal lubrication may still occur in response to either touch or mental stimuli, there can be no orgasmic response arising from or detected in the genitalia" (25). However, sensory input from the sexual system can gain access to the brain, even in women with "complete" SCI (26).

In studies of orgasms in women with complete SCI, using positron-emission tomography scans of the brain coupled with magnetic resonance imaging, sensory pathways from the sexual system to the brain that bypass the spinal cord (the sensory vagus nerves) have been detected. These findings support the presence of multiple sensory pathways from the genital system to the brain (27,28). Perhaps, as demonstrated in these studies, in women with complete SCI with no input from the genitospinal nerves, the sensory vagus

nerve may play a role in stimulating orgasm. Based on these data, it seems likely that there can exist nerve pathways from the sexual system to the brain that are functional in women with complete SCI and that these may mediate orgasm in response to genital stimulation (27,28).

Based on a qualitative study of women with complete SCI, it was reported that after injury to the spinal cord, there are three stages of sexual readjustment: cognitive genital dissociation, sexual disenfranchisement, and sexual recovery (29,36).

Research has found that immediately after a disability or chronic illness, there seems to be a shutting down or closing up of sexuality for many women (29). A woman may become depressed and pessimistic about the future. Sometimes the woman has serious doubts as to whether her partner will accept her with a disability or chronic illness. She may lose interest in her grooming and may feel unattractive (29). During this early phase of sexual recovery, the health care provider can explore the woman's previous level of sexual interest and activity and let her know that a temporary shelving of sexual interest is predictable. Women need to be supported in terms of their own priorities, not those of the health care provider (1,29).

During the second phase of "sexual disenfranchisement," the participants in the study reported that between 3 months and 3 years post-SCI, they experienced sexual intercourse. They stated that they were curious about what the experience would be like. The experience generally resulted in sexual dissonance, a comparison between pleasure (what was) and disappointment (what is). This experience activated a lengthy sexual readjustment and reevaluation of the nature of sexual pleasure (29).

A period of "sexual rediscovery" emerged following sexual disenfranchisement. For some women, significant life events (such as a fortieth birthday) or situation events (such as a new sexual partner) were turning points. Affirming relationships characterized by open communication, creativity, and resourcefulness played a key role in positive sexual self-concept. There was also a reevaluation of the meaning of sexual pleasure and an exploration of alternative approaches to sexual arousal and orgasm (29).

It may be possible that the stages of sexual recovery identified in this qualitative study with women with complete SCI also may emerge from studies of women with other disabilities or chronic illness. It is important to note that anecdotal and case study reports from sex therapists support these stages in women with various disabilities and chronic illnesses (1).

CONCLUSION

It is essential for health care providers and sex therapists to understand the impact of the disability or chronic illness on the woman, rather than impose preconceived ideas of limitations that the disability or chronic illness places on the woman or the couple. This increased sensitivity can foster a positive therapeutic relationship between all members of the health care team and assist women with disabilities or chronic illness to achieve sexual fulfillment.

REFERENCES

1. Whipple B, McGreer KB. Management of female sexual dysfunction. In: Sipski ML, Alexander CJ, eds. *Sexual function in people with disability and chronic illness.* Gaithersburg, MD: Aspen Publishers, 1997: 511–536.
2. Stephen I. Sexual equality: How enlightened have we become? *Disabil Rehab* 1996 Dec;18(12):627–628.
3. Whipple B. Female sexuality. In: Leyson JFJ, ed. *Sexual rehabilitation of the spinal-cord injured patient.* Clifton NJ: Humana Press, 1990:19–38.
4. Whipple B, Gick R. A holistic view of sexuality: Education for the health professional. *Topics Clin Nurs* 1980:91–98.
5. Whipple B. Sexual counseling of couples after a mastectomy or a myocardial infarction. *Nurs Forum* 1987; 23(3):85–91.
6. Koch PB. *Exploring our sexuality.* Dubuque, IA: Kendall/Hunt, 1995.
7. Timmers PO. Treating goal-directed intimacy. *Social Work* 1976:401–402.
8. Masters WH, Johnson VE. *Human sexual response.* Boston: Little Brown, 1966.
9. Kaplan HS. *The new sex therapy.* New York: Brunner/ Mazel, 1974.
10. Perry JD, Whipple B. Pelvic muscle strength of female ejaculators: Evidence in support of a new theory of orgasm. *J Sex Res* 1981;17:22–39.
11. Ladas AK, Whipple B, Perry JD. *The G spot and other recent discoveries about human sexuality.* New York: Holt, Reinhart and Winston, 1982; Dell 1983.
12. Whipple B, Ogden G, Komisaruk BR. Relative analgesic effect of imagery compared to genital self-stimulation. *Arch Sex Behav* 1992;21:121–133.
13. Kaplan HS. *Disorders of sexual desire.* New York: Simon and Schuster, 1979.
14. Rieve JE. Sexuality and the adult with acquired physical disability. *Nurs Clin North Am* 1989 Mar;24(1): 265–276.
15. Boggs JA. *Living and loving: information about sex.* Boston: The Arthritis Foundation, 1982.
16. Smith J, Bullough B. Sexuality and the severely disabled person. *Am J Nurs* 1975 Dec;75(12):2194–2195.
17. Rothrock RW, D'Amore G. *The illustrated guide to better sex for people with chronic pain.* Morrisville, PA: Rothrock & D'Amore, 1992.
18. Szasz G. Sex and disability are not mutually exclusive—evaluation and management. *West J Med* 1991; 154:560–563.
19. Neistadt ME. Sexuality counseling for adults with disabilities: A module for an occupational therapy curriculum. *Am J Occup Ther* 1986;40(8):542–545.
20. Welner SL. Caring for the woman with a disability. In: Wallace L, ed. *Textbook of women's health.* Philadelphia: Lippincott-Raven Publishers, 1998:87–92.
21. Blackburn M. Sexuality, disability, and abuse: advice for life ... not just for kids. *Child Care Health Dev* 1995; 21(5):351–361.
22. Kaplan HS. Sex, intimacy, and the aging process. *J Am Acad Psychoanal* 1990;18(2):185–205.
23. Conine TA, Evans JH. Sexual reactivation of chronically ill and disabled adults. *J Allied Health* 1982; 261–270.
24. Sipski ML, Alexander CJ, Rosen RC. Physiological parameters associated with psychogenic sexual arousal in women with complete spinal cord injuries. *Arch Phys Med Rehabil* 1995;76(9):811–818.
25. Szasz G. Sexual health care. In: Zejdlik CP, ed. *Management of spinal cord injury.* Boston: Jones and Bartlett Publishers, 1992:175–201.
26. Whipple B, Komisaruk BR. Sexuality and women with complete spinal cord injury. *Spinal Cord* 1997;35: 136–138.
27. Whipple B, Gerdes CA, Komisaruk BR. Sexual response to self-stimulation in women with complete spinal cord injury. *J Sex Res* 1996;33(3):231–240.
28. Komisaruk BR, Gerdes C, Whipple B. "Complete" spinal cord injury does not block perceptual responses to genital self-stimulation in women. *Arch Neurol* 1997; 54:1513–1520.
29. Whipple B, Richards E, Tepper M, et al. Sexual response in women with complete spinal cord injury. In: Krotoski DM, Nosek M, Turk M, eds. *Women with physical disabilities: Achieving and maintaining health and well-being.* Baltimore: Paul H. Brookes, 1996:69–80.
30. Sugrue DP, Whipple B. The consensus-based classification of female sexual dysfunction: Barriers to universal acceptance. *J Sex Marital Ther* 2001;27: 221–226.

31. Annon JS. *The behavioral treatment of sexual problems,* Vol. 1. Brief Therapy. Hawaii: Enabling Systems, Inc., 1974.

32. Tepper MS. Providing comprehensive sexual health care in spinal cord injury rehabilitation: Implementation and evaluation of a new curriculum for health professionals. *Sex Disabil* 1997;15(3):271–283.

33. Drugs that cause sexual dysfunction: An update. *Med Lett Drugs Ther* 1992;34(876):73–78.

34. Mona LR, Gardos PS, Brown RC. Sexual views of women with disabilities: The relationship among age-of-onset, nature of disability and sexual self-esteem. *Sex Disabil* 1994;12(4):261–277.

35. Nosek MA. Primary care issues for women with severe physical disabilities. *J Womens Health* 1992;1(4): 245–248.

36. Richards E, Tepper M, Whipple B, et al. Women with complete spinal cord injury: A phenomenological study of sexuality and relationship experiences. *Sex Disabil* 1997;15(4):271–283.

RESOURCES

American Association of Sex Educators, Counselors, and Therapists (AASECT)
P. O. Box 5488
Richmond, VA 23220-0488
Phone: 804-644-3288
Fax: 804-644-3290
www. AASECT.org

Well Spouse Foundation
P.O. Box 801
New York, NY 10023
Phone: 800-838-0879
Fax: 212-724-5209

Pain: Gender Differences, Psychosocial Factors, and Medical Management

Roger B. Fillingim and Iqbal H. Jafri

Pain is a complex personal experience that includes sensory, emotional, and behavioral dimensions. It is as ubiquitous as it is difficult to define. It is estimated that at any one time 20% of the United States adult population experience some form of chronic pain, and pain is estimated to cost society more than $100 billion annually (1). Pain is even more pervasive among patients with disabilities. In addition to arthritic and other rheumatologic conditions, which virtually always are accompanied by pain, two-thirds of patients with multiple sclerosis will experience pain (2). Diabetic neuropathy, which can produce debilitating pain, occurs in approximately one-third of patients with diabetes (3). In addition, lesions of the central nervous system, including cerebrovascular accidents and spinal cord injury, frequently cause pain that is recalcitrant to treatment (4,5). Thus pain is a major public health issue and is highly prevalent in patients with various disabilities.

The nature of the pain accompanying chronic disabling conditions is quite variable and can be categorized broadly as nociceptive or neuropathic. Nociceptive pain typically emanates from somatic structures, such as skin, muscle, or joint, or from visceral structures, such as the internal organs. Neuropathic pain is produced by damage to or dysfunction of the central or peripheral nervous system. These distinctions are important because effective treatments can differ for nociceptive versus neuropathic pain.

Of course, patients often have multiple sources of pain, and many conditions are associated with both nociceptive and neuropathic pain. For example, patients with spinal cord injury commonly experience neuropathic pain as a result of their central lesions, but nociceptive pain as a result of muscle spasm and visceral pain are also frequent manifestations (6).

NEURAL MECHANISMS OF PAIN TRANSMISSION

The pain processing system is quite complex and highly dynamic, and the precise neural circuitry of nociceptive transmission has not been characterized fully. Historically, theories of pain transmission emphasized ascending pathways in which primary afferent nerve fibers activated spinal cord and brainstem neurons, which then simply conveyed the information to higher brain structures. Since the publication of the gate control theory (7) more than three decades ago and the discovery of endogenous opiates in the 1970s (8), the importance of central nervous system pain-modulatory systems increasingly has been recognized. Early efforts were focused on inhibitory systems that actively reduced pain responses by diminishing pain-related input to brain structures (9). In more recent years, systems that augment pain transmission have been investigated widely. These include peripheral (10) and central sensitization (11) as well as descending facilitatory systems originating in higher brain structures that serve to enhance ascending pain transmission (12,13). These sensitization processes and facilitatory systems likely contribute to many chronic painful conditions. In addition, nociceptive activity arising from deep tissues may be under greater inhibitory influence than activity from cutaneous sites (14). This is important because chronic pain associated with disability typically emanates from deep tissues (e.g., muscle, joints, and the viscera), and failure of inhibitory systems may play a particularly important role in these types of pain. In summary, the experience of pain is sculpted by complex and dynamic interactions among peripheral and central sensitization processes counterbalanced by inhibitory control systems, and dysfunction in inhibitory and/or facilitatory systems likely contributes to many chronic pain disorders.

PAIN ASSESSMENT

Pain is an internal and personal experience; therefore pain assessment is heavily dependent on the patient's description of pain. The severity of clinical pain most often is assessed with numeric or visual analog scales (VAS). Numeric scales (e.g., 0 to 10) have the advantage of convenience and familiarity, and most patients find them easy to use, but they may not have ratio properties, meaning that a rating of 6/10 is not necessarily twice as severe as 3/10 (15). Visual analog scales consist of a line of predetermined length (e.g., 10 cm) flanked at either end by anchors such as "no pain" and "most intense pain imaginable." VAS offer ideal statistical properties and relatively continuous response categories; however, they take longer to administer and score and some patients have difficulty using these scales (15). Another method of assessing pain severity is by measuring observable pain behavior. Valid and reliable systems for assessing pain behavior have been described (16), and they have the advantage of not relying on the patient's self-report; however, implementing these systems can be impractical in many clinical settings. Nonetheless, clinical observation of patients' behaviors can provide an important source of additional information regarding pain.

In addition to pain severity, several other pain-related constructs should be assessed, including the temporal characteristics of the pain, the sensory qualities of the pain, the pain location, pain-related disability, and pain-related affective distress. Regarding temporal characteristics, the duration of the pain (i.e., time since first onset) as well as whether the pain is episodic or continuous should be evaluated. The sensory qualities of the pain can be assessed using multiple item measures, such as the McGill Pain Questionnaire (17). Patients choose from lists of adjectives (e.g., sharp, burning, dull, aching) that most accurately describe the nature of their pain, which can provide clinicians with important information regarding the quality of the pain. Pain location can be assessed conveniently and reliably using a Pain Drawing (18), which can specify the location(s) of pain and provide information regarding how widespread the pain is. In patients with chronic conditions that produce disability, it can be difficult to differentiate pain-related disability from disability caused by other aspects of their condition. Nonetheless, pain-related disability is an important clinical issue. Optimally, pain-related disability would be assessed via functional testing (19); however, this is more time consuming than questionnaire-based assessment. Several paper and pencil measures are available for assessing pain-related disability and interference of pain in activities, and these have been reviewed (15). Pain-related affective distress is also an important clinical variable. Anxiety, depression, and anger are the most common affective states associated with chronic pain, and multiple psychometrically sound instruments are available for assessing these mood states (20).

PSYCHOLOGIC FACTORS AND PAIN

The biopsychosocial model of pain posits that the experience of pain is determined by complex and dynamic interactions among biomedical, psychologic, and sociocultural factors (21). Among patients experiencing pain associated with chronic disabling conditions, the identification of contributing psychosocial factors is necessary to provide optimal treatment. Several studies have discussed the role of psychologic factors in chronic pain (22–24). Some aspects of psychologic functioning are important in chronic pain. Personality characteristics may predict the development of chronic pain, and there is evidence that personality disorders are more common in patients with chronic pain (25). In addition, depression, anxiety, and anger commonly are associated with chronic pain, and these affective factors may enhance sensitivity to pain (20,26). A variety of cognitive variables are important predictors of pain-related adjustment. For example, pain beliefs and expectancies, cognitive coping strategies, and one's perceived ability to manage pain can have important influences on clinical outcomes (27,28). Thus psychologic factors can affect adjustment to pain significantly. It is important to note, however, that much of the research in this area has been conducted in populations in which chronic pain is the primary disorder, and the extent to which these findings generalize to patients with pain resulting from other disabling conditions is not known.

Given the interactions between psychosocial factors and pain, it should not be surprising that psychologic treatments are important components of pain management. Cognitive–behavioral treatment has been found efficacious for many pain disorders, including (but not limited to) arthritis and other rheumatic conditions (29,30), musculoskeletal pain (23,31–33), headache (34), and temporomandibular disorders (35). Cognitive–behavioral treatment usually includes several components, such as relaxation training, education, cognitive restructuring to reduce maladaptive thinking, training in the use of distraction, and activity modification/scheduling. These treatments can be administered in group or individual format, and they often are part of a multidisciplinary treatment approach that also includes medical management and physical rehabilitation. In addition to general cognitive–behavioral treatment, both hypnosis (36) and biofeedback (37) are specific psychologic interventions that are effective in pain management.

PAIN AS A WOMEN'S HEALTH ISSUE

Pain in patients with disabilities could be considered a women's health issue because of several factors. First, there is evidence that in general women are at greater risk for experiencing clinical pain. For example, several common chronic pain disorders are more prevalent in women than men (Table 27-1)

Table 27-1. *Common pain disorders that are more prevalent in women compared to men*

Pain disorder	Overall prevalence (%)	Female: male ratio
Migraine headache	15–20	2:1–3:1
Chronic tension-type headache	4–5	2:1
Temporomandibular disorders	4–12	1.5:1
Irritable bowel syndrome	15–20	2:1
Rheumatoid arthritis	1	2.5:1
Osteoarthritis	80 (>age 65)	1.5:1–4:1
Fibromyalgia	2–3	6:1

(From Unruh AM. Gender variations in clinical pain experience. *Pain* 1996;65:123–167; Buckwatter JA, Lappin DR. The disproportionate impact of chronic arthralgia and arthritis among women. *Clin Orthop* 2000;25:159–168; Crombie IK, Croft PR, Linton SJ, et al. *Epidemiology of pain.* Seattle: IASP Press, 1999.)

and population-based studies generally have demonstrated more frequent pain-related symptoms among women relative to men (38–43). Second, proportionately more older women than men are disabled (44); therefore the possibility of disability-associated pain is greater among women. Indeed, some disabling conditions that are associated with pain are more common in women, including arthritis and multiple sclerosis. Finally, because the incidence of pain increases with age (45,46), women's greater longevity places them at increased risk of disability-associated pain (or pain-associated disability).

SEX DIFFERENCES IN PAIN PERCEPTION

In addition to the greater prevalence of clinical pain and disability among women, there is evidence that women and men may perceive pain differently, which could contribute to increased risk of disability-associated pain in women. Laboratory-based research suggests that women exhibit greater sensitivity to experimentally induced pain than men do across a variety of stimulus modalities and assessment methods (47–49). Some of these findings are based on subjective responses, such that women have lower pain thresholds and tolerances and generally describe noxious stimuli as more painful. However, sex differences have been reported for less subjective measures as well. For example, women showed greater temporal summation of thermal pain, which is thought to reflect increasing responses to repeated pain as a result of sensitization in central neurons (50). Also, the nociceptive flexion reflex, which is a spinal pain–related muscle response, occurs in women at a lower stimulus intensity than in men (51), and women exhibited greater pupil dilation in response to painful pressure than men (52). It also has been demonstrated that some brain regions show greater activation during painful stimulation among women than men (53). However, another group of investigators reported more robust cerebral activation among males in responses to non-painful rectal stimulation (54). Thus, the bulk of

the experimental evidence suggests enhanced pain sensitivity among females.

MECHANISMS UNDERLYING SEX DIFFERENCES IN PAIN RESPONSES

The potential mechanisms underlying sex differences in clinical and experimental pain responses have been reviewed elsewhere (48,55,56) and will be discussed briefly here. Hormonal factors often are proposed to account for sex differences in both clinical and experimental pain responses. In this regard, several pain disorders show menstrual cycle–related exacerbations (56a,b,c), and exogenous hormone use is associated with increased risk of some forms of clinical pain (57–60). Experimental pain perception also is influenced by the menstrual cycle in healthy women (55,61), and postmenopausal women taking hormone replacement have lower pain thresholds and tolerances than their counterparts who are not receiving hormone replacement (62).

Other possible contributing factors include several psychosocial variables. It has been suggested that sex roles may be important because stereotypic male roles discourage the reporting of pain, whereas female stereotypes may encourage women to admit pain. In an experimental study, Otto and Dougher (63) found that high masculinity scores were associated with higher pain thresholds among males, but neither masculinity nor femininity was associated with pain threshold for females. However, even after accounting for masculinity–femininity scores, the sex difference in pain threshold remained significant. In another study males reported significantly less pain in the presence of a female experimenter, whereas females' ratings did not differ as a function of experimenter gender. In contrast, other studies have not found significant effects of experimenter gender (63,64). Thus empirical support for a mediating influence of sex role expectancies is not strong, and minimal clinical research has investigated this issue. It is also plausible that cognitive–affective factors including emotional distress, pain coping strategies, and pain-related expectancies may contribute to sex differences in pain. Clinically, affective states such as depression and anxiety are more prevalent among females than males and are associated with increased pain and other physical symptoms (43,65,66), and emotional distress has been associated with greater experimental pain sensitivity (67–70). However, we have reported that anxiety is associated with poorer adjustment to chronic pain (71) as well as increased experimental pain sensitivity (72) among males but not females, suggesting that anxiety produces greater effects on pain responses in men than in women.

Additional psychosocial factors such as pain coping may underlie sex-related differences in pain. Catastrophizing has been associated with poorer adjustment to clinical pain (73–75) and decreased tolerance of laboratory pain (76), and females report greater catastrophizing than males (77–79), which may contribute to their increased risk for experiencing pain. Familial factors also could contribute to sex differences in the experience of pain. A self-reported family history of pain has been related to increased pain complaints in community-based samples (38,42,80,81), and the relationship between family history and pain complaints was stronger for females than males in one study (80). Also, we found that a self-reported familial pain history was associated with increased clinical pain and greater experimental pain sensitivity for females but not males (82). The extent to which such familial influences reflect genetic (83) versus environmental factors has yet to be determined.

SEX DIFFERENCES IN PAIN TREATMENT SETTINGS

The previous discussion indicates that sex differences in the experiences of clinical and experimental pain exist, and multiple mechanisms likely interact to produce such differences. Additional data suggest that there are sex differences in the delivery of and re-sponses to pain treatment. First, women seek more pain-related health care than men (84,85), and in the general population women are more likely to use prescription and non-prescription analgesic medication (86,87). There is also evidence that the prescription of pain treatment may differ for female and male patients. Several reports have documented that both invasive and noninvasive cardiac procedures are prescribed more often for men than for women presenting with chest pain (88–90). In a study using clinical vignettes of patients with back pain, male physicians prescribed higher doses of hydrocodone, an opioid analgesic, to men than women, whereas the reverse was true for female physicians (91). Thus women and men with similar presentations may be treated differently. The reasons for these differences remain unknown and require further investigation.

Another important question regarding treatment is whether the effectiveness of treatment varies as a function of sex. In reviewing the literature, Miaskowski and Levine (92) found that women demanded less postoperative opioid medication; however, because pain relief was not assessed in many of the studies, sex differences in analgesic responses could not be determined directly. These investigators also have reported greater analgesic responses among women compared to men following administration of opioids thought to produce analgesia by activating the kappa-opioid receptor (for review see Miaskowski and Levine [92]). Another study using experimentally induced pain reported greater morphine analgesia among women (93,94). Regarding nonopioid pain medications, analgesic responses to spinally administered neostigmine were greater for women (95), whereas the antiinflammatory ibuprofen produced greater analgesia for men (96). Robinson and colleagues (97) found that Lidocaine produced greater cutaneous anesthesia in men than women. Thus pharmacologic interventions for pain may produce different effects in women and men; however, the pattern of results is not consistent across drugs and test conditions.

Fewer studies have addressed sex differences in the efficacy of nonpharmacologic interventions for pain. In a study of physical medicine treatments for back pain, conventional physical therapy was more effective for men, whereas intensive dynamic back exercises produced greater improvements in pain among women (98). Another study reported that women with pain resulting from temporomandibular disorder showed significant decreases in pain 2 years after conservative multidisciplinary treatment, whereas pain reports among men remained unchanged (99). Similarly, a trial in 2001 demonstrated that women undergoing either cognitive behavioral treatment or the combination of cognitive behavioral treatment plus physical therapy reported improved health-related quality of life, whereas no such improvements were evident for men (100). In addition, for women but not men both treatments reduced the likelihood of being placed on permanent disability (see Table 27-1).

MEDICAL AND PHARMACOLOGIC MANAGEMENT OF MALIGNANT AND NONMALIGNANT CHRONIC PAIN

Selection of the appropriate analgesic therapy is based on the intensity of each patient's pain and type of pain. Pain intensity can be measured reliably with use of written or verbal numeric rating scales (101,102). Pain that is rated 5 or higher on a scale of 0–10 interferes substantially with the quality of life and is defined as substantial pain (101). Pain ratings of 1–4 correspond to mild pain; ratings of 5–6 correspond to moderate pain; and ratings of 7–10 correspond to severe pain (103).

According to several studies (103a,104), 90% of patients with cancer pain can be controlled through relatively simple means. The three-step analgesic ladder of the World Health Organization uses three categories of pain to guide analgesic therapy: Step 1: mild to moderate pain should be treated with nonopioid analgesic drugs (Fig. 27-1). If a patient has mild to moderate pain despite taking a nonopioid analgesic, the dose of nonopioid

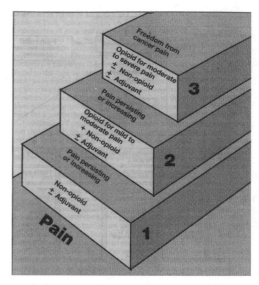

Fig. 27-1. The World Health Organization's three-step analgesic ladder. Reprinted with permission from the World Health Organization.

analgesic should be maximized and a Step 2 opioid analgesic should be added (Table 27-2). Patients who have moderate to severe pain despite therapy with Step 2 opioids require an increase in the dose of the opioids or a change to a Step 3 opioid. Many experts recommend a Step 2 opioid as initial therapy for patients with moderate pain and may initiate therapy with a Step 3 opioid when pain is severe. Patients who have mild to moderate pain while taking a Step 3 opioid should have the dose of that opioid increased to an effective level.

Nonopioid, Step 1 analgesic drugs include acetaminophen, aspirin, and other nonsteroidal antiinflammatory drugs (NSAID) and cyclooxygenase-2 (COX-2) inhibitors. These drugs are of limited value to patients with pain from advanced cancer because of their relatively low maximal efficacy. The dose of acetaminophen should not exceed 4 to 6 grams/day to prevent liver damage. Patients with cancer are not often given aspirin because of high incidence of gastropathy and aspirin's ability to inhibit platelet aggregation (105). The risk of bleeding problems can be minimized by using nonacetylated salicylates, such as choline magnesium trisalicylate, or a

Table 27-2. *Oral and parenteral dose equivalents of opioid analgesic drugs*

Drug	Dose[a] Oral	Dose[a] Parenteral
RECOMMENDED FOR ROUTINE USE		
Step 2 opioids		
Codeine[b]	100 mg every 4 hr	50 mg every 4 hr
Dihydrocodeine	50–75 mg every 4 hr	NA
Hydrocodone	15 mg every 4 hr	NA
Oxycodone[c,d]	7.5–10 mg every 4 hr	NA
Step 3 opioids		
Morphine[d]	15 mg every 4 hr	5 mg every 4 hr
Oxycodone[c,d]	7.5–10 mg every 4 hr	NA
Hydromorphone[e]	4 mg every 4 hr	0.75–1.5 mg every 4 hr
Fentanyl[f]	NA	50 µ/m every 72 hr
NOT RECOMMENDED FOR ROUTINE USE		
Propoxyphene	180 mg every 4–6 hr	NA
Meperidine	150 mg every 2–3 hr	50 mg every 2 hr
Methadone	10 mg every 6–8 hr	5 mg every 6 hr
Levorphanol	2 mg every 6–8 hr	1 mg every 6–8 hr

NA, not available.

[a]Values are dose equivalents for around-the-clock analgesic therapy for chronic pain.

[b]Doses above 1.5 mg per kilogram of body weight are not recommended because of increased toxicity.

[c]Parenteral oxycodone is available in some countries. The equivalent parenteral dose is 50% of the oral dose.

[d]This drug is available in tablets and liquids taken every 4 hours and in controlled-release tablets every 12 hours. The 12-hour dose is 3 times the 4-hour dose.

[e]The ratio of oral to parenteral doses has been reported to be as high as 2:1.

[f]The microgram-per-hour dose of transdermal fentanyl is equal to one-half of the milligram-per-day dose of oral morphine.

COX-2 inhibitor that do not interfere with platelet function (106,107). Patients taking NSAIDs should be monitored for gastropathy, renal failure, hepatic dysfunction, and bleeding (108). Tramadol, a centrally acting analgesic that binds µ-opioid receptors and inhibits the reuptake of norepinephrine and serotonin, has been approved in the treatment of moderate to moderately severe pain. Patients with cancer who are most likely to benefit from tramadol are those who cannot tolerate NSAIDs and those who wish to defer opioid therapy.

The Step 2 opioids used to treat moderate pain include codeine, dihydrocodeine, hydrocodone, oxycodone, and propoxyphene (see Table 27-2). Step 2 opioids are restricted to the treatment of moderate pain because of dose-limiting side effects or because they are prepared in fixed combination with nonopioid analgesics. Propoxyphene is not recommended for routine use because of its long half-life and the risk of accumulation of nonpropoxyphene, a toxic metabolite.

Step 3 opioids commonly prescribed for the relief of moderate to severe cancer pain include morphine, oxycodone, hydromorphone, and fentanyl (see Table 27-2). Morphine is the Step 3 opioid most commonly used to control severe pain because of its wide availability, varied formulations, and well-characterized pharmacologic properties (108a,109). Controlled-release formulations of morphine for oral administration have been the mainstay in the control of chronic cancer pain because of the ease of their administration and titration. Oxycodone is a step 3 opioid. A controlled- release formulation of oxycodone administered at 12-hour intervals is also available and is a useful alternative to controlled-release morphine (110). Fentanyl delivered by means of transdermal patches can control chronic cancer pain for 72 hours and is particularly useful in patients with stable pain who cannot take oral medications (111,112). Methadone and levorphanol also may be considered for the relief of severe cancer pain but are not recommended for initial therapy because of their long half-lives and the risk of drug accumulation.

Opioids not recommended for use in the control of moderate to severe pain include meperidine, buprenorphine, pentazocine, butorphanol, dezocine, and nalbuphine. Meperidine should not be given because its half-life is short and its metabolite, normeperidine, is toxic (108a,109). Partial opioid agonists such as buprenorphine are of limited benefit because of their low maximal efficacy; also, above a certain dose, they are toxic without additional analgesia. Mixed-opioid agonist–antagonists such as pentazocine, butorphanol, dezocaine, and nalbuphine are not recommended because of their low maximal efficacy and their potential to reverse analgesia and even cause a physical withdrawal syndrome when taken by patients already receiving full agonists such as morphine.

There is no one optimal or maximal dose of a Step 3 opioid analgesic drug (113–115). The appropriate dose is one that relieves a patient's pain throughout its dosing interval without causing unmanageable side effects.

ROUTE OF ADMINISTRATION OF ANALGESIC DRUGS

Most patients with cancer who have chronic pain should receive oral analgesic therapy. If a patient cannot swallow tablets or liquids, transdermally administered fentanyl is an excellent alternative. Subcutaneous or intravenous administration of morphine or hydromorphone is preferable to transdermal administration of fentanyl in patients who are unable to take oral medications for 24–48 hours; patients with frequent episodes of incident pain; and patients with acute, severe pain in whom injections or infusions facilitate escalating the dose. This is preferable because the bioavailability of parenterally administered morphine is three times that of oral mor-

phine (see Table 27-2) (113–116). The dosage must be changed when the route is switched from one to the other. Subcutaneous or intravenous administration of opioid analgesics by means of patient-controlled analgesia pumps expedites individual pain relief. Intramuscular opioid therapy is not recommended because it is painful and harder for family caregivers to administer.

Spinal administration of opioid, alone or in combination with local anesthetics, should be reserved for patients for whom systemic analogous therapy is unacceptably or unmanageably toxic. The potency of opioids administered epidurally is five to 10 times that of opioids administered parenterally. The intrathecal route is 10 times more potent than the epidural route. Intraventricular administration can be advantageous in patients with pain from head and neck cancers.

ADJUVANT THERAPY

Adjuvant drug therapy enhances the analgesic efficacy of opioids. Adjuvant drug therapy also treats concurrent symptoms that exacerbate pain or produces independent analgesia for specific types of pain (113). The drugs most commonly used in adjuvant therapy for the treatment of cancer pain are NSAIDs, corticosteroids, tricyclic antidepressant drugs, and anticonvulsant drugs (Table 27-3). NSAIDs are effective in the treatment of pain from bone metastasis, soft-tissue infiltration, arthritis, serositis and recent surgery. Corticosteroids can be helpful in patients with pain resulting from acute nerve compression, visceral distention, increased intracranial pressure, and soft-tissue infiltration (108a,116a,117).

Patients with pain caused by bone metastasis may benefit from adjuvant therapy with pamidronate, strontium chloride Sr89, or calcitonin (118). Pamidronate has been approved for adjuvant therapy in patients with multiple myeloma to reduce bone pain and the incidence of fractures (119). Strontium chloride Sr89, a beta-particle–emitting calcium analog selectively taken up by osteoblasts, relieves

TABLE 27-3. *Drugs commonly used in combination with analgesic drugs for cancer pain*

Type of pain	Drugs
Bone metastasis, soft-tissue infiltration, serositis, arthritis	NSAIDs: 1,500 mg of choline magnesium trisalicylate orally twice a day, 800 mg of ibuprofen orally every 8 hr, 550 mg naproxen sodium orally two to three times a day, 150–200 mg of sulindac orally every 12 hr
Postoperative pain	NSAIDs: 50 mg of indomethacin rectally every 6–8 hr, 15–30 mg of ketorolac intravenously every 6 hr[a]
Soft-tissue infiltration, acute nerve compression, visceral distention, increased intracranial pressure	Corticosteroids.[b] 4–8 mg of dexamethasone orally two to three times a day, 16–32 mg of methylprednisone orally two to three times a day, 20–40 mg of prednisone orally two to three times a day
Acute spinal cord compression; acute, severe increased intracranial pressure	Corticosteroids.[b] 10–20 mg of dexamethasone intravenously every 6 hr[c], 40–80 mg of methylprednisone intravenously every 6 hr
Neuropathic pain	Tricyclic antidepressant drugs[d,e] 50–150 mg of amitriptyline orally at bedtime, 50–150 mg of nortriptyline orally at bedtime, 50–200 mg of desipramine orally at bedtime Anticonvulsant drugs: 200 mg of carbamazepine[d,e] two to four times a day, 0.5–1.0 mg of clonazepam[d] orally three times a day

NSAIDs, nonsteroidal antiinflammatory drugs.

[a]Ketorolac should be given for no more than 5 days.

[b]Dose recommendations are based on uncontrolled, anecdotal reports and clinical experience. After successful adjuvant therapy, the corticosteroid dose should be tapered to the lowest possible effective dose or discontinued, if possible, to avoid long-term adverse effects.

[c]Doses may be as high 40–100 mg of dexamethasone when given as loading doses or when given every 6 hours for the first 24–72 hours of treatment.

[d]Therapy should be initiated at 50% of the lowest dose, and the dose should be titrated every few days until the optimal effect is achieved.

[e]Serum drug concentrations should be monitored to assess compliance and to prevent unexpected toxicity.

(From Levy MH. Pharmacologic treatment of cancer pain. *N Eng J Med* 1996;335:1124–1132, with permission.)

pain and reduces the need for analgesic drugs in 60% to 95% of patients with osteoblastic bone metastasis (118,120). Calcitonin, a polypeptide hormone that inhibits the activity of osteoclasts, may reduce pain from bone metastasis and phantom limb pain.

NEUROPATHIC PAIN

Neuropathic pain is best treated with the use of antidepressant or anticonvulsant medications. Tricyclic antidepressants in dosages between 75 and 200 mg/day relieve pain in 55% to 67% of patients with diabetic neuropathy (113,121). Also, in patients with herpes zoster, treatment with amitriptyline (Elavil) 25 mg/day for 3 months reduces the risk of later development of postherpetic neuralgia (122). Use of the selective serotonin reuptake inhibitors sertraline (Zoloft), 150 mg/day, and paroxetine (Paxil), 30 to 70 mg/day, can reduce neuropathic pain by 75% to 80% (116). Antidepressants also improve the sleep disturbance, depression, and anxiety that often accompany chronic pain. Anticonvulsant drugs have been used in pain management since the 1960s and are effective in trigeminal neuralgia, diabetic neuropathy, and migraine prophylaxis (122a). Antiepileptic medications are also helpful in the treatment of neuropathic pain. Carbamazepine (Tegretol) has a well-established efficacy in the management of trigeminal neuralgia, and case reports show a positive effect on neuropathic pain (123). Gabapentin (Neurontin) has demonstrated efficacy in reducing pain from moderate to mild in patients with diabetic neuropathy (900 to 3,600 mg/day) and in postherpetic neuralgia (2,400 to 3,600 mg/day). Lamotrigine (Lamictal) has been reported to reduce neuropathic pain in case reports, but controlled studies are not yet available (115). Less-effective medications for neuropathic pain include mexiletine (Mexitil), 675 mg/day (124), capsaicin cream (Zostrix), 0.075% four times a day (125), and long active opioids.

Fibromyalgia

The treatment of fibromyalgia may involve a variety of modalities including the use of trigger point injections, antidepressant drugs, and physical modalities including spray and stretch techniques as well as aqua therapy and some forms of physical therapy. The therapeutic use of heat and cold often is combined with trigger point injections and antidepressant compounds to provide pain relief. Some patients will experience decreased pain with the use of transcutaneous nerve stimulation or the use of electrical stimulation to fatigue affected muscles. Massage and myofascial release techniques are beneficial in those patients suffering from myofascial pain syndrome, in which spasms are a significant problem. Massage also provides tactile desensitization that is beneficial in reducing the allodynia associated with sympathetically maintained pain.

Physical Exercise

All patients with chronic pain should engage in some form of physical exercise. Certainly with respect to fibromyalgia, the evidence is clear that a properly supervised aerobic exercise program can be at least temporarily beneficial for a majority of patients. The exercise should be designed to improve cardiovascular activity, range of motion, and muscle tone (126,126a). Exercising too aggressively will increase pain and may restrict mobility around a joint.

Medications

Research on the effectiveness of various medications in the treatment of fibromyalgia indicates amitriptyline (Elavil, 10 to 50 mg/hs) and cyclobenzaprine (Flexeril, 10 to 30 mg/day) as the most consistently beneficial (126b, 126c, 126d).

Occupational Therapy

The occupational therapist's specific role is to adapt activities of daily living to improve patient dysfunction. Focusing on the area of rest, positioning is taught to encourage correct alignment, protect joints, and decrease pain. Body mechanics are taught for getting in and out of bed and proper lifting techniques as well as proper sitting posture.

Electrotherapy: Transcutaneous Electrical Nerve Stimulation

One theory on how transcutaneous electrical nerve stimulation (TENS) works is that it blocks pain in the spinal cord. Another is that stimulation with TENS causes natural pain-relieving substances to be released, thereby reducing pain. TENS has proved to be useful in the treatment of various types of chronic and acute pain. TENS is noninvasive, inexpensive, safe, and easy to use. TENS alone may not provide complete inhibition of hyperalgesia and pain and so will probably not be the only method used clinically for pain relief. However, as an adjunct to existing pain relief methods, TENS may have a number of benefits. Several studies show the intake of opioid analgesics is reduced in patients using TENS (127–131). Other noninvasive devices that use electrotherapy are interferential stimulation, microcurrent therapy, neuromuscular stimulation, and high-voltage pulsed galvanic therapy.

SUMMARY AND CONCLUSIONS

Pain is a major public health issue and a substantial clinical challenge in patients with disabilities. A variety of biopsychosocial factors influence the experience of pain, and the patient's gender may be an important moderating variable. A substantial body of research now strongly indicates that both clinical and experimental pain responses differ significantly in women and men. Thorough assessment of pain and potential contributing psychosocial factors will provide the basis for rational pain treatment. Multiple psychologic and medical interventions are available for pain, and treatment must be tailored to the individual patient. In most cases, a combination of medical and psychologic treatments will provide optimal benefits. Evidence has emerged suggesting that the effectiveness of pharmacologic and nonpharmacologic interventions for pain may differ for women and men. Clearly, additional research in this area is warranted. An improved understanding of gender and other organismic variables that may moderate treatment effects ultimately will lead to enhanced treatment outcomes for all patients.

ACKNOWLEDGMENTS

This material is the result of work supported with resources and the use of facilities at the Malcom Randall VA Medical Center, Gainesville, FL (RBF). This work was supported by NIH/NINDS grant NS41670 (RBF).

The support of JFK Johnson Rehabilitation Institute, JFK Medical Center, Edison, New Jersey, is greatly appreciated.

The authors gratefully acknowledge the assistance of Heather Platt in the preparation of this manuscript.

REFERENCES

1. Gallagher RM. Primary care and pain medicine. A community solution to the public health problem of chronic pain. *Med Clin North Am* 1999;83:555–583, v.
2. Maloni HW. Pain in multiple sclerosis: an overview of its nature and management. *J Neurosci Nurs* 2000;32:139–144, 152.
3. Sugimoto K, Murakawa Y, Sima AA. Diabetic neuropathy—a continuing enigma. *Diabetes Metab Res Rev* 2000;16:408–433.
4. Nicholson K. An overview of pain problems associated with lesions, disorder or dysfunction of the central nervous system. *Neurorehabilitation* 2000;14:3–13.
5. Schott GD. Delayed onset and resolution of pain: some observations and implications. *Brain* 2001;124 1067–1076.
6. Siddall PJ, Loeser JD. Pain following spinal cord injury. *Spinal Cord* 2001;39:63–73.
7. Melzack R, Wall PD. Pain mechanisms: A new theory. *Science* 1965;150:971–979.
8. Hughes J, Smith TW, Kosterlitz HW, et al. Identification of two related pentapeptides from the brain with potent opiate agonist activity. *Nature* 1975;258:577–579.
9. Basbaum AI, Fields HL. Endogenous pain control systems: brainstem spinal pathways and endorphin circuitry. *Annu Rev Neurosci* 1984;7:309–338.
10. Perl ER. Cutaneous polymodal receptors: characteristics and plasticity. *Prog Brain Res* 1996;113:21–37.
11. Dubner R, Basbaum A. Spinal dorsal horn plasticity following tissue or nerve injury. In: Wall P, Melzack R, eds. *Textbook of pain.* Edinburgh: Churchill Livingstone, 1994:225–241.
12. Vanderah TW, Suenaga NM, Ossipov MH, et al. Tonic descending facilitation from the rostral ventromedial medulla mediates opioid-induced abnormal pain and antinociceptive tolerance. *J Neurosci* 2001;21:279–286.
13. Porreca F, Burgess SE, Gardell LR, et al. Inhibition of neuropathic pain by selective ablation of brainstem medullary cells expressing the micro-opioid receptor. *J Neurosci* 2001;21:5281–5288.
14. Mense S. Structure-function relationships in identified afferent neurones. *Anat Embryol (Berl)* 1990;181:1–17.
15. Von Korff M, Jensen MP, Karoly P. Assessing global pain severity by self-report in clinical and health services research. *Spine* 2000;25:3140–3151.
16. Keefe FJ, Dunsmore J. Pain behavior: concepts and controversies. *APS Journal* 1992;1:92–100.
17. Melzack R. The McGill Pain Questionnaire: major properties and scoring methods. *Pain* 1975;1:277–299.
18. Ohnmeiss DD. Repeatability of pain drawings in a low back pain population. *Spine* 2000;25:980–988.
19. Lee CE, Simmonds MJ, Novy DM, et al. Self-reports and clinician-measured physical function among patients with low back pain: a comparison. *Arch Phys Med Rehabil* 2001;82:227–231.
20. Robinson ME, Riley JLI. The role of emotion in pain. In: Gatchel RJ, Turk DC, eds. *Psychosocial factors in pain.* New York: Guilford Press, 1998:74–88.
21. Turk DC. Biopsychosocial perspective on chronic pain. In: Gatchel RJ, Turk DC, eds. *Psychological approaches to pain management: a practitioner's handbook.* New York: Guilford Press, 1996:3–32.
22. Gonzales VA, Martelli MF, Baker JM. Psychological assessment of persons with chronic pain. *Neurorehabilitation* 2000;14:69–83.
23. Linton SJ. A review of psychological risk factors in back and neck pain. *Spine* 2000;25:1148–1156.
24. Eccleston C. Role of psychology in pain management. *Br J Anaesth* 2001;87:144–152.
25. Weisberg JN, Keefe FJ. Personality, individual differences, and psychopathology in chronic pain. In:

Gatchel RJ, Turk DC, eds. *Psychosocial factors in pain.* New York: Guilford Press, 1998:56–73.

26. Keefe FJ, Lumley M, Anderson T, et al. Pain and emotion: new research directions. *J Clin Psychol* 2001;57: 587–607.

27. Jensen MP, Turner JA, Romano JM, et al. Relationship of pain-specific beliefs to chronic pain adjustment. *Pain* 1994;57:301–309.

28. Sullivan MJ, Thorn B, Haythornthwaite JA, et al. Theoretical perspectives on the relation between catastrophizing and pain. *Clin J Pain* 2001;17:52–64.

29. Keefe FJ, Caldwell DS. Cognitive behavioral control of arthritis pain. *Med Clin North Am* 1997;81: 277–290.

30. Bradley LA, Alberts KR. Psychological and behavioral approaches to pain management for patients with rheumatic disease. *Rheum Dis Clin North Am* 1999;25:215–232, viii.

31. Moore JE, Von Korff M, Cherkin D, et al. A randomized trial of a cognitive-behavioral program for enhancing back pain self care in a primary care setting. *Pain* 2000;88:145–153.

32. Marhold C, Linton SJ, Melin L. A cognitive-behavioral return-to-work program: effects on pain patients with a history of long-term versus short-term sick leave. *Pain* 2001;91:155–163.

33. Linton SJ, Ryberg M. A cognitive-behavioral group intervention as prevention for persistent neck and back pain in a non-patient population: a randomized controlled trial. *Pain* 2001;90:83–90.

34. Lake AE III. Behavioral and nonpharmacologic treatments of headache. *Med Clin North Am* 2001;85: 1055–1075.

35. Mishra KD, Gatchel RJ, Gardea MA. The relative efficacy of three cognitive-behavioral treatment approaches to temporomandibular disorders. *J Behav Med* 2000;23:293–309.

36. Holroyd J. Hypnosis treatment of clinical pain: understanding why hypnosis is useful. *Int J Clin Exp Hypn* 1996;44:33–51.

37. Arena JG, Blanchard EB. Biofeedback and relaxation therapy for chronic pain disorders. In: Gatchel RJ, Turk DC, eds. *Psychological approaches to pain management: a practitioner's handbook.* Guilford Press, New York, 1996:179–230.

38. Sternbach RA. Survey of pain in the United States: The Nuprin Pain Report. *Clin J Pain* 1986;2:49–53.

39. Andersson HI, Ejlertsson G, Leden I, et al. Chronic pain in a geographically defined general population: studies of differences in age, gender, social class, and pain localization. *Clin J Pain* 1993;9:174–182.

40. Forgays DG, Rzewnicki R, Ober AJ, et al. Headache in college students: a comparison of four populations. *Headache* 1993;33:182–190.

41. Skovron ML, Szpalski M, Nordin M, et al. Sociocultural factors and back pain. A population-based study in Belgian adults. *Spine* 1994;19:129–137.

42. Lester N, Lefebvre JC, Keefe FJ. Pain in young adults: I. Relationship to gender and family pain history. *Clin J Pain* 1994;10:282–289.

43. Rajala U, Keinanen-Kiukaanniemi S, Uusimaki A, et al. Musculoskeletal pains and depression in a middle-aged Finnish population. *Pain* 1995;61:451–457.

44. Leveille SG, Resnick HE, Balfour J. Gender differences in disability: evidence and underlying reasons. *Aging (Milano)* 2000;12:106–112.

45. Kahana B, Kahana E, Namazi K, et al. The role of pain in the cascade from chronic illness to social disability and psychological distress in later life. In: Mostofsky D, Lomranz J, eds. *Handbook of pain and aging.* New York: Plenum Press, 1997.

46. Scudds RJ, Robertson MD. Empirical evidence of the association between the presence of musculoskeletal pain and physical disability in community-dwelling senior citizens. *Pain* 1998;75:229–235.

47. Fillingim RB, Maixner W. Gender differences in the responses to noxious stimuli. *Pain Forum* 1995;4: 209–221.

48. Berkley KJ. Sex differences in pain. *Behav Brain Sci* 1997;20:371–380.

49. Riley JL, Robinson ME, Wise EA, et al. Sex differences in the perception of noxious experimental stimuli: a meta-analysis. *Pain* 1998;74:181–187.

50. Fillingim RB, Maixner W, Kincaid S, et al. Sex differences in temporal summation but not sensory-discriminative processing of thermal pain. *Pain* 1998;75: 121–127.

51. France CR, Suchowiecki S. A comparison of diffuse noxious inhibitory controls in men and women. *Pain* 1999;81:77–84.

52. Ellermeier W, Westphal W. Gender differences in pain ratings and pupil reactions to painful pressure stimuli. *Pain* 1995;61:435–439.

53. Paulson PE, Minoshima S, Morrow TJ, et al. Gender differences in pain perception and patterns of cerebral activation during noxious heat stimulation in humans. *Pain* 1998;76:223–229.

54. Berman S, Munakata J, Naliboff BD, et al. Gender differences in regional brain response to visceral pressure in IBS patients. *Eur J Pain* 2000;4:157–172.

55. Fillingim RB, Ness TJ. Sex-related hormonal influences on pain and analgesic responses. *Neurosci Biobehav Rev* 2000;24:485–501.

56. Dao TT, LeResche L. Gender differences in pain. *J Orofac Pain* 2000;14:169–184.

56a. Anderberg U, Marteinsdottir I, Hallman J, et al. Symptom perception in relation to hormonal status in female fibromyalgia syndrome patients. *J Musculoskel Pain* 1999;7:21–38.

56b. Heitkemper MM, Jarrett M. Pattern of gastrointestinal and somatic symptoms across the menstrual cycle. *Gastroenterology* 1992;102:505–513.

56c. Keenan PA, Lindamer LA. Non-migraine headache across the menstrual cycle in women with and without premenstrual syndrome. *Cephalagia* 1992;12: 356–359.

57. LeResche L, Saunders K, Von Korff MR, et al. Use of exogenous hormones and risk of temporomandibular disorder pain. *Pain* 1997;69:153–160.

58. Brynhildsen JO, Bjors E, Skarsgard C, et al. Is hormone replacement therapy a risk factor for low back pain among postmenopausal women? *Spine* 1998;23: 809–813.

59. Wise EA, Riley JLI, Robinson ME. Clinical pain perception and hormone replacement therapy in postmenopausal females experiencing orofacial pain. *Clin J Pain* 2000;16:121–126.

60. Musgrave DS, Vogt MT, Nevitt MC, et al. Back prob-

lems among postmenopausal women taking estrogen replacement therapy. *Spine* 2001;26:1606–1612.

61. Riley JLI, Robinson ME, Wise EA, et al. A meta-analytic review of pain perception across the menstrual cycle. *Pain* 1999;81:225–235.

62. Fillingim RB, Edwards RR. The association of hormone replacement therapy with experimental pain responses in postmenopausal women. *Pain* 2001;92:229–234.

63. Otto MW, Dougher MJ. Sex differences and personality factors in responsivity to pain. *Percept Mot Skills* 1985;61:383–390.

64. Feine JS, Bushnell MC, Miron D, et al. Sex differences in the perception of noxious heat stimuli. *Pain* 1991;44:255–262.

65. Kroenke K, Spitzer RL. Gender differences in the reporting of physical and somatoform symptoms. *Psychosom Med* 1998;60:150–155.

66. Moldin SO, Scheftner WA, Rice JP, et al. Association between major depressive disorder and physical illness. *Psychol Med X* 1993;23:755–761.

67. Graffenried BV, Adler R, Abt K, et al. The influence of anxiety and pain sensitivity on experimental pain in man. *Pain* 1978;4:253–263.

68. Dougher MJ, Goldstein D, Leight KA. Induced anxiety and pain. *J Anxiety Dis* 1987;1:259–264.

69. Cornwall A, Donderi DC. The effect of experimentally induced anxiety on the experience of pressure pain. *Pain* 1988;35:105–113.

70. Zelman DC, Howland EW, Nichols SN, et al. The effects of induced mood on laboratory pain. *Pain* 1991;46:105–111.

71. Edwards RR, Augustson E, Fillingim RB. Sex-specific effects of pain-related anxiety on adjustment to chronic pain. *Clin J Pain* 2000;16:46–53.

72. Fillingim RB, Keefe FJ, Light KC, et al. The influence of gender and psychological factors on pain perception. *J Gender Cult Health* 1996;1:21–36.

73. Lester N, Lefebvre JC, Keefe FJ. Pain in young adults—III: Relationships of three pain-coping measures to pain and activity interference. *Clin J Pain* 1996;12:291–300.

74. Keefe FJ, Kashikar-Zuck S, Robinson E, et al. Pain coping strategies that predict patients' and spouses' ratings of patients' self-efficacy. *Pain* 1997;73:191–199.

75. Kashikar-Zuck S, Keefe FJ, Kornguth P, et al. Pain coping and the pain experience during mammography: a preliminary study. *Pain* 1997;73:165–172.

76. Geisser ME, Robinson ME, Pickren WE. Differences in cognitive coping strategies among pain-sensitive and pain-tolerant individuals on the cold pressor test. *Beh Ther* 1992;23:31–42.

77. Fillingim RB, Wilkinson CS, Powell T. Self-reported abuse history and pain complaints among healthy young adults. *Clin J Pain* 1999;15:85–91.

78. Osman A, Barrios FX, Gutierrez PM, et al. The Pain Catastrophizing Scale: further psychometric evaluation with adult samples. *J Behav Med* 2000;23:351–365.

79. Keefe FJ, Lefebvre JC, Egert JR, et al. The relationship of gender to pain, pain behavior, and disability in osteoarthritis patients: the role of catastrophizing. *Pain* 2000;87:325–334.

80. Edwards PW, Zeichner A, Kuczmierczyk AR, et al. Familial pain models: the relationship between family history of pain and current pain experience. *Pain* 1985;21:379–384.

81. Koutantji M, Pearce SA, Oakley DA. The relationship between gender and family history of pain with current pain experience and awareness of pain in others. *Pain* 1998;77:25–31.

82. Fillingim RB, Edwards RR, Powell T. Sex-dependent effects of reported familial pain history on clinical and experimental pain responses. *Pain* 2000;86:87–94.

83. Mogil JS, Flodman P, Spence MA, et al. Oligogenic determination of morphine analgesic magnitude: a genetic analysis of selectively bred mouse lines. *Beh Gen* 1995;25:397–406.

84. Unruh AM. Gender variations in clinical pain experience. *Pain* 1996;65:123–167.

84a. Crombie IK, Croft PR, Linton SJ, et al. *Epidemiology of pain*. Seattle: IASP Press, 1999.

85. Barsky AJ, Peekna HM, Borus JF. Somatic symptom reporting in women and men. *J Gen Intern Med* 2001;16:266–275.

86. Eggen AE. The Tromso Study: frequency and predicting factors of analgesic drug use in a free-living population (12–56 years). *J Clin Epidemiol* 1993;46:1297–1304.

87. Simoni-Wastila L. The use of abusable prescription drugs: the role of gender. *J Womens Health Gend Based Med* 2000;9:289–297.

88. Maynard C, Beshansky JR, Griffith JL, et al. Influence of sex on the use of cardiac procedures in patients presenting to the emergency department. A prospective multicenter study. *Circulation* 1996;94:II93–II98.

89. Schulman KA, Berlin JA, Harless W, et al. The effect of race and sex on physicians' recommendations for cardiac catheterization. *N Engl J Med* 1999;340:618–626.

90. Roger VL, Farkouh ME, Weston SA, et al. Sex differences in evaluation and outcome of unstable angina *JAMA* 2000;283:646–652.

91. Weisse CS, Sorum PC, Sanders KN, et al. Do gender and race affect decisions about pain management? *J Gen Intern Med* 2001;16:211–217.

92. Miaskowski C, Levine JD. Does opioid analgesia show a gender preference for females?. *Pain Forum* 1999;8:34–44.

93. Sarton E, Teppema L, Dahan A. Sex differences in morphine induced ventilatory depression reside in the peripheral chemoreflex loop. *Anesthesiology* 1999;90:1329–1338.

94. Sarton E, Olofsen E, Romberg R, et al. Sex differences in morphine analgesia: an experimental study in healthy volunteers. *Anesthesiology* 2000;93:1245–1254.

95. Eisenach JC, Hood DD. Sex differences in analgesia from intrathecal neostigmine in humans. *Anesthesiology* 1998;89:A1106.

96. Walker JS, Carmody JJ. Experimental pain in healthy human subjects: gender differences in nociception and in response to ibuprofen. *Anesth Analg* 1998;86:1257–1262.

97. Robinson ME, Riley JL, Brown FF, et al. Sex differences in response to cutaneous anesthesia—a double blind randomized study. *Pain* 1998;77:143–149.

98. Hansen FR, Bendix T, Skov P, et al. Intensive, dynamic back-muscle exercises, conventional physiotherapy, or placebo-control treatment of low-back pain. A randomized, observer-blind trial. *Spine* 1993;18:98–108.

99. Krogstad BS, Jokstad A, Dahl BL, et al. The reporting of pain, somatic complaints, and anxiety in a group of patients with TMD before and 2 years after treatment: sex differences. *J Orofac Pain* 1996;10:263–269.

100. Jensen IB, Bergstrom G, Ljungquist T, et al. A randomized controlled component analysis of a behavioral medicine rehabilitation program for chronic spinal pain: are the effects dependent on gender? *Pain* 2001;91:65–78.

101. Cleeland CS. The impact of pain on the patient with cancer. *Cancer* 1984;54(11 Suppl):2635–2641.

102. Au E, Loprinzi CL, Dhodapkar M, et al. Regular use of a verbal pain scale improves the understanding of oncology inpatient pain intensity. *J Clin Oncol* 1994;12(12):2751–2755.

103. Serlin RC, Mendoza TR, Nakamura Y, et al. When is cancer pain mild, moderate or severe? Grading pain severity by its interference with function. *Pain* 1995;61(2):277–284.

104. Zech DF, Grond S, Lynch J, et al. Validation of World Health Organization Guidelines for cancer pain relief: a 10-year prospective study. *Pain* 1995; 63(1):65–76.

105. Stuart MJ, Murphy S, Oski FA, et al. Platelet function in recipients of platelets from donors ingesting aspirin. *N Engl J Med* 1972;287(22):1105–1109.

106. Stuart JJ, Pisko EJ. Choline magnesium trisalicylate does not impair platelet aggregation. *Pharmatherapeutica* 1981;2(8):547–551.

107. Laine L, Harper S, Simon T, et al. A randomized trial comparing the effect of rofecoxib, a cyclooxygenase 2-specific inhibitor, with that of ibuprofen on the gastoduodenal mucosa of patients with osteoarthritis. Rofecoxi Ostwoarthritis Endoscopy Study Group. *Gastroenterology* 1999;117(4):776–783.

108. *Principals of analgesic use in the treatment of acute and chronic cancer pain,* 3rd ed. Skokie, Il: American Pain Society, 1992.

108a.Jacox A, Carr DB, Payne R, et al. Management of cancer pain: clinical practice guidelines No. 9. Rockville, MD: Agency for Healthcare Policy and Research; 1994: Publication 94-0592.

109. Cherny NI, Portenoy RK. The management of cancer pain. *CA Cancer J Clin* 1994;44(5):263–303.

110. Sunshine A, Olson NZ, Colon A, et al. Analgesic efficacy of controlled-release oxycodone in postoperative pain. *J Clin Pharmacol* 1996;36(7):595–603.

111. Payne R. Transdermal fentanyl: suggested recommendations for clinical use. *J Pain Symptom Manage* 1992;7(3 Suppl):S40–44. Review.

112. Hanks GE, Fallon MT. Transdermal fentanyl in cancer pain: conversion from oral morphine. *J Pain Symptom Manage* 1995;10(2):87.

113. Young RJ, Clarke BF. Pain relief in diabetic neuropathy: the effectiveness of imipramine and related drugs. *Diabet Med* 1985;2(5):363–366.

114. Rosner H, Rubin L, Kestenbaum A. Gabapentin adjunctive therapy in neuropathic pain states. *Clin J Pain* 1996;12(1):56–58.

115. Di Vadi PP, Hamann W. The use of lamotrigine in neuropathic pain. *Anaesthesia* 1998;53(8):808–809.

116. Goodnick PJ, Jimenez I, Kumar A. Sertraline in diabetic neuropathy: preliminary results. *Ann Clin Psychiat* 1997;9(4):255–257.

117. Watanabe S, Bruera E. Corticosteroids as adjuvant analgesics. *J Pain Symptom Manage* 1994;9(7): 442–445. Review.

118. Quilty PM, Kirk D, Bolger JJ, et al. A comparison of the palliative effects of strontium-89 and external beam radiotherapy in metastatic prostate cancer. *Radiother Oncol* 1994;31(1):33–40.

119. Berenson JR, Lichtenstein A, Porter L, et al. Efficacy of pamidronate in reducing skeletal events in patients with advanced multiple myeloma. Myeloma Aredia Study Group. *N Engl J Med* 1996;334(8):488–493.

120. Robinson RG, Preston DF, Schiefelbein M, et al. Strontium 89 therapy for the palliation of pain due to osseous metastases. *JAMA* 1995;274(5):420–424.

121. Max MB, Kishore-Kumar R, Schafer SC, et al. Efficacy of desipramine in painful diabetic neuropathy: a placebo-controlled trial. *Pain* 1991;45(1):3–9; discussion 1–2.

122. Bowsher D. The effects of pre-emptive treatment of postherpetic neuralgia with amitriptyline: a randomized, double-blind, placebo-controlled trial. *J Pain Symptom Manage* 1997;13:327–331.

122a.McQuay H, Carroll D, Jadad AR, et al. Anticonvulsant drugs for management of pain: a systematic review. *BMJ* 1995;311(7012):1047–1052.

123. Rizzo MA. Successful treatment of painful traumatic mononeuropathy with carbamazepine: insights into a possible molecular pain mechanism. *J Neurol Sci* 1997;152(1):103–106.

124. Oskarsson P, Ljunggren JG, Lins PE. Efficacy and safety of mexiletine in the treatment of painful diabetic neuropathy. The Mexiletine Study Group. *Diabetes Care* 1997;20(10):1594–1597.

125. Ellison N, Loprinzi CL, Kugler J, et al. Phase III placebo-controlled trial of capsaicin cream in the management of surgical neuropathic pain in cancer patients. *J Clin Oncol* 1997;15(8):2974–2980.

126. Mindell E, Hoppkins V. Prescription alternatives. New Canaan, CT.: Keats Pub., 1998.

126a.McCain GA, Bell DA, Mai FM, Halliday PD. A controlled study of the effects of a supervised cardiovascular fitness training program on the manifestations of primary fibromyalgia. *Arthritis Rheum* 1988;31(9): 1135–1141.

126b.Carette S, Bell MJ, Reynolds WJ, et al. Comparison of amitriptyline, cyclobenzaprine, and placebo in the treatment of fibromyalgia. A randomized, double-blind clinical trial. *Arthritis Rheum* 1994;37(1):32–40.

126c. Santandrea S, Montrone F, Sarzi-Puttini P, et al. A double-blind crossover study of two cyclobenzaprine regimen in primary fibromyalgia syndrome. *J Int Med Res* 1993;21(2):74–80.

126d. Carette S, McCain GA, Bell, DA, Fam AG. Evaluation of amitriptyline in primary fibrositis. A double-blind, placebo-controlled study. *Arthritis Rheum* 1986;29(5): 655–659.

127. Ghoname FA, Craig WF, White PF. Use of percutaneous electrical nerve stimulation (PENS) for treating ECT-induced headaches. *Headache* 1999;39(7): 502–505.

128. Rosenberg M, Curtis L, Bourke DL. Transcutaneous electrical nerve stimulation for the relief of postoperative pain. *Pain* 1978;5(2):129–133.

129. Smith CR, Lewith GT, Machin D. TNS and osteo-arthritic pain. Preliminary study to establish a controlled method of assessing transcutaneous nerve stimulation as a treatment for the pain caused by osteoarthritis of the knee. *Physiotherapy* 1983;69(8): 266–268.

130. Solomon RA, Viernstein MC, Long DM. Reduction of postoperative pain and narcotic use by transcutaneous electrical nerve stimulation. *Surgery* 1980;87: 142–146.

131. Wang B, Tang J, White PF, et al. Effect of transcutaneous acupoint electrical stimulation on the postoperative analgesic requirement. *Anesth Analg* 1998;85: 406–413.

Appendix

Health of Women with Disabilities: From Data to Action

JoAnn M. Thierry and Juliana K. Cyril

In recent years, women's health has emerged as a prominent public health priority. Research focused on women's health has led to important information about how and why certain diseases affect women disproportionately, predominantly, or differently than men. It also has led to a better understanding of the differential health risks faced by certain subpopulations of women, such as those who are members of racial and ethnic minority groups. Yet despite the heightened attention to women's health, research to date has not adequately addressed the health concerns of women with disabilities. Research indicates that women with disabilities encounter many of the same problems as women who are not disabled, yet they report overall poorer health (1,2). Many also face substantial physical, economic, social, and attitudinal barriers to accessing care and have the extra responsibility of dealing with health concerns related to their disability (3–5).

Although studies of people with disabilities have included information about women, population-based data on the causes, risks, and consequences of disability among women were not widely available until 1996 (6). A 1999 study compiled information from multiple data sources on the demographics, education, employment, and health status of girls and women with disabilities (7). However, this report addressed only a few health-related questions and many of its comparisons focused on differences between disabled women and men. Women with disabilities are just as likely to be at risk for health problems as women without disabilities, yet comparisons between these groups are

sparse. Population-based studies are needed to accurately compare differences between women with disabilities and women without disabilities on a number of leading health indicators.

The public health community has started to recognize the health concerns of women with disabilities. Since the mid 1990s the Centers for Disease Control and Prevention (CDC), the National Center on Medical Rehabilitation and Research (NCMRR), the National Institute on Disability and Rehabilitation Research (NIDRR), and a few other agencies have funded a small number of research projects addressing the health needs of women with disabilities. However, coordination, long-term planning activities, and available funding within these agencies have been limited. As a result, there is a need to assess current activities related to the health of women with disabilities and to develop a plan for the future. This chapter describes the current data sources available for assessing the health needs of women with disabilities, the necessity to develop a public health agenda, and the steps required to improve the future health and well-being of women with disabilities.

DEFINITIONS, CAUSES, AND PREVALENCE OF DISABILITY AMONG WOMEN

In general terms, disability refers to "limitations in physical or mental function, caused by one or more health conditions, in carrying out socially defined tasks or roles" (8). Commonly accepted measures of disability have

373

focused on functional limitations, activity limitations, and work limitations. These definitions allow for the inclusion of people with many disabling conditions, including sensory, cognitive, emotional, or physical impairments, and various chronic health conditions. However, use of these multiple definitions has resulted in varying prevalence estimates of disability in women. For example, estimates from the National Health Interview Survey–Disability Supplement (NHIS–D) indicate that 16% of women 18 years of age or older had at least one functional limitation (2). In comparison, state-based estimates from the Behavioral Risk Factor Surveillance System suggest the overall prevalence of disability among women is 18% (9).

Depending on the definition used, overall estimates of disability among women in the United States range from 19.9 to 28.6 million (10,11), or approximately one in every five women. Disorders of the back and spine are the most prevalent conditions associated with disability among women, followed by arthritis and heart disease (12). Together, these conditions represent approximately 38% of all conditions causing limitations among women. Conditions generally thought to have a high risk for causing severe disability among women, such as multiple sclerosis, spinal cord injury, and mental retardation, have small prevalence rates yet often are associated with greater severity of disability and increased need for specialized services (6).

SOURCES OF DATA ON DISABILITY AND HEALTH

There are several national data sets that contribute to our knowledge of disability in the United States. Health surveys, such as the ones listed here, can provide valuable information for assessing the prevalence of heath conditions and potential risk factors over time. The Behavioral Risk Factor Surveillance System (BRFSS), for example, has been used to assess knowledge, attitudes, and health practices in relation to certain conditions affecting women's health. This and other useful sources of data on disability and health are briefly described below.

National Health Interview Survey

The National Health Interview Survey (NHIS) is a nationwide survey of the U.S. civilian noninstitutionalized population and is considered to be a primary source of health information in the United States. The survey has been conducted annually since 1957 by the National Center for Health Statistics (NCHS) of the CDC. The survey consists of two parts: a core set of basic health and demographic questions and supplemental questions addressing specific health topics of concern. Additional information about the NHIS may be found at www.cdc.gov/nchs.

National Health Interview Survey Disability Supplement

In 1994 and 1995, the NHIS included a Disability Supplement. The goal of the NHIS–D was to develop a series of questions that would provide a useful set of measures while maintaining a balance between the social, administrative, and medical considerations involved in disability measurements. Data collected as part of the NHIS–D include sensory, communication, and mobility problems; health conditions; activities of daily living; functional limitations; mental health; services and benefits; education; and perceived disability. Because the NHIS–D was not limited to one definition of disability, it allows researchers from a variety of programs to access data important to their specific programmatic needs.

The NHIS–D was administered in two phases. The Phase I Disability questionnaire, which was conducted in 1994 and 1995, was obtained by personal interview and provides basic information regarding disability. Phase II, which began in 1994 and continued through 1996, reinterviewed individuals with disabilities to obtain supplementary information. Additional information about the NHIS–D may be found at www.cdc.gov/nchs/about/major/nhis_dis/nhis_dis.htm.

Behavioral Risk Factor Surveillance Survey

The Behavioral Risk Factor Surveillance System (BRFSS) is a random-digit-dialed telephone survey of the noninstitutionalized population aged 18 years and older. It is designed to collect uniform, state-specific data on preventive health practices and risk behaviors that are linked to chronic diseases, injuries, and preventable infectious diseases. The BRFSS questionnaire has three parts: (a) the core component, (b) optional modules, and (c) state-added questions. The core includes a standard set of questions asked by all states, including questions about demographic characteristics, health-related perceptions, conditions, and behaviors. In 2001, the BRFSS added two questions on disability to the core questionnaire, one focusing on activity limitation and the other on use of special equipment. The optional modules are sets of questions on specific topics that states elect to use on their questionnaires. For example, in 1998 a special BRFSS Disability Module collected information on disability from 11 states and the District of Columbia, which were used to provide state-specific estimates of disability. Finally, independent, state-added questions may be developed by participating states and added to their state BRFSS questionnaire. Additional information about the BRFSS can be found at www.cdc.gov/brfss.

Medical Expenditure Panel Survey

The Medical Expenditure Panel Survey (MEPS) was designed to provide policymakers, health care administrators, and others with comprehensive information about health care costs and utilization in the United States. MEPS collects data on the specific health-related services that Americans use, how frequently they use them, the costs of these services, and how they are paid for. Additional information about MEPS can be found at www.meps.ahrq.gov.

Census Bureau Data on Disability

The U.S. Bureau of the Census provides data on disability based on three primary sources: the Survey of Income and Program Participation (SIPP), the decennial census of population, and the Current Population Survey (CPS). The SIPP, which began in 1984, is an ongoing study of the economic well-being of U.S. households. This survey collects data on the extent of disability in the civilian noninstitutionalized population. These data include information on (a) functional limitations, (b) work limitations, and (c) receipt of Social Security or veterans' disability benefits. The long-form questionnaire used in the decennial census contained a few questions about disability status. The third data set, the CPS, identifies people who are out of the labor force because of disability and, since 1980, identifies people who have a health problem that "prevents them from working or limits the kind or amount of work they can do." Additional information on Census Bureau data may be found at www.census.gov.

SETTING A PUBLIC HEALTH AGENDA FOR WOMEN WITH DISABILITIES

Healthy People is a national 10-year plan intended to guide federal, state, and local health activities and policies in an effort to improve the health and well-being of Americans (13). The primary goals of Healthy People 2010 (HP 2010) are to increase quality of life and eliminate health disparities. For the first time, HP 2010 includes a chapter that outlines the importance of health promotion and disease prevention for people with disabilities. The new chapter, "Health Promotion and Disease Prevention for People with Disabilities," features 13 objectives targeting disabilities. To promote baseline data collection and provide first-time data about disparities, people with disabilities are included as a special population in several chapters throughout HP 2010. Prior to this, limited information was collected on people with disabilities, particularly women with disabilities.

Current HP 2010 objectives, which include people with disabilities, are outlined in Tables 1 and 2. Table 1 contains information on

Appendix 1. *Health disparities among women for selected Healthy People 2010 focus areas by disability status*

No.	Healthy People 2010 objective	2010 Target	Reference year	With disability	Without disability
Cancer					
3-11a	Increase the proportion of women ages 18+ who have ever received a Pap test	97%	1998	95%	94%
3-11b	Increase the proportion of women ages 18+ who have received a Pap test in preceding 3 yrs	90%	1998	74%	78%
3-13	Increase the proportion of women ages 40+ who have received a mammogram in preceding 2 yrs	70%	1998	55%	61%
NUTRITION AND OVERWEIGHT					
19-1	Increase the proportion of women who are at a healthy weight	60%	1988–1994	35%	45%
19-2	Reduce the proportion of women who are obese	15%	1988–1994	38%	25%
19-12c	Reduce the proportion of women ages 12–49 who have iron deficiency	7%	1988–1994	4%	12%

health indicators that explicitly address women with disabilities. Table 2 includes information for adults with disabilities that pertain to selected HP 2010 focus areas. Although this represents an important first step in addressing disparities for women with disabilities, information needs to be collected on all relevant heath indicators.

Access to Care

All members of the disability community should have access to health promotion, disease prevention, and the direct medical services they need to optimize good health. Yet women with disabilities continue to face substantial barriers that limit their access to health care services (3). This includes physical, attitudinal, and policy barriers; lack of information about how disability affects health; limited finances; and insufficient personal assistance. Health professionals must increase their awareness of the health care issues facing women with disabilities and take an active role in addressing their concerns. All health clinics must be made accessible to women with disabilities. Although many of these bar-

riers are beginning to be addressed through laws such as the Americans with Disabilities Act (PL-101-336), they continue to remain prevalent in our society (14). A recent publication, "Removing Barriers to Health Care: A Guide for Health Professionals," recommends strategies for improving the physical environment for people with disabilities who seek health care services (15). Additional information on the booklet may be found at www.design.ncsu.edu/cud.

Preventive Health Screening

An important aspect of improving the health status of women and achieving the HP 2010 objectives is the provision of clinical preventive services. Although only a few studies have examined the use of preventive health services for women with disabilities, results indicate that these women do not consistently receive preventive health services. A 1998 report on cervical and breast cancer screening among women with functional limitations (FLs) found that older women with FLs were less likely to have received a Papanicolaou (Pap) test or mammogram within the

Appendix 2. *Health disparities among adults for selected Healthy People 2010 focus areas by disability status*

No.	HP 2010 objective	2010 Target	Reference year	With disability	Without disability
DISABILITY AND SECONDARY CONDITIONS					
6-3	Reduce the proportion of adults with disabilities who report sad feelings that prevent them from being active	7%	1997	28%	7%
6-5	Increase the proportion of adults with disabilities reporting sufficient emotional support	79%	1998	71%	79%
6-6	Increase the proportion of adults with disabilities reporting satisfaction with life	96%	1998	87%	96%
EDUCATION AND COMMUNITY-BASED PROGRAMS					
7-12	Increase the proportion of older adults who have participated during the preceding year in at least one organized health promotion activity	90%	1998	10%	12%
IMMUNIZATION AND INFECTIOUS DISEASES					
14-29a	Increase the proportion of noninstitutionalized adults aged 65+ who are vaccinated annually or who have ever been vaccinated against influenza	90%	1998	66%	62%
14-29b	Increase the proportion of noninstitutionalized adults aged 65+ who are vaccinated annually or who have ever been vaccinated against pneumococcal disease	90%	1998	47%	40%
14-29c	Increase the proportion of high-risk noninstitutionalized adults aged 19–64 who are vaccinated annually or who have ever been vaccinated against influenza	60%	1998	28%	23%
14-29d	Increase the proportion of high-risk noninstitutionalized adults aged 18–64 who are vaccinated annually or who have ever been vaccinated against pneumococcal disease	60%	1998	16%	9%
NUTRITION AND OVERWEIGHT					
19-1	Increase the proportion of adults who are at a healthy weight	60%	1988–1994	32%	41%
19-2	Reduce the proportion of adults who are obese	15%	1988–1994	30%	23%
PHYSICAL ACTIVITY					
22-1	Reduce the proportion of adults who engage in no leisure-time physical activity	20%	1997	56%	36%
22-2	Increase the proportion of adults who engage in physical activity for 30 minutes, 5 or more days per week	30%	1997	12%	16%
22-2	Increase the proportion of adults who engage in physical activity for 20 minutes, 3 or more days per week	30%	1997	23%	33%

(Continued

Appendix 2. *(Continued)*

No.	HP 2010 objective	2010 Target	Reference year	With disability	Without disability
PHYSICAL ACTIVITY					
22-3	Increase the proportion of adults who engage in vigorous physical activity that promotes the development and maintenance of cardiorespiratory fitness, 3 or more days per week for 20+ minutes	30%	1997	13%	25%
22-4	Increase the proportion of adults who perform physical activities that enhance and maintain muscular strength and endurance	30%	1998	14%	20%
22-5	Increase the proportion of adults who perform physical activities that enhance and maintain flexibility	43%	1998	29%	31%
TOBACCO USE					
27-1a	Reduction of cigarette smoking in adults aged 18+	12%	1998	33%	23%
27-5	Increase smoking cessation attempts by adult smokers	75%	1998	44%	42%

recommended guidelines (16). A recent study of health care utilization found that although most women with disabilities had seen a general practitioner within the past 6 months, a substantial proportion of these women had not received routine gynecologic care in the preceding 5 years (17). Researchers in Boston found that women with major mobility problems were significantly less likely to receive Pap tests and mammograms than women with no mobility impairments (1). The same study reported that people with mobility impairments were as likely as others to receive pneumococcal and influenza immunizations but were less likely to receive additional services such as tetanus immunization.

These studies confirm that more attention should be given to screening and preventive services for women with disabilities. Health care providers must be careful not to overlook the preventive health needs of women with disabilities. Efforts to improve provider training should include examination techniques that can accommodate women with disabilities including any disability-related symptom

that may interfere with their examinations (16,18). To increase the likelihood that women receive appropriate preventive care, accessible equipment such as adjustable-height examination tables and accessible mammography machines must be widely available. As women with disabilities live longer lives, clinicians must recognize that these women also benefit from the full range of preventive services.

Overweight and Obesity

Overweight and obesity are major contributors to morbidity and mortality in the United States (13). Obesity is a well-established risk factor for hypertension, type 2 diabetes, cardiovascular disease, osteoarthritis, sleep apnea, gallstones, and certain types of cancer (13,19,20). Obesity has reached epidemic proportions in our society, particularly among women. Previous studies have shown that 35% of women in the United States are overweight (19). Despite the heightened awareness of obesity in women, few studies have addressed the problem of obesity among women with disabilities.

Estimates from the NHIS–D indicate that obesity is more prevalent among adults with physical, sensory, and mental health conditions (21). These researchers found that nearly 26% of adults with disabilities were obese, compared to approximately 15% of those without disabilities (21). Adults with mobility difficulties were the most likely to be obese.

State-based BRFSS estimates indicate that 27% of adults with disabilities are obese (22). Compared to women without disabilities, a substantially larger percentage of women with disabilities are obese (15% versus 29%, respectively). Effective interventions must address obstacles to weight control and exercise, including barriers such as inaccessible fitness facilities, lack of recreational opportunities, and limited transportation. In addition, guidelines should be developed to improve providers' counseling skills in this area.

Physical Activity

Physical activity plays an important role in improving and maintaining health. The 1996 Surgeon General's report on Physical Activity concluded that moderate physical activity can decrease considerably the risk of developing or dying from heart disease, diabetes, colon cancer, and high blood pressure (23). Despite the numerous benefits of physical activity, few individuals, including people with disabilities, engage in regular physical activity. Data show that people with disabilities are more likely to report no leisure time physical activity and are less likely to participate in regular physical activity than people without disabilities (13,23). Similar to overweight and obesity, intervention strategies that improve access and facilitate participation should be used to increase physical activity among women with disabilities. Health care providers can obtain additional information on physical activity for people with disabilities by contacting the National Center on Physical Activity and Disability (NICPAD) at www.ncpad.org.

Violence Against Women with Disabilities

Violence is a serious problem for many women with disabilities. Population studies of violence against women with disabilities are lacking. Results of one cross-sectional study showed that women who are physically disabled have the same risk for physical and sexual abuse as able-bodied women but experience abuse over longer periods and have fewer resources by which to leave an abusive environment (24,25). Women with cognitive, psychiatric, or sensory impairments may be at even greater risk because of the nature of their disabilities. In addition to the types of abuse experienced by all women, abuse of women with disabilities may include withholding of needed orthotic equipment, medications, transportation, or the personal assistance required for essential activities of daily living. Screening of all women for abuse, and in particular women with disabilities, must be a routine part of clinical health care practice. Researchers in Houston found that adding two disability-specific questions to a standardized abuse screening instrument improved detection of abuse among women with disabilities (26). For more information on this assessment tool, the Abuse Assessment Screen–Disability, contact the Center for Research on Women with Disabilities at www.bcm.tmc.edu/crowd.

FUTURE DIRECTIONS

Over the last 20 years, advances in medical care have improved greatly the longevity and quality of life of people with disabilities. As a result, there has been a considerable increase in the number of people who live with disabilities throughout their lifespan. National survey data indicate that nearly 16% of the U.S. population have a limitation in one or more activities (28). Results of an analysis of data from the National Medical Expenditure Survey suggest that people with disabilities account for a disproportionate amount of medical expenditures (28). In combination, these data present a strong case for addressing the public health needs of people with disabilities, including women with disabilities.

Until recently, most public health activities have centered on the prevention of disability in the general population, not on activities promoting the health of those who already experience disability. The Institute of Medicine's 1991 report, "Disability in America: Toward a National Agenda for Prevention," made a clear and coherent argument for addressing the public health needs of people living with disabilities (8). Since then, a growing number of researchers have worked to examine the health of people with disabilities, including the prevention of secondary conditions, health promotion, and access to care (1,17,29–34).

One of every five women living in the United States is disabled (7,11). Everyone knows someone who has a disability. Nevertheless, the health needs of women with disabilities are not fully acknowledged by the health care system. Although there is a growing interest in women's health, research addressing the health and well-being of women with disabilities is long overdue. For the first time objectives on the public health needs of people with disabilities are reflected in HP 2010. To attain these objectives, a public health agenda for women with disabilities is essential. Increased collaboration among multiple federal, state, and local partners is a key component to reaching national consensus regarding priority research areas and program responsibilities. Implementing long-term strategies for addressing health disparities among women with disabilities requires the unified efforts of all partners. Women with disabilities are the most knowledgeable source of information about their own health care needs and must participate in setting these research and programmatic priorities.

Setting a public health agenda for women with disabilities requires national and state-level survey data. Health survey data are used to assess public health status, identify health disparities, define public health priorities, identify areas of future research, and monitor progress toward achieving improved health of the population. However, the limitations of existing data that describe the needs of women with disabilities should be recognized. At present disability is not uniformly included in national/statewide surveys and surveillance tools. Thus the true magnitude of the health issues facing women with disabilities cannot be described fully. Accurate population-based data on which to base future policies and interventions for women with disabilities is imperative. Disability must be included as a demographic variable in all national and state-level surveys.

Health promotion for women with disabilities is a new and emerging science. Women with disabilities must be integrated into ongoing prevention initiatives whenever possible. More importantly, it is critical that they become the focus of new health promotion strategies and interventions designed to eliminate existing disparities. Successful intervention strategies require a multifaceted approach that includes behavioral and environmental components. Of particular interest are evidence-based interventions addressing access to care, clinical preventive services, physical activity, and violence against women with disabilities. Initiatives that include funding for research priorities with an emphasis on intervention research must be created.

Health communication increasingly is recognized as an important part of public health that can help increase awareness of potential health risks, motivate individuals to change unhealthy behaviors, and influence attitudes and beliefs (13). Nevertheless, health communication alone cannot change health behavior. A comprehensive approach combining policies and interventions will contribute to behavior change.

Few health messages exist that target women with disabilities. Research to determine the most effective methods for delivering health messages to women with disabilities is critical and also should explore the impact of the information they receive.

Improving the health of women with disabilities is an enormous challenge requiring collaboration at the federal, state, and local level. Developing a public health agenda, including disability in major surveys, emphasizing intervention research, and effectively communicating health messages are key to assuring the health of women with disabilities.

Disability is an issue that increasingly will touch the lives of all Americans. Each of us has a responsibility to better understand the complex issues and barriers that contribute to health disparities among women with disabilities. Better understanding of these barriers will lead to improved interventions directed at reducing morbidity and mortality among this underserved population of women. Addressing the needs of women with disabilities must become a priority of public health professionals and medical care providers at all levels of society.

REFERENCES

1. Iezzoni LI, McCarthy EP, Davis RB, et al. Mobility impairments and use of screening and preventive services. *Am J Public Health* 2000;90:955–961.
2. Chevarley FM, Thierry JM, Gill CJ, et al. Health and well-being for women with disabilities: United States, 1994–1995. Unpublished data.
3. Thierry JM. Promoting the health and wellness of women with disabilities. *J Womens Health* 1998;7(5):505–507.
4. Veltman A, Stewart D, Tardif G, et al. Perceptions of primary healthcare services among people with physical disabilities. Part 1: Access Issues. MedGenMed [serial online]. April 2001. Available at: *www.medscape.com/viewarticle/408122*. Accessed May 30, 2003.
5. Becker H, Stuifbergen A, Tinkle M. Reproductive health care experiences of women with physical disabilities: A qualitative study. *Arch Phys Med Rehabil* 1997;78(Suppl):S-26.
6. Altman BM. Causes, risks, and consequences of disability among women. In: Krotoski DM, Nosek MA, Turk MA, eds. *Women with physical disabilities: Achieving and maintaining health and well-being.* Baltimore: Paul H. Brooks; 1996:35–55.
7. Jans L, Stoddard S. *Chartbook on women and disability in the United States: An InfoUse report.* Washington, DC: U.S. Department of Education, National Institute on Disability and Rehabilitation Research, 1999.
8. Pope AM, Tarlov AR. *Disability in America: toward a national agenda for prevention.* Washington, DC: National Academy Press, 1991.
9. Centers for Disease Control and Prevention. State-specific prevalence of disability among adults-11 States and the District of Columbia, 1998. *MMWR* 2000;49:711–714.
10. LaPlante MP, Carlson D. *Disability in the United States: prevalence and causes, 1992.* Disability Statistics Report (7). Washington, DC: U.S. Department of Education, National Center on Disability and Rehabilitation Research, 1996.
11. McNeil JM. *Americans with disabilities: 1997.* U.S. Bureau of the Census. Current population reports, Washington, DC: U.S. Government Printing Office, 2001:70–73.
12. LaPlante MP. Health conditions and impairments causing disability. Disability Statistics Abstract, 1996; 16.
13. U.S. Department of Health and Human Services. *Healthy People 2010,* 2nd ed. With understanding and improving health and objectives for improving health (2 vols). Washington, DC: U.S. Government Printing Office, November 2000.
14. Americans with Disabilities Act of 1990 (ADA), PL-101-336. (July 26, 1990). Title 42, U.S.C. 12101 et seq. U.S. Statutes at Large, 1990;104:327–378.
15. Center for Universal Design. *Removing barriers to health care: A guide for health professionals.* Raleigh, NC: North Carolina State University, 1998.
16. Centers for Disease Control and Prevention. Use of cervical and breast cancer screening among women with and without functional limitations—United States, 1994–1995. *MMWR* 1998;47:L853–856.
17. Coyle CP, Santiago MC. Healthcare utilization among women with physical disabilities. *Medscape Women's Health eJournal* 2000;7(4). Available at: *www.medscape.com/viewarticle/433156*. Accessed May 30, 2003.
18. Thierry JM. Increasing breast and cervical cancer screening among women with disabilities. *J Womens Health Gend Based Med* 2000;9(1):9–12.
19. Mason JE, Colditz GA, Stampfer MJ, et al. A prospective study of obesity and risk of coronary heart disease in women. *N Engl J Med* 1990;322:882–889.
20. Solomon CG, Manson JE. Obesity and mortality: A review of the epidemiologic data. *Am J Clin Nutr* 1997;66:1044–1050.
21. Weil E, Wachterman M, McCarthy EP, et al. Obesity among adults with disabling conditions. *JAMA* 2002;288:1265–1268.
22. Centers for Disease Control and Prevention. State-specific prevalence of obesity among adults with disabilities—Eight States and the District of Columbia, 1998–1999. *MMWR* 2002;51:805–808.
23. U.S. Department of Health and Human Services. *Physical activity and health: A report of the surgeon general.* Atlanta: U.S. Department of Health and Human Services, Centers for Disease Control and Prevention, National Center for Chronic Disease Prevention and Health Promotion, 1996.
24. Young M, Nosek MA, Howland C, et al. Prevalence of abuse of women with physical disabilities. *Arch Phys Med Rehabil* 1997;78:34.
25. Nosek MA, Hughes RB, Taylor HB. *Violence against women with physical disabilities.* Houston, TX: Baylor College of Medicine, 2002.
26. McFarlane J, Hughes RB, Nosek MA, et al. Abuse assessment screen–disability (AAS–D): Measuring fre-

quency, type, and perpetrator of abuse toward women with physical disabilities. *J Womens Health Gend Based Med* 2001;10(9):861–865.

27. Kaye HS, LaPlante MP, Carlson D, et al. *Trends in disability rates in the United States, 1970–1994.* Disability Statistics Abstracts, No. 17. Washington: Department of Education (U.S.), National Institute on Disability and Rehabilitation Research, 1996.

28. Rice DP, LaPlante MP. Medical expenditures for disability and disabling comorbidity. *Am J Public Health* 1992;82(5):739–741.

29. Vines CL, Shackelford M. *Identifying secondary conditions in women with spinal cord injury.* Little Rock: Arkansas Spinal Cord Commission, 1996.

30. Turk MA, Geremski, CA, Rosenbaum PF. *Secondary conditions of adults with cerebral palsy.* Syracuse, NY: State University of New York, Health Science Center at Syracuse, 1997.

31. Turk MA, Rosenbaum PF, Scandale J. *Project W.E.A.L.T.H. Women empowered, aware, and learning through health education: A health promotion project for women with disabilities.* Syracuse, NY: State University of New York, Health Science Center at Syracuse, 2001.

32. Rimmer JH, Liu Y. *Center on health promotion research for persons with disabilities.* Chicago: University of Illinois at Chicago, 2001.

33. White GW, Figoni S, Froehlich K, et al. *Health promotion for persons with disabilities and prevention of secondary conditions.* Lawrence, KS: University of Kansas, 2001.

34. Ravesloot C, Seekins T, Ipsen C, et al. *A cost effective analysis of a community-based health promotion intervention for adults with mobility impairments: living well with a disability.* Missoula, MT: University of Montana, 2003.

Subject Index